Applied Anatomy & Physiology for Speech–Language Pathology & Audiology

Applied Anatomy & Physiology for Speech–Language Pathology & Audiology

Donald R. Fuller, Ph.D., CCC-SLP, ASHA Fellow

Professor of Communication Disorders
Department of Communication Disorders
Eastern Washington University
Spokane, WA

Jane T. Pimentel, Ph.D., CCC-SLP

Associate Professor of Communication Disorders
Department of Communication Disorders
Eastern Washington University
Spokane, WA

Barbara M. Peregoy, Au.D., CCC-A

Senior Lecturer in Communication Disorders
Department of Communication Disorders
Eastern Washington University
Spokane, WA

Wolters Kluwer | Lippincott Williams & Wilkins
Health

Philadelphia • Baltimore • New York • London
Buenos Aires • Hong Kong • Sydney • Tokyo

Acquisitions Editor: Peter Sabatini
Product Manager: Paula C. Williams
Marketing Manager: Allison Powell
Designer: Teresa Mallon
Compositor: Aptara, Inc.

351 West Camden Street   Two Commerce Square
Baltimore, MD 21201   2001 Market Street
                                Philadelphia, PA 19103

Printed in China

9 8 7 6 5 4 3 2 1

Library of Congress Cataloging-in-Publication Data

Fuller, Donald (Donald R.), author.
  Applied anatomy and physiology for speech-language pathology and audiology / Donald Fuller, Ph.D., CCC-SLP, Jane Pimentel, Ph.D., CCC-SLP, Barbara M. Peregoy, Au. D., CCC-A.
      p. ; cm.
  Includes bibliographical references and index.
  ISBN 978-0-7817-8837-3 (hardback : alkaline paper)
  1. Communicative disorders—Pathophysiology. 2. Human anatomy.
3. Human physiology. I. Pimentel, Jane, author. II. Peregoy, Barbara M., author. III. Title.
  [DNLM: 1. Language Disorders—physiopathology. 2. Hearing Disorders—physiopathology. 3. Nervous System—anatomy & histology.
4. Respiratory System—anatomy & histology. 5. Speech—physiology.
6. Speech-Language Pathology—methods. WL 340.2]
  RC423.F824 2010
  616.85′5—dc22

                                                    2010044328

DISCLAIMER

To my wife, Zhe Qu ("Joyce"), and our daughter, Ersi Nie ("Sisi"), two intellectually superior women who understand the importance of life-long learning; and to our younger children—Destiny, Richard, and Aidan—may the love of learning be just as important to them. Finally, to my mother, Hannah Louise Bridges, and father, Roy Fuller, Sr., both now deceased, who instilled within me the need to never stop learning.

Donald R. Fuller

To my husband, Paul, for his limitless patience and support and to my late mother, Ramona, for her incredible enthusiasm for my professional pursuits.

Jane T. Pimentel

To my husband, Bob, for his patience and for encouraging me to continue when I wanted to quit; to my sons, Stephen and William, for understanding when I told them, "I can't right now, I have a deadline"; and to my big brother, Steve, for teaching me by example that life's challenges are "do-able" even if you just pick your way down the mountain.

Barbara M. Peregoy

REVIEWERS

Jillian G. Barrett, Ph.D., CCC-A, FAAA
Private Practice
Danville, California

James Feuerstein, Ph.D., CCC-A, FAAA
Professor of Audiology
Department of Communication Sciences &
 Disorders
Nazareth College
Rochester, New York

Eric W. Healy, Ph.D.
Associate Professor
Department of Speech and Hearing
 Science
The Ohio State University
Columbus, Ohio

Rajinder Koul, Ph.D., CCC-SLP
Professor and Chair, Associate Dean
 (Research)
Department of Speech, Language, and Hear-
 ing Sciences
Texas Tech University Health Sciences Center
Lubbock, Texas

Thomas Littman, Ph.D., CCC-A
Audiologist
Factoria Hearing Center
Bellevue, Washington

Beverly Miller, M.A., CCC-SLP
Assistant Professor
Department of Communication Disorders
Marshall University
Huntington, West Virginia

Amy T. Neel, Ph.D., CCC-SLP
Associate Professor
Department of Speech and Hearing
 Sciences
University of New Mexico
Albuquerque, New Mexico

Shawn L. Nissen, Ph.D., CCC-SLP
Associate Professor
Department of Communication Disorders
Brigham Young University
Provo, Utah

Sarah Poissant, Ph.D., CCC-A
Associate Professor
Department of Communication Disorders
University of Massachusetts
Amherst, Massachusetts

Tracie Rice, Au.D., CCC-A
Clinical Director
Department of Communication
 Sciences and Disorders
Western Carolina University
Cullowhee, North Carolina

Howard Rothman, Ph.D.
Professor Emeritus
University of Florida
Gainesville, Florida

CONTRIBUTOR

Charles L. Madison, Ph.D., CCC-SLP
Professor
Department of Speech and Hearing Sciences
Washington State University
Spokane, Washington

PREFACE

"Why do we need to know all of this anatomy?"

It's a question for the ages. Every instructor who has ever taught anatomy and physiology of the speech and hearing mechanism has heard that question at least once—if not several times—in his or her career. Too often, and for various reasons, anatomy and physiology is taught separately from the disorders in the typical communication disorders curriculum. For those of us who are "purists," there is a belief that the foundational courses for the profession should be taught before the applied courses are introduced. This is reinforced by the classification of anatomy and physiology as one of the "basic human communication processes." The assumption for many is that applied coursework is not appropriate until the underlying basic processes are understood. For others, the logistical nightmare of trying to coordinate anatomy and physiology with the disorders within a 3-, 4-, or even 5-credit course has precluded the introduction of applied information with the information pertaining to anatomy and physiology. The problem is exacerbated by the fact that the most commonly used textbooks on anatomy and physiology of the speech and hearing mechanism provide very little, if any, applied information. Other than the occasional "clinical application" box or short paragraph, one would be hard pressed to find any substantive information about how anatomy and physiology is used clinically to govern the decision-making process regarding diagnosis or potential intervention strategies.

The reality is that for whatever reason we choose not to integrate anatomy and physiology with their clinical relevance, students are not provided the "big picture." At least while they are taking the course, most students do not fully comprehend how anatomy and physiology fits into this big picture. Most of us try to provide clinically relevant examples while we are teaching the course, but too often, the few examples we provide are simply not enough. The industrious student may take the initiative and seek out that information independently. Most students, however, wait until they take the applied courses and hope that at that point they will begin to see the big picture. From these students who no doubt make up the majority, those often said words are uttered:

"Why do we need to know all of this anatomy?"

Throughout the many years we have taught anatomy and physiology of speech and hearing, we must have heard that question a thousand times. Even in light of our attempts to provide clinically relevant examples to illustrate the importance of understanding the anatomy and physiology, that question kept rearing its ugly head. We are happy to report that the vast majority of students who have taken an anatomy course under us went on to make the connection later in their studies. However, we have always had the nagging feeling that students needed to make that connection much sooner in their undergraduate careers.

We have never been overly enamored with the textbooks in anatomy and physiology that have been published over the years. Some of them were too technical or advanced for the typical undergraduate student, bogging the student down in detail after detail to the point that comprehension was minimal. Other textbooks were too simplistic, not providing enough detail to be meaningful to the student. With the exception of one or two, most textbooks provided very little in the way of ancillary materials. All of them provided too little information about the clinical relevance of anatomy and physiology. The more and more we taught anatomy and physiology over the years, the more we thought about what we would like to see in an anatomy textbook: a good balance in terms of the complexity of the information provided; ancillary materials to assist the student in further understanding the material; and most importantly, a good, healthy dose of applied clinical information to assist the student in making the critical connection between anatomy/physiology and its clinical application. Such a textbook, and a course built around it, would hopefully eliminate the need for students to ask:

"Why do we need to know all of this anatomy?"

Enter the American Speech-Language-Hearing Association (ASHA). When ASHA introduced its new standards for certification in January 2005, we saw it as an opportunity. With the new certification standards being knowledge- and skills-based as opposed to course-based, we realized that professional programs were freed from counting academic credits in various areas such as basic human communication processes, professional courses, etc. Instead, programs could concentrate on ensuring that students acquire certain knowledge and skills outcomes. Such a shift in focus allows professional programs to redesign their curricula to meet knowledge and skills outcomes instead of counting academic credits. Other than the general requirement that graduates have 75 semester hours credit of coursework in the profession (with 36 of those credits being earned at the graduate level), there are no longer specific academic credit requirements. An obvious benefit of this is that the need to separate the anatomy and physiology from the clinical application no longer exists. Both could be taught in parallel since professional programs are no longer required to "bean count" the academic credits.

This textbook represents the culmination of the ideas we have had for the last 20 years. First, a conscious attempt was made to present the anatomy and physiology of speech and hearing in a manner that is not too complex, but also not too simplistic. The critical information is here. The terminology is here. The detail is also here. The writing style is what possibly separates this textbook from the other texts available on the market. An attempt was made to write in a style that invites the reader on a tour of anatomy and physiology.

Second, ancillary materials are available to assist the student in understanding the anatomy and physiology and also to assist the instructor in presenting the material. In our opinion, the artwork (both drawings and photographs) in this textbook is superior by comparison with the artwork in other textbooks on the market. Case studies, clinical "tie-in" boxes, a large glossary, references to research, study questions, and terminology "hint" boxes are used liberally to assist the reader's comprehension. A companion Web site is also available; this includes a library of images and other pedagogical materials to further reinforce the concepts learned. This textbook is possibly the first one in our profession to link the information contained within to the pertinent knowledge outcomes of ASHA's certification standards (see the section Addressing Knowledge and Skills [KASA] Outcomes later).

Third, and most importantly, this textbook includes chapters on pathology and its relationship to anatomy and physiology. Each major part of this book (articulatory/resonance system, auditory/vestibular system, nervous system, phonatory system, and respiratory system) consists of two chapters. The first chapter in each unit provides the relevant information pertaining to anatomy and physiology. The second chapter in each unit provides an in-depth discussion of pathology and its relationship to the anatomy and physiology. Although these chapters do not provide an exhaustive list of all the possible pathologies, sufficient detail is provided about a large number of organic and nonorganic disorders to allow the student to see the big picture. This textbook is organized in such a manner that it can be used in a stand-alone anatomy and physiology course or as the primary text in a combined undergraduate anatomy/pathology course.

Speaking of the organization of this textbook, one may note that it differs from the other anatomy textbooks. After an introductory section on terminology and basic concepts, most other textbooks present the anatomy and physiology in the following order: respiratory system, phonatory system, articulatory/resonance system, nervous system, and auditory system. This textbook organizes the anatomy/physiology information in a slightly altered sequence: nervous system, respiratory system, phonatory system, articulatory/resonance system, and finally the auditory/vestibular system. The rationale for this sequence is that since the nervous system underlies all other processes in speech and hearing, it should be presented first. It should be presented first also because information presented in later chapters (e.g., physiology of muscles) is dependent upon the student's understanding of the neurological bases. Once the student has been introduced to the nervous system, the traditional sequence of respiration, phonation, and articulation/resonance is presented. As a somewhat independent system, the auditory/vestibular system is presented last.

We have told our students over the years, "If you understand the anatomy and physiology, you're more than half-way to understanding the pathology." Many of these students have come back to us years later and affirmed that observation. These same former students have almost invariably mentioned that it would have been more helpful had they made that connection earlier in their academic careers. Hopefully, this textbook represents a successful attempt to align the basic science of anatomy and physiology with the applied art and science of communication disorders. We will know that this attempt was successful if we no longer hear students ask:

"Why do we need to know all of this anatomy?"

Additional Resources

Applied Anatomy and Physiology for Speech–Language Pathology and Audiology includes additional resources for both instructors and students that are available on the book's companion Web site at http://thePoint.lww.com/Fuller.

INSTRUCTOR RESOURCES

Approved adopting instructors will be given access to the following additional resources:

- Test bank
- Answers to Part Questions that are within the textbook
- Image bank to assist in creating Powerpoint slides
- Acland Human Anatomy videos related to speech and hearing

STUDENT RESOURCES

- Interactive student quiz bank
- Animations on the workings of anatomical and physiological structures of the body as they relate to speech and hearing
- Acland Human Anatomy videos related to speech and hearing

In addition, purchasers of the textbook can access the searchable Full Text On-line by going to the *Applied Anatomy and Physiology for Speech–Language Pathology and Audiology* Web site at http://thePoint.lww.com/Fuller. See the inside front cover of this textbook for more details, including the passcode you will need to gain access to the Web site.

Donald R. Fuller
Jane T. Pimentel
Barbara M. Peregoy
February 2011

ADDRESSING KNOWLEDGE AND SKILLS (KASA) OUTCOMES

This textbook may be the first of its kind to indicate which knowledge outcomes of the *Knowledge and Skills Acquisition (KASA)* form are addressed through the content found within its pages. On January 1, 2005, the American Speech-Language-Hearing Association (ASHA) revised its certification standards. These are standards every student must meet to earn the Certificate of Clinical Competence (CCC). The old standards were based upon the student taking certain courses in specific domains. For example, the Basic Human Communication Sciences domain required that the student earn 15 semester credit hours in such courses as anatomy and physiology of speech and hearing; phonetics; speech and language development; and speech and hearing science. The new standards are no longer primarily based upon the student earning a set number of academic credits but instead are primarily competency-based. Now, the student must demonstrate competence in certain knowledge and skills.

Table P-1 indicates the *KASA* knowledge outcomes that are addressed in this textbook. Up to 25 knowledge outcomes may be addressed by this textbook, depending on

TABLE P-1

KASA KNOWLEDGE AND SKILLS OUTCOMES ADDRESSED BY THE CONTENT OF THIS TEXTBOOK

Knowledge Outcome	Addressed to What Extent?	Addressed in Chapter(s)
1. Biological basis of the basic human communication processes (III-B)	80%	2, 3, **6, 8, 10, 12**
2. Neurological basis of the basic human communication processes (III-B)	30%	2, 3, **4**, 6, 8, 10, 12
3. Acoustic basis of the basic human communication processes (III-B)	20%	**8, 10,** 12
4. Psychological basis of the basic human communication processes (III-B)	10%	**4**
5. Developmental and life span bases of the basic human communication processes (III-B)	20%	4, 8, 13
6. Linguistic basis of the basic human communication processes (III-B)	10%	**4**
7. Biological basis of swallowing processes (III-B)	80%	**8, 10**
8. Neurological basis of swallowing processes (III-B)	30%	**4**
9. Etiologies of articulation disorders (III-C)	10%	**11**
10. Characteristics of articulation disorders (III-C)	10%	**11**
11. Etiologies of fluency disorders (III-C)	10%	5, 9, 11
12. Characteristics of fluency disorders (III-C)	10%	5, 9, 11
13. Etiologies of voice and resonance disorders (III-C)	20%	**9**
14. Characteristics of voice and resonance disorders (III-C)	20%	**9**
15. Etiologies of receptive and expressive language disorders (III-C)	10%	**5,** 13
16. Characteristics of receptive and expressive language disorders (III-C)	10%	**5**
17. Etiologies of hearing disorders (III-C)	80% SLP/50% Aud.	**13**
18. Characteristics of hearing disorders (III-C)	60% SLP/30% Aud.	**13**
19. Etiologies of swallowing disorders (III-C)	10%	5, 9, 11
20. Characteristics of swallowing disorders (III-C)	10%	5, 9, 11
21. Etiologies of cognitive aspects of communication (III-C)	10%	**5**
22. Characteristics of cognitive aspects of communication (III-C)	10%	**5**
23. Prevention of voice and resonance disorders (III-D)	10%	9
24. Prevention of hearing disorders (III-D)	50% SLP/10% Aud.	13
25. Prevention related to the cognitive aspects of communication (III-D)	10%	5

how the textbook is used. It should be noted that the items in this table are numbered consecutively from 1 to 25; these numerals were arbitrarily assigned by the authors of this textbook solely for the purpose of organization and reference, and do not correspond to any numbering system developed by ASHA.

The reader will note right away that a horizontal line separates the first eight knowledge outcomes from the remaining outcomes. If this textbook is used as the primary source of information for a stand-alone course in anatomy and physiology of the speech and hearing mechanism, then only knowledge outcomes 1 through 8 are applicable. However, if this textbook is used as the primary source of information in a course having greater content than simply anatomy and physiology (e.g., the anatomy and physiology are presented within a larger course on organic speech, language, and hearing disorders), all 25 knowledge outcomes are applicable.

Table P-1 also provides information as to the relative extent a particular knowledge outcome is being addressed. It should be emphasized that these are *relative* percentages based upon the expected amount of information that would be provided in an anatomy and physiology and/or an organic disorders course and the amount of information that would be provided elsewhere in a typical communication disorders curriculum. To illustrate, the relative extent to which a stand-alone anatomy and physiology course would address the biological basis of the basic human communication processes (outcome 1) has been estimated at 80%. In other words, one would expect that approximately 80% of the information provided within a typical communication disorders curriculum related to outcome 1 would come from a basic, stand-alone course in anatomy and physiology of the speech and hearing mechanism. The remaining 20% is typically addressed in disorders courses, where a review of the anatomy and physiology may be provided as part of the course. For outcomes 17, 18, and 24, relative percentages are provided separately for speech–language pathology and audiology majors. For example, this textbook provides approximately 80% of the information in a typical communication disorders curriculum related to etiologies of hearing disorders for speech–language pathology majors, but only 50% of the same information for audiology majors because they'd more likely receive more extensive information in other courses within their major. Once again, it should be emphasized that these are *relative* percentages. The actual extent to which this textbook addresses the knowledge outcomes in Table P-1 will likely differ from academic program to academic program. It is up to the individual program to determine that extent.

Finally, Table P-1 indicates the chapter or chapters in which the individual knowledge outcomes are addressed. This column is provided as a means of cross-referencing the content of the textbook to the specific knowledge outcomes. The reader will note that in some instances the chapter number has been boldfaced in the table. Chapter numbers that are boldfaced provide the greatest amount of information relative to the knowledge outcome in question. When no chapter number is boldfaced for a corresponding KASA outcome, the information provided in this textbook for that outcome should be considered minimal. Relative percentages are provided in Table P-1 to guide academic programs as they determine how the KASA outcomes are to be addressed within their own unique curriculum.

CONTENTS

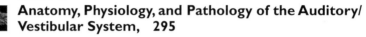

PART I
Terminology, Nomenclature, and Basic Concepts

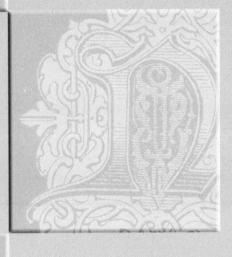

CHAPTER 1

An Overview of this Textbook

"Why do we have to learn all of this anatomy and physiology?"

It is a question for the ages. Speech–language pathology and audiology students have asked this question practically since the beginning of the professions. Although many come to appreciate the relationship between speech perception and production and the concomitant anatomy and physiology, there oftentimes seems to be a disconnect between the two for most clinicians in training. It is not until much later in their education that the link is solidified in the minds of these future professionals.

The answer is simple, yet complex at the same time. To understand what may be pathological, one must first know what is "normal" or "typical." Many of the so-called organic disorders of speech, language, and hearing have an etiology that points toward aberrations in the anatomy and/or physiology of the speech or hearing mechanism. An anatomical or physiological etiology will likely provide the clinician with clues as to the expected signs and symptoms associated with a given disorder, and may also indicate what course of intervention to take.

The complexity of the answer lies in the complexity of the human body. There are literally hundreds of anatomical structures (e.g., bones, cartilages, muscles, organs, and nerves) involved in the speech perception and production processes. Likewise, many laws, principles, and theories of physical science are involved in the physiology of speech and hearing. The prospect of learning all of the terminology and concepts related to speech perception and production can be overwhelming to many students. However, the learning process can seem more manageable (and for many students downright fun!) if one understands that there is actually a method to the madness. More information will be provided about this method in a later section of this chapter.

The authors of this textbook have a combined experience in anatomy and physiology reaching into decades.

Hundreds of students have passed through our classes in anatomy and physiology of speech and hearing. Although we have used clinical examples to some degree in our classes, most of the class time involved the presentation of anatomical and physiological concepts and nomenclature. We suspect this is true for most academic programs in communication disorders.

Because of this, many students simply cannot see a clear relationship between anatomy and physiology and disorders of speech and hearing. The anticipation is that students will come to understand the relationship when coursework in the disorders is taken. The problem with this is that by the time most students take the disorders courses, they have forgotten the anatomy and physiology because a solid link was never established early on. This textbook attempts to alleviate this problem by offering not only the concepts and nomenclature associated with the anatomy and physiology of the speech and hearing mechanism but also in-depth information about a variety of disorders of speech and hearing so that you can understand the link between the two early in your educational experience.

A Quick Tour of this Textbook

Traditionally, speech perception and production have been described according to several components: articulatory/resonance, auditory/vestibular, neural, phonatory, and respiratory. This textbook will not deviate from organizing the anatomy and physiology of speech and hearing according to this well-established scheme. However, we refer to each of these components as a *system*. By definition, a system is a group of independent but interrelated elements comprising a unified whole. The processes of articulation/resonance, hearing, phonation, and respiration are indeed anatomically independent from each other, but they are also composed of interrelated elements that come together for a specific purpose—that purpose being speech perception and production. Although the nervous system is not involved mechanically in speech perception and production in the way the other systems are, without the nervous system the processes of speech perception and production would not be possible. We view the nervous system as the overriding system that coordinates and controls all other systems.

Because we refer to these components of speech perception and production as *systems*, you should not confuse them with the systems that comprise the human body. Depending on the anatomist, the human body may be organized into as few as nine and as many as twelve body systems. Some of these body systems include the circulatory (or vascular) system, digestive system, muscular system, nervous system, reproductive system, respiratory system, and skeletal system. As Table 1-1 illustrates, the systems that are mechanically involved in speech perception and production (i.e., the articulatory/resonance, auditory/vestibular, phonatory, and respiratory systems) are in turn composed of structures from several body systems. Right away, you may note that the muscular, nervous, skeletal, and vascular body systems are all components of every system that is mechanically related to speech perception and production. Using the auditory/vestibular system to illustrate, the contribution of the muscular system comes in the form of several muscles such as the stapedius and tensor tympani muscles. The nervous system contributes by way of the vestibulocochlear nerve and the auditory pathway. The skeletal system is represented by bones (e.g., the ossicles: malleus, incus, and stapes) and cartilages (e.g., the ear canal and pinna). Finally, the vascular system contributes several arteries and veins to the auditory/vestibular system to provide nutrients and to take away waste products.

It is interesting to note that not only is respiration considered a body system but is also considered a system of speech production. Defined as a body system, the respiratory system typically includes only the trachea, bronchial tree, and lungs. When viewed as a system of speech production, respiration also draws upon the muscular, nervous, skeletal, and vascular systems. This points up the fact that when one refers to body systems, one is generally referring to an *anatomical* organization of the human body. It becomes apparent that when one considers the *physiology* of the human body, the body systems overlap considerably. Therefore, although this textbook will describe the articulatory/resonance, auditory/vestibular, nervous, phonatory, and respiratory systems in terms of their anatomy, these systems of speech perception and production are organized primarily according to their *physiological function*.

TABLE I-I

THE SYSTEMS OF COMMUNICATION AND THE HUMAN BODY SYSTEMS (WITH EXAMPLES IN ITALICS) THAT COMPRISE THEM

Communication System	Human Body Systems
Speech Perception	
Auditory system	Muscular system
	Stapedius muscle; tensor tympani muscle
	Nervous system
	Facial nerve; vestibulocochlear nerve
	Skeletal system
	Temporal bone of the skull
	Vascular system
	Anterior inferior cerebellar artery
Speech Production	
Respiratory system	Muscular system
	Diaphragm; external intercostals
	Nervous system
	Phrenic nerve
	Respiratory system
	Lungs
	Skeletal system
	Cervical, thoracic, lumbar vertebrae; ribs
	Vascular system
	Pulmonary artery
Phonatory system	Muscular system
	Cricothyroid; posterior cricoarytenoid
	Nervous system
	Recurrent laryngeal nerve
	Skeletal system
	Hyoid bone
	Vascular system
	Inferior laryngeal artery
Articulatory/resonance system	Digestive system
	Oral cavity; pharynx
	Muscular system
	Levator veli palatini; palatoglossus
	Nervous system
	Mandibular branch of the trigeminal nerve
	Skeletal system
	Ethmoid; mandible; vomer
	Vascular system
	Lingual artery

Although this textbook will not deviate from the established organizational scheme of articulatory/resonance, auditory/vestibular, nervous, phonatory, and respiratory systems, these systems of speech perception and production will be presented in a slightly different order than they typically appear in most anatomy textbooks. Traditionally, the nervous system tends to be presented after the three systems of speech production (respiration, phonation, and articulation/resonance). However, we feel that since the nervous system coordinates and controls all of the other systems of speech perception and production, it should be presented first. Therefore, the nervous system is presented in this textbook in Part II. Following the nervous system will be the three systems involved in speech production. Part III will present the respiratory system, Part IV will present the phonatory system, and Part V will present the articulatory and resonance systems. Finally, the auditory/vestibular system will be presented last, in Part VI. It should be noted that although the auditory system is of primary interest to speech perception, information about the vestibular system is also provided because the audiologist or speech–language pathologist is very likely to encounter patients who exhibit disturbances in balance and equilibrium.

Part I consists of three chapters. The purpose of the present chapter is to orient you to the general organization and intended use of this textbook. Chapter 2 provides basic information to orient you to the anatomical position; planes of reference; terminology describing spatial relationships between and among structures; and other nomenclature related to anatomy, physiology, and pathology. Chapter 3 provides you with basic information concerning the organization of the human organism: cells, tissues, organs, and systems. Upon completion of the first part, you will have the basic building blocks to assist in understanding the information presented in the remaining parts. For the remaining parts of this textbook, not only will anatomy and physiology be presented but information about the relationship between anatomy and physiology and many disorders of speech, language, and hearing will also be presented. For Parts II through VI, the anatomy and physiology of each of the five systems mentioned earlier will be presented first in a stand-alone chapter (Chapters 4, 6, 8, 10, and 12). Following each chapter on anatomy and physiology, a separate chapter will include information relative to certain disorders affecting those systems (Chapters 5, 7, 9, 11, and 13). It is hoped that taken together, the two chapters within each part will provide you with that elusive link between anatomy and physiology and the disorders that may occur when abnormal structures or conditions exist.

A Quick Overview of Speech Perception and Production

As mentioned previously in this chapter, the processes of speech perception and production are quite complex, enlisting the participation of literally hundreds of anatomical structures such as bones, cartilages, muscles, organs, and nerves. In addition, the various anatomical parts are bound together by different types of connective tissue such as fascia, ligaments, membranes, and tendons. In general, the various systems involved in speech perception and production require that you know the entire human body except for the upper and lower extremities (i.e., arms, legs, hands, feet, fingers, and toes).

To illustrate, speech perception involves the auditory and nervous systems. Acoustic energy in the form of sound waves (whether speech or environmental sounds) are collected by the pinna and directed into the ear canal. At the terminus of the ear canal resides the tympanic membrane (eardrum), which converts the acoustic energy into mechanical energy. The mechanical energy is then transmitted through the middle ear cavity by way of the ossicular chain (the malleus, incus, and stapes). To protect the inner ear from being excessively driven, the acoustic reflex may enter the picture. This reflex is accomplished through the contraction of muscles. As mechanical energy is transmitted through the middle ear, the stapes acts upon the oval window of the cochlea, which is in the inner ear. Housed within a chamber of the cochlea is the essential organ of hearing (the organ of Corti) that contains fluid and is also surrounded by two other chambers filled with fluid. The rocking action of the stapes causes the fluid inside these chambers to vibrate. Vibration of the fluid within the cochlea sets up a receptor potential from the organ of Corti. Sensory nerve impulses then travel to fibers of the cochlear portion of cranial nerve VIII (the vestibulocochlear or auditory nerve), where the impulses are then relayed through the auditory pathway. The auditory pathway includes portions of the lower brain stem, upper brainstem (i.e., the midbrain), and cerebral cortex. It is at the cerebral cortex where sound is finally perceived and interpreted. Separate from the acoustic and vestibular functions of the hearing mechanism, the Eustachian tube assists in regulating air pressure within the middle ear cavity. When air pressure within the middle ear cavity becomes negative in relation to atmospheric pressure, the Eustachian tube opens to equalize pressure. This is accomplished in part through muscle contraction.

In total, a very large number of anatomical structures make up the auditory/vestibular system. These include bones, cartilages, ligaments, membranes, muscles, neurons, organs, and tendons.

By the same token, the process of speech production is equally complex. This process requires coordinated activity of the nervous, respiratory, phonatory, and articulatory/resonance systems. To an extent, the auditory system is also involved, as it is used by individuals who can hear as a means of acquiring speech and language. Further, once speech and language have been acquired, the auditory system is used by persons with normal hearing to monitor their own speech.

Proper timing of the events that make up speech production is essential. Neural impulses will regulate the various aspects of speech production such as respiration, phonation, and articulation/resonance, and will also provide the brain with sensory information related to tactile and kinesthetic feedback during the speech production process. Respiration will serve as the energy source for speech production. Expired air will be used to set the vocal folds into vibration to produce voicing. Neural impulses will cause certain muscles to contract, thereby resulting in respiration. The process of inhalation—whether for the purpose of speech production or not—is always active; that is, muscle contraction is always necessary to effect this process. On the other hand, normal exhalation is passive (i.e., no muscle contraction), while exhalation for vocal activity is typically active. Once the vocal folds are adducted (i.e., brought together or "closed") by muscles of the larynx, the air trapped below the closed vocal folds must be pressurized by active muscle action in the abdomen and thorax. The vocal folds must also be abducted (i.e., separated or "opened") for the production of voiceless speech sounds and to replenish air during vocal activity. The abductor muscles of the larynx are needed for this action. In turn, neural impulses are needed to contract the abductor and adductor muscles of the larynx.

Upon adduction of the vocal folds, exhaled air coming up from the lungs gets trapped below the vocal folds, creating air pressure (referred to as subglottic pressure). Subglottic pressure will eventually force an opening between the vocal folds, setting them into vibration as the air passes through (a process referred to as phonation). During phonation, only a buzzing sound is produced. This buzzing sound is then shaped and molded (i.e., articulated and resonated) as it proceeds up through the pharynx and into the oral and/or nasal cavities. When oral speech sounds are produced, the soft palate will raise and seal off the nasal cavity from the oral cavity so that all of the resonating sound passes through the oral cavity and out through the lips. When the nasal speech sounds (i.e., /m/, /n/, and /ŋ/) are produced, the soft palate will lower, creating an opening between the oral and nasal cavities so that part of the vocal tone can resonate within the nasal cavity. Action of the soft palate is mediated through muscle activity. The tongue is the primary structure involved in articulation and resonance. All vowel sounds and most of the consonant sounds of English are created by placement and/or movement of the tongue. The tongue consists of muscle tissue. For some speech sounds, there may be rounding of the lips (e.g., the /w/ sound). Shaping of the lips is accomplished by muscle action. Once again, muscle activity is accomplished via neural impulses from the nervous system.

The entire speech production mechanism is overlaid either upon or within the skeletal system. For example, the thoracic region is primarily associated with respiration and consists of the ribs, sternum, and thoracic vertebrae of the spinal column. In addition, the bones of the pectoral (i.e., shoulder) and pelvic (i.e., hip) girdles serve as a point of attachment for many of the muscles involved in respiration. The trachea (a structure made of cartilage) and the lungs (which are organs) are also involved in the respiratory process.

In terms of the phonatory system, the primary structure is the larynx, which is composed of a series of cartilages interconnected by membranes and ligaments. The hyoid bone serves as the superior attachment for the larynx as well as the skeletal base for many of the muscles of the tongue. The pharynx, soft palate, and tongue consist of connective tissue, muscles, and mucous membrane. Many of the bones of the skull serve as points of attachment for muscles involved in articulation and resonance. The bones of the cranium house the brain.

In all, it should be apparent to you that a study of the anatomy and physiology of speech and hearing will require extensive knowledge of the human body and its components. In the parts that follow, each of the various systems (nervous, respiratory, phonatory, articulatory/resonance, and auditory/vestibular) will be provided in greater detail. You will learn the various components that make up each of the systems (e.g., bones, cartilages, muscles, organs, and nerves) and will also gain knowledge of the normal physiology of the various systems individually, as well as the physiology of the various systems collectively as they are used for the purpose of speech perception and production. However, before engaging in the study of the various systems involved in speech perception and production, you should have a solid understanding of the basic terminology and concepts that are used in the study of anatomy, physiology, and pathology. The remaining chapters of this part provide you with a basic foundation of terminology and concepts related to anatomy, physiology, and pathology so that learning of the various systems will be facilitated. We now turn our attention specifically to the nomenclature of anatomy, physiology, and pathology.

CHAPTER 2

Understanding Orientation and Nomenclature

Knowledge Outcomes for ASHA Certification for Chapter 2

- Demonstrate knowledge of the biological basis of the basic human communication processes (III-B)
- Demonstrate knowledge of the neurological basis of the basic human communication processes (III-B)

Learning Objectives

- You will be able to recite the definitions of biology, anatomy, physiology, and pathology.
- You will describe the anatomical position, planes of reference, and spatial terminology used to denote the position and orientation of anatomical structures of interest to speech perception and production.
- You will determine the meaning of unfamiliar terminology by analyzing the meaning of the root and any affixes that may be attached.

Basic Concepts, Terminology, and Nomenclature

ANATOMY, PHYSIOLOGY, AND PATHOLOGY

Anatomy and physiology are both branches of **biology**. You may recall from a high school biological science course that biology is the scientific study of living organisms. A living organism is anything that exhibits the properties of life, including but not limited to:

- *Cell structure*—the cell is the basic unit of the organism, and in many organisms can create more complex structures like tissues and organs.
- *Metabolism*—the organism captures energy to be used to maintain itself.
- *Reproduction*—the production of offspring to perpetuate the species.
- *Mutation*—random changes in the structure or composition of the organism.
- *Death*—eventually, the organism will die.

Living organisms can range from single-celled creatures (e.g., bacteria) to more complex structures such as plants and animals. The human being, of course, is a complex animal, and therefore is a living organism.

Anatomy and physiology both fall under the umbrella of biology. Anatomy is the scientific study of the structure and organization of living organisms. The term comes from the Greek words "anatomia" and "anatemnein," meaning to cut up or cut open. Years ago, in order to study the structure and organization of the human body it would have had to have been dissected. Since not too many human beings want to be cut up so that someone else can study them, anatomical studies were accomplished through the use of cadavers (an acronym of the Latin phrase "*caro data vermibus*," which translated means "flesh given to worms"), deceased human bodies that have been donated to science for the purpose of study. Although cadavers are still used today to study the anatomical structure of the human body, modern technology such as positron emission tomography allows us to study these structures without dissecting the body. The advantage of imaging technology is that anatomy can be studied on living human beings.

Physiology is the study of the functions of living organisms and their parts. Physiology cannot be studied using a cadaver since a deceased organism does not function. Instead, physiology must be studied by using a living human being, by using an animal that is similar in structure to a human being, or by using a model of the particular anatomical part of interest to the scientist. Taken together, anatomy and physiology are biological sciences that examine the living organism in terms of its parts and the functions of those parts and of the organism as a whole.

Pathology is the scientific study of the nature of diseases and of the structural and functional changes that are imposed upon the living organism as a result. In other words, pathology is concerned with conditions or processes that are outside the realm of typical or normal, whether the aberration is associated with anatomical structure or physiological function. One should note that a good understanding of pathology and its effect on the organism cannot be fully realized until the individual has an equally good understanding of the anatomy and physiology of the organism.

ORIENTATION TO THE HUMAN BODY

The Anatomical Position

To understand the human body and the spatial relationships among the various bones, cartilages, muscles, organs, nerves, and other structures, one must have a general point of reference. In the study of anatomy, this point of reference is known as the anatomical position. You should always remember that the anatomical position is in reference to the body being observed (whether a living human or a cadaver), not the observer. For illustrative purposes, a cadaver will be the body being observed. Thus, when one refers to the left side of the body, it is the left side of the *cadaver's* body. If the cadaver is facing the observer, its left side will be on the right side to the observer. If you always remember that spatial terminology is used in reference to the cadaver, you will have little difficulty in understanding the terminology associated with positioning and orientation.

The anatomical position is illustrated in Figure 2-1. Note that the body being observed is standing upright, facing the observer, with its eyes straight ahead, arms at its side with the palms of the hands and toes of the feet facing forward. All of the terminology that will be used in this textbook, including terms associated with planes of reference and spatial orientation, will be in reference to the anatomical position.

Planes of Reference

The internal structures of the human body can be viewed from several different perspectives. For example, one can look at a particular organ from any angle, or

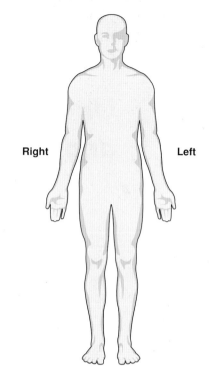

Right   **Left**

Figure 2-1   The anatomical position used as the general point of reference for describing the spatial orientation of the various parts of the body. (Reprinted with permission from Cohen, B.J. (2008). *Memmler's the human body in health and disease* (11th ed.). Baltimore: Lippincott Williams & Wilkins.)

the organ can be dissected in a horizontal, vertical, or other plane. When anatomical structures are photographed or drawn, it is important to note the plane of reference in which the structure is being presented. An anatomical structure may look quite different depending on its plane of reference. As you view the photographs and drawings in this textbook (and in other media as well), it is important that the figure caption be read and the plane of reference be noted.

There are three planes of reference that will be used throughout this textbook; these are illustrated in Figure 2-2 and defined in Table 2-1. These planes of reference include *coronal, sagittal,* and *transverse.* The coronal plane of reference is a vertical plane that separates the body or body part into anterior (front) and posterior (back) sections. It is called the coronal plane in reference to the coronal suture, a suture of the skull immediately above the forehead, running from temple to temple and separating the frontal bone of the skull from the parietal bones. This plane of reference is also sometimes referred to as the frontal plane.

The sagittal plane is also a vertically oriented plane of reference, although the orientation is a bit different than the coronal plane. In the case of the sagittal plane, the body or body part is separated into a left and a right portion. This plane is named in reference to the sagittal suture that runs lengthwise down the

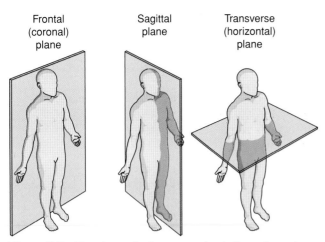

Frontal
(coronal)
plane

Sagittal
plane

Transverse
(horizontal)
plane

Figure 2-2 The planes of reference used to indicate the angle at which the observer is viewing the anatomy. (Reprinted with permission from Cohen, B.J. (2008). *Memmler's the human body in health and disease* (11th ed.). Baltimore: Lippincott Williams & Wilkins.)

center of the top of the skull, where the two parietal bones articulate with each other. If one were to divide the body or a body part right down the middle so that there is a left and right portion of relatively equal size, this is referred to as the *midsagittal* plane. The term *parasagittal* is often used in reference to any section that is parallel to the midsagittal plane.

Finally, the transverse plane is a horizontal plane of reference that separates the body or body part into an upper and a lower portion. When a magician performs the trick where the assistant lies down in a box and is supposedly cut in half, essentially the assistant is being divided in a transverse plane. It should be noted that in neuroanatomy, the term *horizontal plane* is used more often than transverse plane.

Other Terminology Associated with Spatial Orientation

Now that the anatomical position and planes of reference have been established, your attention is directed toward more specific terminology that is associated with the spatial relationships that exist between and among the various structures of the body. Although not an exhaustive list, Table 2-1 provides a "survival list" of terms that will help you understand the relationships various body parts have to each other. Figure 2-3 also illustrates some of the more commonly used terms to describe spatial position and orientation. It is imperative that you become comfortable using these terms. Learning these terms is half the battle when it comes to understanding the relationships between and among the various anatomical structures of the human body.

The terms and affixes in Table 2-1 are presented in alphabetic order. However, one should note that many of the terms describing spatial position or orientation come in pairs, in which the two terms have opposite meanings. These include:

- Anterior/posterior (i.e., front/back)
- Caudal/cranial or rostral (i.e., closer to the tail/closer to the head)
- Central/peripheral (i.e., located centrally/located in the periphery)
- Contra-/ipsi- (i.e., opposite side/same side)
- Deep/superficial (i.e., away from the body surface/toward the body surface)
- Distal/proximal (i.e., away from the point of origin/toward the point of origin)
- Dorsal/ventral (i.e., toward the back/toward the belly)
- Ecto-/endo- (i.e., outer/inner)
- External/internal (i.e., outside/inside)
- Extra-/intra- (i.e., outside/inside)
- Extrinsic/intrinsic (i.e., coming from the outside/coming from within)
- Inferior/superior (i.e., below/above)
- Infra-/supra- (i.e., below/above)
- Lateral/medial (i.e., toward the side/toward the middle)
- Post-/pre- (i.e., after/before)
- Prone/supine (i.e., face down/face up)

It should also be noted that Table 2-1 contains several prefixes. These are placed at the beginning of root words to indicate direction, position, or spatial orientation. For example, take the prefixes "infra-" and "supra-." When placed in front of the root word *hyoid*, they literally mean "below the hyoid" and "above the hyoid," respectively. In Chapter 8, you will be presented the anatomy and physiology of the phonatory system. In that chapter, a discussion will center on the extrinsic muscles of the larynx (note the term *extrinsic* here, which is defined in Table 2-1 as "external or coming from the outside"). Muscles of the larynx are classified as either intrinsic or extrinsic. The extrinsic muscles are subdivided into *suprahyoid* and *infrahyoid* muscles. All of these muscles make an attachment to the hyoid bone (hence the root word *hyoid*). The suprahyoid muscles come from anatomical structures located above the hyoid bone, whereas infrahyoid muscles come from anatomical structures located below the hyoid.

As a second example, consider the prefixes "pre-" and "post-." When used in conjunction with the term

TABLE 2-1

TERMS AND PREFIXES USED TO DESCRIBE PLANES OF REFERENCE AND SPATIAL RELATIONSHIPS

Term	Definition
Ante-	Situated before or in front of
Anterior	One structure is situated closer to the front of the body than another structure; sometimes the term *ventral* is used; opposite of *posterior*
Anteroposterior	Situated in an anterior-to-posterior (front-to-back) plane
Anti-	Situated against or on the opposite side
Bilateral	Pertaining to both sides of the body or an anatomical structure
Caudal	One structure is situated closer to the tail than another structure; opposite of *cranial* and *rostral*
Central	Pertaining to the center, or composing the primary part; opposite of *peripheral*
Contra-	Pertaining to the opposite side; opposite of *ipsi-*
Coronal	Vertical plane of reference that divides the body or a structure into an anterior and a posterior part; also known as the *frontal* plane
Cranial	One structure is situated closer to the head than another structure; used synonymously with *rostral*; opposite of *caudal*
Deep	One structure is situated further away from the body surface than another structure; opposite of *superficial*
Distal	Situated away from the center of the body or from the point of origin; opposite of *proximal*
Disto-	Pertaining to *distal*
Dorsal	Pertaining to the back; opposite of *ventral*
Dorsi-	Toward the *dorsal* (back) direction
Ecto-	Outer or on the outside; opposite of *endo-*
Endo-	Inner or on the inside; within; opposite of *ecto-*
Ento-	Inner or within
Epi-	Situated upon, following, or subsequent to
External	Situated on the outside; one structure is situated to the outside of another structure; opposite of *internal*
Extra-	Situated to the outside; opposite of *intra-*
Extrinsic	External or coming from the outside; opposite of *intrinsic*
Frontal	Situated in front of or relating to the anterior part of the body; also used synonymously with *coronal* as a plane of reference
Hypo-	Situated below; used sometimes instead of *sub-* or *infra-*
Inferior	Situated below or in a downward direction; opposite of *superior*
Infra-	Situated below; used sometimes instead of *sub-* or *hypo-*; opposite of *supra-*
Inter-	Situated between
Internal	Situated on the inside; one structure is situated to the inside of another structure; opposite of *external*
Intra-	Situated within or inside; opposite of *extra-*
Intrinsic	Internal or completely within; opposite of *extrinsic*
Ipsi-	Pertaining to the same side; opposite of *contra-*
Lateral	Situated to the side or farther from the *midsagittal* plane; opposite of *medial*
Longitudinal	Situated lengthwise or in the direction of the axis of the body or any of its parts
Medial	Situated toward the middle or center, or closer to the *midsagittal* plane; opposite of *lateral*
Mes-, Mesio-, Meso-	Situated in the middle; intermediate
Mesial	Toward the median or *midsagittal* plane
Met-, Meta-	After, behind, or hindmost; see also *post-*
Midsagittal	Vertical plane of reference through the midline of the body, dividing the body into left and right halves
Oblique	Situated in a slanting or diagonal direction
Palmar	Pertaining to the palm of the hand

TABLE 2-1

TERMS AND PREFIXES USED TO DESCRIBE PLANES OF REFERENCE AND SPATIAL RELATIONSHIPS (Continued)

Term	Definition
Para-	Adjacent, alongside, or near
Peri-	Around, about, or near
Peripheral	Pertaining to the periphery, or composing the secondary part; opposite of *central*
Plantar	Pertaining to the sole of the foot
Post-	After, behind, or posterior to; see also *meta-*; opposite of *pre-*
Posterior	One structure is situated closer to the back of the body than another structure; sometimes the term *dorsal* is used; opposite of *anterior*
Pre-	Before, in front of, or anterior to; opposite of *post-*
Prone	Body lying face down; opposite of *supine*
Proximal	Situated toward the center of the body or close to the point of origin; opposite of *distal*
Rectus	Straight, usually in a longitudinal direction
Retro-	Situated behind or in a backward direction
Rostral	One structure is situated closer to the head than another structure; used synonymously with *cranial*; opposite of *caudal*
Sagittal	Vertical plane of reference that divides the body or a structure into a left and a right part
Sub-	Situated beneath
Superficial	One structure is situated closer to the body surface than another structure; opposite of *deep*
Superior	Situated above or in an upward direction; opposite of *inferior*
Supine	Body lying face up; opposite of *prone*
Supra-	Situated above; used sometimes instead of *epi-*; opposite of *infra-*
Transverse	Horizontal plane of reference that divides the body or a structure into upper and lower parts
Unilateral	Pertaining to one side of the body or an anatomical structure
Ventral	Pertaining to the front or belly; opposite of *dorsal*
Version	Deviation of a body part from its normal axis

central and in reference to gyri (convolutions of the cerebrum), these terms denote two very important gyri of the brain. The *precentral gyrus* is the primary motor area and the *postcentral gyrus* is the primary somatosensory area. In this example, the root word *central* is in reference to the *central sulcus,* a narrow trough that separates the frontal lobe from the parietal lobe. The precentral gyrus is located immediately anterior to the central sulcus, whereas the postcentral gyrus is located immediately posterior to the central sulcus.

In the chapters that follow, the position of a particular body part may be described in reference to its spatial relationship to another body part. As you read these chapters and attempt to make sense of the anatomy, it is important to note the spatial terminology that is being used. These are not trivial terms. To the contrary, these terms allow you to pinpoint the exact location or orientation of a body part. You cannot have a complete understanding of anatomy without knowing where the various parts are located, especially in reference to other body parts.

A METHOD TO THE MADNESS

At the beginning of this chapter, it was mentioned that although the prospect of learning all of the anatomy and physiology of speech and hearing may cause anxiety on your part, there is a method to the madness that can make the learning process much easier than it first appears. There is no getting around it; to become a competent clinician you must learn the anatomy and physiology of speech perception and production. In part, this will involve committing a huge body of terminology to memory. How can one be expected to remember the vast nomenclature associated with anatomy and physiology? If you take each individual term and attempt to commit it to memory without really thinking about what the term really *means,* then the process of memorizing the vast amount of terminology will indeed be nearly impossible. However, if you analyze each term by considering the root and any affixes that may be attached, the learning process can be a lot less taxing.

In addition to the terminology presented in Table 2-1, you are referred to the appendix at the end of this

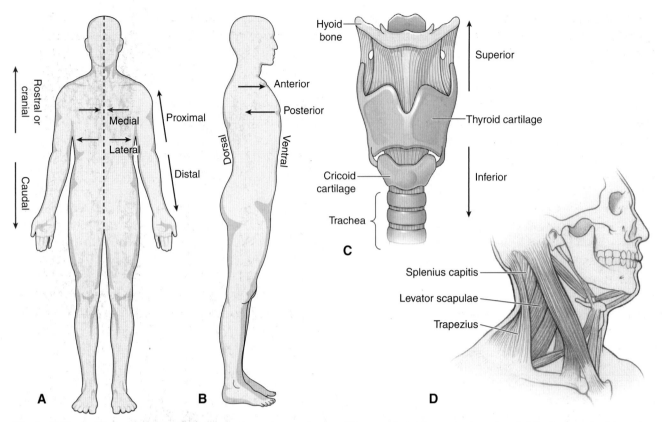

Figure 2-3   An illustration of the more commonly used terms for describing spatial position and orientation. **A**. Distal vs. proximal; lateral vs. medial; rostral (cranial) vs. caudal. **B**. Anterior vs. posterior; dorsal vs. ventral. **C**. Superior vs. inferior (note that the hyoid bone and thyroid cartilage are superior to the cricoid cartilage, and the trachea is inferior to the cricoid). **D**. Deep vs. superficial (note that the levator scapulae and splenius capitis are deep to the trapezius). (**A** and **B**: Modified with permission from Cohen, B.J. (2008). *Memmler's the human body in health and disease* (11th ed.). Baltimore: Lippincott Williams & Wilkins. **C**: Reprinted with permission from Cohen, B.J. (2008). *Memmler's the human body in health and disease* (11th ed.). Baltimore: Lippincott Williams & Wilkins. **D**: Reprinted with permission from Scheuman, D.W. (2006). *The balanced body: A guide to deep tissue and neuromuscular therapy* (3rd ed.). Baltimore: Lippincott Williams & Wilkins.)

book. The appendix contains seven tables that present terms and affixes that are used extensively in describing the anatomy, physiology, and pathology of the speech and hearing mechanisms. Although you would certainly be in a better position if you committed to memory the vocabulary and affixes found within these tables, the tables are provided primarily as a reference for you as you encounter the vast nomenclature of anatomy and physiology throughout the remainder of this textbook. Many of the terms and affixes presented in the appendix will also be included in the individual chapters that follow. It is hoped that by presenting the terminology numerous times throughout the book, you will be more likely to learn the nomenclature.

How to Use the Appendix

As mentioned above, the appendix is organized into seven tables. Each table presents vocabulary and affixes that are related in terms of what they describe. These include:

- Table A-1: Terms and affixes associated with movement
- Table A-2: Terms and affixes associated with anatomical structures or their parts
- Table A-3: Terms and affixes associated with color, form, general location, relative size, or shape
- Table A-4: Terms and affixes associated with bones, cartilages, cavities, membranes, or spaces
- Table A-5: Terms and affixes associated with the nervous system
- Table A-6: Terms and affixes associated with the auditory/vestibular system
- Table A-7: Miscellaneous terms and affixes used in anatomy, physiology, and pathology

With the exception of Table A-1 (which provides definitions only), the tables in the appendix provide definitions of the terms and affixes as well as an example of the use of each term or affix. The paragraphs that follow also provide more detailed information as to how knowledge of these terms and affixes can assist you in developing a deeper understanding of the anatomy, physiology, and pathology of the speech and hearing mechanisms.

Table A-1 presents terms and prefixes that are used to describe movement. In terms of muscle activity, the terms *extension* and *flexion* are used to denote how muscle contraction affects the movement of the body part being acted upon. The terms *abduction* and *adduction* are also very important. Although a single anatomical structure can abduct or adduct, these terms are used most often to describe the movement of two structures. For example, humans have two vocal folds. When the vocal folds are abducted (moved away from midline), the glottis—a variable-sized aperture between the vocal folds—opens so that air can flow in and out of the lungs. When the vocal folds are adducted (moved toward midline), they come together so that expired air can be used to vibrate them to produce voicing.

The terms *depressor, levator,* and *tensor* are also used to describe the action that occurs when muscles contract and act upon an anatomical structure. These terms are sometimes used as part of the name of a muscle, and therefore describe the action that particular muscle makes. For example, the *tensor tympani* muscle tenses the eardrum (tympanic membrane) by pulling inward on the malleus, to which the eardrum is attached. The *depressor anguli oris* is a muscle of the lips that pulls the corner of the mouth downward, as in frowning. Finally, the *levator veli palatini* muscle elevates or raises the soft palate (i.e., the velum, where according to Table A-2 the term *veli palatini* comes).

In reference to pathology, the prefixes "hyper-" and "hypo-" are often used to describe movement disorders. For example, a *hyperkinetic* movement disorder means that the patient exhibits involuntary, excessive, extraneous movements. By the same token, a patient with a *hypokinetic* movement disorder exhibits paucity of movement (i.e., the movements tend to be difficult to initiate and are very slow).

Table A-2 provides terms and affixes whose meanings are related to specific body parts. For example, upon first encountering the *omohyoid* muscle, you may scratch your head in wonder. However, if the term was analyzed into its components "omo-" and *hyoid,* one would be able to discern very quickly that the omohyoid muscle runs from the shoulder area to the hyoid bone. Similarly, by understanding the root terms and affixes, one can readily understand that cranial nerve III, the *oculomotor* nerve, is responsible for movements of the eyeball ("oculo-" meaning eye, and *motor* referring to activity resulting in movement).

What does *sternocleidomastoid* mean? By knowing the terminology in Table A-2, you can determine that it is a muscle that has three attachments. "Sterno-" refers to the sternum, "-cleido-" refers to the clavicle, and *mastoid* refers to the mastoid process, which is the rounded part of the base of the skull right behind the ear. Therefore, the sternocleidomastoid is a muscle that attaches to the sternum, clavicle, and mastoid process.

Table A-3 provides terms and prefixes associated with general location, size, shape, color, or general form. For example, the *serratus posterior superior* muscle can be found in the upper part (*superior*) of the back (*posterior*) and has a jagged or sawtooth (*serratus*) appearance. In Chapter 8, while learning about the cricoid cartilage (one of the cartilages of the larynx), you will encounter the term *posterior quadrate lamina*. From Table 2-1, you know that *posterior* refers to the back. Table A-3 defines *quadrate* as something that is somewhat square- or rectangular-shaped. Finally, according to Table A-4 *lamina* is a thin plate or flat layer of bone or cartilage. Taken together, you will correctly deduce that the posterior quadrate lamina is the back plate of the cricoid cartilage that is somewhat square-shaped.

Table A-4 includes terms and affixes that are used in reference to bones, cartilages, membranes, or cavities. For example, "cerato-" refers to a horn of some sort. The thyroid cartilage has two sets of cornua (horns) along its posterior margin. The superior cornua articulate with the greater cornua of the hyoid bone. The inferior cornua of the thyroid cartilage articulate with the cricoid cartilage, forming the cricothyroid joint. This joint is held in place by a series of ligaments known as the *ceratocricoid ligaments*. The term *ceratocricoid* refers to the two parts that make up the joint—the inferior cornua of the thyroid cartilage and the cricoid cartilage. Similarly, the *mental symphysis* refers to the fusion of the two halves of the mandible (jaw). During fetal development, the two halves of the mandible fuse to form a singular bone. The point where the two halves meet is the *mentum,* which is the protruding part of the chin. A *symphysis* is a union of two structures, in this case the two halves of the mandible.

Table A-5 provides terms and affixes associated primarily with the nervous system, and Table A-6 provides terms and prefixes associated with the auditory/vestibular system. (It should be noted here that although the respiratory, phonatory, and articulatory/resonance systems have their own unique nomenclature, many of the terms and affixes provided in Table 2-1 in this chapter and Tables A-1 through A-4 in the appendix are also used to describe structures and functions pertaining to these systems.)

In reference to the nervous system, the terms *afferent* and *efferent* are often used to describe nerves and nerve pathways. Afferent nerves are also known as sensory nerves because the impulses originate in the periphery (where the sense organs are located) and then are sent toward the central nervous system for interpretation. On the other hand, the impulses of efferent (or motor) nerves originate in the central nervous system and then proceed to the various muscles and viscera located in the periphery. The purpose of these nerves is to effect movement.

Many of the structures of the brain have peculiar names: *caudate nucleus, corpus striatum, olives,* and *pyramids* to name a few. Once again, by analyzing these names you can remember something about each of them. *Caudate* means tail (see Table A-5 of the appendix). A nucleus is a collection of gray matter— nerve cell bodies. Therefore, the caudate nucleus is a mass of gray matter that has a head and a long slender tail. *Corpus* means body. *Striatum* refers to a striped appearance. The corpus striatum then is a series of bodies deep within the brain that has a striped appearance. Finally, the olives (technically, the olivary complex) and pyramids can be seen on the ventral surface of the medulla oblongata. They each get their name from their general shape. To carry this thought out a bit further, when one encounters the term *pyramidal motor tract,* one should not be alarmed. The astute observer will note that another term for motor is efferent. The pyramidal motor tract is a tract of efferent nerve fibers that passes through the pyramids on the way to the spinal cord, which is immediately below the medulla oblongata. In fact, the pyramidal motor tract is the primary motor tract, as opposed to the *extrapyramidal motor tract,* which is a secondary motor tract whose nerve fibers also pass down to the spinal cord, but do not make a stop at the pyramids along the way. Remember from Table 2-1, "extra-" means situated to the outside, so extrapyramidal means "situated to the outside of the pyramids."

In regard to the auditory/vestibular system (see Table A-6), terms and prefixes can also be analyzed to provide meaning to the nomenclature. For example, *incudostapedial* refers to the incus and stapes, and in fact, the incudostapedial joint is formed by the articulation of the incus with the stapes. As another example, a pathological condition of the middle ear, *otitis media,* can easily be remembered if the term is analyzed into its individual parts: "ot-" means ear; "itis-" means inflammation; and *media* refers to the middle. Therefore, otitis media is an inflammation of the middle ear cavity.

The last table in the appendix (Table A-7) provides a list of miscellaneous terms and affixes that can also be used to assist you in retaining the nomenclature of anatomy, physiology, and pathology. Although many of the terms and affixes in this table are pertinent to anatomy and physiology, a large number of them are used in reference to pathology. Once again, the terms and affixes presented in this table can be considered a "survival set" of vocabulary for you. For example, a *tracheotomy* is a procedure in which an incision is made in the anterior wall of the trachea through the outer neck to assist the patient in breathing (usually due to some type of upper airway obstruction). You know from Table A-2 that "tracheo-" refers to the trachea or windpipe. Table A-7 shows that "-otomy" means an operation involving cutting. As a second example, Table A-7 provides the definition for *malacia* (a softening or loss of consistency of tissues or organs). From Table A-4, you can see that "chondro-" is a prefix meaning cartilage. Therefore, *chondromalacia* is a pathological condition in which a cartilage is too soft or underdeveloped.

As a final word, it should be noted that the terms presented in Table 2-1 of this chapter and Tables A-1 through A-7 in the appendix are not an exhaustive list but are presented as a starter set for you. You are encouraged to consult a dictionary when an unfamiliar term is encountered. Pay particular attention to the root and any affixes that may be attached. Clues often exist to assist you in learning the nomenclature. Also, it should be emphasized that many of the terms presented in this chapter were placed in a particular table because of the *primary* context in which the term is used. There are many terms and affixes in these tables that could just as well be presented in another table. For example, the prefixes "ary-," "crico-," and "thyro-" were all placed in Table A-2 because they refer to specific parts of the human body (i.e., the arytenoid cartilages, cricoid cartilage, and thyroid cartilage, respectively). However, all of them could just as easily have been placed in Table A-4 because they are associated with cartilages. You are discouraged from relying too heavily on how these terms and affixes are organized in the tables. Instead, your focus should be simply on the terminology.

It should be readily apparent from all of these examples that the process of learning anatomy, physiology, and pathology is not as difficult as one may first imagine. Learning anatomy and physiology should not be an exercise in rote memorization of terms. Instead, by focusing more on the meanings of a relatively small, finite set of terms and affixes, you have nearly the entire world of anatomy, physiology, and pathology within grasp. As you proceed through the remaining chapters of this textbook and encounter terminology that is unfamiliar to you, the last thing you should do is panic. Step back, think of the meanings of the root and affixes, and

the meaning of the unfamiliar term may very well present itself.

Now that you have an understanding of the basic nomenclature in terms of the anatomical position, planes of reference, spatial terminology, and more specific vocabulary related to anatomy, physiology, and pathology, it is time to turn your attention to the structural organization of human beings.

CHAPTER 3

The Structural Organization of Humans

Knowledge Outcomes for ASHA Certification for Chapter 3
- Demonstrate knowledge of the biological basis of the basic human communication processes (III-B)
- Demonstrate knowledge of the neurological basis of the basic human communication processes (III-B)
- Demonstrate knowledge of the biological basis of swallowing processes (III-B)

Learning Objectives
- You will define cell types and organelles.
- You will describe the four tissue types and subclassifications.
- You will discuss the organ systems most pertinent for speech and swallow function.

MEDICAL TERM PART BOX

TERM	MEANING	EXAMPLE
-arthrodial	joint	di**arthrodial**
bi-	two or double	**bi**polar
cellular	related to a cell	intra**cellular** movement
chondrium	related to cartilage	peri**chondrium**
cyto-	pertaining to a cell	**cyto**plasm
endo-	toward the interior	**endo**mysium
epi-	upon or above	**epi**mysium
extra-	outside of	**extra**cellular
inter-	between	**inter**cellular
intra-	within	**intra**cellular
meatus	an opening	external auditory **meatus**
meso-	middle or intermediate	**meso**thelial tissue
micro-	small size	**micro**tubule
-mysium	pertaining to muscle	peri**mysium**
os	bone	**os**sicles
-osteum	pertaining to bone	peri**osteum**

TERM	MEANING	EXAMPLE
peri-	around	**peri**mysium
-plasm	cellular substance	cyto**plasm**
proto-	first	**proto**plasm
uni-	one or single	**uni**polar

The complexity of human communication is largely what sets human beings apart from other vertebrate species. Thought, language, and speech are all necessary for effective verbal communication. Speech, our primary mode of expressive communication, is the sequential production of sounds to represent our thoughts resulting in a comprehensible auditory signal for a listener to perceive. Furthermore, the ability to produce speech relies on the coordination of multiple speech processes: respiration, phonation, and articulation/resonance. In order to better understand these speech processes, they can be broken down by reducing them to their structural makeup. For example, the process of respiration relies on the thoracic skeletal framework of the ribcage and vertebral column upon which the muscles attach to enact the movement necessary to breathe for speech. In addition, each speech process includes organs, such as lungs, and each organ has a predominant tissue type. Tissues are defined by their cellular makeup. Thus, the cell is our most basic component of life.

Cells

There are more than 100 trillion cells in the human body. Some cells live the life span of the body such as those in the central nervous system; some live a moderate amount of time such as blood cells, and some cells are continuously dying and being replaced such as those that comprise the epithelium—otherwise known as skin.

A cell possesses five characteristics, making it a living organism. These characteristics are (1) irritability, (2) growth, (3) spontaneous movement, (4) metabolism, and (5) reproduction. Irritability refers to the cell's ability to respond to stimulation. A cell, in most cases, goes through a life process of birth, development, and death; this is considered growth. Spontaneous movement is characterized by movement that originates and occurs within the cell; that is, **intracellular** movement. Metabolism refers to the cell's capability to take in raw products, break down these products, and utilize the "food" in the form of usable energy to carry out its life support roles. Lastly, cells have the ability to reproduce themselves.

Cells are formed out of **protoplasm** which is the basic living substance that comprises all cells. This protoplasm subdivides into the cell nucleus and the surrounding **cytoplasm**, the fluid outside the nucleus (see Figure 3-1). The outer membrane surrounding the cell is referred to as the **plasma membrane**. It is composed of a double layer of molecules that exhibits *selective permeability*; that is, some materials are allowed to enter or exit the cell whereas other materials are prohibited. Essentially, the plasma membrane controls the exchange of molecules and ions between the cell and its external environment (i.e., **extracellular** space). Further explanation and illustration of this double-layered membrane is presented in Chapter 4. The **nucleus** is considered the "control center" of the cell. It is usually found toward the center of the cell and is separated from other cellular material by the nuclear membrane. The nucleus contains the genetic material of the cell in the form of threadlike structures termed chromosomes, which are double strands of deoxyribonucleic acid. The most prominent structure within the nucleus is the nucleolus, the genetic control center for ribosome synthesis.

Inside each cell are a number of structures called **organelles** ("cell organs") found within the cytoplasm (see Figure 3-1). Each organelle performs a specific task necessary for the functioning and survival of the cell. For example, **mitochondria** provide energy and serve as a power source for the cell. The **Golgi apparatus** serves to store materials and is responsible for packaging substances for intracellular transport. The **endoplasmic reticulum** (granular or agranular) synthesizes, stores, and releases various substances such as fatty acids, protein, and calcium. **Lysosomes** break down and digest bacterial and cellular debris that have been ingested by the cell; they are considered the "garbage can" of the cell. **Microtubules** and **microfilaments** assist with cell movement as well as provide for intracellular transport of substances. **Centrioles** are fused sets of microtubules that participate in nuclear and cell division (i.e., reproduction). Refer to Table 3-1 for further descriptions of these organelles.

Figure 3-1   A generic human cell illustrating the plasma membrane, cilia, nucleus, and organelles found within the cytoplasm. (Reprinted with permission from Cohen, B.J. (2008). *Memmler's the human body in health and disease* (11th ed.). Baltimore: Lippincott Williams & Wilkins.)

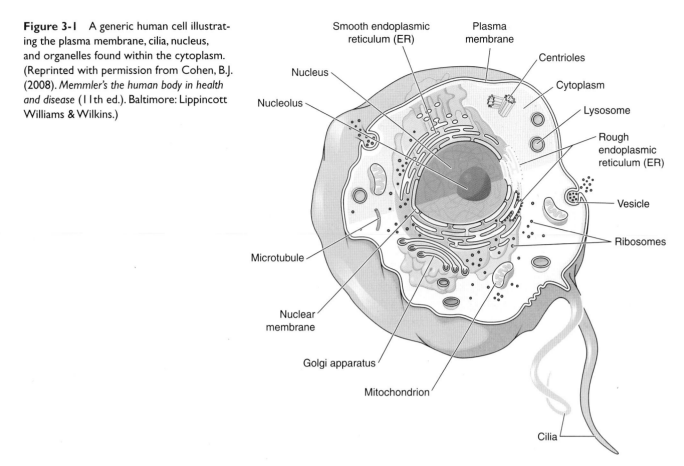

Cells can be classified into four types specialized for specific functions: **epithelial cells**, **muscle cells**, **connective tissue cells,** and **nerve cells** or neurons. Epithelial cells are specialized for the selective secretion and absorption of molecules and ions; they cover surfaces and form selective barriers. Muscle cells, synonymous with muscle fibers, are specialized for the production of mechanical forces, which produce movement. Connective tissue cells are specialized for the formation and secretion of various types of extracellular connecting and supporting elements—connecting, anchoring, and supporting structures of the body. Nerve cells (i.e., neurons) are specialized for the initiation and conduction of electrochemical

TABLE 3-1	
PARTS OF A TYPICAL CELL	
Cell Part	**Function**
Centrioles	Assist in cell division, microtubule formation
Chromosomes	Store and pass on genetic information
Golgi apparatus	Stores and delivers various proteins
Lysosomes	Digest cell debris and bacteria
Microfilaments	Support cytoplasm, cell movement
Microtubules	Provide cell framework and movement of parts of cells
Mitochondria	Produce energy for the cell
Nucleus	Genetic control center via both deoxyribonucleic acid and ribosome synthesis
Plasma membrane	Surrounding barrier of a single cell; separates intracellular material from extracellular material and dictates entry and exit of material from the cell
Ribosomes	Synthesize protein as directed by genetic information
Rough (granular) endoplasmic reticulum	Protein production, stored and released
Smooth (agranular) endoplasmic reticulum	Stores and releases enzymes and calcium for muscle contraction

information traveling over distances; they are the basic functional unit of the nervous system. Aggregates of cells form the four different tissue types. It is important for groups of cells to join and cooperate for the good of the organism as a whole. Thus, groups of cells similar in structure, function, and embryonic origin band together with varying amounts of extracellular material to form tissues. An organization of these tissue types and subclassifications is presented in Table 3-2.

Tissues

EPITHELIAL TISSUE

Epithelial tissue refers to "tissue upon tissue"; thus, by definition this tissue lines the surface of the body and those passages communicating with the external environment (e.g., the ear canal) and the cavities of our body. Epithelium has very little extracellular material, so the cells lie adjacent to one another. This tissue is often described on the basis of cell shape and number of cell layers. Epithelial cells can be flat or plate-like (i.e., squamous), cube-shaped (i.e., cuboidal), or oblong (i.e., columnar). In addition, epithelial cells may have **cilia** (short, hairlike structures) protruding from their surface to provide a transport mechanism to move materials over the surface of the cells (e.g., respiratory tract). Tissue is made up of these different cell shapes organized in one or more layers. Where transport of material occurs, the cells are arranged in one layer; this is referred to as "simple." Multiple cell layers are referred to as "stratified" or "compound." Hence, the terms can be combined to describe both cell shape and layers—for example, simple columnar or stratified squamous (see Figure 3-2).

Epithelial tissue can also be classified into three groups based on location. **Epithelial tissue proper** is tissue forming the skin (i.e., epidermis) and the internal membranes continuous with the skin. This tissue comprises various layers and shapes of cells that line the digestive, respiratory, urinary, and reproductive tracts and tubes. **Endothelial tissue** makes up the linings of blood and lymph vessels. Simple squamous cells comprise this tissue because of the necessity to have extremely smooth surfaces to reduce the possibility of fragmenting blood cells. It should be noted here that arteries and veins also require elastic tissue (a type of connective tissue) and smooth muscle (a type of muscle tissue). Lastly, **mesothelial tissue** lines the internal body cavities. Mesothelial tissue is often referred to as serous membrane because the cells secrete a serous fluid or serum, which has a thin,

TABLE 3-2

TYPES OF TISSUES WITH SUBCLASSIFICATIONS

I. Epithelial tissue
  A. Shape
    1. Squamous
    2. Cuboidal
    3. Columnar
  B. Number of cell layers
    1. Simple
    2. Stratified/compound
  C. Location
    1. Epithelial tissue proper
    2. Endothelial
    3. Mesothelial
      a. Peritoneal
      b. Pleural
      c. Pericardial
II. Connective tissue
  A. Loose
    1. Areolar
    2. Adipose
  B. Dense
    1. Tendons
    2. White fibrous
      a. Ligaments
      b. Fascia
  C. Specialized
    1. Cartilage
      a. Hyaline
      b. Fibrous (fibrocartilage)
      c. Elastic (yellow)
    2. Blood
    3. Bone
      a. Compact
      b. Spongy
III. Muscle tissue
  A. Striated/skeletal (voluntary)
  B. Smooth (involuntary)
  C. Cardiac (striated, involuntary)
IV. Nervous tissue
  A. Neurons
  B. Glial cells

watery constitution. There are a total of four body cavities that are lined with serous membrane (see Figure 3-3). Three are located in the thorax: the **pericardial cavity** housing the heart and the two **pleural cavities** housing each lung. The fourth cavity, in the abdomen, is the **peritoneal cavity** housing the viscera (i.e., abdominal organs). The pleural cavities will be discussed in more detail in Chapter 6.

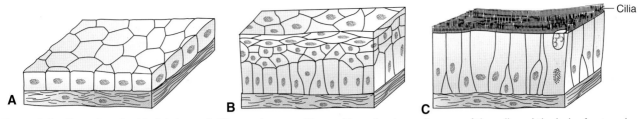

Cilia

A **B** **C**

Figure 3-2 Examples of epithelial tissue of different shapes and layers. Note the close adjacency of the cells and the lack of extracellular material. **A.** Simple cuboidal. **B.** Stratified squamous. **C.** Pseudostratified ciliated columnar. (Reprinted with permission from Porth, C.M., & Matfin, G. (2008). *Pathophysiology: Concepts of altered health states* (8th ed.). Philadelphia: Lippincott Williams & Wilkins.)

CONNECTIVE TISSUE

Tissues which combine or hold together structures, support the body, and aid in body maintenance are referred to as **connective tissues**. In contrast to epithelial tissue, there are fewer cells making up connective tissue but much more extracellular substance. The extracellular components of connective tissue are collectively called **matrix**. Matrix is formed by protein fibers such as collagen, nonprotein molecules such as ground substance, and fluid. Connective tissue can be classified according to the make-up of its extracellular matrix as connective tissue proper or specialized connective tissue (see Table 3-2).

Connective tissue proper is further classified into loose or dense connective tissue. Loose connective tissue fills spaces and is considered the "packing material of the body." Loosely packed fibers are distributed throughout the body to bind parts together. Just deep to the skin are two loose connective tissue types: **areolar**, which forms the "bed" for the skin,

and **adipose**, which includes a number of fat-storing cells. Dense connective tissue is characterized by an abundance of tightly packed extracellular fibers, either collagen or elastic. Collagen is a fibrous protein with great strength; therefore, these tissues are able to tolerate high degrees of tension. Furthermore, there are three types of dense connective tissues: **tendons**, **ligaments**, and **fascia**. Tendons are tough, nonelastic cords that are associated with muscle as they attach muscle to bone, muscle to cartilage, or muscle to another muscle. Broad tendinous sheets are called **aponeuroses**. Ligaments are also tough cords but, in contrast to tendons, they have an abundance of elastic fibers and they join bone to bone, bone to cartilage, or cartilage to cartilage; thus, they are a critical part of joints. Finally, fascia makes up fibrous tissue underlying the skin or covers and separates muscle into functional groups.

Cartilage and bone make up specialized connective tissue; their hardness is imposed by solid or rigid extracellular substance. Cartilage is characterized by its rigidity, flexibility, and varying amounts of elasticity depending on the type of cartilage. Cartilage is further subdivided into **hyaline**, **elastic** or **fibrous**. Hyaline cartilage is the most abundant type of cartilage in the human body. It has a bluish-white translucent appearance and is found primarily in places where strong support is needed with some flexibility as well. Hyaline makes up most of the embryonic skeleton, which later turns to bone. In regard to structures critical for speech production, hyaline cartilage is found in the rib cage, the larynx, and the nose. Figure 3-4 illustrates the nasal septum; the most anterior part comprises hyaline cartilage. Elastic cartilage appears yellow and opaque and is extremely flexible. This cartilage is the basis of the outer ear, comprising the *pinna* and the cartilaginous portion of the *external auditory meatus* (i.e., ear canal; see Figure 3-5). The *epiglottis* and small cartilages of the larynx (i.e., *corniculates* and *cuneiforms*) also comprise elastic cartilage. Fibrous cartilage has a coarse appearance

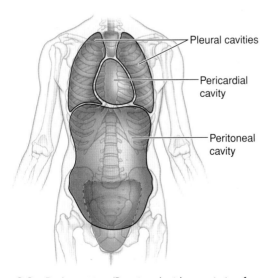

Pleural cavities

Pericardial cavity

Peritoneal cavity

Figure 3-3 Body cavities. (Reprinted with permission from Nath, J.L. (2005). *Using medical terminology: A practical approach.* Baltimore: Lippincott Williams & Wilkins.)

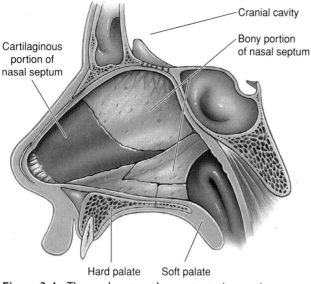

Figure 3-4   The nasal septum; the most anterior portion comprises hyaline cartilage. (Reprinted with permission from Anatomical Chart Company.)

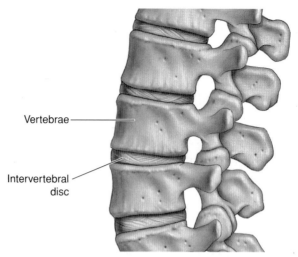

Figure 3-6   A segment of the vertebral column; note that the intervertebral discs are made up of fibrous cartilage. (Reprinted with permission from Anatomical Chart Company.)

as fibers are arranged in thick parallel bundles. This cartilage is slightly compressible and can withstand great amounts of pressure; therefore, it is found in regions that support body weight such as the *intervertebral discs* (see Figure 3-6) and some joints of the body such as the *temporomandibular joint* (which will be described more fully in Chapter 10).

Bone is a specialized connective tissue that provides the framework for other tissues of the body.

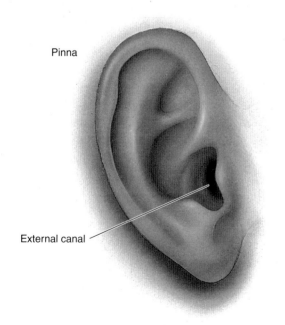

Figure 3-5   The external ear; note that the pinna and external ear canal are made up of elastic cartilage. (Reprinted with permission from Anatomical Chart Company.)

Bone is unique in that the collagen and matrix are intermixed with minerals (i.e., calcium phosphate and calcium carbonate salts) that impart rigidity and hardness. Each bone has a dense, outer, compact layer surrounded by a fibrous membrane termed **periosteum**. Each bone also has a porous, inner, spongy layer where bone marrow is found for the production of red and white blood cells.

The adult, human skeleton has approximately 206 bones, depending how they are counted, and is broadly divided into the axial and appendicular skeleton (see Figure 3-7). The axial skeleton is most relevant to speech and hearing anatomy as it consists of the skull which includes the *ossicles* (bones of the middle ear) and the facial bones, as well as the hyoid bone, the ribcage, and the vertebral column. The appendicular skeleton refers to the pectoral girdle (shoulder) and bones of the arms and hands (upper extremities) as well as the pelvic girdle (hip) and bones of the legs and feet (lower extremities). It should be noted that both the pectoral girdle and pelvic girdle are connection points for muscles involved in breathing. These will be described more completely in Chapter 6.

Bones join other bones at joints, as do some cartilages. These joints are held together by ligaments. Joints may be described on the basis of their anatomy or their function (see Table 3-3). Anatomically, **fibrous joints** are united by fibrous connective tissue. These joints are considered **synarthrodial** as they are only slightly movable or totally immovable. Cranial sutures that join the bones of the cranium are one example of a class of fibrous joints that are immovable. **Cartilaginous joints** are considered **amphiarthrodial** or as joints that yield. These joints utilize either hyaline

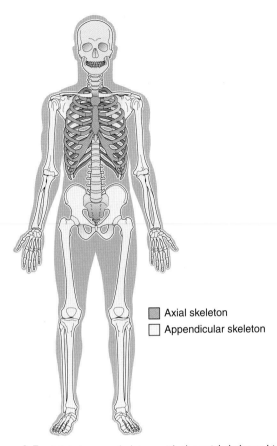

Figure 3-7 Adult, human skeleton with the axial skeleton highlighted. (Reprinted with permission from Cohen, B.J. (2008). *Memmler's the human body in health and disease* (11th ed.). Baltimore: Lippincott Williams & Wilkins.)

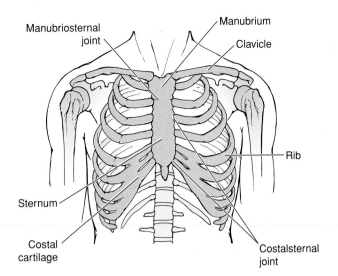

Figure 3-8 Anterior view of the ribcage illustrating the costalsternal joint and the manubriosternal joint. (Modified with permission from Hendrickson, T. (2009). *Massage and manual therapy for orthopedic conditions* (2nd ed.). Baltimore: Lippincott Williams & Wilkins.)

or fibrocartilage to unite bone to bone. If hyaline is the cartilage involved, the joint is referred to as a **synchondrosis** joint. An example of this type of joint pertinent to speech is found within the ribcage between the bony ribs and the sternum via the costal cartilages (see Figure 3-8). A synchondrosis joint allows for some movement given the flexibility inherent in hyaline cartilage. This is imperative to breathing as the ribcage must be able to expand in order to inhale and, conversely, get smaller to exhale. The most common joint is the **synovial joint** that is considered **diarthrodial**, which means freely moving. The synovial joint is anatomically more complex than fibrous or cartilaginous joints.

The synovial joint itself is enclosed by a fibrous capsule called the articular capsule that is lined by a

TABLE 3-3

ANATOMICAL AND FUNCTIONAL TERMS FOR COMMON JOINTS SEEN IN THE ANATOMY OF THE SPEECH AND HEARING MECHANISM WITH EXAMPLES

Functional Name	Anatomical Name	Example
Synarthrodial	Fibrous	
	Syndesmosis	Stylohyoid syndesmosis
	Sutures	Coronal suture
	Gomphosis	Dentoalveolar joint
Amphiarthrodial	Cartilaginous	
	Synchondrosis	Costosternal synchondrosis
	Symphysis	Manubriosternal symphysis
Diarthrodial	Synovial	
	Plane (gliding)	Costovertebral joint
	Saddle	Malleoincudal joint
	Hinge	Genu (knee)
	Pivot	Atlas (C1) and axis (C2)
	Ball-and-socket	Humeral (shoulder) joint
	Ellipsoid (condyloid)	Temporomandibular joint

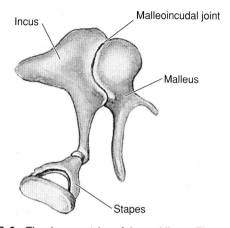

Figure 3-9   The three ossicles of the middle ear. The malleoincudal joint is a saddle joint, a type of synovial joint. (Reprinted with permission from Anatomical Chart Company.)

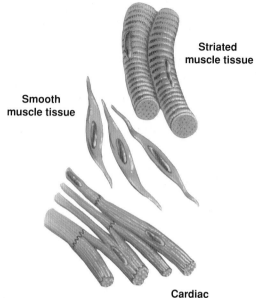

Figure 3-10   Three types of muscle tissues: cardiac, smooth, and striated (skeletal). (Reprinted with permission from Anatomical Chart Company.)

membrane called the **synovial** membrane. The synovial membrane secretes synovial fluid which (1) lubricates the joint, (2) provides nourishment to the articular cartilages (which are hyaline), and (3) protects the joint from impact and friction. There are six types of synovial joints which are classified according to the shape of their articulating surfaces: plane, saddle, hinge, pivot, ball-and-socket, and ellipsoid (or condyloid). An example of a saddle joint, which allows for all types of movement except rotation, is the *malleoincudal joint*, which joins two of the ossicles in the middle ear, the malleus and the incus (see Figure 3-9). Table 3-3 provides examples of amphiarthrodial, diarthrodial, and synarthrodial joints.

MUSCLE TISSUE

Muscle cells, which are also called muscle fibers, come together to form muscle tissue. Muscle tissue has the important property of contractility—the ability to change shape, becoming shorter and thicker thus enabling movement of bones and other structures. Muscle tissue is described in terms of its anatomy, being striated or nonstriated, and function, being voluntary or involuntary. There are three types of muscle tissues: cardiac, smooth, and striated or striped (see Figure 3-10). Cardiac muscle forms the walls of the heart and is responsible for pumping blood; it is under involuntary control. Each cardiac muscle cell has one nucleus, appears striated, and branches to connect with adjacent cells. This branching is significant in regard to the type of communication that occurs between cardiac cells, allowing for continuous heart muscle contraction.

Smooth muscle forms the muscular portion of the visceral organs (e.g., lower esophagus, stomach, intestines) and is also found within blood vessels. Smooth muscle controls the size, shape, and movements of these visceral organs. It is nonstriated and is under involuntary control (i.e., it contracts without the individual having conscious control over it).

Striated muscle tissue is also referred to as skeletal muscle. Skeletal muscle is easiest to envision as it connects to our skeletal framework and contraction results in body movement. Skeletal muscle can contract to about one-half its original length. The larger the diameter of the muscle, the greater its strength. As the name implies, cells making up skeletal muscle tissue appear striated and its function is under voluntary control. Skeletal muscle is the predominant type of muscle involved with speech production. Speech production is, indeed, a voluntary behavior and is mediated by the contraction and relaxation of skeletal muscles.

Skeletal muscle is attached to bone or cartilage and occasionally inserts into another muscle (i.e., muscles of the tongue) or to the epidermis (e.g., eyelids, lips). Muscle is attached via a tendon to the periosteum of the bone or the **perichondrium** of the cartilage. Muscle may also be attached via an aponeurosis (a broad tendinous sheet).

The microscopic structure of skeletal muscle is very organized with the help of connective tissue. Muscle consists of bundles of muscle fibers (recall that a muscle fiber is a muscle cell). Each bundle is termed a **fasciculus**. Each muscle fiber in the fasciculus is surrounded by a thin layer of delicate connective tissue called **endomysium**. Each fasciculus is, in turn, surrounded by a sheath of fibrous connective tissue called **perimysium**, which serves to separate groups of muscle fibers from each other to enable muscle to function as a unit. A group of fasciculi is encased in a coarser connective tissue called **epimysium**. Finally, the entire outer surface of each muscle is enclosed with fascia, a dense connective tissue which is continuous with the connective tissue of the tendons and periosteum or perichondrium. Figure 3-11 illustrates this organization.

NERVOUS TISSUE

Nervous tissue consists of nerve cells (i.e., neurons) and support cells called **glial cells**. This tissue is found in the brain, spinal cord, and peripheral nervous system, and relays information to and from the head, neck, and body. Nervous tissue is specialized to transmit information across distances. This information is passed on through both chemical (e.g., *neurotransmitters*) and electrical (e.g., *action potentials*) means. Neurons are composed of four parts—dendrites, cell body (i.e., soma), axon, and terminal (see Figure 3-12). In general, the dendrites receive electrical signals and conduct them toward the cell body. The cell body houses the nucleus and a number of organelles critical to the function of the neuron. The axon projects off the cell body and is key in transmitting the electrical signal (i.e., impulse) in one direction, down the axon toward the terminal. The terminal, if adequately stimulated, then releases a chemical to carry the message to the next neuron in line. In the case of muscle in the periphery, the neuron releases a chemical that directs the muscle to contract.

Neurons are classified according to number of processes (i.e., axons and dendrites), function, and speed of information transfer. Neurons with multiple dendrites and a single axon are called *multipolar neurons*; these are the most commonly seen in illustrations of neurons. The majority of the neurons in the brain are multipolar, often having a motoric function. Those with a single dendrite and a single axon are *bipolar neurons* and those with only a single axon emerging from the cell body are *unipolar neurons*. Bipolar neurons are found in systems involved with special senses. For example, the cells of the sensory cochlea and the vestibular ganglia are bipolar. Unipolar neurons are found in the dorsal root ganglia next to the spinal cord. Neurons function in sensory, motor, or integrative (i.e., association neurons) capacities. Speed of transfer is dependent on the covering of the axon (i.e., myelin) and the diameter of the axon.

Axons are also referred to as nerve fibers. Nerve fibers are classified as Type A, Type B, or Type C based on their diameter. Type A fibers transfer information most rapidly, as they are large diameter, myelinated axons. Type B fibers have a medium diameter and are slightly myelinated resulting in a slower speed of information transfer as compared with Type A. Finally, Type C fibers are relatively slow as they are small in diameter and are nonmyelinated. Speech processes rely on Type A nerve fibers for rapid sensory input to the brain and for rapid motor impulses to the muscles of respiration, phonation, and articulation/resonance.

An example of Type A nerve fibers is the motor neurons that inform muscles whether to contract and how much to contract; this occurs at the **neuromuscular junction**. The neuromuscular junction is the point of communication and information transfer between the terminal branches of an axon and the muscle fibers it innervates. This junction is also referred to as the myoneural junction as "myo-" refers to muscle and "neural" refers to the nerve fiber. This point of information transfer between the nerve fiber and its muscle fibers is a synapse. Synapses also take place between neurons but here the synapse is specific to the neuron and the muscle. The terminal branches from a single neuron synapse with many muscle fibers. A motor unit is one motor neuron and all the muscle fibers it innervates.

Similar to muscle, nerves of the peripheral nervous system have an organization imposed by their connective tissue coverings (see Figure 3-11). A delicate connective tissue called **endoneurium** surrounds the individual nerve fibers (i.e., axons). These nerve fibers run in bundles called **fascicles**; each fascicle is encased in **perineurium**. Fascicles, in turn, are bundled in groupings that form a nerve which is wrapped by **epineurium**. These connective tissue coverings allow a peripheral nerve, such as the hypoglossal cranial nerve, to function as a unit with a specific responsibility. For instance, the hypoglossal cranial nerve provides impulses to muscles of the tongue for movement.

Organs

Organs are the result of a combination of two or more tissue types that come together to form a functional unit. A functional unit refers to tissues working together to perform a specific function. Examples pertinent to speech production and swallowing include the lungs, which function to provide breath support for speech. The larynx is also an organ that provides

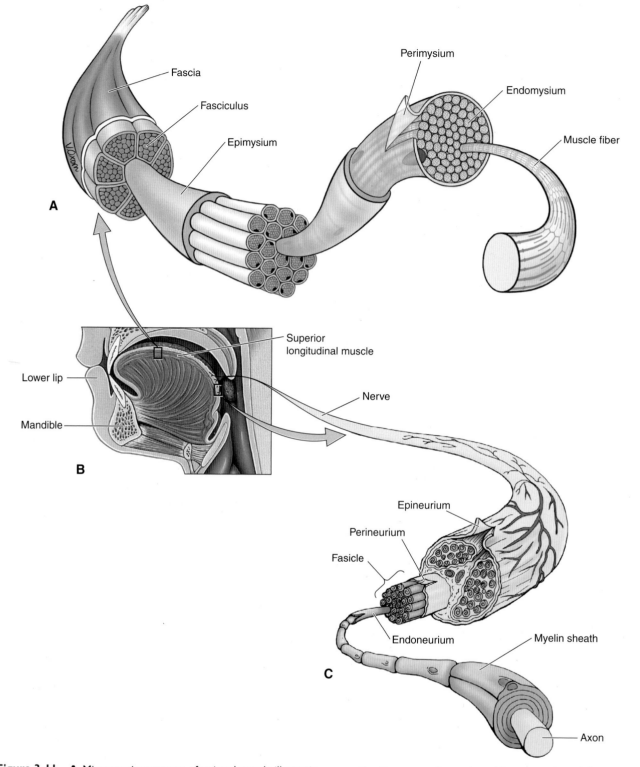

Figure 3-11   **A**. Microscopic structure of striated muscle illustrating connective tissue coverings enlarged from a section of the superior longitudinal tongue muscle. **B**. Tongue muscles. **C**. Microscopic structure of peripheral nerves illustrating connective tissue coverings of the nerve innervating the superior longitudinal tongue muscle. (**A**: Reprinted with permission from Moore, K.L., Agur, A.M., & Dalley, A, F. (2010). *Essential clinical anatomy* (4th ed.). Baltimore: Lippincott Williams & Wilkins. **B**: Reprinted with permission from Anatomical Chart Company. **C**: Reprinted with permission from Moore, K.L, Agur, A.M., & Dalley, A.F. (2009). *Clinically oriented anatomy* (6th ed.). Baltimore: Lippincott Williams & Wilkins.)

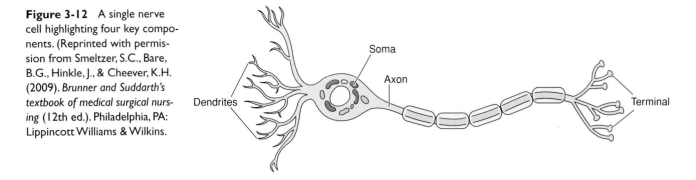

Figure 3-12 A single nerve cell highlighting four key components. (Reprinted with permission from Smeltzer, S.C., Bare, B.G., Hinkle, J., & Cheever, K.H. (2009). *Brunner and Suddarth's textbook of medical surgical nursing* (12th ed.). Philadelphia, PA: Lippincott Williams & Wilkins.

airway protection during swallow and provides a critical sound source, that is, the voice. The tongue is an organ that provides movement necessary for mastication (i.e., chewing) and for sound production and resonation. An organ usually has a predominant tissue type. In the case of the tongue, muscle tissue is predominant, with supporting connective tissue (e.g., the hyoid bone for attachment), vascular tissue (blood supply), and nervous tissue (e.g., motor neurons to innervate tongue muscles). In the case of the larynx, connective tissue (by way of the cartilages that comprise it) is the predominant tissue type.

Systems

Two or more organs combine to form a functional unit called a system. There are 9 to 12 systems in the human body, depending on the anatomist. The most important body systems for speech production and swallowing function are the following six: circulatory (or vascular); digestive; muscular; nervous; respiratory; and skeletal (see Table 3-4). The circulatory system includes the blood vessels, the blood itself, and the cardiac muscle that comprises the heart. The skeletal system includes the human body's bony framework inclusive of cartilage and the connecting elements of joints, ligaments, and tendons. The muscular system includes the striated muscle of the body, which attaches to the skeletal framework. The respiratory system includes organs and structures of both the upper and lower respiratory airways. Thus, the nasal and oral cavities, the pharynx (throat), the larynx (as a passageway), the trachea, the bronchi and all their branches, and the lungs themselves are included. The digestive system is included for its pertinence in swallowing function; it includes again the oral cavity, the pharynx, the larynx (as a protective mechanism), the esophagus, and the lower digestive tract (e.g., stomach, intestines). Structures of the oral cavity

TABLE 3-4

BODY SYSTEMS THAT HAVE A FUNCTION IN SPEECH PRODUCTION

System	Major Organs and Tissues	Primary Function	Professional Relevance
Circulatory (vascular)	Heart, blood vessels, blood	Provide oxygen and nutrients to the body	Blood supply to the brain and other parts of the speech mechanism
Digestive	Lips, teeth, tongue, velum, pharynx, esophagus, stomach, intestines	Take in and process nutrients, eliminate byproducts	Mediate articulation and resonance of the vocal tone
Muscular	Skeletal muscle	Enact movements on the skeletal framework and maintain posture	Movement for speech production
Nervous	Brain, spinal cord, peripheral nerves, ganglia, sensory receptors	Control and regulate internal environment and interaction (sensory and motor) with the external environment	Innervation of muscles and mucosa associated with speech
Respiratory	Nasal passages, pharynx, larynx, trachea, bronchi and branches, lungs	Exchange of O_2 and CO_2	Power source for speech production
Skeletal	Cartilages, bones, ligaments, tendons, joints	Provide structure and support, and to mediate movement	Framework for the speech production mechanism

(e.g., teeth, tongue, soft palate) are also involved in articulation and resonance, and the larynx is the primary organ of phonation.

Speech Processes

The mechanism for speech production requires the coordinated effort of multiple systems functioning together to produce speech. As mentioned previously, these speech processes are respiration, phonation, and articulation/resonance. Each process is supported by the various organ systems just discussed. Each of these processes will be presented in detail in the coming chapters. Following is a brief description of each.

RESPIRATION

The respiratory system is necessary to provide the power behind our speech signal (see Figure 3-13A). The breath we take in is converted to energy to produce both the voiced and unvoiced sounds for speech. Furthermore, control over our breath stream influences pitch, loudness, and timing of our speech. Necessary to understanding the respiratory system is the bony and cartilaginous framework of the ribcage including the ribs, the sternum, and the vertebral column. Upon this framework are the muscles critical for expanding or contracting the size of the lungs for inspiration and expiration, respectively. The anatomy

and physiology of the respiratory system is presented in detail in Chapter 6.

PHONATION

The phonatory system provides the sound source for voicing (see Figure 3-13B). All speech processes interact but the interaction here between the respiratory and phonatory system is especially evident. It is the power generated by the breath rising from the respiratory system along with the movement and the properties of the muscles and connective tissues of the vocal folds that is responsible for producing voice. Necessary to understanding the function of the phonatory system is the largely cartilaginous framework of the larynx along with the hyoid bone and the muscles and connecting structures that allow the larynx to function as a unit. The anatomy and physiology of the phonatory system is presented in detail in Chapter 8.

ARTICULATION/RESONANCE

The articulatory/resonance system modifies the sound produced at the larynx into the sounds that are heard and perceived as speech (see Figure 3-13C). This is done by changing the configuration of the vocal tract. The vocal tract includes the nasal and oral cavities and the pharynx. For example, resonance is significantly affected when the back and upper part of the pharynx is opened to the nasal cavity. In this case, the sounds produced have a nasal resonance to them;

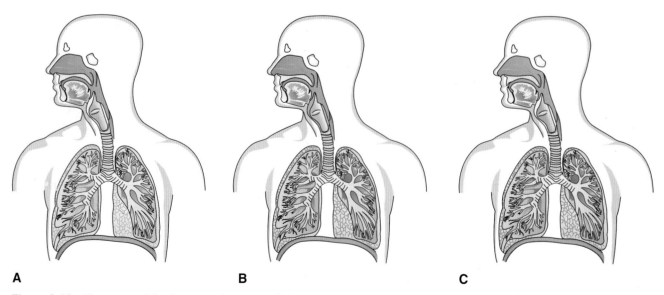

A   **B**   **C**

Figure 3-13   Illustration of the three speech systems. **A**. Respiratory speech system. **B**. Phonatory speech system. **C**. Articulatory/resonance speech system. (Reprinted with permission from Cohen, B.J. (2008). *Memmler's the human body in health and disease* (11th ed.). Baltimore: Lippincott Williams & Wilkins.)

such is the case for the sounds /m/, /n/, and /ŋ/. Necessary to understanding the function of the resonatory system is learning the bony framework of the cranial and facial bones (i.e., the skull) and the bony processes that project and serve as attachment points for muscle. In regard to resonance, many muscle groups are involved including muscles of the pharynx, muscles of the velum or soft palate, muscles of the tongue, and muscles of the mouth and cheeks.

The articulatory system acts as both a sound source and a resonator of sound. Articulation refers to movement; in this case, movement and placement of the articulators. The articulators include the lips and tongue and their interaction with the hard palate, teeth, and velum. It is the process of articulation that the layperson commonly thinks of as speech. While critical, articulation alone cannot produce speech. Consider an individual without a larynx as in the case of someone who had laryngeal cancer (i.e., a laryngectomee). Without the power of the respiratory system (the individual with the laryngectomee must breathe directly in and out of the trachea through an opening in the neck) and the voice source from the phonatory system, effective speech cannot be produced. Again, knowledge of the bony framework of the skull is necessary to understanding the functioning of this system. In addition, many of the same muscle groups involved in resonance are involved in articulation. These include muscles of the mouth and the tongue. Because of this overlap of anatomical structures the processes of articulation and resonance are often considered together as is the case in this textbook.

The anatomy and physiology of the articulatory system is presented in detail in Chapter 10 along with the resonatory system.

Summary

In order for you to understand the systems involved with speech and swallowing these systems are reduced to the basic components of cells and tissues. Cells of a particular type come together to comprise tissues of the same name: epithelial, connective, muscle, and nervous. Each of these tissue types has subclassifications based on location and/or function. These tissues then come together to form an organ; an organ has a predominant tissue type with other tissues for support and life functioning. Finally, the organs come together in functional groupings to form systems. There are a number of these systems; those most pertinent to speech and swallowing are circulatory (or vascular); digestive; muscular; nervous; respiratory; and skeletal systems. These systems are called upon to support the processes of speech. Speech processes are also referred to as speech systems. The process of respiration relies on the respiratory system, the process of phonation relies on the phonatory system, the process of resonance relies on the resonatory system, and the process of articulation relies on the articulatory system. These systems are the focus of the three units of this textbook that immediately follow the next unit on the nervous system.

PART I SUMMARY

In Chapter 2, you were presented the basic nomenclature associated with the study of human anatomy, physiology, and pathology. First, a definition was provided for the anatomical position, the general point of reference for all terminology associated with spatial orientation and positioning. Second, you were exposed to the planes of reference and more specific terminology associated with spatial relationships among the various body parts. Finally, as preparation for the remaining chapters of this textbook, you were provided with information pertaining to how you can understand unfamiliar terminology by analyzing specific terms into their roots and affixes.

In Chapter 3, you were provided basic information about the organization of the human organism. To understand the systems involved with speech and swallowing, these systems are reduced to the basic components of cells and tissues. Cells of a particular type come together to comprise tissues of the same name: epithelial, connective, muscle, and nervous. Each of these tissue types has subclassifications based on location and/or function. These tissues then come together to form an organ; an organ has a predominant tissue type with other tissues for support and life functioning. Finally, the organs come together in functional groupings to form systems. There are a number of these systems. Those most pertinent to speech and swallowing are circulatory (or vascular); digestive; muscular; nervous; respiratory; and skeletal. These systems are called upon to support the processes of speech. Speech processes are also referred to as speech systems. The process of respiration relies on the respiratory system, the process of phonation relies on the phonatory system, the process of resonance relies on the resonatory system, and the process of articulation relies on the articulatory system.

PART I REVIEW QUESTIONS

1. Refer back to Table 1-1 in Chapter 1. Describe specifically how the body systems on the right side of the table contribute to the systems of speech perception and production (i.e., auditory, articulation/resonance, phonation, and respiration) on the left side of the table. In other words, name a few specific structures from each of the body systems that can be found in each of the systems of speech perception and production, other than the ones provided in the table as examples.

2. Without returning to Chapter 2, assume the anatomical position and describe it as accurately as possible.

3. Without returning to Chapter 2, name and describe as accurately as possible the three planes of reference.

4. Use your knowledge of terminology to decipher the general meaning of each of the following terms.
   - Hypothalamus
   - Epidural space
   - Pneumotachygraph
   - Laryngoplasty
   - Tympanosclerosis
   - Subclavius
   - Suprasternal notch
   - Cricotracheal ligament

- Chondro-osseous junction
- Subglottic pressure

5. Describe the four tissue types discussed in Chapter 3 and give one specific example of each.

6. Name the three types of muscle tissue. Of the three, which is involved predominantly in speech production? What does this indicate about the process of speech production?

7. Both muscle and nerves are organized by connective tissue coverings. List the names for some of these coverings for both muscle and nerves using the prefixes endo-, epi- and peri-. What do these prefixes mean?

8. Indicate the speech system that is being described:
   - Speech sound production source for speech
   - Energy source for speech
   - Sound modifier for speech
   - Voice source for speech
   - Source of speech reception and interpretation

9. With the limited information you've been provided up to this point, try to describe one situation in which damage to any of the body systems (e.g., circulatory, digestive, muscular, nervous, respiratory, skeletal) may have a negative impact on speech perception or production.

PART 2

Anatomy, Physiology, and Pathology of the Nervous System

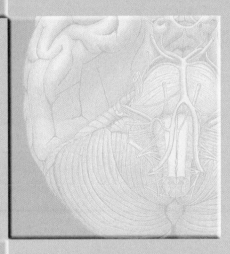

CHAPTER 4

Anatomy and Physiology of the Nervous System

Knowledge Outcomes for ASHA Certification for Chapter 4

- Demonstrate knowledge of the neurological basis of the basic human communication processes (III-B)
- Demonstrate knowledge of the neurological basis of swallowing processes (III-B)

Learning Objectives

- You will be able to outline nervous system organization.
- You will be able to explain the neurodevelopment of the central nervous system.
- You will be able to list surface anatomy of the brain including gyri and sulci most pertinent to speech, language, and hearing.
- You will be able to describe the supporting systems of the central nervous system including meninges, ventricles, cerebrospinal fluid and blood supply.
- You will be able to explain the basic microscopic nervous system anatomy and will demonstrate preliminary understanding of neural function.

AFFIX AND PART-WORD BOX

TERM	MEANING	EXAMPLE
aráchn-	spider's web	**arachn**oid
brachium	arm	**brachium** of inferior colliculus
colliculus	bump	inferior **colliculus**
cortex	outer "bark" or covering	cerebral **cortex**
di-	through	**di**encephalon
dura	hard, tough	**dura** mater
-encephalon	pertaining to the brain	di**encephalon**
falx	sickle-shaped	**falx** cerebelli
fasciculus	bundle	dorsal **fasciculus**
glosso-	tongue	**glosso**pharyngeus
lemniscus	ribbon	lateral **lemniscus**
mes-	middle	**mes**encephalon
met-	after	**met**encephalon
myel-	marrow	**myel**encephalon
peduncle	bridge	cerebral **peduncle**
phagein	to eat	**phag**ocyte

TERM	MEANING	EXAMPLE
pros-	at	**pros**encephalon
radiation	fanning out	auditory **radiation**s
rhomb-	diamond shaped	**rhomb**encephalon
sub-	below	**sub**cortical
tel-	end	**tel**encephalon
trigone	triangular ridge	hypoglossal **trigone**

Clinical Teaser

Sisi, an elderly woman age 82, enjoyed a quiet evening with her spouse and retired to bed early. Sometime in the early hours of the morning (around 2:00 AM), she awoke thinking she needed to use the bathroom. As she swung her legs over the edge of the bed she noticed her right leg seemed particularly heavy. She attempted to assist her leg with her right arm but realized she could no longer move her right arm. She laid back down and tried to go back to sleep in hopes that these symptoms would resolve. The symptoms did not resolve and some time later, with some alarm, she used her left arm to wake her husband. When she tried to tell him what was happening, she found she could not speak although it seemed to her that her thoughts were quite clear. Her husband immediately called 911 and the paramedics were on the scene as promptly as possible given that they lived in a rural area of Washington. After initial assessment, Life Flight was called and Sisi was taken to an urban center for evaluation and treatment.

On admission to the emergency room, around 7:00 AM, the physician conducted a basic neurology exam and sent her off for a computed tomography (CT) scan. No evidence of hemorrhage was found, so the physician administered tissue plasminogen activator to break up what was inferred to be a clot or plug in the arterial circulation of the brain. The neurologist diagnosed this at this early stage as a thromboembolic stroke minimally involving the frontal cortex of the left cerebral hemisphere. Sisi was admitted to the hospital for observation with referral to the speech–language pathologist for evaluation the following day.

The speech–language pathologist conducted a brief speech–language examination at bedside across all language modalities and speech functions. A cranial nerve exam revealed a right facial droop (cranial nerve VII—the **facial**) and a slight slurring of any speech she did have (cranial nerve XII—the **hypoglossal**) with no other significant cranial nerve involvement regarding speech production. Verbal output was limited to automatic speech (e.g., counting, reciting the days of the week) and vocalizations. Written output was extremely limited although she did attempt to write her name albeit illegibly. Sisi's writing was further confounded by the fact that she is right-handed and she had right hemiparesis of the upper (and lower) extremities. Auditory comprehension and reading comprehension were determined to be language strengths.

Note any terms or concepts in the above case study that are unfamiliar to you. As you read the first chapter of this part, pay particular attention to the anatomy and physiology pertinent to this case. We will return to this case at the conclusion of this part.

Introduction

The nervous system of a human is both simple in its organization and amazing in its complexity. In a simple model of speech production, we can see that the nervous system directs all the activity that occurs; it does this by both receiving information from the external (the world around us) and internal (our body) environments. This applies equally to swallowing. Without the nervous system, nothing happens. Understanding nervous system organization along with key terminology will assist you in mastering the basics of the neuroanatomy and neurophysiology of the human nervous system.

The central nervous system (CNS) is made up of the brain and spinal cord and all the structures and spaces within. The brain itself has over 100 billion neurons and has been likened to the consistency of jello but is probably more like tofu in substance (Firlik, 2006). The brain constitutes about 2% of an individual's weight, yet it is a demanding oxygen consumer as it requires 20% of the body's blood supply. In fact, it could be argued that the functions of the rest of the body's organs are devoted to keeping the brain alive (Goodman, 2003). In turn, the brain makes our reality conscious and allows us to respond in thought, planning, and action.

TERMINOLOGY

The importance of understanding critical terms in neuroanatomy and neurophysiology cannot be stressed enough, as these terms form the foundation to build

TABLE 4-I

NEUROSCIENCE TERMS, DEFINITIONS, AND EXAMPLE(S)

Terms	Definition	Example
Neuron	Basic cell of the nervous system	Multipolar neuron
Glial cell	Support cell of the nervous system	Oligodendroglia
Afferent	Coming toward the CNS or a given structure	Sensory spinal nerves
Efferent	Going away from the CNS or a given structure	Motor spinal nerves
Tract	Bundle of axons in the CNS	Corticospinal tract
Nerve	Bundle of axons in the PNS	Facial cranial nerve
Nuclei	Cluster of neuronal cell bodies in the CNS	Caudate nucleus
Ganglia	Cluster of neuronal cell bodies in the PNS	Dorsal root ganglia
Gyrus	Mound of cortical surface nervous tissue	Postcentral gyrus
Sulcus	Groove or depression between gyri	Central sulcus
Cortical	Pertaining to the outer surface of the brain	Cerebral cortex
Subcortical	Deep to the cortex	Subcortical nuclei (e.g., putamen)
Gray matter	General term for any collection of neuronal cell bodies in the CNS	Cerebral cortex Basal ganglia
White matter	General term for any axonal bundle in the CNS	Internal capsule Corpus callosum

upon and provide the critical information necessary to apply reasoning to determine the location and function of structures and systems. The terms presented in Table 4-1 provide a foundation for understanding the information presented in this chapter. You are strongly encouraged to attend to these terms, as they will arise repeatedly in this chapter.

ANATOMICAL ORIENTATION

In Chapter 2, you were introduced to anatomical directional terms and planes or views of anatomy. A few of these terms take on a different meaning when referring to the CNS. During development of the CNS, the front end of the encephalon (brain) undergoes elaboration and takes a sharp turn, which alters spatial orientation and thus the anatomical terms used to refer to the CNS above the spinal cord. As illustrated in Figure 4-1, above the **diencephalon** (central region of the brain), the term *rostral* means toward the nose, caudal toward the back of the head, ventral toward the jaw, and dorsal toward the top of the skull. This is a little different as compared with the spinal cord extending down the vertebral canal where rostral means toward the head, caudal toward the tail (e.g., tail bone), ventral toward the belly, and dorsal toward the back.

Directional terms can be combined in different ways to very specifically describe a location. It may be helpful to review the definitions of these terms in Chapter 2. The directional terms that may be combined include medial, lateral, superficial, deep, and, as just discussed, dorsal, ventral, rostral, and caudal. For example, consider the **thalamus**, which is a mass of gray matter located in the center of the brain. This mass of gray matter is comprised of a number of nuclei. Many of these nuclei are named for their location relative to the thalamus itself. For example, the nucleus responsible for acting as a relay station for body sensations of pain, temperature, and touch is the ventrolateral nucleus found on the bottom (ventral) side (lateral) of the thalamus.

Anatomical planes of reference are also worthy of a brief review, as these different planes are used

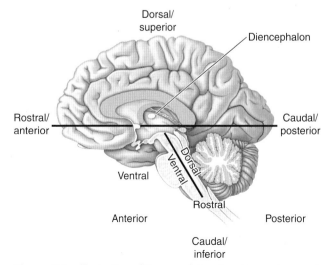

Figure 4-I Illustration of the use of directional terms in regard to the central nervous system.

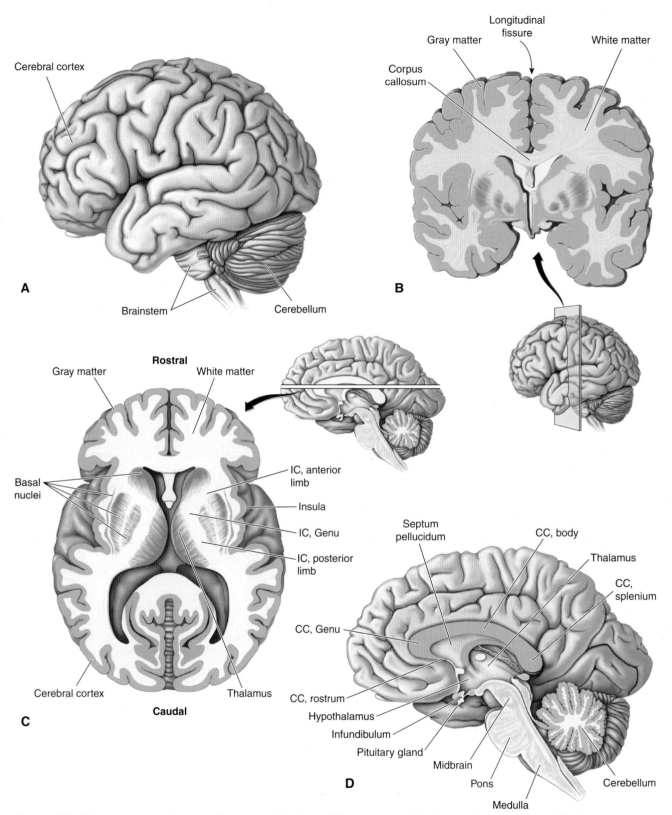

Figure 4-2   Different anatomical views and sections of the brain. (**A**) Lateral view of the left cerebral hemisphere. (**B**) Coronal section illustrating gray and white matter. (**C**) Horizontal section illustrating gray and white matter (IC, internal capsule). (**D**) Midsagittal view of the right cerebral hemisphere (CC, corpus callosum). (**A**. Reprinted with permission from Bear, M.F., Connors, B.W., Paradiso, M.A. (2007). *Neuroscience: Exploring the brain* (3rd ed.). Baltimore, MD: Lippincott Williams & Wilkins. **B**. Reprinted with permission from Bear, M.F., Connors, B.W., Paradiso, M.A. (2007). *Neuroscience: Exploring the brain* (3rd ed.). Baltimore, MD: Lippincott Williams & Wilkins. **C**. Reprinted with permission from Premkumar, K. (2004). *The massage connection anatomy and physiology*. Baltimore, MD: Lippincott Williams & Wilkins. **D**. Reprinted with permission from Bear, M.F., Connors, B.W., Paradiso, M.A. (2007). *Neuroscience: Exploring the brain* (3rd ed.). Baltimore, MD: Lippincott Williams & Wilkins.)

repeatedly in the study of neuroanatomy. A coronal (frontal) section is perpendicular to midline and splits a structure into front and back. A horizontal section is literally taken "across the horizon" resulting in top and bottom sections of the structure. A sagittal section is parallel to midline and splits a structure into left and right parts. Sagittal sections can be right at midline (i.e., midsagittal) or off midline (i.e., parasagittal). Figure 4-2 illustrates a lateral view and a coronal, a horizontal, and a midsagittal section of the brain with various structures labeled for future reference in the chapter. Each time you view a figure illustrating an anatomical plane, take the time to determine the specific plane being viewed as well as gain your directional bearings (e.g., where is rostral?) prior to locating specific structures in the figure.

Neurodevelopment

There are four general stages of nervous system growth: **induction, proliferation, migration**, and **differentiation**. The nervous system develops from ectodermal tissue (i.e., the outermost layer of the three germ layers). This ectoderm changes around the 18th day of gestation through a critical event known as induction. Induction refers to the interaction of ectoderm with the underlying mesoderm causing a commitment of tissue to become neural tissue; this new tissue is termed *neuroectoderm*. Following induction, the nerve cells increase their rate of production and proliferate. Nuclear movement of these cells occurs via migration where the cells travel from where they originated to the region of the nervous system where they will end up. Differentiation refers to cell specialization and the formation of the parts of the neuron and early synaptic patterns.

Once induction occurs, the development of the nervous system is rapid. At 21 days, a **neural plate** develops and, as this plate thickens via cell proliferation, it folds upon itself and a **neural tube** is created by 25 days growing rostrally and caudally like a zipper going in both directions (see Figure 4-3). This neural tube develops into all the neurons and glial cells in the CNS. Pinched off from this neural tube is the neuroectoderm, now called the **neural crest**, that will develop into the neurons and glial cells comprising the peripheral nervous system (PNS).

Through this rapid period of growth, the CNS further differentiates into vesicles with spaces (i.e., lumen) surrounded by walls (nervous tissue). As illustrated in Figure 4-3, by 28 days, three vesicles are formed: **prosencephalon, mesencephalon**, and **rhombencephalon**. These vesicles further differentiate 1 week later with the prosencephalon dividing into the **telencephalon** and the diencephalon and the rhombencephalon further dividing into the **metencephalon** and the **myelencephalon**. The mesencephalon remains and the lumen becomes the ventricular spaces discussed later in this chapter.

The spinal cord is also undergoing development, dividing into two plates (see Figure 4-4). The **alar plate** is found dorsally and develops into nervous tissue serving sensory purposes, whereas the **basal plate** is found ventrally and develops into nervous tissue for motor functions. A dividing point between these two plates is the **sulcus limitans**; lateral to the sulcus limitans is the area devoted to development of nervous tissue supporting autonomic functions.

ORGANIZATION

The nervous system is divided into two parts, the CNS and the PNS as schematized in Figure 4-5. These two parts are separated by the meninges, which are

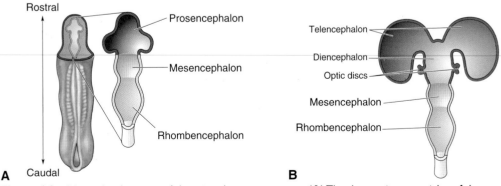

Figure 4-3 Neurodevelopment of the central nervous system. (**A**) The three primary vesicles of the neural tube. (**B**) The five secondary vesicles of the neural tube that further develop into the structures of the brain. The optic discs of the diencephalon develop into the retina of the eyes. (Reprinted with permission from Bear, M.F., Connors, B.W., Paradiso, M.A. (2006). *Neuroscience exploring the brain* (3rd ed.). Baltimore, MD: Lippincott Williams & Wilkins.)

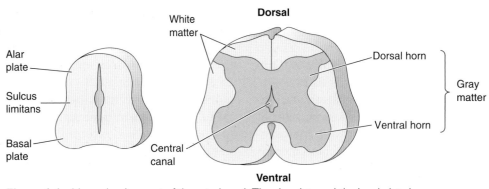

Figure 4-4   Neurodevelopment of the spinal cord. The alar plate and the basal plate become sensory and motor regions of the mature spinal cord. (Reprinted with permission from Bear, M.F., Connors, B.W., Paradiso, M.A. (2006). *Neuroscience exploring the brain* (3rd ed.). Baltimore, MD: Lippincott Williams & Wilkins.)

connective tissue coverings of the CNS. The PNS is connected to the CNS via nerves: **cranial nerves** at the **brainstem** and **spinal nerves** at the spinal cord. These nerves take information to and from the CNS in regard to our head and neck (i.e., cranial nerves) and our body (i.e., spinal nerves).

The developed human brain has five divisions: the telencephalon, diencephalon, mesencephalon, metencephalon, and myelencephalon. The organizational

flowchart (see Figure 4-5) under each encephalon area shows the general brain structures for that region. For example, the telencephalon includes the left and right cerebral hemispheres and all cortical and subcortical structures, that is, both gray and white matter. The diencephalon is the thalamic region and the mesencephalon is composed of those structures making up the midbrain. The metencephalon includes part of the brainstem (i.e., pons) and the cerebellum, whereas

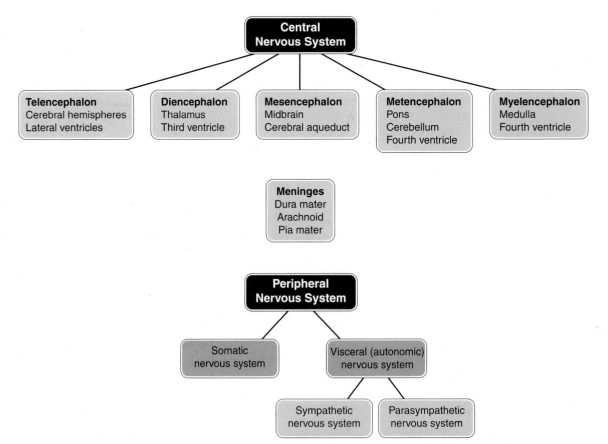

Figure 4-5   The organization of the nervous system. The meninges divide the central nervous system from the peripheral nervous system.

the myelencephalon is the most caudal portion of the brain—the medulla oblongata. The medulla is continuous with the spinal cord.

The spinal cord is necessary for the control of our body's sensations and movements. The spinal cord is connected to the brain at the brainstem in the region of the **foramen magnum**. The spinal cord is organized into two axes: longitudinal and transverse (or segmental) axes. The longitudinal axis runs up and down the spinal cord carrying information via tracts. The segmental axis runs perpendicular to the longitudinal axis at each segment of the spinal cord and receives or sends out information via the spinal nerves. The spinal cord is further organized by segments that correspond to the sections of the vertebral column: cervical, thoracic, lumbar, sacral, and coccygeal.

The PNS is also further subdivided. The two components of the PNS are the **visceral nervous system** and the **somatic nervous system**. The visceral nervous system is considered involuntary and carries information to organs, glands, and blood vessels to regulate arousal and body functions; this is our **autonomic nervous system (ANS)**, which is further subdivided into the **sympathetic division** and the **parasympathetic division** (see Figure 4-5). The ANS carries **afferent** information regarding visceral function (e.g., oxygen content of blood) and sends **efferent** commands (e.g., secretion from glands). The sympathetic division expends energy during body responses in stressful situations such as in fight or flight scenarios. The projections from this system arise from the thoracic and lumbar spinal cord. On the other hand, the parasympathetic nervous system conserves body energy and works to maintain the internal balance of our body systems (i.e., **homeostasis**). Many projections from the parasympathetic division arise from the brainstem as well as from the sacral region of the spinal cord. Thus, a number of the cranial nerves have parasympathetic components; this will be returned to later in the chapter. The neurons of the ANS, regardless of division, are made up of a two-neuron chain. The first neuron has its cell body in the CNS (either spinal cord or brainstem) and is called the preganglionic neuron. The preganglionic neuron synapses at the ganglia found in the PNS. The ganglia for the sympathetic division are quite near the spinal cord, whereas the parasympathetic division's ganglia are located near the organ to be innervated.

The somatic nervous system has both motor and sensory functions carrying information to and from skeletal muscle via the cranial nerves and the spinal nerves. The motor or efferent fibers innervate the skeletal muscles of the body; these include those responsible for speech and hearing function. The sensory or afferent fibers transmit head, neck, and body sensations for touch, pain, temperature, and body position.

> ### Why You Need to Know
> *These sensory and motor systems work together to perform functions such as speech production. Although we may look at speech production as primarily a result of motor movement (e.g., moving our tongue to shape sounds, moving our vocal folds to produce voice), our brains must receive sensory information to plan and produce speech. Exactly how body sensation contributes to speech production is not well understood. Minimally, it appears that sensory feedback regarding where articulatory structures are (i.e., proprioception) is necessary for optimal speech production. As an example, consider the effects Novocain can have on your ability to clearly articulate following a dentist appointment.*

Gross Anatomy

Gross anatomy refers to what can be identified with the naked eye. In the case of the CNS, this gross anatomy will include the surface features of the brain and spinal cord as well as the internal anatomy of the same. The following section of the chapter presents the gross anatomy most relevant to speech, language, and hearing function for the five divisions of the CNS.

TELENCEPHALON

The telencephalon is made up of two symmetrical cerebral hemispheres, a right and a left. In each hemisphere are four lobes that correspond to the bones of the skull. These are the *frontal, parietal, temporal,* and *occipital;* sometimes a fifth lobe is named—the *limbic* lobe (see Figure 4-6). Each lobe has surface features and outer "bark" (i.e., the cortex) and structures deep to the cortex including both gray and white matter. The lobes are separated from one another on the surface by grooves or **sulci**.

Most obvious upon inspection of the brain are the grooves and mounds of the cortex. The cortical mounds are called gyri and the cortical grooves are referred to as sulci (sulcus if singular) or, if they are large, fissures. Each of these gyri and sulci has a particular name and is associated with one of the lobes

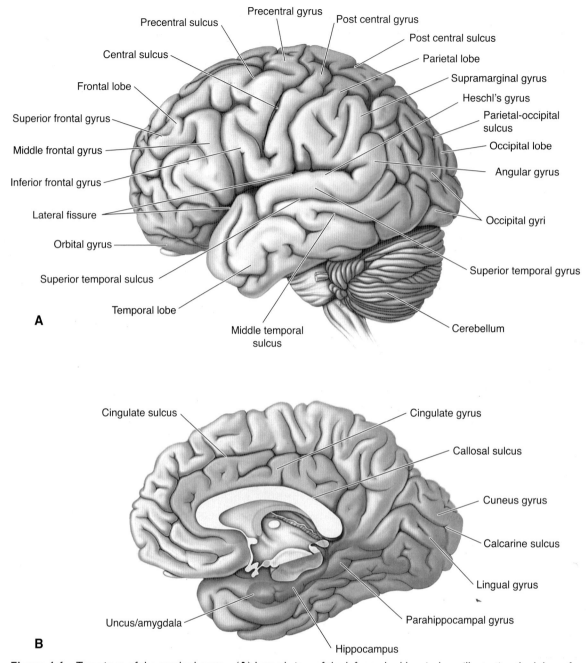

Figure 4-6   Two views of the cerebral cortex. (**A**) Lateral view of the left cerebral hemisphere illustrating the lobes of the brain and prominent sulci and gyri. (**B**) Midsagittal view of the right cerebral hemisphere with the brainstem and cerebellum removed to reveal the limbic lobe and prominent sulci and gyri. (Reprinted with permission from Bear, M.F., Connors, B.W., Paradiso, M.A. (2006). *Neuroscience exploring the brain* (3rd ed.). Baltimore, MD: Lippincott Williams & Wilkins.)

(see Table 4-2). For our purposes, those areas of the cortex most significant to speech, language, and hearing are illustrated in Figures 4-6A and 4-6B and are presented here. The largest of these grooves is the **longitudinal fissure** (refer back to Figure 4-2B), which divides the cerebrum into right and left halves: the right cerebral hemisphere and the left cerebral hemisphere. Furthermore, the longitudinal fissure is deep extending all the way down to the **corpus callosum** (a major tract). Another prominent groove is

the **central sulcus**; it divides the frontal lobe from the parietal lobe in each hemisphere. The precentral sulcus is found immediately anterior to the gyrus of the same name in the frontal lobe, whereas the postcentral sulcus is found immediately posterior to the gyrus of the same name in the parietal lobe. The **lateral sulcus** (also known as the Sylvian fissure) is also deep, separating the frontal and parietal lobes from the temporal lobe. The temporal lobe is demarked with anatomically labeled sulci, the superior temporal

TABLE 4-2

GYRI (WITH BRODMANN NUMBERS AND GENERAL FUNCTION) AND SULCI PERTINENT TO SPEECH, LANGUAGE, AND HEARING SPECIFIC TO EACH LOBE

Lobe	Gyri	Function	Sulci
Frontal lobe	Inferior frontal gyrus (44, 45)	Expressive language	Longitudinal fissure
	Precentral gyrus (4)	Volitional movement	Central sulcus
	Middle frontal gyrus (46)	Motor planning	Precentral sulcus
	Orbital gyrus (11)	Cognition	Lateral fissure
	Superior frontal gyrus (10)	Cognition	
Parietal lobe	Postcentral gyrus (3, 1, 2)	Conscious sensation	Longitudinal fissure
	Supramarginal gyrus (40)	Language[a]	Central sulcus
	Angular gyrus (39)	Language[a]	Postcentral sulcus
			Lateral fissure
Temporal lobe	Heschl's gyrus (41)	Audition	Lateral fissure
	Superior gyrus (22)	Receptive language	Superior temporal sulcus
			Middle temporal sulcus
Occipital lobe	Cuneus gyrus (17, 18)	Vision	Longitudinal fissure
	Lingual gyrus (17)	Vision	Calcarine sulcus
	Occipital gyri (17, 18, 19)	Visual recognition and association	Parietal–occipital sulcus
Limbic lobe	Cingulate gyrus (24, 23)	Emotion	Callosal sulcus
	Parahippocampal gyrus (28)	Memory	Cingulate sulcus
	Uncus (34)	Emotion, fear, and aggression	

[a]Part of the multimodal association cortex integrating auditory, visual, and somatosensory inputs for language activities such as word retrieval, reading, and writing.

sulcus is found toward the top and the middle temporal sulcus is found in the middle of the temporal lobe. The most prominent sulcus of the occipital lobe is the **calcarine sulcus**, which is located centrally on the medial aspect of the lobe (see Figure 4-6B). The parietal lobe is separated from the occipital lobe by the aptly named parietal–occipital sulcus. The limbic lobe also has prominent sulci. These are seen on a midsagittal view (see Figure 4-6B) and include the **callosal sulcus** running the length of the corpus callosum along its superior border and the **cingulate sulcus** found superior to the gyrus of the same name.

Similar to sulci, particular gyri are found in the lobes of the cerebral hemispheres; these also have names (see Table 4-2). Processing of neural information occurs at the gyri for various functions, which will be elucidated later in the chapter. For now, the primary focus is on the location of these various gyri as seen in Figure 4-6A. The **precentral gyrus** is the mound of gray matter anterior to the central sulcus extending from the longitudinal fissure superiorly to the lateral fissure inferiorly. The **inferior frontal gyrus** is located anterior to the inferior end of the precentral gyrus and the middle frontal gyrus is located anterior

to the precentral gyrus. These three gyri, found in the frontal lobe, are involved with motor function. More anterior areas of the frontal lobe are involved with cognitive processes (e.g., attention, memory, and reasoning) and our personality. These areas include the orbital gyrus found immediately superior to our eye orbits inside the cranium and the superior frontal gyrus located above the orbital gyrus; these two areas together make up the bulk of the prefrontal cortex that we will return to later.

The parietal lobe is responsible for the conscious reception and integration of various sensations. Immediately behind the central sulcus is the postcentral gyrus. Like the precentral gyrus, it extends from the longitudinal fissure down to the lateral fissure. Two complex areas associated with the parietal lobe critical to language function are the supramarginal gyrus and the angular gyrus. The supramarginal gyrus is found superior to the posterior end of the lateral fissure (see Figure 4-6A) with the angular gyrus inferior to it.

The temporal lobe is critical for auditory function and language comprehension. Heschl's gyrus is found at the very superior aspect of the superior temporal gyrus; this is the primary auditory cortex where signals from the cochleae in the inner ears end up. The remainder of the superior temporal gyrus is known as Wernicke's area, an area specific to language comprehension.

A midsagittal view of the occipital lobe reveals the cuneus gyri and the lingual gyri surrounding the calcarine fissure (see Figure 4-6B). The occipital gyri make up the remainder of the lobe given the lateral view (see Figure 4-6A).

Why You Need to Know

The cerebral hemispheres are largely mirror images of one another with the same sulci and gyri; however, functions differ across the hemispheres especially in regard to the way the hemispheres process information. A good example of this is our auditory processing. Auditory processing occurs in both the left and right cerebral hemisphere temporal lobes (superior and middle temporal gyri) communicating with one another via the corpus callosum. In general, the left cerebral hemisphere processes speech and language, whereas the right cerebral hemisphere processes speech prosody (e.g., melody, rate, and stress), environmental sounds, and certain musical elements. For instance, Gazzaniga, Ivry, and Mangun (1998) found that when listening to a lyrical song, the perception of the words is a left hemisphere function while perception of the song's melody is a right hemisphere function. Of course, it is important to note that the hemispheres communicate with one another and share functions to some extent.

Finally, the *limbic lobe* has three gyri associated with it: the cingulate, the parahippocampal, and the **uncus**. The cingulate gyrus is large, surrounding the corpus callosum at its anterior, superior, and posterior aspects. The **parahippocampal gyrus** is nearly continuous with the cingulate gyrus at its posterior inferior site (see Figure 4-6B). The parahippocampal gyrus continues inferiorly and anteriorly on the medial aspect of the temporal lobe. At its most anterior end, this gyrus folds back on itself at a point called the uncus. Two important nuclei of the limbic system are deep to these gyri; the **hippocampus** is deep to the parahippocampal gyrus and the **amygdala** is deep to the uncus.

A part of the cerebral cortex hidden from external view is the insular cortex. The **insula** can be viewed when portions of the frontal and temporal lobe are pulled away from each other as can be seen in Figure 4-7. Those cortical areas that overlie the insular cortex are referred to as opercular regions associated with the various lobes. Hence, there is a frontal **operculum**, a temporal operculum, and a parietal operculum.

At this point, we move from a presentation of the external anatomy of the telencephalon to the internal anatomy which includes both nuclei and tracts. The most prominent subcortical nuclei are clusters of gray matter collectively referred to as the **basal ganglia**. Here is one of those instances when the use of "ganglia" is technically in error as we are referring to a collection of neuronal cell bodies deep to the telencephalon (part of the CNS); thus, the appropriate terminology is nuclei. Indeed, it is more appropriate to refer to the basal ganglia as basal nuclei but old

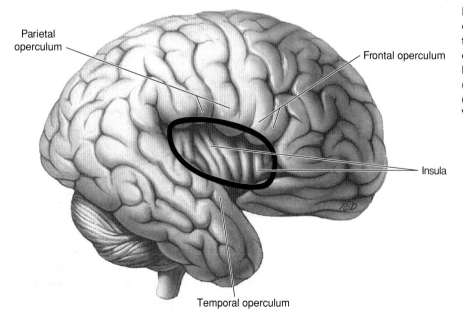

Figure 4-7   Lateral view of the right cerebral hemisphere with the lateral fissure opened to reveal the insular cortex. (Reprinted with permission from Bear, M.F., Connors, B.W., Paradiso, M.A. (2007). *Neuroscience: Exploring the brain* (3rd ed.). Baltimore, MD: Lippincott Williams & Wilkins.)

Parietal operculum

Frontal operculum

Insula

Temporal operculum

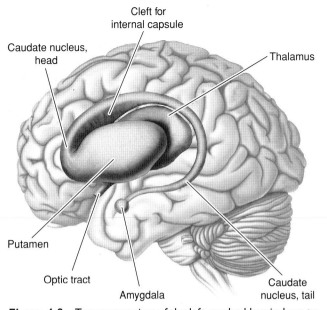

Cleft for
internal capsule

Caudate nucleus,
head

Thalamus

Putamen

Optic tract

Amygdala

Caudate
nucleus, tail

Figure 4-8   Transparent view of the left cerebral hemisphere to illustrate the location of the subcortical basal nuclei. (Reprinted with permission from Bhatnagar, S.C. (2008). *Neuroscience for the study of communicative disorders* (3rd ed.). Baltimore, MD: Lippincott Williams & Wilkins.)

terminology dies hard. Nonetheless, the individual nuclei making up the telencephalic basal ganglia are the **putamen**, the **globus pallidus**, and the **caudate nucleus**; these are paired nuclei found in each cerebral hemisphere. The putamen and the caudate nucleus together are collectively called the **striatum**. Figure 4-8 shows these nuclei via a lateral transparent drawing of the cerebral hemisphere. In neuroimaging studies (e.g., CT scans or magnetic resonance imaging [MRI]) or gross dissections, the basal ganglia are best viewed with coronal or horizontal slices because they are deep to the cerebral cortex (see Figures 4-2B and 4-2C). Two other prominent nuclei lie deep to the temporal lobes and are part of the limbic system; these are the hippocampus and the amygdala; again, one in each hemisphere. The hippocampus is an outgrowth of the medial wall of the temporal lobe, folding back on itself and roughly resembling a seahorse in shape; it is deep to the parahippocampal gyrus. The almond-shaped amygdala is found rostral to the hippocampus and deep to the uncus in the anterior medial portion of the temporal lobe. These structures of the basal ganglia and limbic system communicate with one another and/or other areas of the brain by way of tracts or fibers.

Collectively, the white matter fiber systems in the cerebral hemispheres are called **medullary centers**. The three medullary centers are **commissural fiber tracts, projection fiber tracts**, and **association fiber tracts**. You will recall that tracts are bundles of axons found in the CNS; furthermore, these tracts connect nuclei with each other and provide a means of information transfer throughout the CNS. Commissural fiber tracts connect the hemispheres of the brain and can be roughly visualized as horizontal connections; there are three of these. The largest is the corpus callosum, which is large enough to require labeling of distinct regions. From rostral to caudal, these are the rostrum, genu, body, and splenium (refer back to Figure 4-2D). Much smaller commissural tracts include the anterior commissure found ventral to the rostrum of the corpus callosum and the hippocampal commissure connecting the left hemisphere hippocampus with the right hemisphere hippocampus in the temporal lobes.

Projection fiber tracts establish connections between higher and lower parts of the CNS and can be roughly visualized as vertical connections. The telencephalic projection tract is the **internal capsule**. The internal capsule carries motor and sensory information to and from the cerebral cortex as well as information traveling between the nuclei of the basal ganglia and the thalamus. It is an incredibly busy expressway of multidirectional information flow with particular information traveling in specific lanes. As expected, there are different areas of the internal capsule—the anterior limb, the genu, and the posterior limb (refer back to Figure 4-2C). Similar to the basal ganglia, areas of the internal capsule are usually viewed via coronal or horizontal planes.

Association fiber tracts connect different cortical areas within the same hemisphere. These tracts can be very short or very long. Notable examples of long association tracts are the **arcuate fasciculus** connecting the frontal lobe speech and language centers with the temporal lobe language centers and the **uncinate fasciculus** connecting the orbital gyri of the frontal lobe with the anterior region of the temporal lobe.

DIENCEPHALON

The diencephalon is found deep in the center of the brain extending down to the ventral medial surface. The thalamus and all other anatomical regions with "thalamus" in their name are part of the diencephalon. This includes the **epithalamus**, **subthalamus**, and **hypothalamus**. In addition, the mammillary bodies, part of the limbic system, are included here. The thalamus is often viewed on a midsagittal brain section as can be seen in Figure 4-2D. Only one-half of the thalamus is seen in this view, as the thalamus has a right and left half that correspond to the cerebral

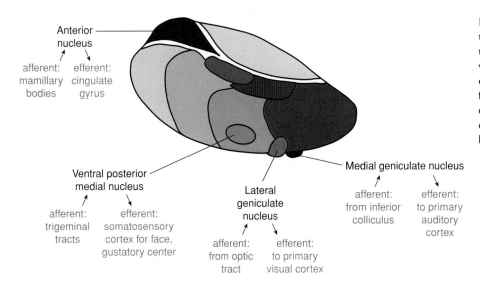

Figure 4-9 The nuclei of the thalamus. Those nuclei discussed in the chapter are labeled here along with their afferent input and efferent output. (Reprinted with permission from Bhatnagar, S.C. (2008). *Neuroscience for the study of communicative disorders* (3rd ed.). Baltimore, MD: Lippincott Williams & Wilkins.)

hemispheres. The halves are connected by the **interthalamic adhesion** (or massa intermedia). The thalamus itself is made up of multiple nuclei coming together to form a gray mass that resembles a small egg sitting in the center of the brain. Some of the more significant of these nuclei for speech, language, and hearing include the anterior nucleus, the ventrolateral nucleus, the ventroposterior medial nucleus, the **lateral geniculate nucleus (LGN)**, and the **medial geniculate nucleus (MGN)**. Figure 4-9 illustrates these thalamic nuclei and their connections to other areas of the nervous system; we will return to these later in the discussion of brain function. The hypothalamus can also be viewed in Figure 4-2D and is anterior and ventral to the thalamus. The hypothalamus is composed of multiple nuclei and directly influences endocrine function via its attachment to the pituitary gland by way of the **infundibulum** (i.e., pituitary stalk; refer back to Figure 4-2D). Finally, the mamillary bodies, of which there are two, are seen superficially on the ventral surface of the brain; a tract runs between these bodies to the anterior nuclei of the thalamus.

METENCEPHALON (CEREBELLAR COMPONENT)

The cerebellum comprises part of the metencephalon and is posteriorly oriented in the cranium just ventral to the occipital lobes. The cerebellum resembles cauliflower when viewed from a midsagittal section with a finely convoluted cortex and intricate weaving of internal white matter (refer back to Figure 4-2D). The cerebellum is divided into right and left lateral hemispheres complete with lobes, cortex, fissures, subcortical nuclei, and tracts (i.e., gray and white matter). The hemispheres are separated at midline by the

vermis, the central area of the cerebellar cortex. The cerebellar hemispheres are divided into three lobes: the posterior lobe, the anterior lobe, and the **flocculonodular lobe**. The primary fissure separates the anterior from the posterior lobe (see Figure 4-10). The flocculonodular lobe comprises the inferior aspect of the cerebellum with the nodular portion at midline (i.e., vermis) and the floccular portion on the sides. The flocculonodular lobe receives afferent information from the vestibular system and is important in assisting in controlling eye movements and postural adjustments secondary to head position and gravity.

A set of deep cerebellar nuclei receives input and sends output via the white matter. As seen in Figure 4-11, the **fastigial nucleus** is found most medially and the **dentate nucleus** is found most laterally, one in each hemisphere of the cerebellum. Between these nuclei lie the **emboliform nucleus** and **globose nucleus,** collectively referred to as the interposed nuclei.

Tracts travel in and out of the cerebellum by way of the **cerebellar peduncles** (see Figure 4-12A). There are three pairs of cerebellar peduncles—the superior, the middle, and the inferior—which connect to the brainstem. Importantly, the cerebellum receives much more neural information that it sends out (by a ratio of approximately 40:1). This large ratio of input to output relates directly to the function of the cerebellum. The cerebellum is responsible for analyzing and synthesizing large amounts of sensory information (input) and then, based on that synthesis, sending out neural impulses to adjust movements by way of motor control centers. The vast majority of neural information comes into the cerebellum through the inferior and middle cerebellar peduncles with the superior cerebellar peduncle reserved primarily for

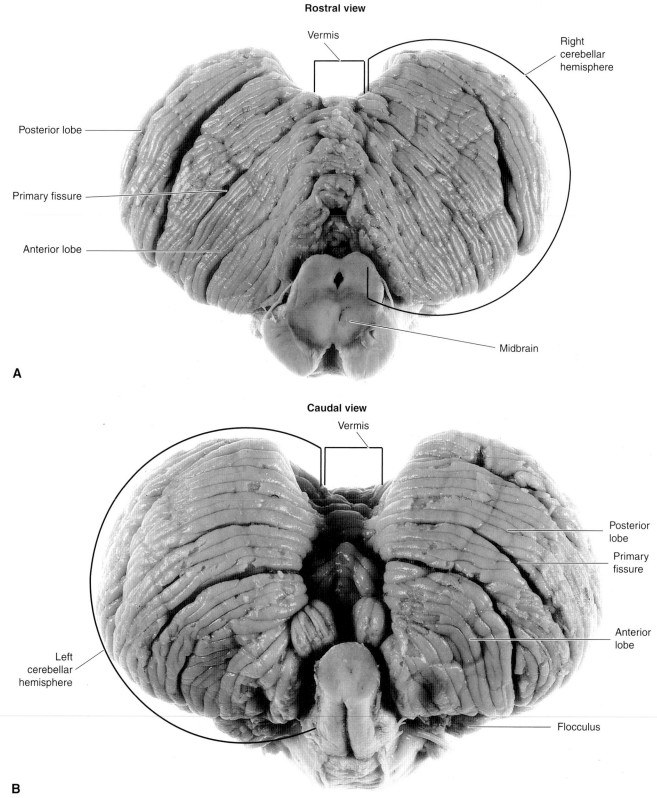

Figure 4-10 External views of the cerebellum. (**A**) The cerebellum viewed from above (i.e., a rostral direction). (**B**) The cerebellum viewed from below (i.e., a caudal direction). Major landmarks are labeled. (Reprinted with permission from Bhatnagar, S.C. (2008). *Neuroscience for the study of communicative disorders* (3rd ed.). Baltimore, MD: Lippincott Williams & Wilkins.)

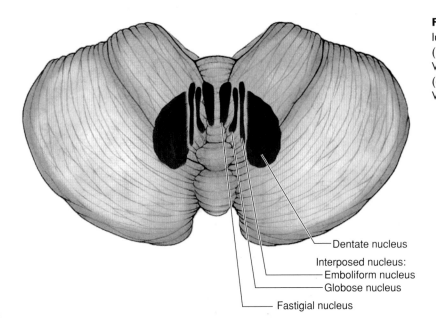

Figure 4-11   Transparent view of the cerebellum to illustrate the deep cerebellar nuclei. (Reprinted with permission from Campbell, W.W. (2005). *DeJong's the neurologic examination* (6th ed.). Philadelphia, PA: Lippincott Williams & Wilkins.)

Dentate nucleus
Interposed nucleus:
Emboliform nucleus
Globose nucleus
Fastigial nucleus

transmitting neural information from the cerebellum.

BRAINSTEM ("M-ENCEPHALON")

The mesencephalon, part of the metencephalon, and the myelencephalon together make up what is known as the brainstem. Figure 4-12 shows a dorsal and ventral view of the external features of the brainstem. The mesencephalon is the midbrain and is the most rostral of the brainstem components being in very close proximity to the thalamus. The midbrain has a number of surface features—the **superior colliculi** and **inferior colliculi**, collectively referred to as the **corpora quadrigemina**, on the dorsal surface and the **cerebral peduncles** on the ventral surface. The colliculi are bumps or swellings that overlie nuclei involved with hearing and vision, whereas the peduncles are home to critical motor pathways. The **cerebral aqueduct**, part of the ventricular system, courses through the midbrain. The **pons** (part of the metencephalon) is found in the middle of the brainstem and acts as a bridge to the cerebellum (the other part of the metencephalon). Ventrally, the pons has a midline pontine sulcus which cradles the **basilar artery**; dorsally, the pons gives rise to the largest of the cerebellar peduncles, the middle cerebellar peduncle. The rostral aspect of the **fourth ventricle** is associated with the dorsal aspect of the pons. Finally, the myelencephalon or **medulla oblongata** makes up the most caudal aspect of the brainstem and is continuous with the spinal cord. The ventral aspect of the medulla hosts connection points for a number of cranial nerves critical for speech, hearing, and swallowing. Also on the ventral surface are areas called the **pyramids** and pyramidal decussation; these regions overlie tracts that carry motor information to cranial and spinal nerves for muscle movement—key for speech production to be discussed later. The dorsal aspect of the medulla houses the caudal portion of the fourth ventricle.

Spinal Cord

The spinal cord is the most caudal part of the CNS extending 42 to 45 cm in length from the foramen magnum down the **vertebral canal** terminating around the first lumbar vertebra (see Figure 4-13). As mentioned previously, the spinal cord is continuous with the medulla at its most rostral connection but tapers off at its most inferior end as the **conus medullaris**. Caudal to this region, a mass of spinal nerves are found which are collectively called the **cauda equina** (horse's tail).

SEGMENTAL (i.e., HORIZONTAL) AXIS

The spinal cord is organized into five segments paired with the corresponding vertebrae, listed here from superior to inferior: **cervical, thoracic, lumbar, sacral**, and **coccygeal segments**. Each segment, in turn, has pairs of spinal nerves numbered and named for the segment they are associated with for a total of 31 pairs of spinal nerves. Specifically, the cervical segment has 8 pairs of spinal nerves (i.e., C1 to C8), the thoracic segment has 12 pairs of spinal nerves (i.e., T1 to T12), the lumbar segment has 5 pairs of spinal nerves (i.e.,

Figure 4-12   External views of the brainstem. (**A**) Dorsal view of the brainstem with major structures labeled. (**B**) Ventral view of the brainstem with major structures labeled. Note the number of cranial nerve rootlets on the ventral aspect of the brainstem. (Reprinted with permission from Bhatnagar, S.C. (2008). *Neuroscience for the study of communicative disorders* (3rd ed.). Baltimore, MD: Lippincott Williams & Wilkins.)

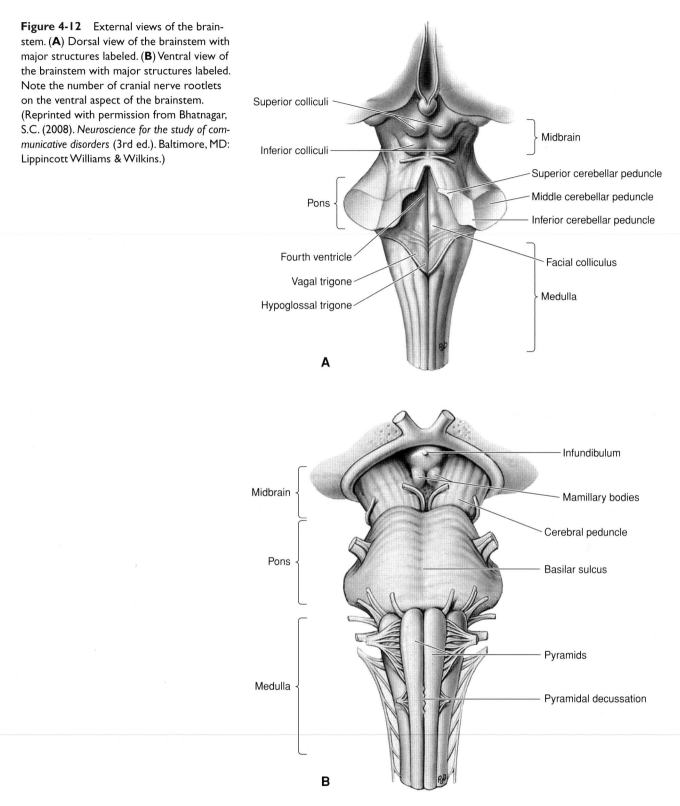

L1 to L5), the sacral segment also has 5 pairs of spinal nerves (i.e., S1 to S5), and finally the coccygeal segment has just 1 pair of spinal nerves (i.e., CO1). All spinal nerves are "mixed" nerves, that is, they carry both sensory and motor information. The sensory component enters the dorsal root of the spinal nerve with its neuronal cell bodies housed in the **dorsal root ganglion** outside the spinal cord. Alternatively, the motor component of the spinal nerve emerges from the ventral root with its neuronal cell bodies in

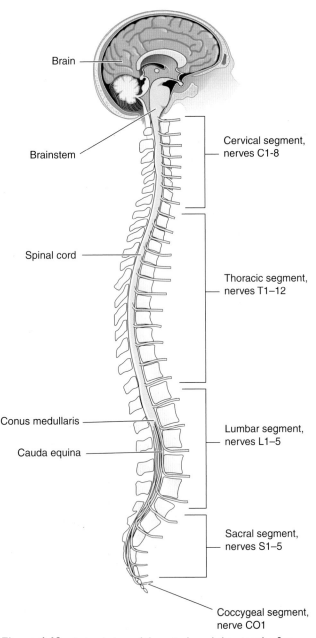

Figure 4-13 Lateral view of the spinal cord showing the five segments and their corresponding spinal nerves. (Reprinted with permission from Cohen, B.J. (2010). *Medical terminology* (6th ed.). Philadelphia, PA: Lippincott Williams & Wilkins.)

the ventral horn of the gray matter of the spinal cord as pictured in Figure 4-14 and discussed next.

A transverse section of the spinal cord illustrates the division of gray and white matter (see Figure 4-14). The posterior aspects of the gray matter are the dorsal horns, whereas the anterior aspects of the gray matter are the ventral horns. Consistent with neurodevelopment of the spinal cord, the dorsal region is involved with sensory functions and the ventral region is involved with motor functions. The amount of gray matter in the ventral horns is related to the amount of skeletal muscle innervated at that level. For instance,

at the cervical and lumbar segments, there is more gray matter to serve the innervation requirements for the muscles of the arms and legs, respectively. Gray matter surrounding the **central canal** is involved with ANS functions. This holds true for the white matter as well. Referring to Figure 4-14, there are three white matter areas that are named for their anatomical location in the spinal cord and for the fact that tracts run up (i.e., ascending tracts) and down (i.e., descending tracts) these "columns." These columns make up the longitudinal axis of the spinal cord and have specific names. They are referred to as the **dorsal fasciculus** (i.e., bundle), **lateral fasciculus**, and **ventral fasciculus**. There is more white matter as you move up the spinal cord because more neural information is traveling there.

LONGITUDINAL AXIS

Numerous tracts run up and down the spinal cord, bringing sensory (i.e., afferent) information in and sending motor (i.e., efferent) information out. Sensory information is brought to the spinal cord or brainstem for reflex reactions, to the cerebellum for integration and adjustments to our movement patterns, or, primarily, to higher cortical centers for conscious perception. Motor tracts transmit neural commands to skeletal muscle for movement. For the most part, these tracts are specific to body sensations (e.g., touch, pain, and temperature) and body movements (e.g., gross and fine motor movement) not specific to speech, language, and hearing. An exception is the tracts and nerves involved with respiratory function to be discussed in the physiology section of this chapter.

Supporting Systems

The CNS could not function without the support of other systems to provide oxygen, nutrients, waste removal, and protection. Protective coverings are provided by the **meninges**. Oxygen and glucose are brought to the nervous tissue by the blood system. The ventricular system produces **cerebrospinal fluid (CSF)** for cushioning and nutrient support both within and enveloping the CNS.

MENINGES

The meninges, shown in Figure 4-15, are connective tissue coverings that surround the CNS; these are the **dura mater** ("tough mother"), the **arachnoid**

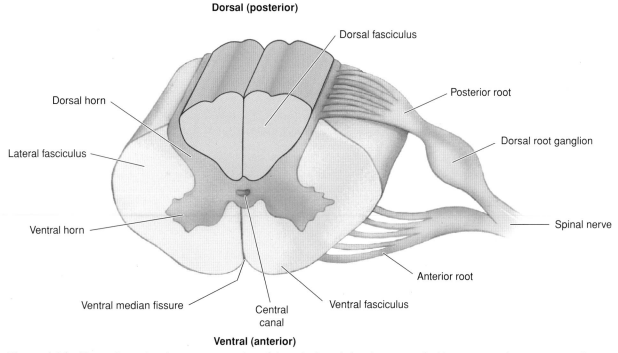

Dorsal (posterior)

Dorsal fasciculus

Dorsal horn

Lateral fasciculus

Posterior root

Dorsal root ganglion

Ventral horn

Spinal nerve

Anterior root

Ventral median fissure

Central canal

Ventral fasciculus

Ventral (anterior)

Figure 4-14   Three-dimensional transverse section of the spinal cord showing gray and white matter and components of a typical spinal nerve. (Reprinted with permission from Premkumar, K. (2004). *The massage connection anatomy and physiology*. Baltimore, MD: Lippincott Williams & Wilkins.)

mater ("web") and the **pia mater** ("tender mother"). The two-layered dura mater, a dense, fibrous connective tissue (tough and inelastic), is the most superficial of these with its outer periosteal layer adhering to the inside of the cranium and its inner meningeal layer immediately below. Between these two layers of dura are sinuses or spaces for venous blood drainage and CSF reabsorption into the blood

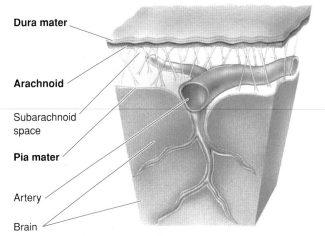

Dura mater

Arachnoid

Subarachnoid space

Pia mater

Artery

Brain

Figure 4-15   A cross section illustrating the three meningeal layers surrounding the central nervous system—the dura mater, the arachnoid, and the pia mater. (Reprinted with permission from Bear, M.F., Connors, B.W., Paradiso, M.A. (2006). *Neuroscience exploring the brain* (3rd ed.). Baltimore, MD: Lippincott Williams & Wilkins.)

stream. In addition, the inner meningeal layer of the dura mater has three dural extensions: (1) the **falx cerebri** which extends into the longitudinal fissure, (2) the **falx cerebelli** which partially separates the cerebellar hemispheres, and (3) the **tentorium cerebelli**, a horizontally oriented extension separating the occipital lobe of the cerebrum from the cerebellum (see Figure 4-16). The dura limits excessive movement of the brain within the skull. The dura surrounding the spinal cord is single layered with only the meningeal layer present (i.e., the periosteal layer remains within the cranium as the meningeal layer passes through the foramen magnum and down the spinal cord).

The arachnoid layer is in direct contact with the dura but is much thinner and more elastic than the dura. The arachnoid is an avascular, continuous, fibrous, and elastic connective tissue membrane running over the sulci of the cerebrum. It can be likened to taking a piece of Saran Wrap® and stretching it over the cerebral cortex and spinal cord making sure it adheres to the gyri but not pressing down into the sulci or spaces. Cisterns exist where the arachnoid bridges over larger spaces. The arachnoid pierces through the dura at the dural sinuses; these are called **arachnoid granulations** (or singularly arachnoid villi; see Figure 4-17). This is where CSF diffuses into the venous blood. An important space lies immediately

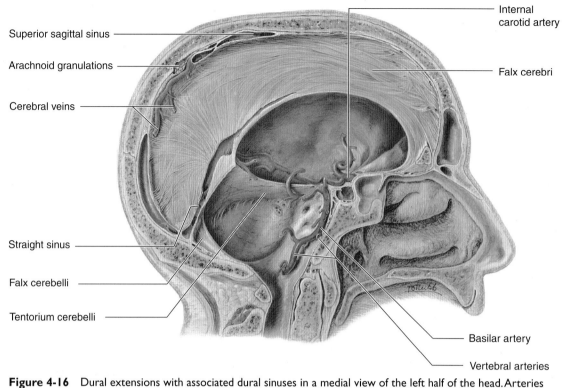

Figure 4-16   Dural extensions with associated dural sinuses in a medial view of the left half of the head. Arteries supplying blood to the brain are also labeled. (Reprinted with permission from Moore, K.L., Agur, A.M., Dalley, A.F. (2009). *Clinically oriented anatomy* (6th ed.). Baltimore, MD: Lippincott Williams & Wilkins.)

below the arachnoid called the **subarachnoid space**. In this space, CSF flows and cerebral arteries travel (refer back to Figure 4-15).

The pia mater is the third meningeal layer, adhering closely to the cortical tissue running down into sulci and fissures following the contour of the brain and spinal cord. The pia is a very delicate and thin collagenous connective tissue membrane. The pia serves as a protective barrier and is involved in the production of CSF. A sleeve of pia encapsulates blood vessels as they travel from the subarachnoid space to pierce the cerebral cortex.

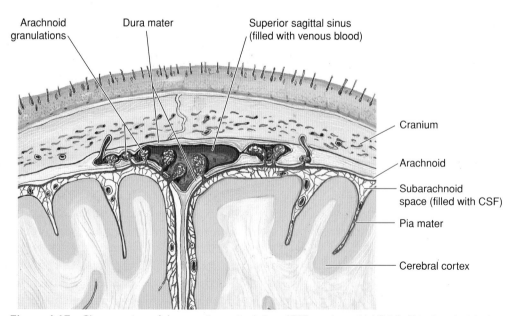

Figure 4-17   Close-up view of the superior sagittal sinus (CSF, cerebrospinal fluid). (Reprinted with permission from Anatomical Chart Company.)

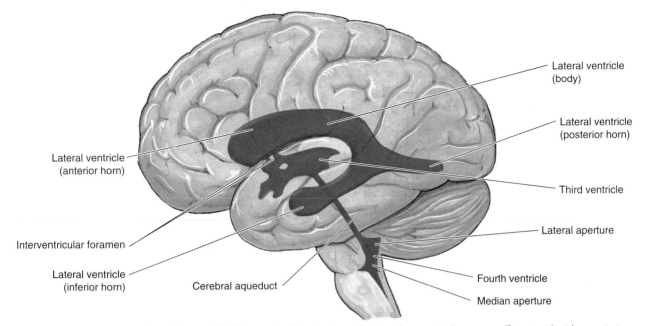

Lateral ventricle
(body)

Lateral ventricle
(posterior horn)

Third ventricle

Lateral aperture

Fourth ventricle

Median aperture

Cerebral aqueduct

Lateral ventricle
(inferior horn)

Interventricular foramen

Lateral ventricle
(anterior horn)

Figure 4-18 Transparent lateral view of the left cerebral hemisphere showing the ventricular system. (Reprinted with permission from Anatomical Chart Company.)

VENTRICULAR SYSTEM

The ventricles and associated canals and passageways are developmentally derived from the cavity or lumen of the neural tube. The ventricles are spaces that are lined with **ependymal cells** (a type of epithelial tissue) and filled with CSF. There are four ventricles: two **lateral ventricles** (one in each cerebral hemisphere), one third ventricle, and one fourth ventricle. As seen in Figure 4-18, the ventricles communicate with each other through passages. The lateral ventricles are connected to the third ventricle by the **interventricular foramen** and the third ventricle is connected to the fourth ventricle by the cerebral aqueduct.

Each ventricle has a unique configuration. The two lateral ventricles are symmetrical and are found deep in the telencephalon. Each of these ventricles has horns that extend into the lobes—anterior horn in the frontal lobe, posterior horn in the occipital lobe, and inferior horn in the temporal lobe. The parietal lobe houses the body of the lateral ventricles with the corpus callosum forming the roof of the body. A membranous partition, the **septum pellucidum**, forms the medial wall of the lateral ventricles. The single third ventricle looks like a slit-like cleft between the two halves of the thalamus and may be interrupted by the interthalamic adhesion. The fourth ventricle is found between the cerebellum and the pons and medulla and resembles a diamond shape. The caudal end of the fourth ventricle is continuous with the central canal that runs the length of the spinal cord. The fourth ventricle also has the openings from the ventricles to the subarachnoid space via three apertures. One median aperture (also referred to as the foramen of Magendie) and two lateral apertures (also referred to as the foramen of Luschka) allow for CSF to flow into the subarachnoid space to surround and cushion the brain and spinal cord.

CSF is produced by **choroid plexus** found in the walls of the ventricles. Production is continuous, with approximately 130 ml being produced each 3 to 4 hours. The choroid plexus consists of an intertwined mass of pia, capillaries, and ependymal cells and, on dissection, looks like soft and delicate strands of red-colored tissue. As schematized in Figure 4-19, the CSF then flows through the ventricles, out the median and lateral apertures into the **cisterna magna** and **pontine cisterns** (part of the subarachnoid space) and flows superiorly toward the **superior sagittal sinus** via arterial pulsations with an ebb and flow. Some CSF flows inferiorly to the **lumbar cistern** around the spinal cord. A small amount of CSF flows into the central canal of the spinal cord from the fourth ventricle. The absorption of the majority of the CSF occurs through the arachnoid granulations into the venous blood found in the dural sinuses. A blockage in this system of production to absorption can result in a condition called hydrocephalus, which will be discussed in Chapter 5.

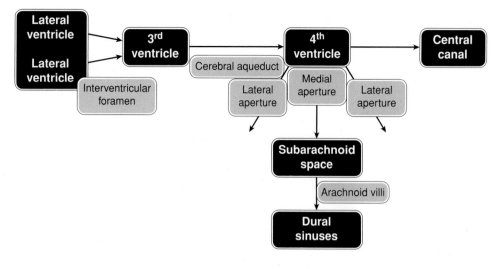

Figure 4-19 Flowchart of the flow of cerebrospinal fluid beginning at the lateral ventricles and ending in the dural sinuses.

BLOOD SUPPLY

Nervous tissue is incapable of storing essential nutrients yet has the highest metabolic rate of any tissue in the human body. Metabolism is aerobic which means nervous tissue requires a constant supply of oxygen via the blood stream. The brain itself comprises about 2% of an individual's body weight yet requires around 20% of available oxygen. Without this constant supply of oxygen by way of the blood stream, the brain ceases to function and dies. In fact, if blood circulation is disrupted for only 10 seconds, a loss of consciousness occurs; extend that time to 3 to 4 minutes and brain damage occurs.

Recall that arteries bring oxygenated blood from the heart and veins return deoxygenated blood to the heart. This is a continuous system with oxygen exchanged in the capillary beds. This occurs for the entire nervous system, but the focus of this section of the chapter is on the arterial blood supply to the brain as this is most pertinent to speech, language, and hearing.

Why You Need to Know

Nervous tissue is incapable of storing oxygen; for that reason, the brain is fully reliant on the blood supply to bring a continuous supply of oxygen. When that oxygen supply is disrupted, an ischemic event occurs. If the disruption of oxygen is of short duration and any behavioral symptoms resolve quickly, this is termed a transient ischemic attack. A stroke, or cerebro-vascular accident (CVA) occurs when a disruption of oxygen extends over a longer period of time due to a clot or plug (e.g., plaque build-up) in the arteries of the brain. This results in nervous tissue dying and the resultant behavioral symptoms associated with that tissue death such as body weakness and slurred speech.

Origin of Blood to the Brain

The blood to the brain comes from two systems: (1) the internal carotid arteries and (2) the vertebral basilar arteries. Both of these systems originate with blood from the aorta (see Figure 4-20). The **subclavian arteries** arise from the aorta and, in turn, give rise to the **vertebral arteries**. The vertebral arteries ascend through the transverse foramen of the upper six cervical vertebrae and enter the base of the skull at the foramen magnum. Here, they join together to form the basilar artery, which lies on the ventral aspect of the pons. The **common carotid arteries** also extend off the aorta and bifurcate (i.e., split in two) into the **external carotid artery** and **internal carotid artery**.

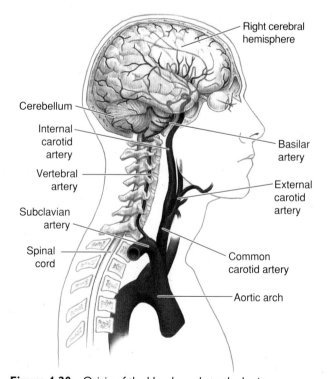

Figure 4-20 Origin of the blood supply to the brain. (Reprinted with permission from Anatomical Chart Company.)

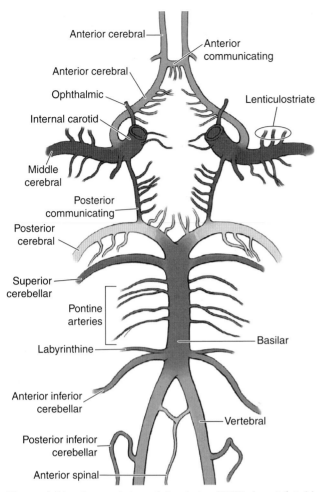

Figure 4-21   A ventral view of the circle of Willis (*arterial circle*) and arteries arising from it, and the vertebral basilar system that supplies blood to the brain and spinal cord. (Reprinted with permission from Agur, A.M., Dalley, A.F. (2008). *Grant's atlas of anatomy* (12th ed.). Baltimore, MD: Lippincott Williams & Wilkins.)

The internal carotid arteries ascend the anterior lateral neck to the base of the skull where they enter the cranium through the carotid canal in the petrous portion of the temporal bone. These systems join at the large **anastomoses** called the circle of Willis (i.e., arterial circle) found on the ventral aspect of the brain superficial to the midbrain. This is an uninterrupted circle of blood vessels that the two internal carotid arteries and the one basilar artery feed into. Three small communicating arteries (one anterior communicating and two posterior communicating) and proximal parts of two cerebral arteries complete the circle (see Figure 4-21). This arterial circle provides a safety mechanism for the blood supply to the brain as blockage below the circle (e.g., internal carotid **arteriosclerosis**) can be compensated for by the other arteries that feed into the circle.

Cerebral Arteries

Three pairs of cerebral arteries arise from the circle of Willis to supply blood to the telencephalon. These are the anterior cerebral arteries (ACAs), middle cerebral arteries (MCAs), and posterior cerebral arteries (PCAs). Although all of these arteries are critical to brain function, the MCAs are especially important as they supply blood to cortical areas critical for speech, language, and hearing. The MCAs are the largest of these paired cerebral arteries and originate at the termination of the internal carotid arteries as they come into the circle of Willis. The MCAs then turn laterally to course through the lateral sulci. As they course through, the MCAs give off small arterial branches referred to as the **lenticulostriate arteries** to supply blood to parts of the basal ganglia and parts of the internal capsule. The MCAs emerge from the lateral sulcus to fan out and supply the majority of the lateral surface of the cerebral hemispheres via a multitude of branches as seen in Figure 4-22. Most of these branches are logically named according to the part of the cortex they supply blood to such as the orbito-frontal branch or the posterior temporal branch as seen in the figure. All the branches off the MCA supply critical areas for language and cognition. The ACAs and PCAs also give rise to multiple branches. The cortical region that is at the distal reaches of the arterial branches is referred to as the **watershed area** (see Figure 4-22). The overlap of blood supply that occurs in the watershed area is called collateral circulation.

Cerebellum, Brainstem, and Spinal Cord Arteries

Arterial branches arise from the vertebral basilar system to supply blood to the cerebellum, brainstem, and spinal cord (refer back to Figure 4-21). Direct from the vertebral arteries arises a singular anterior spinal artery that runs along the ventral midline of the spinal cord and two posterior spinal arteries found on the other side of the spinal cord. In addition, the vertebral arteries give rise to the paired posterior inferior cerebellar arteries. Branches off the basilar artery also supply blood to the cerebellum in addition to the brainstem. The paired anterior inferior cerebellar arteries emerge from the most caudal aspect of the basilar artery, whereas the paired superior cerebellar arteries emerge from the basilar artery just before it joins the circle of Willis. At the junction of the basilar artery with the circle of Willis, the PCAs, mentioned earlier, also arise; these supply blood to the midbrain. The basilar artery also gives rise to a number of small pontine arteries to supply this part of the brainstem. Although not associated with brainstem blood supply, the basilar artery gives rise to the **labyrinthine arteries** that pass laterally through the **internal auditory canal** to supply blood to structures of the inner ear for hearing and balance function.

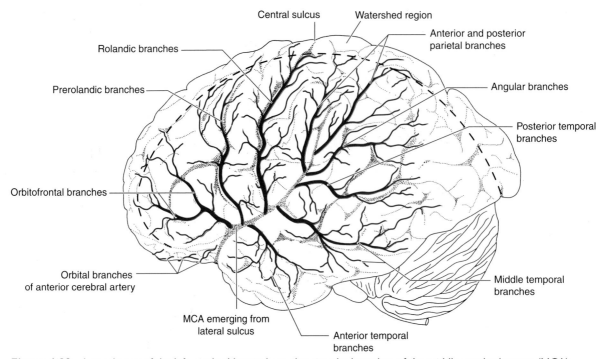

Figure 4-22   Lateral view of the left cerebral hemisphere showing the branches of the middle cerebral artery (MCA) and the watershed area (the border zone between arterial distributions). (Reprinted with permission from Haines, D.E. (2004). *Neuroanatomy: An atlas of structures, sections, and systems* (6th ed.). Baltimore, MD: Lippincott Williams & Wilkins.)

Venous System

The deoxygenated blood needs a way out of the brain to return to the heart. This occurs through the drainage of this venous blood toward the midline of the brain through two sets of veins: (1) deep veins and (2) superficial veins. The deep veins drain into the inferior sagittal sinus and then into the straight sinus. The superficial veins drain into the superior sagittal sinus. Blood from all of these sinuses converge to travel inferiorly to the internal jugular veins (see Figure 4-23).

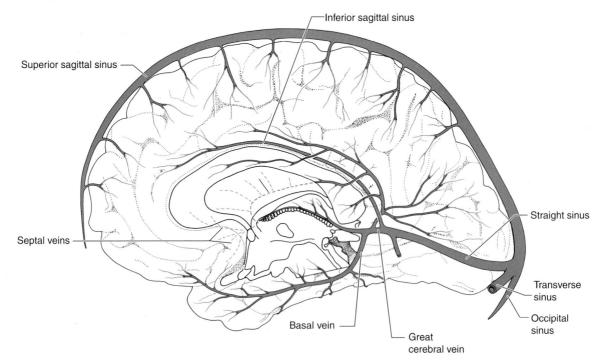

Figure 4-23   Medial view of the right cerebral hemisphere with brainstem and cerebellum removed showing cerebral sinuses for the drainage of venous blood with select veins labeled. (Reprinted with permission from Haines, D.E. (2004). *Neuroanatomy: An atlas of structures, sections, and systems* (6th ed.). Baltimore, MD: Lippincott Williams & Wilkins.)

Microscopic Neuroanatomy

The singular cells that comprise the nervous system cannot be seen with the naked eye; these are the neurons (i.e., nerve cell) and glial cells (i.e., neuroglia) introduced in Chapter 3. There are multiple types of neurons and multiple types of glial cells. The anatomical structure of these different types of cells relate to their function.

Neurons are composed of four parts: **dendrites**, cell body (i.e., soma), **axon**, and terminal (see Figure 4-24). The diameter of the cell body varies from 4 microns to 100 microns (1 micron = 1/1000 mm) and is filled with cytoplasm and organelles. The organelles found in the cell body were covered in Chapter 3; these include the mitochondria, golgi complex, lysosomes, Nissl substance, microtubules, and microfilaments. Also in the cell body is the nucleus and, within that, the nucleolus—the genetic center of the cell. Some of these organelles extend into the neuron's axon and terminal. Extending out from the cell body are dendrites, often viewed as branches of a tree with buds on these branches representing dendritic spines. The dendrites offer expanded surface area for communication between neurons to occur. The singular axon ranges from microns to several feet in length. The connection point of the axon with the cell body is called the **axon hillock**. The distal end of the axon has multiple terminal branches and is often referred to as the presynaptic ending. The branches of the terminal that resemble the arms of an octopus are collectively called **telodendria**. In turn, the end points of each teledendrite are termed **terminal boutons**; the terminal boutons house **neurotransmitters** that are the chemical messengers of the nervous system. The entire neuron is encased in a double-layered plasma membrane with channels that allow certain ions to pass; this is called **selective permeability**. These channels, however, are only available for exchange of ions at certain points called the **nodes of Ranvier**—intervening spaces between myelin segments on an axon where the axon communicates with the extracellular space.

Glial cells are found in both the CNS and PNS and outnumber the neurons by a ratio of 5:1. Those found in the CNS are **oligodendroglia, microglia**, and

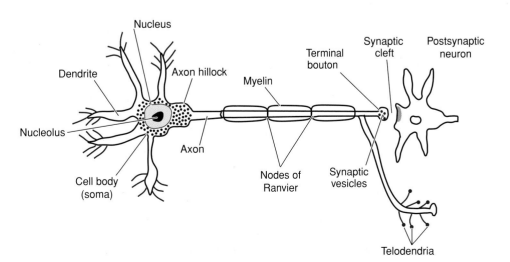

Figure 4-24 A neuron (nerve cell) with its functional components labeled. (Reprinted with permission from Bhatnager, S.C. (2008). *Neuroscience for the study of communicative disorders* (3rd ed.). Baltimore, MD: Lippincott Williams & Wilkins.)

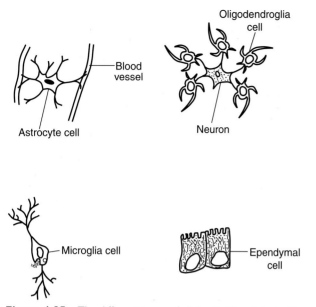

Figure 4-25   The different types of glial cells. (Reprinted with permission from Bhatnagar, S.C. (2008). *Neuroscience for the study of communicative disorders* (3rd ed.). Baltimore, MD: Lippincott Williams & Wilkins.)

astrocytes (see Figure 4-25). Oligodendroglia are found in white matter as they form and maintain **myelin** in the CNS. In fact, each individual oligodendroglia cell is responsible for providing myelin for dozens of axons! Microglia are scattered throughout the CNS often near and around blood vessels and, as the name implies, have a multitude of fine, small processes. Microglia are most active following trauma to the CNS where they will come in and "clean up" neuronal debris, a process referred to as **phagocytosis**, and leaving what is referred to as a glial scar. The star-shaped astrocytes are also involved with phagocytosis after trauma but have many other functions as well. Notably, astrocytes are intricately involved with the **blood–brain barrier** with their processes extending to surround capillaries.

The only glial cell found in the PNS is the **Schwann cell**. Schwann cells form myelin that surrounds the axons that make up our spinal nerves and our cranial nerves. Each Schwann cell wraps around a segment of an axon in a jelly roll fashion. Myelin serves as an insulator for faster conduction and separates the axon from the extracellular tissue fluid except at the nodes of Ranvier. The nodes of Ranvier, then, are the gaps that exist between adjacent Schwann cells in the PNS or oligodendroglia cells in the CNS in a myelinated axon. This turns out to be critical for neuronal impulse conduction, which will be discussed later in the chapter. Finally, ependymal cells are also found in the CNS lining the ventricles and central canal and contributing

to the choroid plexus. Clearly, glial cells support and assist the neurons in both the CNS and PNS in accomplishing their functions.

> ### *Why You Need to Know*
>
> *Brain tumors (i.e., neoplasms) are often due to the abnormal growth of glial cells. The general name for these brain tumors is gliomas but, more specifically, include astrocytomas, ependymomas, and oligodendrogliomas. Of particular interest to current and future audiologists is the inaccurately named acoustic neuroma (another term for neoplasm), which results from the pathological overproduction of Schwann cells surrounding the vestibulocochlear (VIII) nerve. The more accurate name for this tumor is a vestibular schwannoma as the tumor most often surrounds the vestibular portion of cranial nerve VIII.*

Neurons are classified according to their number of processes (i.e., axons and dendrites), function, and speed of information transfer. Neurons with multiple dendrites and a single axon are called *multipolar neurons*; these are the most commonly seen in illustrations of neurons as illustrated in Figure 4-24. The majority of the neurons in the brain are multipolar, often part of a motor system. Those with a single dendrite and a single axon are *bipolar neurons* and are found in systems involved with special senses such as the visual and auditory systems. Those neurons with only a single axon emerging from the cell body are *unipolar neurons*. Unipolar neurons are found in the dorsal root ganglia next to the spinal cord and are involved in the transmission of sensory information from the body. Figure 4-26 illustrates these three types of neurons. Speed of information transfer is dependent on the myelin covering of the axon and the diameter of the axon. Axons are also referred to as nerve fibers.

Nerve fibers are classified as Type A, Type B, or Type C based on their diameter. Type A fibers transfer information most rapidly as they are large diameter, myelinated axons. Type B fibers have a medium diameter and are more finely myelinated resulting in a slower speed of information transfer as compared with Type A; they are involved in smooth muscle innervation. Type C fibers are relatively slow as they are small in diameter and are nonmyelinated; they are involved in the transmission of pain impulses.

An example of Type A nerve fibers are the motor neurons that inform skeletal muscles whether to contract and how much to contract; this occurs at the **neuromuscular junction**. The neuromuscular junction is the point of communication and information

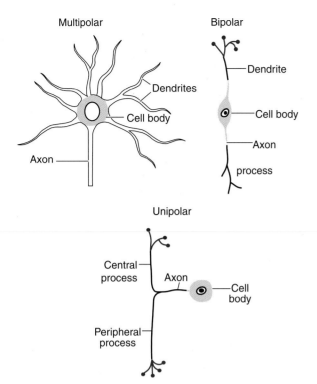

Figure 4-26 Classification of neurons based on their number of processes. (Reprinted with permission from Bhatnagar, S.C. (2008). *Neuroscience for the study of communicative disorders* (3rd ed.). Baltimore, MD: Lippincott Williams & Wilkins.)

transfer between the terminal branches of an axon and the muscle fibers it innervates. This junction is also referred to as the myoneural junction as "myo" refers to muscle and "neural" refers to the nerve fiber. This point of information transfer between the nerve fiber and the muscle fibers is a synapse. Synapses also take place between neurons, but here, the synapse is specific to the neuron and the muscle. The terminal branches from a single neuron synapse with many muscle fibers. A motor unit is one motor neuron and all the muscle fibers it innervates (see Figure 4-27).

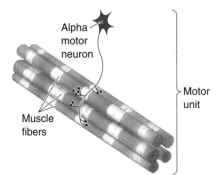

Figure 4-27 A motor unit—a single alpha motor neuron and all the muscle fibers (muscle cells) it innervates. (Reprinted with permission from Bear, M.F., Connors, B.W., Paradiso, M.A. (2007). *Neuroscience: Exploring the brain* (3rd ed.). Baltimore, MD: Lippincott Williams & Wilkins.)

Nerves of the PNS have an organization imposed by their connective tissue coverings as illustrated in Chapter 3 (see Figure 3-11). A delicate connective tissue called endoneurium surrounds the individual nerve fibers (i.e., axons). These nerve fibers run in bundles called fascicles; each fascicle is encased in perineurium. Fascicles, in turn, are bundled in groupings that form a nerve encased in epineurium. These connective tissue coverings allow a peripheral nerve, such as the hypoglossal cranial nerve, to function as a unit with a specific responsibility. For instance, the hypoglossal cranial nerve provides impulses to muscles of the tongue for movement.

Physiology of the Nervous System

The chapter, up to this point, has been primarily concerned with the anatomy, or structure, of the different parts of the nervous system with much new terminology and labels. Now your attention is turned more fully to neurophysiology. First, the means in which neurons communicate with one another will be presented. Then, the general functions of the brain areas will be covered. The bulk of this section of the chapter involves a discussion of cranial nerves which will be guided by a systems approach focusing, again, on those systems most closely tied to speech, language, and hearing functions. These are the visual system, the auditory/vestibular system, and the speech system. Finally, neurophysiology as it relates to swallowing function will be addressed.

ELECTROCHEMICAL COMMUNICATION

Neurons "speak" to one another through two means: electrical changes (measured in millivolts) and chemical changes. These changes relate to moving an "at-rest" neuron to one that is actively engaged with the transmission of a message, more properly called impulse conduction. To understand how this works, the "at-rest" neuron should be explained. As mentioned previously, each neuron is encased in a double-walled plasma membrane that has channels to allow certain ions to come in and certain ions to go out—selective permeability. An at-rest neuron has a particular charge with the interior of the cell being more negative relative to the outside of the cell (see Figure 4-28). This at-rest charge is approximately –70 mv and is referred to as the **resting membrane potential (RMP)**. Thus, an "at-rest" neuron is a polarized cell; this polarization is maintained by concentration gradients (of chemicals), electrical gradients (opposite

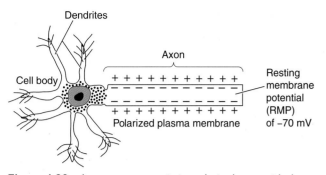

Figure 4-28 An at-rest neuron in its polarized state with the intracellular fluid more negative than the extracellular fluid. (Reprinted with permission from Bhatnagar, S.C. (2008). *Neuroscience for the study of communicative disorders* (3rd ed.). Baltimore, MD: Lippincott Williams & Wilkins.)

charges attract), and the **sodium–potassium pump (SPP)**. This pump exchanges internal sodium (Na^+) for external potassium (K^+) to assist in maintaining the concentration gradient of these two ions, which is necessary for the at-rest charge. Specifically, the at-rest neuron has much more sodium (Na^+) outside the cell than inside (Na^+ has a positive charge) and the plasma membrane channels are closed to Na^+. Inside the at-rest neuron are other ions such as potassium (K^+) and chloride (Cl^-). Even though there are positive ions inside the at-rest neuron, it is the uneven distribution of the ions and their electrical charges that maintain the RMP. All neuronal signals involve changing this membrane potential.

The membrane potential (electrical charge) can become either more positive or more negative. The positive change is referred to as **depolarization** and makes it easier for the neuron to initiate an impulse (called "firing"), whereas a change in the negative direction is referred to as **hyperpolarization** and makes it harder for the neuron to fire. Thus, an impulse is characterized by a sudden depolarization in a section of a neuron. Depolarization can occur at any location on a neuron—a dendrite, a cell body, an axon—however, the initiation of an impulse ("firing" of a neuron) occurs at the axon because its membrane houses Na^+ channels specialized to open when voltage changes occur. These are called voltage-gated channels.

Action Potential

An action potential, the mechanism used by the nervous system to communicate over distances, results from transient changes in membrane permeability. When a segment of an axon is depolarized enough, that is, reaches **threshold**, Na^+ channels open and Na^+ rushes into the cell due to the electrical and chemical concentration gradients (see Figure 4-29). This results in

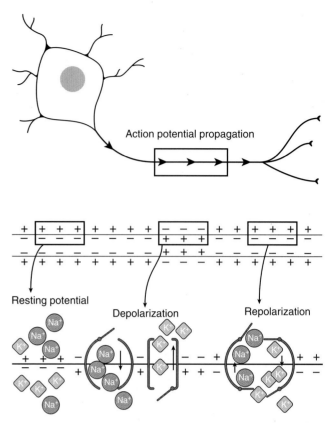

Figure 4-29 A schematic illustration of the propagation of an impulse (action potential) in a segment of an axon from resting potential, to depolarization, to repolarization (Na^+ = sodium; K^+ = potassium).

depolarization of the next segment of the axon continuing down the length of the axon until this wave of depolarization reaches the axon terminal—this is the action potential. If threshold is attained, an action potential occurs; if threshold is not reached, an action potential does not occur; this is referred to as the all or none principle. The movement of the action potential down the axon is called **propagation**. Propagation occurs in one direction only, traveling down myelinated axons at fast speeds up to 120 m/second, due to **saltatory conduction**. Saltatory means "to jump"; thus, the impulse transmitted down the axon "jumps" over sections of myelin. In reality, what is actually occurring is that the changes in membrane potential (in the case of action potentials—depolarization) can only occur at the nodes of Ranvier where the ion channels in the plasma membrane can communicate with the extracellular space; the rest of the axon is insulated by myelin. Nonetheless, the action potential moves down the axon without decrement, that is, the amplitude of voltage change down the length of the axon does not decrease. Immediately following an action potential, for a brief period of time, the cell will not respond to a stimulus to fire or responds only if the stimulus is especially strong; this is termed

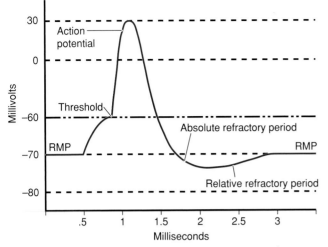

Figure 4-30 A graph depicting the membrane potential changes in millivolts across time during the generation of an action potential (RMP, resting membrane potential).

the **absolute refractory period** and the **relative refractory period**, respectively (see Figure 4-30). The voltage change (in millivolts) and the time involved (in milliseconds) in a single action potential at a segment of an axon is illustrated in Figure 4-30. Following are the key characteristics of an action potential:

- Initiated by membrane depolarization
- Threshold usually 10 to 15 mV depolarized relative to RMP

- All or none principle
- Conducted without decrement
- Refractory period

The initial stimulus for depolarization of a cell is either an external stimulus to our sensory systems or internal stimulus from chemicals called neurotransmitters. External stimuli such as pressure to the tongue tip, light to the retina, or movement of cochlear hair cells act as triggers to initiate enough depolarization to result in an action potential. In the case of neuron to neuron or neuron to muscle communication, the initial stimulus is the chemical transmitted by the neuron terminal. This is the chemical part of the electrochemical communication system.

Synapse

A synapse is an anatomically specialized junction between two neurons or between a neuron and the muscle fibers it innervates. There are multiple neuronal locations where synapses occur, with the most frequent being between an axon and a dendrite, termed axodendritic. At a synapse, the activity of the first neuron influences the excitability of the next neuron. Neurons conducting neural information toward the synapse are called presynaptic cells and neurons conducting neural information away from the synapse are called postsynaptic cells (see Figure 4-31). A presynaptic cell

Figure 4-31 An illustration of a synapse between neurons. (Reprinted with permission from Bear, M.F., Connors, B.W., Paradiso, M.A. (2006). *Neuroscience exploring the brain* (3rd ed.). Baltimore, MD: Lippincott Williams & Wilkins.)

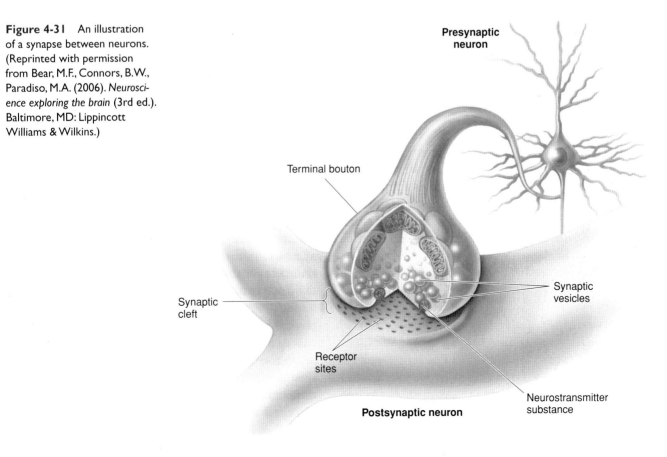

TABLE 4-3

SMALL MOLECULE NEUROTRANSMITTERS, WITH GENERAL LOCATION AND PRIMARY FUNCTION		
Neurotransmitter	**Central Nervous System**	**Peripheral Nervous System**
Acetylcholine (ACh)	Widespread—regulates telencephalic activity, critical for the sleep–wake cycle, influences stereotyped movements	Neuromuscular junction—excitatory for muscle contraction
Norepinephrine	Thalamus, hypothalamus, cerebral cortex—adjusts levels of attention and arousal	
Dopamine	Midbrain, basal ganglia, amygdala, cortex—involved in movement, motivation, and cognition	
Serotonin	Brainstem, diencephalon, hippocampus, amygdala, cerebral cortex—adjusts levels of attention and arousal; involved with pain control	
Gamma-aminobutyric acid (GABA)	Widespread, especially basal ganglia and cerebellum—critical inhibitory function	
Glutamate	Widespread—excitatory; may be involved with learning and memory functions	

produces either an inhibitory or excitatory response in the postsynaptic cell based on the chemical messenger sent across the synaptic cleft. These chemical messengers are called neurotransmitters.

There are a number of chemicals that act as neurotransmitters; the focus here will be on those that are stored in and released from the synaptic vesicles in the terminal boutons of the axon. These are small molecules (see Table 4-3). Small molecule neurotransmitters have fast responses and short-lasting effects; these include glutamate, gamma-aminobutyric acid, acetylcholine (ACh), dopamine, norepinephrine, and serotonin. ACh is responsible for the fast synaptic transmission that happens at the neuromuscular junction. Large molecules (i.e., neuropeptides) have also been found to act as neurotransmitters. The reader is referred to Bear, Connors, and Paradiso (2007) for a detailed discussion of current thinking in regard to neurotransmitters. A presynaptic neuron may have more than one neurotransmitter type and a postsynaptic neuron will have more than one receptor type to receive the neurotransmitter.

The steps involved in neurotransmitter release are listed below:

- Depolarization (action potential) in presynaptic cell results in calcium (Ca^{2+}) channels opening at the axon terminal
- Ca^{2+} influx into the presynaptic cell occurs

- Ca^{2+} mobilizes synaptic vesicles
- Synaptic vesicles fuse to presynaptic terminal bouton membrane
- Exocytosis occurs
- Neurotransmitter substance diffuses across the synaptic cleft
- Neurotransmitter attaches to receptor sites on postsynaptic membrane
- Neurotransmitter affects the chemical gates of the postsynaptic membrane, changing membrane permeability

Calcium (Ca^{2+}) plays a key role, infusing into the presynaptic terminal bouton to mobilize the synaptic vesicles. The vesicles then fuse to the plasma membrane and open to release their contents (i.e., a neurotransmitter such as dopamine) into the extracellular space, a process referred to as **exocytosis**. The neurotransmitter traverses the synaptic cleft to attach to a receptor site, if one is available for it, on the postsynaptic membrane. Here, the neurotransmitter affects the ion channels changing the permeability of the membrane at the localized area. These channels are referred to as chemically gated channels as they respond to the neurotransmitter chemical. Changes in membrane potential at receptor sites are called **graded potentials** and can be added up (i.e., summed) in two ways: temporally and spatially.

These localized or graded potentials can have an excitatory or an inhibitory effect on the postsynaptic neuron. **Excitatory postsynaptic potentials (EPSPs)** have a localized depolarizing effect, increasing the likelihood that the postsynaptic neuron will initiate an action potential. For example, the neurotransmitter glutamate would result in an EPSP. **Inhibitory postsynaptic potentials (IPSPs)** have the opposite effect. An IPSP results in a localized hyperpolarizing of the membrane, decreasing the likelihood for the initiation of an action potential. The neuron can be thought of as a mini processor of information as it integrates the type of message the neurotransmitters are communicating via the receptor sites (i.e., IPSPs and/or EPSPs). Furthermore, the integration of EPSPs necessary to result in a firing of an action potential is referred to as summation, either over time (i.e., temporal) or area (i.e., spatial). **Temporal summation** is the combining of rapid, sequential excitatory potentials generated at the same synapse, whereas **spatial summation** refers to the combining of excitatory potentials generated at different synapses on the same cell.

This electrical–chemical communication system of graded potentials at the sensory receptors or synapse site and the subsequent generation of action potentials results in the transmission of coded neural messages throughout the entire nervous system. Different parts of the nervous system are specialized to communicate specific types of neural information. The various functions of the different areas of the CNS and the PNS (in regard to cranial nerves especially) are covered next.

Functional Neuroanatomy

The study of brain anatomy and its correlates to behavior has been going on for some time. Franz Joseph Gall, an Austrian medical student, proposed one of the early examples of this in the early 19th century. He believed bumps on the skull reflected underlying mounds of brain tissue that correlated with different aspects of personality and other behavioral traits. This was called **phrenology**. The notion of correlating brain regions with particular language behaviors (localization theory) was scientifically corroborated by the observations of Paul Broca (1824–1880) and later, Carl Wernicke (1848–1904). Broca identified a frontal lobe area in the left hemisphere of the brain that, when lesioned, resulted in significant deficits of expressive language. Wernicke observed specific difficulties with the comprehension of language when the superior aspect of the left hemisphere temporal lobe was damaged.

There are distinct types of cerebral cortex in the human brain related to its evolution. The **neocortex** is the "newest" of the cortical areas (making up more than 90% of the cortical area) and has six layers. This vertical organization relates specifically to the type of neuron found in that cellular layer. The six layers are: (I) molecular, (II) external granular, (III) external pyramidal, (IV) internal granular, (V) internal pyramidal, and (VI) multiform layer. Flow of neural information occurs in both the horizontal and the vertical direction across these layers connecting cells to other cortical areas or to subcortical structures. The remainder of the telencephalic cortex, older in regard to evolution, is the two-layered olfactory cortex and the single-layered hippocampal cortex. It is the neocortex that sets humans apart from other mammalian species; in fact, when clinicians and scientists refer to the "cortex," they are most often referring to the neocortex. The cellular makeup (i.e., **cytoarchitecture**) across regions of the cerebral cortex has been well studied.

CEREBRAL FUNCTION

Brodmann investigated the cytoarchitecture of the cerebral hemispheres at the turn of the 20th century and discovered multiple areas with different cellular anatomy that could be related to various human behaviors. He numbered approximately 50 different areas; this cytoarchitectural map and numbering system is often referred to in neurological fields. Table 4-2 lists select **Brodmann areas** for the cortical regions most involved with speech, language, and hearing. Figure 4-32 illustrates this map on both a left hemisphere lateral view and the medial surface of the left hemisphere with select numbers emphasized for their clinical importance to the speech and hearing field. Another way to view the functional neuroanatomy of the brain is in regard to cortical regions associated with particular functions.

The cerebral cortex can be subdivided into **primary areas, association areas** (which are further subdivided into unimodal and multimodal association areas), and **limbic areas** (see Figure 4-32). Primary areas have a one-to-one correlation to motor and sensory functions and receive projections from the thalamic nuclei associated with motor and sensory functions. If a primary area is stimulated (as in the case of cortical mapping studies) or is damaged, then predictable motor and/or sensory behaviors or deficits, respectively, will be seen. Primary areas include the precentral gyrus of the *frontal lobe*, Brodmann area 4, commonly referred to as the motor

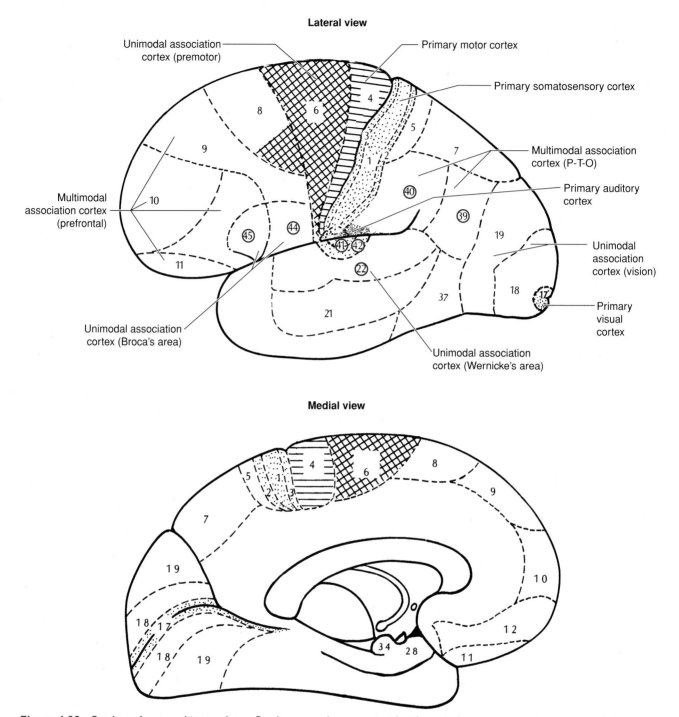

Figure 4-32 Brodmann's cytoarchitectural map. Brodmann numbers associated with cortical areas most pertinent to speech, language, and hearing are circled. Primary, unimodal association, and multimodal association cortical areas are labeled on the lateral view of the left cerebral hemisphere (P-T-O, parietal–temporal–occipital). (Reprinted with permission from Kiernan, J.A. (1998). *Barr: The human nervous system: An anatomical viewpoint* (7th ed.). Philadelphia, PA: Lippincott Williams & Wilkins.)

strip or **primary motor cortex**. The motor cortex gives rise to projection tracts to the brainstem and spinal cord for volitional movement of muscles of the head, neck, and body. Caudal to the motor strip is the postcentral gyrus of the *parietal lobe*, Brodmann areas 3, 1, 2, commonly called the sensory strip or **primary somatosensory cortex**. This area receives

sensory information (i.e., touch, vibration, pain, and temperature) via tracts that travel from the brainstem and spinal cord transmitting conscious sensations from sensory receptors in the head, neck, and body. The special senses of hearing and vision have their own primary cortical regions. Heschls' gyrus, located on the most superior aspect of the superior temporal gyrus in the *temporal lobe*, was numbered by Brodmann as area 41 and 42, and functions as the **primary auditory cortex** (Heschl's gyrus) where sound is consciously perceived. The **primary visual cortex**, Brodmann area 17, is found surrounding the calcarine fissure primarily on the medial aspect of the *occipital lobe*. Note that each of the four lobes of the cerebral hemispheres has one primary cortical region.

Single-function, or unimodal, association areas are adjacent to each of the primary cortical areas and are involved with the same functions and receive or give projections to the corresponding primary area. When stimulated or damaged, these areas reflect behaviors that are related to their sensory or motor function but in a less specific and localized way as compared with their primary counterparts. Five unimodal association areas are shown in Figure 4-32. The premotor cortex, Brodmann area 6, is found rostral to the motor strip and provides projections to the motor strip. The inferior frontal gyrus, Brodmann areas 44 and 45, is found at the inferior end and just anterior to area 6. This area is commonly referred to as **Broca's area** and provides projections to area 4 regarding movement for speech. The somatosensory association area, Brodmann numbers 5 and 7, is immediately caudal to the sensory strip and receives projections from the same. The auditory association cortex is especially important for language and hearing function. This is Brodmann area 22, commonly referred to as **Wernicke's area**. The auditory association cortex is critical for applying meaning to what we hear and receives projections directly from the primary auditory cortex. The visual association cortex takes up the remainder of the occipital lobe; these are Brodmann areas 18 and 19. The visual association cortex receives projections from the primary visual cortex and works to perceive, interpret, and attach meaning to the visual stimuli in our environment. Primary and unimodal association areas take up much of the surface area of the cerebral cortex; what remains are the multimodal association cortices.

The two multimodal association areas receive multiple inputs from the single-function association areas described earlier. The **parietal–temporal–occipital (P-T-O)** region is located at the confluence of those lobes and includes Brodmann areas 39 and 40. The P-T-O is surrounded by sensory areas and provides for the integration and association of multiple sensory inputs. The other complex, multimodal association cortex can be found at the most anterior aspect of the brain and is referred to as the **prefrontal cortex**. The prefrontal cortex is expansive, corresponding to Brodmann areas 8, 9, 10, 11, 12, and 46. The prefrontal cortex receives converging inputs from multiple areas of the brain and thalamus. This area of the brain is responsible for higher cognitive processes such as reasoning and executive function (i.e., planning, organization, monitoring, and controlling of behavior). The prefrontal cortex is also home to our personality.

Limbic areas of the brain include cortical areas (cingulate gyrus, parahippocampal gyrus, and uncus) in addition to the subcortical nuclei of the hippocampus and amygdala. The paired mammillary bodies are also considered part of the limbic system and can be found on the exposed ventral surface of the diencephalon. These structures, along with the tracts that connect them, make up the limbic system. The limbic system is responsible for regulating emotional and motivational aspects of behavior. It is also critically involved in memory, especially as it relates to new learning.

Why You Need to Know

The importance of the hippocampus in memory function was made evident by a famous case—H.M. H.M. underwent surgery for epilepsy in 1953 to remove nervous tissue from both medial temporal lobes (where the hippocampi and their connections are housed). Subsequent to the surgery, H.M. could not form any new memories. For example, H.M. could not recall a conversation he had just had or could not recall a magazine he had just looked at. His memories from before the surgery were intact and he was able to learn new motor activities (although he was not able to consciously recollect doing so).

As presented earlier in this chapter, all of these areas of the cortex, whether primary, association, or limbic, require tracts to communicate with one another and with subcortical structures such as the thalamus. Neural impulses travel along the tracts to communicate across hemispheres (commissural), within hemispheres (association), and at lower brain centers (projection). For example, the left prefrontal cortex communicates with the right prefrontal cortex by way of the corpus callosum, a commissural tract. The left hemisphere primary auditory cortex communicates with Wernicke's area by way of short association fibers, and the somatosensory cortex receives thalamic input via tracts traveling through the internal capsule, a projection fiber system.

NEURAL SYSTEMS

Neural systems refer to the different neural circuitry patterns of the peripheral and central nervous systems working together to achieve a specific function. This section of the chapter focuses on those neural systems key to speech, language, and hearing function. These consist of the visual system, the auditory/vestibular system, and the motor speech system. Also included is the neural circuitry involved in swallow function.

Cranial Nerves

A key part of the neural circuitry for the systems most involved in speech and hearing are the cranial nerves (CNs). Cranial nerves do for the head and neck what the spinal nerves do for the rest of the body: (1) they provide motor and sensory innervation to muscles and structures of the head and neck, (2) they are involved with the innervation of our special senses—most notably vision and audition, and (3) they play an important role in the ANS such as pupil dilation and saliva production. There are 12 pairs of cranial nerves with all but two pairs (CN I and CN II) entering or exiting the brainstem. The cranial nerves are numbered using Roman numerals I to XII. They are named for their function (e.g., **olfactory**), or the part of the head/neck they innervate (e.g., **optic**), or by virtue of the nerve's anatomy (e.g., **trigeminal**—having three parts). Table 4-4 lists each cranial nerve name and number, associated system, general function, and general location of neural cell bodies. The cranial nerves will be discussed in more detail as they relate to each system presented.

TABLE 4-4			
NUMBERS AND NAMES OF CRANIAL NERVES WITH GENERAL FUNCTION AND CELL BODY LOCATION			
Cranial Nerve	**System**	**Function**	**Location of Brainstem Nuclei**[a]
I Olfactory	Olfactory	Sensory	Nasal cavity[a]
II Optic	Visual	Sensory	Retina[a] of the eye
III Oculomotor	Visual	Motor	Midbrain
		Autonomic nervous system	Midbrain
IV Trochlear	Visual	Motor	Midbrain
V Trigeminal	Motor speech and swallowing	Motor	Pons
		Sensory	Pons (extending rostral to midbrain and caudal to medulla)
VI Abducens	Visual	Motor	Pons
VII Facial	Motor speech and swallowing	Motor	Pons
		Sensory	Medulla
		Autonomic nervous system	Pons
VIII Vestibulocochlear (also known as the auditory or acoustic)	Audition and balance	Sensory	Pons/medulla
IX Glossopharyngeal	Motor speech and swallowing	Motor	Medulla
		Sensory	Medulla
		Autonomic nervous system	Medulla
X Vagus	Motor speech and swallowing	Motor	Medulla
		Sensory	Medulla
		Autonomic nervous system	Medulla
XI Spinal accessory	Motor speech and swallowing	Motor	Medulla Cervical spinal cord
XII Hypoglossal	Motor speech and swallowing	Motor	Medulla

[a]Cell bodies for cranial nerves I and II are not located in the brainstem.

Visual System

The visual system is obviously important to language function in regard to reading comprehension and oral reading as well as perceiving and interpreting the non-verbal visual signals relied upon to supplement a communicator's message. Vision begins peripherally with light acting as the stimulus entering the eye and ends centrally with the processing of visual information in the single-modality association cortex and even beyond, to multimodal association areas of the brain.

A brief review of the structure of the eyeball will serve to assist in understanding the input from the visual fields to our retinas. The different parts of the eyeball are labeled in Figure 4-33. The cornea is the transparent covering of the eye that bends and focuses the incoming light rays. The sclera is the lateral continuation of the cornea and is often referred to as "the white of our eye." The lens of the eye inverts the visual image projection onto the retina. The iris is the colored ring that surrounds and controls the size of the pupil, the opening through which light enters. The choroid layer is deep to the sclera and provides vascularization to the eye. The most inner layer of the eye is the retina, which we will return to shortly.

The eye maintains its spherical shape via a liquid filling; the anterior cavity of the eye is filled with aqueous humor (a watery substance) and the posterior cavity is filled with vitreous humor (a jelly-like substance). Furthermore, the anterior cavity has two chambers: an anterior chamber between the cornea and iris and the posterior chamber between the iris and the lens. The canal of Schlemm connects these two chambers for regular drainage of the aqueous humor into the venous system; this is a critical system that regulates intraocular pressure. Glaucoma is a condition of increased intraocular pressure that results from problems with either overproduction of the aqueous humor or dysfunction of this canal.

Returning to the retina, it is here that the nervous system's involvement in vision begins. The retina develops from diencephalic tissue; therefore, it acts in a way like a "mini-brain." The retina is multilayered with three nuclear layers and two synaptic layers (see Bhatnagar, 2008, or Nolte, 1999, for a detailed discussion of the retinal layers). The focus here is on the outer nuclear layer of the retina that houses the sensory receptors for vision—the **rods** and **cones**. Returning to Figure 4-33, it can be seen that the retina is interrupted by the optic disc—a "hole" in the back of our eye. The optic disc is the exit point for the axons making up cranial nerve II (the optic nerve) as well as the entry point for blood vessels supplying the eye. Due to the lack of sensory receptors at the disc, any image falling there will not be perceived and, hence, we have a blind spot. Interestingly, this blind spot goes unnoticed, as our brain makes up for the missing information through perceptual processes in the visual cortex at the occipital lobe. Another key feature of the retina is the **fovea**. At the fovea, intervening neural layers are shifted to the side so that light focuses directly on the sensory receptors there for increased resolution.

The rods and cones are referred to as **photoreceptors**. Rods are sensitive to light and are found in most

Figure 4-33 Anatomical structures of the eyeball. (Reprinted with permission from Bhatnagar, S.C. (2008). *Neuroscience for the study of communicative disorders* (3rd ed.). Baltimore, MD: Lippincott Williams & Wilkins.)

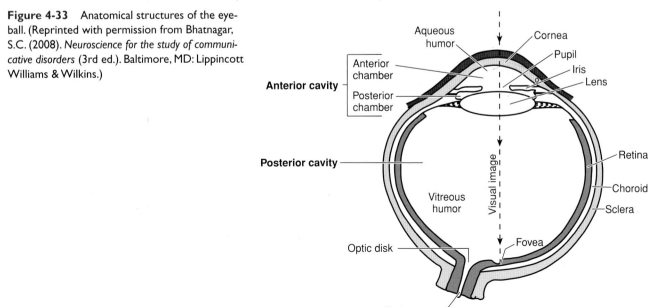

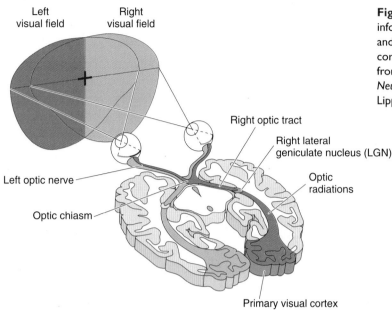

Figure 4-34   Primary visual pathway showing the information from the visual fields coming to the retinas and the projection from the retinas to the primary visual cortex in the occipital lobes. (Reprinted with permission from Bear, M.F., Connors, B.W., Paradiso, M.A. (2007). *Neuroscience: Exploring the brain* (3rd ed.). Baltimore, MD: Lippincott Williams & Wilkins.)

abundance lateral to the fovea. There are around 100 million rods in each retina. Rods assist us greatly in "night vision," helping us to see shades of gray and perceive movement and shapes. The retina also contains cones, found in greatest abundance at the fovea; nonetheless, cones are much less in number as compared with rods. There are around 6 million cones, the photoreceptors responsible for perceiving form and color. Thus, cones are responsible for visual acuity. Light is transferred to neural information by the photoreceptors and passed on to axons making up the optic nerve via the nuclear and synaptic layers of the retina. The optic nerve transmits this neural information toward the CNS.

The **primary visual pathway** is our system for sight and begins with the optic nerve as illustrated in Figure 4-34. The optic nerve from each eye transmits visual information from left and right visual fields (what you see with your eyes straight forward) toward the **optic chiasm**. At the chiasm, the outer fibers of the optic nerves stay ipsilateral while the inner fibers cross, or decussate, to the contralateral hemisphere. It is at the optic chiasm that fibers get "sorted out" so that the fibers carrying information from the right visual field are destined for the left hemisphere and the fibers carrying information from the left visual field are destined for the right hemisphere. The significance of this crossing over will be elucidated in Chapter 5 during the discussion of lesion effects on the visual system following a neurological trauma such as stroke. From the chiasm, the fibers continue back as the **optic tract** to synapse at the LGN of the thalamus. Fibers fan

out from the thalamus as they project back toward the occipital lobe as the **optic radiations**. Finally, synapses occur at the primary visual cortex, Brodmann area 17, at the occipital cortex surrounding the calcarine fissure. The surrounding single-function association areas, 18 and 19, further process visual information.

Small secondary visual pathways exist that send axons to the hypothalamus and midbrain. Those going to the hypothalamus play a role in the sleep–wake cycle by relaying information regarding the amount of light in our environment. Other axons diverge from the optic tract to synapse with the nuclei of the superior colliculi found in the midbrain. Visual reflexes important to maintain the position of our eyes and control the fixation of the eyes to keep objects focused on the fovea for the best resolution are part of this system.

Our eyes move in-synergy to draw attention to visual fields and focus light on our fovea. The cranial nerves responsible for these eye movements are the **oculomotor** (III), **trochlear** (IV), and **abducens** (VI) and are shown in Figure 4-35. Each of these cranial nerves innervates muscles associated with a particular eyeball movement. The oculomotor is responsible for moving our eyes upward, downward, inward, and medially. Importantly, CN III also innervates the muscle responsible for elevating the eyelid (i.e., levator palpebrae superioris). Damage to this cranial nerve, then, results in a droopy eyelid, called **ptosis**. The oculomotor nucleus for CN III is located centrally in the midbrain and its nerve fibers exit from the ventral

Figure 4-35 Ventral aspect of the brain showing cranial nerve locations. (Reprinted with permission from Cohen, B.J., Taylor, J.J. (2009). *Memmler's the human body in health and disease* (11th ed.). Baltimore, MD: Wolters Kluwer Health.)

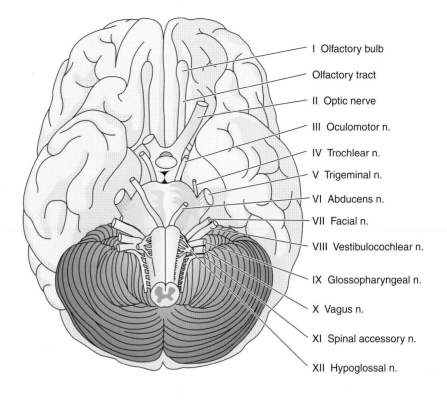

I Olfactory bulb

Olfactory tract

II Optic nerve

III Oculomotor n.

IV Trochlear n.

V Trigeminal n.

VI Abducens n.

VII Facial n.

VIII Vestibulocochlear n.

IX Glossopharyngeal n.

X Vagus n.

XI Spinal accessory n.

XII Hypoglossal n.

surface of the brainstem (see Figure 4-36 for a view of all the brainstem nuclei associated with the cranial nerves). The trochlear cranial nerve enables our eyes to move downward and outward. The trochlear nerve is engaged when we walk downstairs. The motor nucleus for the trochlear is found just caudal to the oculomotor nucleus at the junction of the midbrain and pons. CN IV's fibers emerge from the dorsal surface of the brainstem where they immediately decussate to curve around the brainstem and join the other cranial nerves on the ventral side. The abducens cranial nerve innervates muscles associated with moving the eye laterally (i.e., abduction—away from midline). This is easily tested by visually tracking an object from one side of the visual field to the other. The abducens motor nucleus is found in the caudal pons with its fibers emerging from the ventral surface of the brainstem.

Cranial nerve III, the oculomotor, also has an ANS component. It is part of the parasympathetic system innervating smooth muscle to adjust the lens of the eye for accommodation—to focus and adjust for moving targets and distances. It is also involved in pupil constriction; this is tested by the pupillary light reflex. Any ANS component of a cranial nerve has its own nuclei in the brainstem and CN III is no exception. The Edinger–Westphal nucleus, found next to the motor nucleus of CN III, gives rise to parasympathetic fibers that exit as part of the oculomotor nerve.

These cranial nerves will be returned to in the next section of the chapter, as they are related to the vestibular system as well.

Why You Need to Know

Lesions involving the visual system have varying effects. Damage to the primary visual tract, including the optic nerve, may result in various visual field deficits depending on the extent and site of damage. Damage to the cranial nerves involved in eyeball movement may result in **diplopia** *(i.e., double vision) or* **strabismus** *(i.e., tilting of the eye), what has commonly been referred to as "lazy eye."*

Auditory and Vestibular Systems

A case does not need to be made in regard to the auditory system's involvement in speech, language, and, of course, hearing. The sense of hearing supports our functioning and enjoyment of life. In regard to speech and language, the ability to perceive and understand the acoustic signal generated by the vocal tract provides crucial feedback for learning. Separate chapters (see Chapters 12 and 13) in this text explain the auditory and vestibular system in detail as well as the pathologies associated with damage to those systems. Here, the focus is on cranial nerve VIII, the **vestibulocochlear** nerve, and the tracts associated with

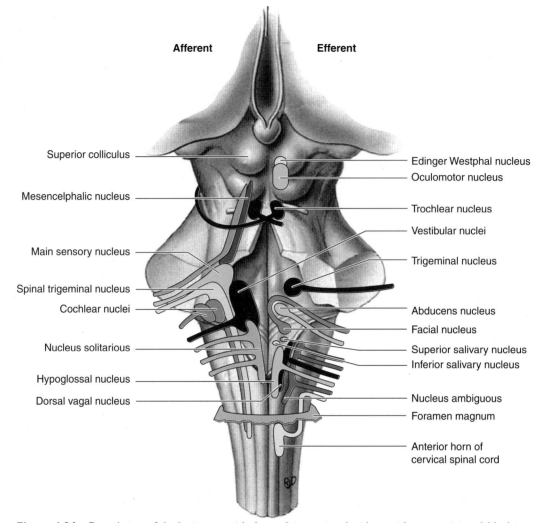

Figure 4-36 Dorsal view of the brainstem with the nuclei associated with cranial nerves pictured. Nuclei receiving afferent projections are illustrated on the left half of the diagram and nuclei giving rise to efferent projections are illustrated on the right half of the diagram. It should be noted that all of these nuclei are paired (i.e., one in each half of the brainstem). For ease of illustration, only one of each nucleus (except the trochlear) is pictured. (Reprinted with permission from Bhatnagar, S.C. (2008). *Neuroscience for the study of communicative disorders* (3rd ed.). Baltimore, MD: Lippincott Williams & Wilkins.)

the auditory and vestibular systems. Cranial nerve VIII divides into two branches in the periphery as its name implies: the vestibular branch and the cochlear branch. We will look first at the auditory component of this system, which includes the cochlear branch of the eighth cranial nerve.

Auditory (Cochlear) Component

The auditory pathway begins at the peripheral sensory receptors for hearing, the hair cells of the cochlea. These are analogous in some ways to the rods and cones of the retina. The stereocilia (thread-like processes) residing on top of the hair cells bend and deflect secondary to basilar membrane movement (and other components of the organ of Corti), thereby generating action potentials. Details

regarding the transduction of mechanical vibrations (i.e., the movements) of the hair cells into neural information are covered in Chapter 12. Processes of these hair cells go to the cell body found in the **spiral ganglion** of the cochlea. Axons from here project through the **modiolus** in the center of the cochlea and proceed through the internal auditory canal (found in the petrous portion of the temporal bone) to the brainstem. Figure 4-37 diagrams the auditory pathway from the brainstem up to primary auditory cortex. Cranial nerve VIII enters the brainstem adjacent to the inferior cerebellar peduncle at the pons-medullary junction where fibers from the cochlear component will synapse at the ipsilateral cochlear nuclear complex—here starts the auditory brainstem. The cochlear complex is composed of a total of four

Figure 4-37 Auditory pathway from the cochlea to the primary auditory cortex. (Reprinted with permission from Bear, M.F., Connors, B.W., Paradiso, M.A. (2007). *Neuroscience: Exploring the brain* (3rd ed.). Baltimore, MD: Lippincott Williams & Wilkins.)

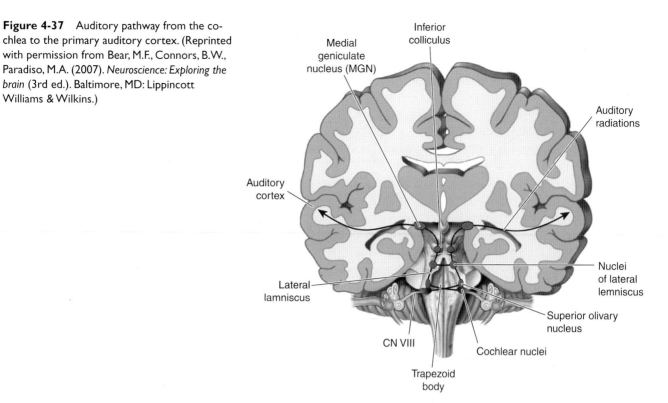

nuclei, one dorsal and one ventral on each side of the brainstem (refer back to Figure 4-36). From here, the auditory pathway becomes more complex due to multiple nuclei for synapses and multiple opportunities for axons to decussate prior to continuing their ascent. Nonetheless, there are four main relay nuclei between the cochlea and the cortex. These are the cochlear nuclei already mentioned followed by the **superior olivary nucleus**, the inferior colliculi, and the MGN of the thalamus.

Figure 4-37 illustrates the auditory pathway and possible crossover points for axons. Fibers of the cochlear branch of CN VIII bifurcate and synapse at the cochlear nuclei. The fibers then travel to synapse at either the ipsilateral superior olive or the contralateral superior olive via the trapezoid body; hence, some fibers decussate at this point. From there, fibers ascend in a tract called the **lateral lemniscus**; the cell bodies along this tract form the nuclei of the lateral lemniscus. Here, some fibers cross over to the other side as well. The fibers then ascend to synapse in the midbrain at the inferior colliculi (recall that the superior colliculi are related to vision). From here, the fibers travel via the brachium of the inferior colliculus to synapse at the MGN of the thalamus (recall that the lateral geniculate nuclei are associated with the visual system). Finally, the fibers travel via the **auditory radiations** (similar to the optic radiations)

to synapse at the primary auditory cortex, Brodmann area 41.

The auditory system is considered redundant with its multiple synapses and decussations. Thus, auditory information from one ear is ultimately shared with each cerebral cortex. Despite this intermixing of auditory signals, there remains what is called a contralateral effect. That is, a majority of auditory information reaching the primary auditory cortex originates in the contralateral ear.

There is now evidence to support the presence of descending, efferent auditory pathways which appear to act as a feedback mechanism. Chapter 12 presents more information specific to the efferent **olivocochlear pathway**. These descending tracts serve to inhibit the reception of sound providing for auditory sharpening of the acoustic signal.

Vestibular Component

The sensory receptors for the vestibular component of the eighth cranial nerve are the hair cells found in the semicircular canals, the utricle and the saccule. The semicircular canals, more specifically the crista ampullaris within the canals, are involved in the perception of angular movements of the head in space (i.e., dynamic equilibrium), whereas the macula within the utricle and saccule of the vestibule are involved in perceiving the position of the head relative to gravity (i.e., static equilibrium). A more thorough discussion of the vestibular apparatus' anatomy and physiology can be found in Chapter 12. The cell bodies for these hair cells are located in the vestibular ganglion found between the vestibular apparatus and the internal auditory canal. The axons making up the central projections for the cell bodies continues as CN VIII's vestibular component to enter the brainstem at the pons-medullary junction.

The fibers from the vestibular component of the eighth cranial nerve synapse at the vestibular nuclei; in turn, projections from these nuclei travel either in an ascending or descending direction as tracts (see Figure 4-38). Indicative to the importance of equilibrium and balance, there are a total of eight vestibular nuclei in the rostral medulla, four on each side of the brainstem. Axons from these nuclei give rise to a tract called the **medial longitudinal fasciculus** (MLF). The ascending fibers of the MLF synapse at the cranial nerve nuclei for those nerves innervating eye movement. Recall from the previous section that these are the oculomotor (CN III), trochlear (CN IV), and abducens (CN VI) nuclei. Thus, the ascending MLF is critical for eye movement reflexes secondary to changes in head position.

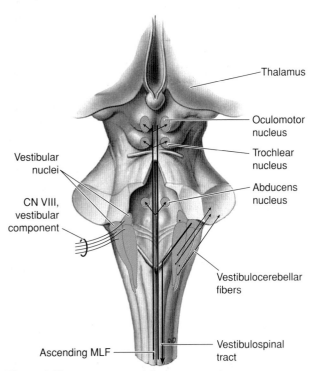

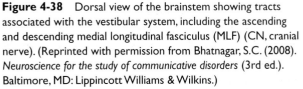

Figure 4-38 Dorsal view of the brainstem showing tracts associated with the vestibular system, including the ascending and descending medial longitudinal fasciculus (MLF) (CN, cranial nerve). (Reprinted with permission from Bhatnagar, S.C. (2008). *Neuroscience for the study of communicative disorders* (3rd ed.). Baltimore, MD: Lippincott Williams & Wilkins.)

> ### Why You Need to Know
>
> *The vestibuloocular reflex allows eye direction to stay stable in space to aid visual focus. In fact, the semicircular canals of our inner ears developed in parallel with the muscles that control the movements of our eyes; these two systems work together for this reflex. You can demonstrate this reflex to yourself by shaking your head while reading this text; although your head is moving your eyes will adjust via reflexive movements. Alternatively, if you shake the text back and forth while reading, it will be much more difficult, if not impossible, to read. This is because your semicircular canals cannot receive any afferent information from the textbook to make the necessary eye movement adjustments!*

The descending fibers of the MLF make up the medial and lateral **vestibulospinal tracts**. The lateral vestibulospinal tract is critical for vestibular reflex reactions (e.g., extensor or antigravity muscles) to maintain body balance and make the appropriate posture adjustments. For example, if you spin until you feel dizzy and then stop, the staggering that follows is a result of exaggerated lateral vestibulospinal tract activity (Nolte, 1999). The medial vestibulospinal tract is responsible for stabilizing head position as we move and to coordinate head position with eye movements as described earlier.

In addition to the ascending and descending tracts described earlier, a number of fibers from the vestibular nuclei travel directly to the cerebellum. These projections travel via the inferior cerebellar peduncle to synapse in the older parts of the cerebellum (i.e., flocculonodular lobe, vermis, and fastigial nucleus) to provide information regarding head position. The cerebellum, in turn, sends projections back out to the vestibular nuclei to influence muscle adjustments required for the maintenance of balance.

Motor Speech System

> ### Why You Need to Know
>
> *The motor speech system involves peripheral and central nervous system mechanisms to literally "produce speech." Although the label "motor speech" emphasizes the motor aspect of speech production, the sensory mechanisms are critical to providing the feedback necessary to coordinate and modulate our musculoskeletal system to produce intelligible and natural sounding speech. The term "motor speech" is apt because it is routinely used to describe communication disorders secondary to disruption in these systems.*

Half of our cranial nerves are involved with speech production. These are the trigeminal (CN V), facial (CN VII), **glossopharyngeal** (CN IX), **vagus** (CN X), **spinal accessory** (CN XI), and hypoglossal (CN XII). As seen in Table 4-4, the majority of these cranial nerves have sensory and motor components. Three of them, the facial, glossopharyngeal, and vagus, also serve the ANS. The last two, spinal accessory and hypoglossal, are motor only.

An idea or "thought" that initiates speech production comes from our cognitive systems that are housed in the multimodal association cortices of our brain. Language is intricately tied to cognition. For example, associating and accessing memories (prefrontal cortex) to word retrieval (P-T-O cortex) requires multiple regions of the brain to work together in a coordinated, parallel fashion. Of course, this whole process of formulating an idea and converting it into language often begins with sensation of the world around us. For example, a particular smell may evoke an image of your grandmother and inspire you to say something about her. This "idea" is then conveyed, via tracts, to language centers of the brain—Wernicke's area (Brodmann area 22) and Broca's area (Brodmann area 44, 45). Recall that these areas are single-function, or unimodal, association cortices. Broca's area, along with other premotor cortices, basal nuclei, cerebellum, and sensory strip send projections to the motor cortex (Brodmann area 4) to direct volitional motor activity. We now turn to the tracts that will bring the messages to the cranial nerves and spinal nerves involved in speech production.

Corticospinal and Corticobulbar Tracts

Motor fibers that direct movements of our body, head, and neck originate in the motor cortex (i.e., precentral gyrus). The fibers that run from the cortex to the spinal cord to innervate efferent fibers of the motor component of the spinal nerves make up the **corticospinal tract**. The emphasis here is on the fibers that run from the motor cortex to the motor nuclei housed in the brainstem that give rise to the cranial nerves referred to as the **corticobulbar tract**. These two tracts together (corticospinal and corticobulbar) are often referred to as the pyramidal tracts. The name pyramidal comes from the fact that these tracts arise from the pyramidal cells (the largest of these are Betz cells), named for their shape, in cortical layer V of the cerebral cortex. In addition, the majority of the corticospinal tract decussates at the denoted area of the *pyramids* in the caudal medulla. This accounts for contralateral control of body movement, that is, the left hemisphere motor cortex controls right body movement and vice versa. Nonetheless, by using the

more anatomical names for these tracts, the tracts' origination and destination becomes transparent. Specifically, the corticospinal tract begins at the cortex ("cortico-") and ends at the spinal cord ("-spinal"), whereas the corticobulbar tract begins at the cortex and ends at the "bulb" ("-bulbar") which refers to the medulla due to its shape.

> ### Why You Need to Know
> Clinicians use the terms upper motor neuron (UMN) and lower motor neuron (LMN) when speaking of the effects of a disruption of the motor system. Basically, UMNs refer to neurons of the corticospinal and corticobulbar tracts and LMNs refer to the neurons of the cranial and spinal nerves including their origination in the brainstem and spinal cord, respectively.

Neural information for respiratory control involves a complex array of neural signals beginning at the motor cortex (i.e., precentral gyrus) and traveling via the corticospinal tract. Neural information flows from the cortex down through the internal capsule, the ventral midbrain (i.e., cerebral peduncle) and through the medulla (i.e., pyramids) to innervate neuronal cell bodies in the anterior horns of the cervical, thoracic, and lumbar regions of the spinal cord for volitional respiratory control. It should be noted that the majority (around 85%) of the corticospinal fibers decussate (crossover) at the pyramidal decussation in the caudal medulla. Again, this means that the majority of neural information directing volitional movement in one half of our body is mediated by the motor signals arising in the contralateral hemisphere. Specifically, corticospinal projections arising from the left hemisphere innervate movement on the right side of the body, whereas projections arising from the right hemisphere innervate movement for the left half of the body.

The corticospinal tract is significant for speech production in regard to respiratory function. Volitional respiratory control occurs during breathing activities such as meditative breathing or voluntarily taking a deep breath; whenever you have conscious control over your breathing, this is volitional. Involuntary, or automatic, respiration is the norm of course. Automatic respiratory control requires constant input from nuclei in the pons and medulla that send projections to the same ventral horn cells in the cervical and thoracic regions of the spinal cord. From these ventral horns, neural projections are sent out via the ventral spinal roots to innervate muscles of respiration. Most notable is spinal nerve C4, part of the phrenic nerve,

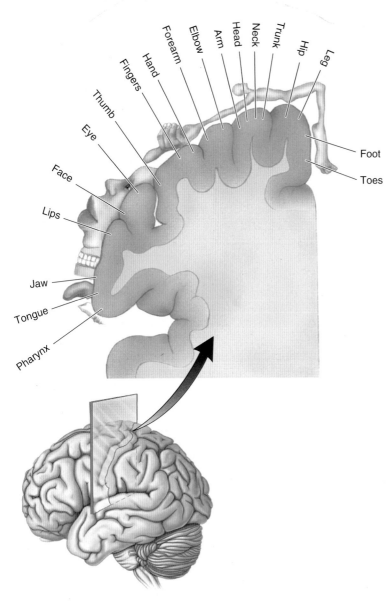

Thumb
Fingers
Hand
Forearm
Elbow
Arm
Head
Neck
Trunk
Hip
Leg

Eye
Face
Lips

Jaw
Tongue
Pharynx

Foot
Toes

Figure 4-39 A coronal section of the motor homunculus showing the topographical representation of the right half of the body in the primary motor cortex of the left cerebral hemisphere. The same representation exists in the right cerebral hemisphere for the left half of the body. A sensory homunculus, not pictured here, represents the body for conscious sensation at the primary sensory cortex. (Reprinted with permission from Bear, M.F., Connors, B.W., Paradiso, M.A. (2006). *Neuroscience exploring the brain* (3rd ed.). Baltimore, MD: Lippincott Williams & Wilkins.)

which innervates the diaphragm muscle, our primary and critical muscle for inspiration.

The corticobulbar tract sends neural commands to the cranial nerve motor nuclei in the brainstem responsible for innervating muscles of the head and neck. Here, we are concerned with motor speech function, but these same neural mechanisms and muscles are involved with swallow function. The corticobulbar tract begins at the lateral aspect of the motor cortex. The motor cortex has a topographical organization referred to as the **motor homunculus** (see Figure 4-39) that very specifically indicates the cortical region, giving rise to neurons controlling particular parts of our face and neck including the vocal tract (i.e., oral cavity, nasal cavity, pharynx, and larynx). Fibers from the motor cortex converge and travel via the anterior limb of the internal capsule, continue to descend through the cerebral peduncle (ventral midbrain) giving off fibers to both sides of

the brainstem to innervate the motor nuclei of cranial nerves V (pons), VII (pons), IX (medulla), X (medulla), XI (medulla), and XII (medulla). Note that four of the six cranial nerves involved with speech house their cell bodies in the medulla with the facial motor nuclei close by at the junction of the pons and medulla (refer back to Figure 4-36). It should be emphasized that the corticobulbar tract from one hemisphere provides neural information to cranial nerve nuclei in both the left and right halves of the brainstem. This "double coverage" serves as an important safety mechanism should one cerebral hemisphere be compromised by neurological insult (e.g., tumor or stroke). An exception to this double coverage rule is discussed later with regard to the facial and hypoglossal motor nuclei.

Trigeminal Nerve

Cranial nerve V, the trigeminal, is the largest of the cranial nerves. It emerges from the lateral ventral aspect of the pons (refer back to Figure 4-35) and has both sensory and motor functions. The trigeminal is responsible for transmitting sensory information regarding touch, pressure, pain, and temperature from the head, face, and teeth including senses from the mucous membranes of the oral and nasal cavities. Next time you get a toothache, you can thank the trigeminal nerve. This cranial nerve also transmits **proprioceptive** information from facial and lingual musculature. Proprioception refers to an internal awareness of muscle movement, position, and posture. Motor function of the trigeminal is primarily responsible for jaw movement: innervating the muscles that open and close the jaw and lateralize movement for chewing or **mastication**. Refer to Chapter 10 for a thorough discussion of the musculoskeletal anatomy associated with jaw movement. In addition, the trigeminal innervates one velar (i.e., soft palate) muscle—the **tensor veli palatini**—and one middle ear muscle—the **tensor tympani**.

The trigeminal has three branches ("tri-" means "three"). The ophthalmic branch is sensory only and transmits information from the forehead, upper eyelid, eyeball, and mucous membranes of the nasal cavity. The maxillary branch is also sensory only, transmitting information from the upper lip, lateral nose, upper cheek, mucous membranes of the nasal cavity, the roof of the mouth (i.e., hard palate), and the upper teeth and jaw. The mandibular branch is sensory *and* motor, transmitting sensory information from the lower lip, chin, posterior cheek and temple, external ear, lower jaw and teeth, inside of the cheeks, floor of the mouth and tactile, pain, and temperature information from the anterior two-thirds of the tongue. However, the mandibular branch does not transmit any taste sensation: that is left to other cranial nerves. As mentioned earlier, motor impulses travel by way of the mandibular branch to muscles of mastication (e.g., masseter, temporalis, mylohyoid), the middle ear (tensor tympani), and velum (tensor veli palatini).

The trigeminal has three brainstem nuclei for sensation associated with it (refer back to Figure 4-36). Fibers from the sensory component of CN V synapse here upon entry into the brainstem; the nuclei where the synapse occurs depends on the sensory information a given fiber is carrying. The **mesencephalic nucleus**, as the name implies, extends into the midbrain and receives proprioceptive information. The **main sensory nucleus**, found in the pons, receives tactile sense information. The **spinal trigeminal nucleus**, located in the pons and medulla and extending into the cervical spinal cord (as the name

indicates), primarily receives information regarding pain and temperature. In this way, sensory information from the head is already being organized but has not reached conscious sensation yet, as that happens in the cortex.

The sensory fibers that arise from the sensory nuclei of the trigeminal ascend to the cortex by way of the thalamus. Fibers from the main sensory nuclei ascend ipsilaterally as part of the **medial lemniscus** pathway or contralaterally as the dorsal trigeminal tract to synapse in the **ventral posterior medial (VPM) nucleus** of the thalamus. Following another synapse, the fibers that arise from the VPM ascend via the internal capsule to the postcentral gyrus (Brodmann areas 3, 1, 2), where conscious sensation occurs for tactile sensation from the head. Fibers from the spinal trigeminal nucleus ascend contralaterally either as the spinal trigeminal tract (and merge with **Lissauer's tract**) or along with the spinothalamic tract (coming from the spinal cord) to synapse again in the thalamus at the VPM. From here, fibers follow the same route through the internal capsule to the cortex for conscious sensation of pain and temperature. Similar to the motor representation at the primary motor cortex, a **sensory homunculus** exists for the somatosensory cortex. Sensations from the head and face are received at the inferior lateral aspect of the sensory strip.

Keeping with one trigeminal motor branch, there is one trigeminal motor nucleus (refer back to Figure 4-36). The motor nucleus of CN V is centrally located in the pons. This motor nucleus receives both ipsilateral and contralateral input (recall "double coverage") from the motor cortex via the corticobulbar tract. A synapse occurs at the motor nucleus and fibers emerge from the lateral aspect of the ventral pons as the motor component of CN V's mandibular branch.

Facial Nerve

Cranial nerve VII, the facial, innervates the muscles of facial expression, among other functions. It emerges from the ventral junction of the pons and medulla just lateral to the abducens nerve (refer back to Figure 4-35) and has components serving all three functions: sensory, motor, and autonomic. Its sensory component is smaller than its motor component but is critical for our enjoyment of life, as it picks up taste sensation from the anterior two-thirds of the tongue. Motorically, CN VII supplies innervation to the many muscles involved with lip movement for speech (see Chapter 10 for detailed information regarding these muscles) such as the orbicularis oris. In addition, this cranial nerve innervates eyelid depressors, so we can sleep and blink to protect the eye and maintain moisture (recall that CN III, the oculomotor, innervates muscles elevating the eyelid). In addition, the facial nerve innervates the tiny stapedius muscle (within the middle ear), which responds to loud noise by dampening excessive movement of the ossicles (see Chapter 12 for more information regarding the stapedial reflex). The autonomic component is part of the parasympathetic nervous system and provides stimulation to glands that produce saliva.

The facial cranial nerve has three brainstem nuclei associated with it, one for sensation, one for motor function, and one for autonomic function (refer back to Figure 4-36). Fibers carrying sensation for taste enter the brainstem to synapse in the nucleus solitarius. The nucleus solitarius, located in the medulla, is a shared nucleus that receives input from afferent fibers of cranial nerves IX and X as well. Fibers from this nucleus ascend to synapse at the VPM nucleus of the thalamus in the same manner as sensations carried by the trigeminal. From here, projections travel via the internal capsule to the **gustatory cortex** located at the anterior insular cortex and the frontal operculum overlying it. Association fibers from here project to the orbital cortex to integrate taste information with olfaction.

The motor nucleus of cranial nerve VII is housed in the rostral medulla (see Figure 4-36). Unique to the facial motor nucleus is that the lower half of the nucleus receives input from *only* the contralateral corticobulbar tract. This lower half has the cell bodies that give rise to the axons innervating muscles of facial expression for the lower half of the face. This is an exception to the "double coverage" safety mechanism, which means that if a lesion occurs (e.g., stroke, tumor) affecting the corticobulbar fibers in one hemisphere, the effects will be seen in the contralateral lower face. This is most clearly manifested as a droopy half of the lower face with marked impairments in raising that lip corner. The motor nucleus that sends projections out to innervate muscles of the upper face receives corticobulbar input from both hemispheres as expected.

Cranial nerves that have ANS components have dedicated nuclei for the particular ANS function. Specifically for the facial cranial nerve, the superior salivary nucleus contains the cell bodies that give rise to its parasympathetic component. This nucleus is found in the rostral medulla adjacent to the motor nucleus of CN VII. Its fibers travel with cranial nerve VII to innervate sublingual and submandibular glands for the production of saliva.

Glossopharyngeal Nerve

Cranial nerve IX, the glossopharyngeal, is involved with the tongue and pharynx as its name implies. It emerges from the lateral ventral aspect of the medulla below cranial nerve VIII (refer back to Figure 4-35) and has all three functions: sensory, motor, and autonomic. It provides sensory information from the upper throat (i.e., pharynx) and completes the special sense of taste by transmitting information from the posterior one-third of the tongue (recall that the facial cranial nerve does the job for the anterior two-thirds). You are able to gag or to be consciously aware of a nasty sore throat, thanks to CN IX! The glossopharyngeal's motor component innervates some pharyngeal (e.g., stylopharyngeus) and lingual (e.g., palatoglossus) muscles (see Chapter 10). Similar to the facial cranial nerve, the glossopharyngeal's autonomic component is part of the parasympathetic nervous system and provides stimulation to the parotid glands that produce saliva.

A brainstem nucleus is associated with each of the glossopharyngeal functions. Fibers carrying sensory information synapse, along with facial nerve sensory fibers, at the nucleus solitarius already described (refer back to Figure 4-36). Fibers from this nucleus ascend to the thalamus to synapse at the VPM nucleus for taste, tactile, pain, and temperature sensations. The fibers then continue on via the internal capsule to terminate at the tongue and pharyngeal regions of the sensory homunculus of the postcentral gyrus for most of these conscious sensations. Projections associated with taste go to the gustatory cortex as described earlier. Efferent projections that comprise the motor component of the glossopharyngeal nerve arise from the rostral end of a shared brainstem nucleus found in the medulla called the nucleus ambiguous (see Figure 4-36). The ANS fibers of the glossopharyngeal nerve that innervate the parotid gland arise from the inferior salivary nucleus.

Vagus Nerve

Cranial nerve X, the vagus, is best known to speech clinicians and speech scientists for its prominent role in voice production, yet, as elucidated later, the vagus is involved with numerous functions in addition to voice. The vagus is a large, prominent cranial nerve emerging from the lateral aspect of the medulla just caudal to the glossopharyngeal nerve (refer back to Figure 4-35). Like the glossopharyngeal nerve, it has all three functions: sensory, motor, and autonomic. The sensory functions are many; those most relevant to speech and swallowing are listed here. The vagus transmits sensation from the mucosal surfaces of the lower pharynx, larynx, trachea and bronchi, esophagus, and stomach. In addition, it conveys information from a small number of taste buds around the

epiglottis. This is thought to have a protective effect from ingesting toxic substances, as these taste buds pick up bitterness.

As alluded to above, cranial nerve X innervates all of the intrinsic muscles of the larynx (e.g., lateral and posterior cricoarytenoids, interarytenoids); these are the muscles that have both their origin and insertion within the larynx itself. Chapter 8 provides detailed coverage of these muscles. The vagus also innervates all the pharyngeal muscles with the exception of one, and all the velar muscles with the exception of one. The stylopharyngeus (a pharyngeal muscle) is innervated by the glossopharyngeal cranial nerve and, as mentioned previously, the tensor veli palatini (velar muscle) is innervated by the trigeminal cranial nerve. The vagus is a critical part of the parasympathetic division of the ANS, innervating glands, cardiac muscle, and the smooth muscle of blood vessels, trachea, bronchi, esophagus, stomach, and intestines. Thus, the vagus is involved with breathing, cardiac function, and digestive function—critical indeed!

The vagus (which means "wanderer") wanders throughout the body by way of multiple branches; three of these branches are particularly relevant to speech production as they innervate the muscles of the velum, pharynx, and larynx. The *pharyngeal branch* provides motor innervation to the velar muscles (with the exception of the tensor veli palatini) and the pharyngeal constrictor muscles. The *superior laryngeal nerve* is a branch of the vagus that further divides into external and internal laryngeal branches. The external branch of the superior laryngeal nerve provides motor innervation to muscles of the inferior pharynx (i.e., inferior constrictor muscle and cricopharyngeus) and to one intrinsic laryngeal muscle—the cricothyroid. As you will learn later (see Chapter 8), the cricothyroid muscle is our primary muscle for changing the pitch of our voice. The internal branch of the superior laryngeal nerve carries sensory information from the larynx above the vocal folds and from the tongue base and epiglottis. The *recurrent laryngeal nerve* (RLN) is the primary cranial nerve branch involved with voice. The name "recurrent" is apt secondary to the fact that the nerve on the left side extends down toward the heart prior to looping under the aortic arch and then ascending back up to innervate muscles on the left side of the larynx. The RLN on the right side extends down and loops under the subclavian artery. Understandably, the RLN is at risk for being damaged during thoracic surgery or secondary to thoracic trauma. The RLN transmits sensation from the larynx below the vocal folds as well as from the superior esophagus.

Importantly, it is this branch of CN X—the RLN—that innervates all the intrinsic laryngeal muscles with the exception of the cricothyroid.

The three different brainstem nuclei associated with the vagus are found in the medulla. Afferent fibers bringing in the variety of sensations the vagus is responsible for go to different nuclei depending on the sensation. The fibers carrying taste information join the afferent fibers from cranial nerves VII and IX to synapse in the nucleus solitarius. As mentioned earlier, these fibers then ascend to synapse in the VPM nucleus of the thalamus. Projections for taste sensation from the thalamus travel to the gustatory center at the insular cortex and frontal operculum for the conscious sensation of taste. The many fibers carrying sensation from the viscera (e.g., organs of the thorax and abdomen) also go to the nucleus solitarius. The fibers transmitting pain, temperature, and touch from the inferior pharynx, larynx, esophagus, and regions of the outer ear join afferent fibers from cranial nerve V to synapse in the spinal trigeminal nucleus. Fibers then ascend to the VPM nucleus of the thalamus and on to the postcentral gyrus as previously described.

Two brainstem nuclei give rise to CN X's efferent projections. The nucleus ambiguous (refer back to Figure 4-36) is a shared nucleus as mentioned earlier, giving rise also to efferent fibers of cranial nerves IX (glossopharyngeal) and XI (spinal accessory). The fibers from this nucleus innervate those skeletal muscles of the velum, pharynx, and larynx served by the branches of the vagus described earlier. The dorsal vagal nucleus (see Figure 4-36) is the major parasympathetic nucleus of the brain. Fibers from this nucleus provide parasympathetic innervation to the thoracic and abdominal viscera.

Spinal Accessory Nerve

Cranial nerve XI is named spinal accessory because it has a spinal component that innervates muscles of the neck and shoulders and a cranial component that provides assistance to the vagus nerve. The spinal accessory cranial nerve has only a motor function. The cranial root is the most caudally located of the cranial nerves, emerging from the lateral aspect of the ventral medulla very near the spinal cord (refer back to Figure 4-35). It serves to assist the pharyngeal and recurrent branches of the vagus in innervating muscles of the velum, pharynx, and larynx with the exception of the palatoglossus muscle. The spinal root arises from the anterior horns of the cervical spinal cord (C1 to C5) to innervate the muscles that turn our head (e.g., sternocleidomastoid) and shrug our shoulders (e.g., trapezius).

Hypoglossal Nerve

Cranial nerve XII, the hypoglossal, is responsible for tongue movement; therefore, it is critical in both speech and swallow function. The hypoglossal also has only a motor component. It emerges from the ventral medulla medial to the other medullary cranial nerves (see Figure 4-35). It provides motor innervation to all the intrinsic and extrinsic muscles of the tongue except for the palatoglossus (CN IX's responsibility). In addition, the hypoglossal nerve also innervates some of the extrinsic laryngeal muscles (also referred to as the strap muscles of the neck), especially those involved with lowering the larynx (i.e., the infrahyoid muscles).

Given its singular function, all efferent fibers that comprise cranial nerve XII arise from a single nucleus. The hypoglossal nucleus is found in the medulla adjacent to midline (refer back to Figure 4-36). This motor nucleus receives the majority of its input from the contralateral cerebral hemisphere via the corticobulbar tract. This, again, is an exception to the "double coverage" rule. This means that a lesion to one cerebral hemisphere can result in significant weakness in the contralateral side of the tongue. For example, a right cerebral hemisphere lesion involving the lateral precentral gyrus (see Figure 4-39) would affect the left side of the tongue.

Swallow Function

The neural circuitry responsible for swallowing has much overlap with the circuitry for motor speech function, although the reflexive nature of swallowing dictates control by the swallow center located in the medulla. Nonetheless, the cranial nerves discussed earlier along with their afferent and efferent innervations are all critical. Thus, the cranial nerves involved with swallow function include the trigeminal (V), facial (VII), glossopharyngeal (IX), vagus (X), spinal accessory (XI), and hypoglossal (XII). A brief presentation of swallow physiology will assist the reader in understanding the importance of these cranial nerves and the structures they innervate. Swallowing, or **deglutition**, occurs in four stages: (1) **oral preparatory stage**, (2) **oral stage**, (3) **pharyngeal stage**, and (4) **esophageal stage** (see Chapter 10).

The oral preparatory stage involves preparing the food and/or drink for swallow. This includes the introduction of food to the oral cavity requiring active involvement of the lips and the manipulation of that food once in the oral cavity requiring additional involvement of the jaw and tongue. Chewing,

TABLE 4-5

CRANIAL NERVES ASSOCIATED WITH SPEECH PROCESSES AND SWALLOW STAGES

Cranial Nerve	Speech Process	Swallow Stage
V. Trigeminal	Articulation Resonance	Oral preparatory
VII. Facial	Articulation	Oral preparatory Oral
IX. Glosso-pharyngeal	Articulation Resonance	Oral Pharyngeal
X. Vagus	Phonation Resonance	Pharyngeal Esophageal
XI. Spinal accessory	Phonation Resonance	Pharyngeal
XII. Hypoglossal	Articulation	Oral preparatory Oral

or mastication, manipulates the food into a **bolus**—a cohesive mass of food in preparation of the swallow. Cranial nerves involved with this stage of the swallow are indicated in Table 4-5 and include the trigeminal (jaw movement), facial (lip seal and cheek tension), and hypoglossal (tongue movement). In addition, the velum is depressed while all this food preparation is going on so nasal breathing can occur. This requires the involvement of the glossopharyngeal, vagus (pharyngeal branch), and spinal accessory cranial nerves. As you can imagine, the time for this stage varies widely and is dependent on how much the food is enjoyed and how quickly the food is ingested.

The oral stage of the swallow starts the moment the bolus begins to move from the anterior to the posterior oral cavity. This stage is quite quick in the normal swallow, averaging about one second; this is referred to as **oral transit time**. Cranial nerves involved with tongue movement are primary during this stage (see Table 4-5). Of course, that means the hypoglossal cranial nerve is heavily involved with assistance from the trigeminal to maintain elevation of the jaw.

The pharyngeal stage of the swallow is largely reflexive and considered involuntary. That is, what we think of as the swallow is automatically initiated once the bolus reaches the posterior oral cavity (near the region of the **posterior faucial pillars**; see Chapter 10). Certainly, a swallow can be voluntarily initiated as well; although you may be surprised that swallowing suddenly becomes more difficult when thinking about it, especially when swallowing your saliva in multiple successions (give this a try). This stage of the swallow involves moving the bolus from the posterior oral cavity into the esophagus. Multiple synchronous events must happen for this swallow reflex to occur. The velum must elevate to close off the nasal cavity requiring innervation of velar muscles from the trigeminal, vagus, and spinal accessory cranial nerves (see Table 4-5). The tongue must continue to be active in propelling the bolus toward the esophagus requiring hypoglossal involvement. Pharyngeal muscles must be active as well, narrowing and constricting the pharynx to assist bolus movement; this requires innervation from the glossopharyngeal, vagus, and spinal accessory cranial nerves. At the same time, the larynx must move up and forward and the vocal folds must close, all to protect the airway from bolus entry (i.e., **aspiration**), requiring major activity from the RLN (recall this is an important branch of cranial nerve X) to close the vocal folds and to draw the epiglottis down and back to cover the opening to the larynx. The hypoglossal cranial nerve is also involved here, as it innervates neck muscles that elevate the larynx.

The cricopharyngeus, along with fibers from the inferior constrictor muscle, make up the sphincter muscle found at the opening to the esophagus, collectively called the **upper esophageal sphincter** or UES. The UES relaxes or opens during the pharyngeal phase to accommodate the incoming bolus. The specific innervation of the UES continues to be studied. The glossopharyngeal nerve, pharyngeal and recurrent branch of the vagus nerve, and the spinal accessory nerve are all involved. Once initiated, the swallow occurs quickly. This timing is referred to as **pharyngeal transit time (PTT)**.

The pharyngeal stage of the swallow is mediated by the swallow reflex center in the brainstem. Sensations are transmitted from the posterior oral cavity to the reticular swallowing center in the pons and medulla. This swallow center then sends input to the motor nuclei of cranial nerves V, VII, IX, X, XI, and XII as well as to the respiratory centers of the medulla to coordinate the reflexive muscle activity for the swallow with a brief cessation of breathing. Once the bolus passes into the esophagus, the pharyngeal stage is completed and breathing resumes.

The esophageal stage of the swallow is involuntary and involves the transport of the bolus from the superior esophagus to the stomach. The movement of the bolus occurs through **peristaltic**, or wavelike, action of the esophagus requiring 10 to 20 seconds depending on the consistency of the food being swallowed.

The parasympathetic component of the vagus is involved with esophageal innervation below the level of the cricopharyngeus muscle (i.e., superior opening of the esophagus).

The special senses of taste and smell influence the swallow through the subjective, conscious experience of taste and the stimulation of saliva production. Taste, or gustation, has been discussed in the previous section by covering the specific functions of each cranial nerve. By way of review, cranial nerves VII, IX, and, to a much lesser degree, X have afferent fibers from taste buds to the nucleus solitarius in the brainstem. From here, fibers travel to the VPM nucleus of the thalamus and on to the gustatory center of the insular cortex. The insular cortex also receives projections from the olfactory system. The olfactory system includes the last cranial nerve to be discussed, cranial nerve I—the olfactory nerve.

The olfactory nerve is responsible for the sense of smell. It has only this sensory function and is one of two cranial nerves that does not enter or emerge from the brainstem (can you recall the other?). The olfactory nerve's cell bodies are located in the olfactory bulbs (refer back to Figure 4-35) on the ventral surface of the frontal lobe. The sensory receptors for smell are found in the epithelium of the nasal cavities. The actual nerve is made up of the unmyelinated short axons projecting through the **cribriform plate** of the **ethmoid bone** (see Chapter 10) to the olfactory bulb. Projections from here travel caudally to multiple areas including the anterior medial temporal poles (primary olfactory cortex) with secondary projections to the limbic system, orbital gyri, insular cortex, and hypothalamus. The limbic system connects smell to emotion and aggressive responses; the orbital gyri of the frontal lobe connects smell to odor discrimination; the insula connects smell to taste (recall that the gustatory center is there); and the hypothalamus connects smell to hunger and thirst signals.

Summary

A foundation was laid in this chapter for you to appreciate the importance of the nervous system in the production of speech, in the sensory ability to hear, and in the reception and expression of language. The chapter began by stressing, again, the necessity to understand and use terminology, in this case neurological terms. The organization of the nervous system into its mature form begins in neurodevelopment with the ultimate differentiation into the cortical and subcortical components of the telencephalon, the different thalamic regions of the diencephalon, the three areas of the brainstem (mesencephalon, metencephalon, and myelencephalon), and the connections to the cerebellum and the spinal cord. The somatic and autonomic divisions of the PNS are also involved with functions important to the speech and hearing professional, most notably the cranial nerves and the cervical spinal nerves. These nerves, with their sensory, motor, and autonomic components, are responsible for the special senses of audition, balance, vision, smell, and taste. They also serve to pick up sensations and provide motor commands for structures and muscles involved in respiration, phonation, resonation, articulation, and swallowing.

CHAPTER 5

Pathologies Associated with the Nervous System

Knowledge Outcomes for ASHA Certification for Chapter 5

- Demonstrate knowledge of the etiologies of fluency disorders (III-C)
- Demonstrate knowledge of the characteristics of fluency disorders (III-C)
- Demonstrate knowledge of the etiologies of voice and resonance disorders (III-C)
- Demonstrate knowledge of the characteristics of voice and resonance disorders (III-C)
- Demonstrate knowledge of the etiologies of receptive and expressive language disorders (III-C)
- Demonstrate knowledge of the characteristics of receptive and expressive language disorders (III-C)
- Demonstrate knowledge of the etiologies of swallowing disorders (III-C)
- Demonstrate knowledge of the characteristics of swallowing disorders (III-C)
- Demonstrate knowledge of the etiologies of cognitive aspects of communication (III-C)
- Demonstrate knowledge of the characteristics of the cognitive aspects of communication (III-C)
- Demonstrate knowledge of the prevention related to cognitive aspects of communication (III-C)

Learning Objectives

- You will be able to relate lesion site(s) with probable communication disorder(s).
- You will be able to describe the medical etiologies associated with neurogenic communication disorders.
- You will be able to define aphasia and differentiate the types of aphasia.
- You will be able to compare and contrast cognitive-communicative impairments associated with traumatic brain injury and dementia.
- You will be able to define the motor speech disorders (dysarthrias and apraxia of speech) and differentiate the types of dysarthria.

AFFIX AND PART-WORD BOX

TERM	MEANING	EXAMPLE
a-	without, absent, negative	**a**phasia
arterio-	artery	**arterio**sclerosis
brady-	slow	**brady**kinesia
dys-	bad or difficult	**dys**arthria
hemi	one-half	**hemi**paresis
hyper	too much	**hyper**tonic
hypo	too little	**hypo**tonic
kinetic/kinesia	movement	hyper**kinetic**

TERM	MEANING	EXAMPLE
neo-	new	**neo**cortex
-oma	tumor, growth	astrocyt**oma**
-osis	state of disease	arterioscler**osis**
-rrhea	flow, discharge	logo**rrhea**
scler-	scar, plaque	multiple **scler**osis
-sia	abnormal or pathological state	dyskine**sia**

Introduction

This chapter now applies your knowledge from Chapter 4. To understand neurological disorders, it is necessary to understand the neurological systems and how a **lesion** to those systems results in various **symptoms**. The term lesion is rather generic, as it applies to any disruption to the nervous system as a result of any **etiology**. As a student of the nervous system, you will soon realize that the behaviors seen with a given disorder are quite closely associated with the site of lesion in the nervous system (Duffy, 2005). The notion of lesion site and its correlation to symptomatology will be returned to in the discussion of the various communication disorders associated with neuropathology. Each of the communication disorders discussed in this chapter has a list of symptoms associated with it. A symptom is a deviation from normal function; a collection of symptoms is called a **syndrome**. These communication disorders include: **aphasia**, **cognitive-communicative disorders**, **apraxia of speech (AOS)**, and **dysarthria**. Prior to discussing the disorders of most pertinence to the field of speech–language pathology, an overview of the many medical etiologies that give rise to these communication disorders is presented. Brookshire (2003) reminds us that clinicians who wish to treat individuals with neurogenic communication disorders must have at least a basic knowledge of the anatomy and physiology of the nervous system and what can go wrong with it.

Neuropathologies

A number of traumas, disorders, and diseases of the nervous system may result in a communication disorder. Various signs (i.e., objective data reported by a physician) and symptoms are associated with disruption to the nervous system (Brookshire, 2003). The signs and symptoms reflect the location of the lesion rather than the cause. Nonetheless, the etiology of nervous system breakdown is important as it directs

medical management and future outcomes. As you can imagine, there are many neurologic problems that can result in symptoms specific to a communication disorder. This chapter will highlight those that are most often seen by speech–language pathologists.

NERVE CELLS AND GLIAL CELLS

Recall that the neuron, or nerve cell, is the basic functional unit of the nervous system. Therefore, all disruptions involving the nervous system impact the neuron. Nonetheless, certain pathologies specifically target certain types of neurons (e.g., motor neurons) or parts of the neuron (e.g., myelin sheath composed of oligodendroglia in the central nervous system [CNS]). Three presented here are the degenerative disorders of **amyotrophic lateral sclerosis** (ALS), **multiple sclerosis** (MS), and **Parkinson's disease** (PD). In addition, various **neoplasms** or tumors can occur that affect nervous system function.

Amyotrophic lateral sclerosis is commonly referred to as "Lou Gehrig's disease," named after the famous baseball player who suffered from it. ALS is a disease of the motor neurons (see Figure 5-1). More specifically, the motor cell bodies in the anterior horns of the spinal cord, the cranial nerve nuclei, and the precentral gyrus are affected, as are the motor neurons comprising the corticospinal and corticobulbar tracts. This results in both upper motor neuron (UMN) and lower motor neuron (LMN) symptoms. Thus, symptoms are motor and progressive in nature. Early symptoms may manifest in limb weakness or in weakness of the muscles of the head and neck resulting in speech and swallowing problems. Onset of the disease is in adulthood and life span ranges, on average, from 1 to 5 years with death usually due to respiratory failure (Duffy, 2005).

Multiple sclerosis is primarily a disease of the white matter. In MS, the myelin sheath degenerates but the axon remains intact as illustrated in Figure 5-2. Recall that myelin in the CNS is made up of a particular type

Normal motor unit   **Motor unit affected by ALS**

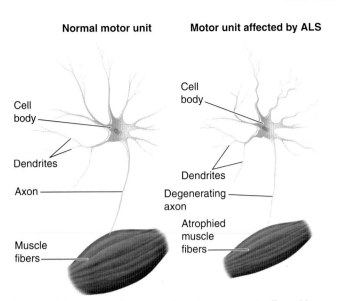

Figure 5-1   A normal motor unit and a motor unit affected by amyotrophic lateral sclerosis (ALS). (Reprinted with permission from Anatomical Chart Company.)

of glial cell, the oligodendroglia. Although neuronal transmission can still occur, it does so in a disrupted manner. The process of demyelination and glial cell proliferation happens concurrently (Bhatnagar, 2008). This results in the forming of plaques in the white matter of the CNS with a predilection for the brainstem, periventricular white matter, spinal cord, and optic nerves (Duffy, 2005). Symptoms reflect the

area of lesion, thus both sensory and motor systems may be affected. MS strikes young adults usually between 20 and 40 years of age. The exact cause is unknown, but MS is thought to be among the auto-immune disorders. There are multiple types of MS based on disease progression: (1) benign with sudden onset but complete or near complete remission; (2) relapsing–remitting with periods of exacerbation followed by incomplete or nearly full remission; (3) chronic progressive with slow onset and continuous symptoms worsening; and (4) malignant with severe, rapid progression (Cobble, Dietz, Grigsby, & Kennedy, 1993; Kraft, Freal, Coryell, Hanan, & Chitnis, 1981; both as cited in Yorkston, Miller, & Strand, 1995).

Parkinson's disease is named for James Parkinson, a British physician who first described it back in 1817. This disease involves the basal ganglia. More specifically, PD is a result of the degeneration of dopamine producing neurons in the substantia nigra. Dopamine is a neurotransmitter that plays a large role in the transmission of neural information regarding movement. Figure 5-3 illustrates that the substantia nigra, located in the midbrain, is functionally a part of the basal ganglia circuit with tracts connecting it to the striatum. In the case of basal ganglia function, dopamine is an inhibitor and works synergistically with acetylcholine (Ach) in the striatum to regulate

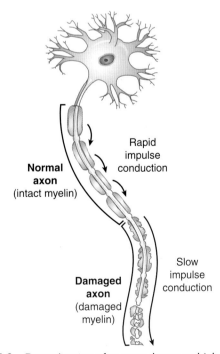

Figure 5-2   Demyelination of an axon due to multiple sclerosis. (Reprinted with permission from Smeltzer, S.C., Bare, B.G. (2000). *Textbook of medical-surgical nursing* (9th ed.). Philadelphia, PA: Lippincott Williams & Wilkins.)

Dopamine system

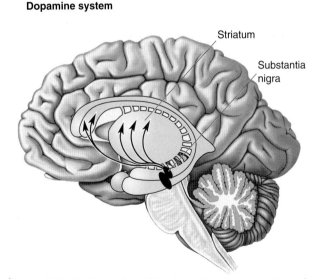

Figure 5-3   An illustration of the dopaminergic connections of the substantia nigra in the midbrain to the rest of the basal ganglia. (Reprinted with permission from Bear, M.F., Connors, B.W., Paradiso, M.A. (2007). *Neuroscience: Exploring the brain* (3rd ed.). Baltimore, MD: Lippincott Williams & Wilkins.)

movement. Cardinal symptoms of PD include **bradykinesia** (i.e., slowness of movement), rigidity, and resting tremor. Diagnosis of PD is usually made later in life, 60 years and older although younger people can get the disease (see Why You Need to Know box).

Why You Need to Know

Parkinson's disease is medically treated and managed through medication such as leva-dopa (L-dopa) used to synthetically replace the diminishing dopamine in the substantia nigra. When the medication is working as it should, the patient is "on;" when it is not, the patient is "off." Following is an excerpt from actor Michael J. Fox's (2002) memoir called Lucky Man describing this "on/off" phenomenon:

When I'm "off," the disease has complete authority over my physical being. I'm utterly in its possession. Sometimes there are flashes of function, and I can be effective at performing basic physical tasks, certainly feeding and dressing myself (though I'll lean toward loafers and pullover sweaters), as well as any chore calling for more brute forces than manual dexterity. In my very worst "off" times I experience the full panoply of classic Parkinsonian symptoms: rigidity, shuffling, tremors, lack of balance, diminished small motor control, and the insidious cluster of symptoms that makes communication—written as well as spoken—difficult and sometimes impossible. (p. 214)

Neoplasms refer to tumors (an abnormal proliferation of cells) of the CNS. Tumors that originate within the CNS are almost always of glial cell origin (called **gliomas**), a common type being **astrocytomas**. These types of tumors are usually benign, meaning they rarely travel away, or metastasize, beyond their place of origin. Alternatively, tumors originating in other areas of the body may well metastasize to the CNS. As can be seen in Figure 5-4, tumor growth in the CNS displaces surrounding nervous tissue resulting in elevated intracranial pressure. Symptoms will reflect the location of the tumor and may include double vision, cognitive impairment, nausea, seizures, and headache (Bhatnagar, 2008). Gliomas are named for the cell that gives rise to them; in addition to astrocytomas, there are oligodendrogliomas and ependymomas. Acoustic **neuromas** are tumors that arise from the Schwann cells that comprise the myelin surrounding the eighth cranial nerve. Lastly, although not glial in origin,

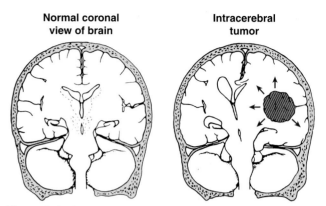

Normal coronal view of brain

Intracerebral tumor

Figure 5-4 Intracerebral tumor resulting in displacement of nervous tissue. Note the mass effect on the ventricle and the herniation of tissue at the brainstem. (Reprinted with permission from Smeltzer, S.C., Bare, B.G. (2000). *Textbook of medical-surgical nursing* (9th ed.). Philadelphia, PA: Lippincott Williams & Wilkins.)

tissue from the dura mater can give rise to **meningiomas**.

DISRUPTION OF SUPPORTING SYSTEMS

Recall that the blood supply, meningeal coverings, and ventricular system all act to support the work of the CNS. These systems do not communicate neural information but are critical to the neuron's ability to do so. Disease and injury can disrupt these support systems and result in damage to the nervous tissue.

Inflammation of the meninges is called **meningitis** which specifically affects the pia mater and the arachnoid mater, collectively referred to as the **leptomeninges**. This includes the subarachnoid space and the cerebrospinal fluid (CSF) traveling in it. Meningitis is caused by the entry of microorganisms by way of the blood stream into the CSF. These microorganisms are typically bacterial or viral. Bacterial meningitis is treated with intravenously administered antibiotics, whereas the treatment for viral meningitis is directed more at the symptoms than the cause because viruses do not respond to antibiotic treatment. The onset of meningitis is rapid, over the course of a few days, with symptoms including headache, fever, vomiting, lethargy, stiff neck, and confusion. **Otitis media**, left untreated, is one of many potential causes of meningitis (see Chapter 13 for a detailed discussion of otitis media). Several different bacteria (e.g., pneumococcal, haemophilus influenzae type B) are responsible for meningitis with meningococcal bacteria being the leading cause of bacterial meningitis in children 2 to 18 years of age (Centers for Disease Control and Prevention, 2007).

Why You Need to Know

Through the practice of immunization, bacterial meningitis has been significantly reduced. Just 20 years ago, Haemophilus influenzae type B (Hib) bacteria was the most common form of life-threatening bacterial meningitis in children younger than 5 years. In 1991, the Hib vaccine was approved for infants 2 months of age. A physician training in pediatrics today will likely never see a case of Hib meningitis. The current incidence of Hib disease is 1.3/100,000 children; 3% to 6% of those cases are fatal and up to 20% of surviving patients have permanent hearing loss or other long-term sequelae. Menactra is a new vaccine that offers protections against the meningococcal bacteria. This vaccine is recommended for children at their routine preadolescent visit (11 to 12 years old) and college freshman living in dorms. "Meningococcal infections can be treated with drugs such as penicillin. Still, about one of every ten people who get the disease dies from it and many others are affected for life. This is why preventing the disease through the use of vaccine is important for people at highest risk" (Center for Disease Control and Prevention, 2007).

The meninges can also be impacted by physical trauma to the head via penetration through the meninges to the brain. This is referred to as open head injury and will be discussed later.

The *ventricular system* includes the choroid plexus, the ventricles, the associated foramen, the subarachnoid space, and the CSF that flows through it all. Any disruption of this system results in a buildup of CSF and associated increase in intracranial pressure. Disruptions can take two forms: a blockage somewhere in the flow of CSF or an inadequate drainage of the CSF into the venous sinuses. Both of these problems result in **hydrocephalus.**

There are two types of hydrocephalus. *Communicating hydrocephalus* refers to a breakdown of the drainage mechanism of the CSF into the sinuses, whereas *noncommunicating hydrocephalus* results from an obstruction to CSF flow from the ventricles to the subarachnoid space (Bhatnagar, 2008). The most common site of occlusion is at the cerebral aqueduct and is typically caused by surrounding brain tissue edema or the presence of tumors (Brookshire, 2003). Regardless of the cause, hydrocephalus results in increased CSF pressure, thereby enlarging the ventricles and shifting the surrounding brain tissue out

of the way. Communicating hydrocephalus is also referred to as "normal pressure hydrocephalus" (Bradley, 2002) because it is not accompanied by increased intracranial pressure. Infantile hydrocephalus results in enlarged head size. In infants, the cranial sutures (see Chapter 10) are not yet fused, so the increased intracranial pressure results in an expansion of the cranium. Hydrocephalus is often surgically treated quite successfully. The typical treatment for noncommunicating hydrocephalus is the placement of an intraventricular shunt that drains excess CSF from the ventricular system to the patient's neck or abdomen as seen in Figure 5-5.

Blood supply to the brain is an absolutely critical supporting system. The most common vascular disease interrupting this blood supply and resulting in communication disorders is **stroke** or **cerebrovascular accident**. Stroke occurs when there is a sudden disruption of blood supply to the brain, thus cutting off oxygen and glucose to the nervous tissue. This decrease in oxygen is called **ischemia**. If the blood supply is returned fairly rapidly (i.e., within hours) and there are no residual symptoms, this is referred to as a **transient ischemic attack** (or event) **(TIA)**. If the loss of blood supply lasts too long, the resulting effect is an area of **infarct**. In regard to the CNS, an infarct is a localized area of dead nervous tissue.

Figure 5-6 illustrates various examples of cardiovascular disease that can lead to stroke. There are different types of strokes related to their etiologies—*ischemic stroke* and *hemorrhagic stroke*. Ischemic stroke is further subdivided as **thrombotic** or **embolic** in nature. Thrombosis refers to the gradual buildup of material, typically plaque on arterial walls that ultimately occludes the artery. This is often a result of **atherosclerosis**, which refers to the process whereby fatty deposits, cholesterol, calcium, and other substances build up within the walls of an artery (American Heart Association, 2007). This buildup first creates a severe narrowing of the artery lumen (called **stenosis**) prior to total occlusion (see Figure 5-6B). Figure 5-6C pictures a thrombus as a result of such plaque buildup on an arterial wall. Illustrated in Figure 5-6D is an embolus, which refers to material traveling in the blood stream until it gets to an artery or capillary too narrow to pass through. Varied embolic material exists such as blood clots due to heart disease or a breaking off of plaque buildup in the carotid or vertebral arteries. Infarcts due to ischemia account for roughly 80% of strokes, the remaining 20% are due to hemorrhage.

Most simply, hemorrhage refers to a burst blood vessel (see Figure 5-6E). Here, we are concerned with

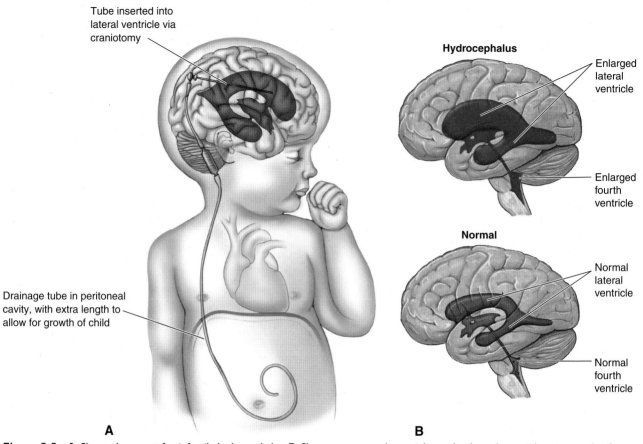

Figure 5-5   A. Shunt placement for infantile hydrocephalus. **B**. Shown are normal ventricles and enlarged ventricles as a result of hydrocephalus. (**A**. Reprinted with permission from Bear, M.F., Connors, B.W., Paradiso, M.A. (2007). *Neuroscience: Exploring the brain* (3rd ed.). Baltimore, MD: Lippincott Williams & Wilkins. **B**. Reprinted with permission from Anatomical Chart Company.)

a burst blood vessel in the CNS. The impact of this bleeding is twofold: (1) the nervous tissue beyond the point of hemorrhage does not receive its oxygen and glucose and (2) the pooling of blood puts pressure on surrounding nervous tissue and shifts it out of the way; this is referred to as a **mass effect**. Hemorrhages are labeled according to where they occur; three locations of hemorrhage are shown in Figure 5-7. Hemorrhages can occur within the meningeal layers, that is, epidural, subdural, and subarachnoid. Those associated with the dura are typically caused by blows to the head as in traumatic brain injury (TBI). Hemorrhages can also occur subcortically; these are called intracerebral (or **parenchymal**) hemorrhages. Frequent sites of intracerebral hemorrhage include the thalamus, basal ganglia, cerebellum, or brainstem (Duffy, 2005). A common precursor to this type of hemorrhage is chronic high blood pressure (hypertension). Another antecedent to hemorrhage is the presence of an **aneurysm** (see Figure 5-8). An aneurysm is a weakening of the arterial walls so that they begin ballooning out over time. A ruptured aneurysm is often the cause of subarachnoid hemorrhage (Duffy, 2005). Lastly, abnormally formed capillary beds (arteries and veins) called **arteriovenous malformations** can result in weakened vessel walls and become enlarged to the point of rupture.

Why You Need to Know

Risk factors for stroke fall into treatable and untreatable categories. Untreatable risk factors include the greatest risk factor, age. Males and females have similar rates of stroke once women are postmenopause. Family history and race play a role especially in blood clotting disorders. Race also influences dietary habits. Medical conditions such as a previous stroke or heart attack also increase risk. Treatable risk factors are those variables that can be changed or controlled; changing certain behaviors can help to prevent stroke from occurring. These include treating medical conditions such as high blood pressure, cardiac arrhythmia, and the occurrence of TIAs. Lifestyle factors that increase stroke risk include smoking, type II diabetes, hyperlipidemia (too much fatty tissue in the blood stream), and obesity (Reinmuth, 1994).

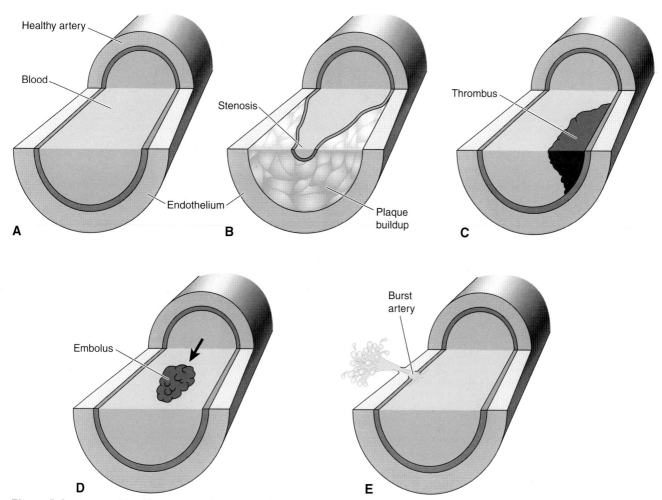

Figure 5-6 A normal, healthy artery and cutaways of arteries illustrating cardiovascular disease. **A**. Normal, healthy artery. **B**. Buildup of plaque within an artery. **C**. Thrombosis. **D**. Embolus. **E**. Hemorrhage.

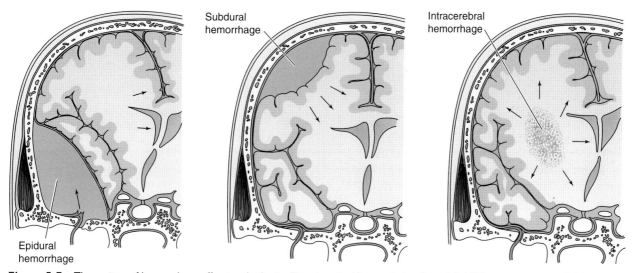

Figure 5-7 Three sites of hemorrhage affecting the brain. (Reprinted with permission from LifeART image copyright © 2010. Lippincott Williams & Wilkins. All rights reserved.)

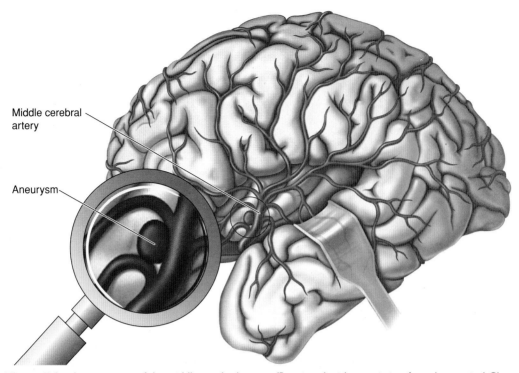

Middle cerebral artery

Aneurysm

Figure 5-8 An aneurysm of the middle cerebral artery. (Reprinted with permission from Anatomical Chart Company.)

CEREBRAL HEMISPHERES

A number of neuropathologies cross neural systems and affect multiple nervous system functions. Three of these will be discussed here: **encephalitis, TBI**, and **dementia**. In all cases, cognitive and limbic system functions are especially vulnerable to disorder.

Generalized brain tissue inflammation most often due to viral causes is termed *encephalitis*. This viral infection of the brain tissue causes swelling, especially in the temporal lobes. A common viral cause is the Herpes simplex virus, but there are a number of other viruses that may result in encephalitis. Symptoms are similar to meningitis including severe headache, confusion, and fever sometimes accompanied by drowsiness, irritability (in children), and seizures. Medical treatment for encephalitis involves the administration of antiviral agents if the cause is Herpes simplex; otherwise, the treatment is primarily symptomatic. Survivors of encephalitis may have neurological deficits in the areas of cognition, motor abilities, vision, and epilepsy as well as associated behavioral and emotional changes.

Brain damage refers to any type of injury to the brain from any cause and at any age, whereas TBI refers to brain damage as a result of physical trauma. There are two categories of TBI: *open (penetrating) head injury* and *closed (nonpenetrating) head injury* (see Table 5-1). Open head injury results from a penetrating wound to the head that pierces through the protective meningeal layers and impacts brain tissue. Examples of this type of injury include gunshot wounds or depressed skull fractures. The effects of penetrating head injuries are largely focal, but the physical force of the trauma to the brain also sets up impact-induced shock waves that propagate through nervous tissue (Kirkpatrick & DiMaio, 1978).

TABLE 5-1

MECHANISMS OF TRAUMATIC BRAIN INJURY

1. Penetrating (open) head injury
2. Nonpenetrating (closed) head injury
   - i. Discrete lesions
     - (a) Concussion
     - (b) Contusion
       - 1. Coup
       - 2. Contrecoup
     - (c) Hematoma
     - (d) Ischemic brain damage
   - ii. Diffuse lesions
     - (a) Diffuse axonal injury
     - (b) Hypoxia

Closed head injuries (CHIs) are the result of blunt trauma to the head along with linear and rotational acceleration of the brain within the skull. This movement results in the stretching of axons and blood vessels (Strich, 1961) as well as the back and forth movement of the brain within the cranial cavity. As a result, lesions due to CHI can be focal or diffuse. Focal damage is most likely to occur when the brain is in motion due to the mechanical forces associated with the brain shifting forward into the anterior and middle cranial fossa (see Chapter 10; Adams, Graham, Murray, & Scott, 1982).

Concussion, contusion, hematoma, and ischemic brain damage are among the discrete effects of CHI. A concussion is the most minor of brain injuries. It results in an alteration of consciousness for a short period of time and may be accompanied by a disturbance of vision or equilibrium. A contusion is a more serious consequence of head injury caused by the impact of the brain and skull during trauma. Contusions result from minor hemorrhages or tearing of blood vessels at the site of impact and are generally associated with blows or falls. The most vulnerable areas for contusion are the orbitofrontal, anterotemporal, and lateral temporal cortices (Sohlberg & Mateer, 2001). The TBI term **coup** refers to the contusion at the site of impact, and the term **contrecoup** refers to the contusion opposite the site of impact as illustrated in Figure 5-9. For example, if the site of impact is the left hemisphere orbitofrontal cortex, the expected contrecoup contusion would be the right hemisphere posterior occipital lobe. Another discreet lesion as a result of TBI is a hematoma, an accumula-

tion of blood. Hematomas are named for their location such as "epidural" or "subdural." Lastly, areas of brain tissue can be affected by ischemia with the most susceptible areas being boundary zones between the anterior cerebral artery (ACA) distribution and the middle cerebral artery (MCA) distribution.

Although there are a number of discreet or focal lesions that may occur as a result of TBI, the diffuse lesions may have the most lasting impact on function. Diffuse lesions refer to damage to the brain that is not localized to one particular region. These lesions are the result of damage to the nerve fibers (i.e., axons) or the generalized effect of hypoxia. The damage and shearing of CNS white matter is referred to as diffuse axonal injury (DAI). Hypoxia refers to decreased oxygenation of neural tissue resulting from systemic hypotension (low blood pressure), increased intracranial pressure, or secondary to seizure activity or cardiopulmonary compromise (e.g., heart attack). Patients typically present with a mixed type of damage, that is, both focal and diffuse, although one type usually predominates.

Why You Need to Know

Computerized tomography (CT) and magnetic resonance imaging (MRI) are the primary neuroimaging tools used for diagnostic purposes in clinical settings. In addition, newer technologies are built upon these imaging techniques. CT scans make use of a series of x-ray images or slices allowing for different cross sections of the live brain, or body, to be viewed. Although CT scans do not produce pretty pictures, they are incredibly useful in detecting abnormalities such as an infarct following a stroke or the occurrence of a hemorrhage. Alternatively, MRIs produce an image that has much better resolution, or picture, using an imaging technique that draws upon magnetic properties of hydrogen atoms in our body to, again, view sections of the live brain or body. In the case of TBI, the x-rays used with CT are preferable to detect skull fractures while MRI is preferable to detect DAI.

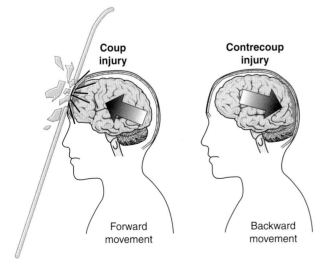

Figure 5-9 Coup and contrecoup focal areas of contusion in head injury. (Reprinted with permission from LifeART image copyright © 2010. Lippincott Williams & Wilkins. All rights reserved.)

Dementia is a disorder characterized by a progressive decline in cognitive abilities that typically strikes in later years. Difficulty with memory is typically one of the earliest and most devastatingly affected of the cognitive processes. In addition to memory, an individual must evidence other deficits including at least one of the following: apraxia, **agnosia**, aphasia, or **executive function** impairment. In turn, these multiple deficits impact the individual's ability to carry out social and occupational roles (American Psychiatric

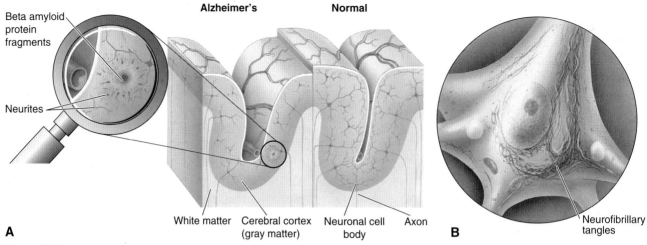

Figure 5-10 Microscopic brain tissue changes in Alzheimer's disease. **A**. Amyloid plaques. **B**. Neurofibrillary tangles. (Reprinted with permission from Anatomical Chart Company.)

Association, 1994). Dementias can be grouped as *cortical dementias* or *subcortical dementias* according to the primary locale of brain damage. Dementia of the Alzheimer's type is classified as a cortical dementia and accounts for approximately 50% of the cases seen (Katzman & Bick, 2000). It is progressive and irreversible. Life expectancy after diagnosis ranges from 3 to 23 years with an average of 8 years (Lubinski, 2005).

Alzheimer's dementia results in progressive atrophy of the cerebral cortex due to the breakdown of neurons at the cellular level. Predominate pathologies at the cellular level include the presence of neuritic plaques and neurofibrillary tangles which are shown in Figure 5-10. Neuritic, or amyloid, plaques are a result of clumps of beta-amyloid protein fragments that congregate in the extracellular space throughout the CNS. These plaques are thought to stimulate free radical production and, in turn, cause neuronal cell death (Cummings, Vinters, Cole, & Khachaturian, 1998). The tangles refer to intracellular twisted strands of tau protein. Tau protein functions in normal cells to promote axonal growth and development (Cummings et al., 1998). Even though AD is classified as a cortical dementia affecting neurons in the medial temporal lobe and widespread association cortices, these histologic changes also occur subcortically, particularly in the hippocampus. Neuronal cell death in certain nuclei leads to a disruption of neurotransmitter production particularly affecting the cholinergic system. ACh is the neurotransmitter of the cholinergic mechanism. ACh in the CNS is involved with learning and memory. This has become a promising area of neuropharmacological research and therapy (Massey, 2005). This combination of neuronal cell death and ACh depletion leads to the dementia syndrome of the Alzheimer's type.

More recent research has explored the role of genes in causation of **Alzheimer's disease (AD)**. Genetics is a predominant factor in early-onset AD, also referred to as familial AD, which typically affects individuals from 30 to 60 years of age. The genetic difference is due to a mutation of specific genes resulting in an individual having a 50/50 chance of getting the disease if their parent had it. The **genetic mutation** causes abnormal proteins to be formed in a cell; in the case of AD, more beta-amyloid protein is formed and, as indicated earlier, this protein is part of the plaques leading to cell breakdown. More common, however, is late-onset AD, occurring after the age of 60. Genetics still play a role but not nearly as strong. In this case, **genetic variants** increase the risk of developing the disease. This risk is related to a gene called the apolipoprotein E gene (APOE); there are three forms of this gene with APOE €4 most directly related to increasing the risk of developing AD. Better understanding of the role of genes in AD is a priority of research. For more on the role of genes and other causative factors associated with this devastating disease, access the information provided by the National Institutes of Health (www.nih.org).

Why You Need to Know

The exact cause, and therefore prevention, of AD is unknown at this time. However, research has discovered associated risk factors. Like heart disease and stroke, there are untreatable risk factors such as age and genetics. Treatable risk factors include overall cardiovascular health (e.g., cholesterol levels, blood pressure) and diabetes control. Nonmedical variables under our control include educational level, social engagement, cognitive stimulation (e.g., doing puzzles, reading the newspaper, going to museums), and aerobic exercise to increase oxygen to the brain. Although it is not known whether any of these activities will actually prevent the onset and progression of AD, it certainly will not hurt and will definitely help decrease risk of other health conditions such as heart disease or depression.

Pick's disease is another type of cortical dementia and is grouped under a broader heading of dementias called **frontotemporal dementias**. Pick's disease is named for the neurologist, Arnold Pick, who first identified the pathology back in 1892. Thus, the abnormal cells involved with this disease are referred to as Pick cells; these cells include abnormal deposits of the tau protein which are referred to as Pick bodies. Interestingly, in this dementia, the affected areas of the cortex remain localized to the frontal and anterior temporal lobes, which is different from the diffuse cortical atrophy associated with dementia of the Alzheimer's type. Because of this localized damage, early symptoms are associated with emotion and language functions.

A type of dementia that can be cortical, subcortical, or a combination is that resulting from vascular disease. In fact, this type of dementia is referred to as *vascular dementia* or multi-infarct dementia. This type of progressive cognitive loss is a result of multiple "mini-strokes" throughout the brain having a cumulative effect on function.

Dementias of the subcortical classification are associated with degenerative diseases of the basal ganglia. **Huntington's disease** affects the telencephalic basal ganglia and results in devastating movement disorders and, ultimately, dementia. As already discussed, Parkinson's disease (PD) is primarily a movement disorder but, in some cases, the disease can also be accompanied by an associated dementia.

All of the neuropathologies just reviewed may result in a communication disorder. These communication disorders may be due to a breakdown or damage to cortical language regions (e.g., aphasia), to various motor nuclei and tracts (e.g., apraxia or dysarthria), or to widespread cortical and subcortical mechanisms supporting cognitive and limbic functions (e.g., cognitive-communicative impairments). It should be noted here that an individual may present with multiple communication disorders at a given time. The next section of the chapter presents each of these disorders by making reference to typical neuropathologies resulting in the disorder, defining the disorder, and explaining its subtypes.

Neurologic Communication Disorders

APHASIA

Aphasia refers to language impairment as a result of brain damage to the language dominant hemisphere, almost always the left hemisphere. The language problems are primarily in form (phonology, morphology, and syntax) and in content (semantics) for both expression and reception. The pragmatic function of language is largely intact for individuals with aphasia, as many skills that govern and regulate language use are housed in the right hemisphere of the brain. The brain damage is typically due to an ischemic stroke to the language-dominant hemisphere. However, aphasia can also be the result of any lesion affecting the perisylvian region, referred to as the language zone (see Figure 5-11). Stroke due to hemorrhage, tumors such as gliomas, or focal lesions due to TBI can also result in aphasia.

A stroke can occur anywhere within the CNS, but the middle cerebral artery (MCA) is particularly at risk for embolic ischemic strokes. This is due to the MCA being almost a direct continuation of the internal carotid system and, therefore, any plaque or clots moving in the blood stream up toward the brain tend to travel this path prior to becoming lodged and occluding an artery. Recall that the arterial distribution of the MCA includes the majority of the lateral cortex of the frontal, parietal, and temporal lobes for both right and left hemispheres. In the language-dominant hemisphere, such a stroke results in language impairment. The type of impairment depends on where along the arterial distribution the stroke occurs.

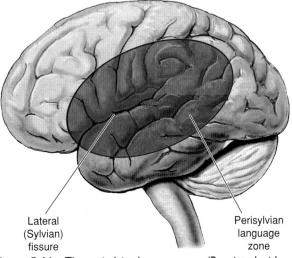

Lateral
(Sylvian)
fissure

Perisylvian
language
zone

Figure 5-11 The perisylvian language zone. (Reprinted with permission from Anatomical Chart Company.)

Aphasia can be further defined as an acquired language impairment affecting both expressive and receptive abilities. Expressive modalities of language include verbal (i.e., spoken) and graphic (i.e., written) expression. Receptive modalities of language include auditory and reading comprehension. In addition, the interpretation and use of gestures for communication are affected. All of these language modalities are affected to some degree in aphasia, although the severity across modalities is influenced by the size and site of the lesion (i.e., brain damage). In fact, aphasias are classified into subtypes based on effects to the various modalities. For example, an individual with an ischemic stroke involving the left hemisphere inferior frontal gyrus would likely evidence significant deficits in expression and less severe deficits in comprehension. Conversely, a stroke affecting the left hemisphere superior temporal gyrus would likely result in significant deficits in comprehension but better verbal expression skills. Nonetheless, both scenarios would show problems across all modalities.

The most basic way to classify the aphasias is into nonfluent and fluent types. These types are correlated to a general site of lesion and broadly differentiated by symptomatology (see Table 5-2). Persons presenting with **nonfluent aphasias** have lesions to the inferior frontal lobe involving Broca's area, the anterior insular cortex, and surrounding tissues. These individuals have concomitant motor symptoms of contralateral hemiparesis of the limbs; typically right-side hemiparesis, as the left hemisphere is language dominant in the vast majority of people. In addition, due to unilateral upper motor neuron (UUMN) involvement, a contralateral lower facial droop and tongue weakness is expected. Persons with **fluent aphasias** have lesions involving the superior temporal lobe often extending into the inferior parietal lobe. These individuals do not show motor impairment but may have visual field deficits consistent with a lesion involving the optic radiations of the primary visual pathway.

Nonfluent versus fluent distinctions are made based on characteristics of verbal output. A nonfluent speaker uses language the way a text message via a cell phone may be written—with the fewest words, grammatical markings, and punctuation to get the message across. Hence, a nonfluent speaker has more content (e.g., nouns and verbs) than functor words (e.g., conjunctions, prepositions, and articles) present in their speech. This symptom of aphasia is referred to as **agrammatism**, which literally means "without grammar." As the nonfluent label implies, their speech is effortful with many hesitations, revisions, and interrupted melody. These speakers are usually quite aware of their errors, which may in turn increase frustration or decrease their willingness to attempt to speak. Alternatively, fluent speakers sound good. Their speech is produced without effort and has appropriate melodic contours. Grammatical markings are present although their use may be in error; this symptom is called **paragrammatism**. Inferred from verbal output and lesion site, the symptom that most impacts the communication of fluent speakers is their decreased comprehension. They may manifest this by behaviors such as failing to respond appropriately to verbal input, being unable to follow commands, giving quizzical facial expressions, and/or making requests for repetition. Also evident is their decreased ability to monitor their own speech and make self-corrections. Table 5-2 provides a summary list of the expected language characteristics associated with the nonfluent and fluent classifications.

Multiple types of aphasia fall under these broad categories of nonfluent and fluent. Traditionalists in aphasia use a classification scheme developed by Geschwind and others out of the Boston School of Medicine (Goodglass, 1993). This scheme further classifies aphasia into syndromes (a collection of symptoms) based on (1) lesion site, (2) fluency, (3) speech, (4) word retrieval, (5) repetition, and (6) comprehension (Brookshire, 2003). Symptom patterns across these categories result in the classification. The different aphasia syndromes broken down according to their fluent or nonfluent verbal output are *Nonfluent:* Broca's aphasia, transcortical motor aphasia, and global aphasia; *Fluent:* Wernicke's aphasia, conduction aphasia, transcortical sensory aphasia, and anomic aphasia. Each type is briefly discussed next, but you are referred to texts devoted to aphasia for further discussion of this classification scheme

TABLE 5-2

SPEECH AND LANGUAGE CHARACTERISTICS ASSOCIATED WITH NONFLUENT AND FLUENT APHASIA

Nonfluent Aphasia	Fluent Aphasia
Decreased melodic line	Adequate melodic line
Decreased utterance length	Normal or extended utterance length
Text message speech	Adequate grammar (may have errors in use)
Effortful articulation	Effortless articulation
Word retrieval difficulties	Word retrieval difficulties
Better comprehension than expression	Better expression than comprehension

and the use of these labels to describe aphasia (e.g., Brookshire, 2003; Goodglass, 1993)

Nonfluent Aphasias

Broca's aphasia is named for the physician, Paul Broca, who first documented speech and language deficits due to brain damage involving the language dominant hemisphere. This syndrome results from a lesion to Brodmann areas 44 and 45. Verbal output is nonfluent and agrammatic with effortful and halting speech, most likely due to a motor programming disorder called apraxia of speech (AOS) that often co-occurs with Broca's aphasia (AOS will be discussed later in this chapter). Word retrieval is considered fair for content words but often masked by speech difficulty. Speech repetition (i.e., immediately repeating a word or phrase) is marked by misarticulated and halting speech. Writing abilities may be the stronger output modality, as graphic language abilities will not be compromised by AOS but the dominant writing hand may be motorically involved. Auditory and reading comprehension is fair to good as compared with expressive abilities.

Transcortical motor aphasia is the result of white matter tracts being disconnected from cortical language centers in the frontal lobe; hence, this is often referred to as anterior isolation syndrome (Brookshire, 2003). Lesions are to the anterior superior frontal lobe, Brodmann areas 8 and 9. Individuals with this type of aphasia are nonfluent speakers who lack initiation exemplified by severely impaired spontaneous speech (LaPointe, 1994). Speech abilities and word retrieval are variable while repetition abilities are remarkably strong. Comprehension is good relative to expression.

Global aphasia, as the name implies, is a result of a large, widespread lesion to the perisylvian language zone as a result of blockage at the proximal MCA. Individuals with this type of aphasia are nonfluent and may have severely limited verbal output called verbal stereotypes (e.g., "where where," "da wanni," "nuts"), overlearned or automatic phrases ("one, two, three . . .") or expletives. Written output is also extremely limited. Word retrieval is poor as is their ability to repeat. In keeping with the global nature of the deficit, comprehension is also poor.

Fluent Aphasias

Wernicke's aphasia, a type of fluent aphasia, was named for Karl Wernicke, an early localizationist, who, like Paul Broca, found particular language symptoms associated with damage to the brain. In contrast to Broca's area, Wernicke's area is located in the posterior superior temporal gyrus of the language dominant hemisphere, Brodmann area 22. Damage to this region results in fluent, yet empty, verbal productions with unintended word substitutions. These substitutions are called **verbal** (or **semantic**) **paraphasias**, and may or may not be related to the target word (e.g., television/computer vs. fork/computer). Word retrieval is poor as is repetition with the presence of these paraphasias. In fact, individuals with Wernicke's aphasia may produce words not found in their language called **neologisms**. A string of neologisms along with inappropriate use of real words is referred to as **jargon**. As expected, comprehension is poor; therefore, awareness of these errors is often not present. This decreased awareness may result in effusive output of speech, referred to as **press of speech** or **logorrhea**.

Similar to the transcortical motor aphasia described earlier, *transcortical sensory aphasia* results from damage to white matter tracts cut off from posterior language zones and has been referred to as a posterior isolation syndrome. Site of lesion is associated with the posterior superior parietal lobe, Brodmann area 7 or around the complex association areas of the parietal–temporal–occipital (P-T-O) lobes. Verbal output is fluent but empty with variable speech; they may evidence verbal paraphasias. Word retrieval is poor but repetition skills are remarkably intact. Comprehension is poor.

Conduction aphasia is most likely a result of a lesion impacting the arcuate fasciculus, the tract connecting Wernicke's to Broca's area. Verbal output is fluent and good but may include **literal** (or **phonemic) paraphasias**. In literal paraphasia, an individual unintentionally substitutes phonemes in the target word or transposes phonemes in the target word (e.g., *domtutor* for *computer* or *comtuper* for *computer*). The production of literal paraphasias impacts a fair ability to retrieve words. Interestingly, repetition is significantly impacted because of the disconnection between the comprehension and formulation/production centers for language. That is, problems with repetition are due to the disconnection rather than comprehension as these individuals have relatively intact comprehension abilities.

Anomic aphasia is the mildest of the aphasia syndromes and is associated with ". . . lesion sites that are remote from each other" (Goodglass, 1993, p. 214). Goodglass indicates possible lesion sites resulting in anomic aphasia to include the frontal lobe, the angular gyrus, or the inferior temporal gyrus, with each of

TABLE 5-3

DISTINGUISHING LANGUAGE CHARACTERISTICS OF APHASIA SYNDROMES

Aphasia Syndrome	Distinguishing Features
Broca's	Agrammatism
Transcortical motor	Preserved repetition ability
Global	Profound impairment across all language modalities
Wernicke's	Empty speech
Transcortical sensory	Preserved repetition ability
Conduction	Marked impairment of repetition
Anomic	Primary difficulty in word retrieval

these sites resulting in slightly different versions of anomia. Verbal output is fluent, but word retrieval is only fair with verbal paraphasias evident. This impaired word retrieval is also apparent in writing. Repetition and comprehension is fair to good relative to verbal expression.

Table 5-3 highlights a language characteristic of each syndrome that assists in making an accurate classification. That said, it should be noted that even experienced diagnosticians often cannot classify an individual's aphasia into a syndrome type. In fact, the accuracy of identified syndrome is quite dependent on the rigor of the classification criteria used and ranges from 30% to 80% accuracy (Goodglass, Kaplan, & Barresi, 2001).

COGNITIVE-COMMUNICATIVE DISORDERS

"Cognitive-communicative disorders encompass difficulty with any aspect of communication that is affected by disruption of cognition" (American Speech-Language-Hearing Association, 2005, p.1). Disrupted cognitive processes that can impact communication abilities include attention, memory, reasoning, and executive function. The neurologic underpinnings for these functions rely on complex association areas, that is, the prefrontal cortex and P-T-O cortex and their connections to one another and the limbic system. Thus, any pathology that impacts these systems can result in a cognitive-communicative disorder. These pathologies include stroke, TBI, dementia, anoxia, meningitis, encephalitis, tumors, and hydrocephalus. Although many types of trauma or disease may result in disrupted cognition, the expected pattern of disruption differs. Following is a discussion of the cognitive deficits associated with communicative breakdown due to right hemisphere brain damage, TBI, and dementia.

Right Hemisphere Syndrome

Similar to aphasia, right hemisphere syndrome (RHS) results from a collection of symptoms displayed following damage to a cerebral hemisphere. In this case, the damage is to the nondominant hemisphere for language, most often the right hemisphere. In most of the patients seen, the damage is due to stroke. However, right hemisphere damage can be incurred due to other causes such as focal brain injury, tumor, or other disease processes.

Much has been written about hemispheric differences. For example, analytical and logic-oriented people have been referred to as "left hemisphere thinkers," whereas more creative and intuitive people have been called "right hemisphere thinkers." This tendency to categorize people according to hemispheric dominance is associated with their style of thinking. Although oversimplified, there is some truth to this notion. The left hemisphere is associated with more linear processing, perceiving detail, and being heavily involved in linguistic encoding and decoding and the motor planning for speech. Alternatively, the right hemisphere processes information more holistically with parallel processing, enabling us to see the gestalt or "big picture." Thus, the right hemisphere excels in the simultaneous integration of information and is heavily involved in visual perception and spatial relationships. As the famed author Carl Sagan (1977) reminds us, we need both hemispheres to function optimally as human beings:

> There is no way to tell whether the patterns extracted by the right hemisphere are real or imagined without subjecting them to left hemisphere scrutiny. On the other hand, mere critical thinking, without creative insights, without the search for new patterns, is sterile and doomed. To solve complex patterns in changing circumstances requires the activity of both hemispheres: the path to the future lies through the corpus callosum. (p. 191)

Individuals with RHS have been described as having language without communication (Burns, 1985). These individuals have most of their linguistic abilities intact, masking what can be more subtle cognitive deficits. The problems associated with damage to the nondominant hemisphere for language, most typically the right hemisphere, fall under the broad categories of visuospatial deficits, affect and prosody, and higher cognitive functions. The cognitive functions impacted are most likely grounded in difficulties with attention and integration (Myers, 1999). Myers has characterized a "typical" individual with RHS as displaying the following: (1) adequate superficial conversation; (2) flat voice or affect; and (3) communication partner perceptions of inattention, insensitivity, and poor pragmatics or use of language (e.g., eye contact, turn taking).

Visuospatial Deficits

One of the most interesting deficits seen following right hemisphere damage is that of *neglect*. Neglect is defined as the failure to report, respond, or orient to novel or meaningful stimuli contralateral to the side of lesion; hence, *left* **hemispatial neglect** may be present with *right* cerebral hemisphere damage. What makes this complex disorder fascinating is the interplay of multiple perceptual and cognitive systems including attentional mechanisms, intention, awareness, and internal mental representations (Brookshire, 2003). The most severe neglect has been associated with lesions to the right parietal lobe especially posterior inferior lesions (Mesulam, 1981), but the frontal lobes are also implicated. Individuals present with many behavioral symptoms of neglect including (1) failure to respond to stimuli in the left hemispace (i.e., to the left of body midline); (2) attending only to the right side during activities of daily living such as dressing the right half of their body or only eating food from the right side of their plate; and (3) motor behaviors such as bumping into doorways and walls to their left (Myers, 1999). Neglect can also directly affect the communicative acts of writing and reading with writing oriented on the right side of the page or reading only the words presented to right of midline.

A number of other perception-based impairments can be part of RHS. **Constructional impairments** reflect difficulty in drawing, copying, or utilizing objects in constructing figures and products. Constructions evidence distortion and disorganization and may reflect impairments in attention, perception, and neglect. **Prosopagnosia** refers to an inability to recognize familiar faces and is associated with right temporal occipital lesions with long-term difficulties associated with bilateral lesions (Benson, 1989). Denial of illness, termed **anosognosia**, is a common sequela of right hemisphere damage and is correlated with parietal lobe damage. The extent of denial varies among patients, ranging from indifference toward their deficits to complete denial of ownership of their very own limbs (Brookshire, 2003).

Affect and Prosody

Individuals with RHS may exhibit symptoms of flat affect exhibited in decreased facial expression as well as lack of prosodic contours in their speech. Interestingly, these problems are not only expressive but also receptive. That is, individuals with RHS also exhibit difficulties "reading" facial cues, body language, and the prosodic features of others' speech. Hence, many adults with RHS have difficulty using and appreciating emotion in daily life situations (Brookshire, 2003). Emotional competence involves both mood and affect. Mood is the inner emotional state, whereas affect is the external manifestation of mood. The limbic system is clearly involved with emotion and mood, but the ability to appropriately express emotion (via affect) and to interpret others' emotions seems to be mediated by the nondominant hemisphere for language, that is, the right hemisphere for most adults (Tucker & Frederick, 1989).

The prosodic disturbances often seen are referred to as **aprosodia**—deficits in the ability to both understand and produce prosodic features. Prosody is part of speech production. It includes the perceptual features of pitch, loudness, and duration in speech. Acoustically, the speech signal is altered in frequency, intensity, and timing, respectively. These alterations come together to provide the contour or intonation of speech that, in turn, signals meaning. The combination of aprosodia and disturbed emotional expression and interpretation is a part of the matrix of RHS.

Higher Cognitive Functions

Individuals with RHS exhibit impairment in attention and integration. In fact, Myers (1999) postulates that difficulties in attention and integration may be at the root of many of the symptoms individuals with RHS manifest.

The right hemisphere is dominant for arousal mechanisms that direct us to *attend* to important stimuli in our environment. For example, the frontal eye fields (represented in Brodmann area 8 in the superior frontal lobe) are involved in orienting the movement of the eyes and head to the contralateral space (Bhatnagar, 2008). Following right hemisphere damage, many individuals evidence problems with focusing, sustaining, and shifting (i.e., alternating and dividing) attention. Because attention is a fundamental cognitive process that supports other cognitive and language tasks, the impact of deficits here can be seen in issues of neglect, emotion, reading, writing, and pragmatics.

The diminished ability to pull together relevant details while ignoring irrelevant details to *integrate* information and draw inferences is a distinguishing feature of RHS. The impact of this lack of integration on discourse abilities was noted in 1979 when Myers described the discourse of individuals with right hemisphere damage as "... wend*ing* [italics added] their way through a maze of disassociated detail, seemingly incapable of filtering out unnecessary information" (cited in Myers, 2005, p. 1147). She further described the communication deficits of individuals with RHS, when they exist, as being irrelevant and often peppered with excessive information and literal responses to questions and events. Further research has determined that these individuals are able to make simple inferences, but difficulty is seen with generating inference in less predictable and novel situations.

Pragmatics refers to the social use of language and follows conventional rules in a given society. These rules include use of personal space, appropriate turn taking and eye contact, and maintaining topic and appropriate topic switching. Pragmatic problems are not always present following right hemisphere damage (Lehman-Blake, Duffy, Myers, & Tompkins, 2002). When they are, these individuals exhibit problem behaviors such as decreased eye contact, giving up their conversational turn, inappropriately terminating conversations, and engaging in excessive and ego-oriented speech (Kennedy, Strand, Burton, & Peterson, 1994; Prutting & Kirchner, 1987). Nonetheless, as Lehman-Blake et al. (2002), Kennedy et al. (1994), and Brookshire (2003) remind us, pragmatic impairments may or may not be present. Therefore, it is important to (1) understand the individual's pragmatic style prior to injury and (2) undertake a careful analysis of pragmatic skills.

Traumatic Brain Injury

The deficits seen following TBI are as widespread and varied as the injury itself. Recall from a previous section that TBI is a result of a combination of focal and diffuse damage to the brain due to some outside force. The damage can be further complicated by the body's reaction to the trauma (e.g., intracranial pressure) and other secondary factors (e.g., anoxia). Although focal effects of TBI can result in the communication disorders of aphasia, dysarthria, and those associated with RHS, the focus here will be on the cognitive sequelae most often noted with TBI. Alternatively, other pathologies can result in similar cognitive symptomatology as in TBI. These include meningitis, encephalitis, and anoxic events (e.g., near drowning or excessive bleeding). Attention, memory, and executive functions are nearly always affected with associated problems in speed of processing, reasoning, and problem solving. Although not focused on here, personality changes and behavioral symptoms (e.g., impulsivity) are also common following TBI. Attention, memory, and executive functions share neural systems and are especially vulnerable to injury in TBI (Sohlberg & Mateer, 1989). These are the anterior frontal and temporal brain regions mentioned earlier. Recall, however, that these areas connect to other brain regions via tracts. For example, connections between limbic system structures such as the cingulate gyrus and subcortical systems such as the thalamus have been implicated in higher level attentional mechanisms (Mateer & Ojemann, 1983).

Medical recovery following TBI occurs in more of a stepwise fashion as compared with vascular disease such as stroke (Brookshire, 2003). Recovery following TBI has a predictable course, but time to move through stages of recovery varies and is dependent on a number of variables such as severity of injury and secondary effects. A common scale utilized to make gross judgments of recovery level is the *Rancho Los Amigos Levels of Cognitive Functioning Scale*, traditionally an eight-point descriptive scale (revised to include two advanced levels of recovery) to determine functional severity based on behavioral symptoms and to denote amount of assistance required to function (Bushnik, 2000; see Table 5-4).

> ### Why You Need to Know
>
> The best way to "treat" TBI is to prevent it from happening or at least decrease the impact of injury. One way to do this is to put laws in place that require the use of protective equipment such as child safety seats, seat belts, and compulsory helmet use for motorcycle and bicycle riders. Improving highway safety and imposing speed limits also prevents or lessens the impact of TBI. Special playground surfaces help as well. When a brain injury does occur, improved emergency technology and paramedic skill along with swift medical response such as helicopter transport work to lessen the effects of the injury.

Attention, or the ability to concentrate, refers to one's ability to scan, select out, and respond to relevant stimuli in the environment and maintain this behavior over time. Ability to focus, screen out distractions, and sustain attention is foundational to other cognitive processes. For example, if you do not attend to new information in the classroom you

TABLE 5-4

RANCHO LOS AMIGOS REVISED LEVELS OF COGNITIVE FUNCTIONING SCALE

Level	Descriptor
I	No response Total assistance required
II	Generalized response Total assistance required
III	Localized response Total assistance required
IV	Confused, agitated Maximal assistance required
V	Confused, inappropriate, nonagitated Maximal assistance required
VI	Confused, appropriate Moderate assistance required
VII	Automatic, appropriate Minimal assistance required for activities of daily living
VIII	Purposeful, appropriate Stand-by assistance required
IX	Purposeful, appropriate Stand-by assistance on request
X	Purposeful, appropriate Modified independence

From Hagen, C. (1998). *The Rancho levels of cognitive functioning: The revised levels* (3rd ed.). www.rancho.org/patient_education/cognitive_levels.pdf

Retrieved August 27, 2010 from Rancho Los Amigos hospital website: www.rancho.org/patient_education/cognitive_levels.pdf

TABLE 5-5

THE FIVE COMPONENTS OF ATTENTION

Component	Description
Focused attention	Gross attention to environmental stimuli
Sustained attention	Maintaining attention over time to repetitive stimuli (i.e., vigilance) Holding and manipulating sensory information (i.e., working memory)
Selective attention	Focusing on relevant stimuli while filtering out irrelevant stimuli (i.e., freedom from distraction)
Alternating attention	Switching attention across different stimuli requiring different cognitive mindset (i.e., mental flexibility)
Divided attention	Ability to simultaneously respond to multiple tasks

Adapted from Sohlberg, M.M., & Mateer, C.A. (1989). *Introduction to cognitive rehabilitation: Theory and practice.* New York, NY: Guilford Press.

will not be able to encode ("store") that information for future retrieval. As alluded to, there are different attentional components. Some of these components are more foundational (e.g., focused, sustained, and selective attention), while others require control and manipulation (e.g., alternating and divided attention) (Sohlberg & Mateer, 2001; see Table 5-5). The interested reader is referred to Sohlberg and Mateer (1989, 2001) for a detailed explanation of their clinical model of attention.

Memory relates closely to attention and can be defined as stored knowledge and the processes for making and manipulating that stored knowledge (Bayles, 2006). Various memory models have been postulated based on stages of memory or content of memory. In the stage model, memory is thought of as having different levels. *Attention* to the stimuli to be remembered is the first step. *Encoding* is the next step which refers to the ". . . level of analysis performed on material to be remembered" (Sohlberg & Mateer, 2001, p. 163). This analysis may be phonological in the case

of verbal material or graphic in the case of visual material. Transferring new information for retention and later access is referred to as *storage. Retrieval* refers to the ability to search, find, and activate existing memories. Different types of memory exist and are stored.

These stored memories are referred to as **retrospective** (or **long-term**) **memories** and can be described based on the content recalled. **Declarative memory** refers to memory for consciously recalled facts (also referred to as *explicit memory*). There are three types of declarative memory: **episodic memory, semantic memory**, and **lexical memory**. Memories of events that are time and place specific are episodic memories, such as recalling your dinner experience last night (e.g., when you ate, who was there, what you had). Semantic memories are the long-term storage of concepts and general world knowledge. These types of memories are made throughout life experiences and cannot be equated with a specific time or place, for example, "knowing" that a garden is composed of plants cared for by people. Lexical memory refers to memory for words such as word meaning, spelling, and pronunciation (Bayles, 2006).

Nondeclarative memory refers to unconscious recall (also referred to as *implicit memory*). Two types of nondeclarative memory are procedural memory and priming. Procedural memory can be roughly equated with "motor memory," as it refers to one's ability to carry out overlearned motor sequences such as driving a stick shift, planting a flower, or carrying out computer command sequences without thinking. Priming refers to the notion that previous exposure to information readies the brain to recall associated information.

Some types of memory are interdependent on executive functions, to be discussed in the next section. One is **prospective memory** or "remembering to remember," that is, remembering to carry out a task in the future. The second type is called **metamemory** and can be thought of as "memory about memory" or having knowledge and making judgments about one's own memory abilities. This type of memory is called upon when learning new information as personal judgments are made regarding acquisition of knowledge. For example, this type of memory is used when studying for an exam. Another type of memory that requires executive functions is **working memory**. Working memory takes information from the senses (e.g., auditory, visual) and relates that to stored semantic memories that are retrieved for comparison purposes. In addition, working memory is involved in making judgments about the worthiness of encoding incoming sensory information to store long term. The location of memory in the brain is widespread and dependent on specific type of memory. Table 5-6 lists areas of the brain associated with various types of memory.

Executive functions allow us to put our thoughts and desires into action. Consider the job of a good company executive; that executive generates plans and actions to reach certain company goals. To do that the executive delegates tasks and oversees, or monitors and controls, progress toward goals, making adjustments when necessary. Executive functioning can be viewed as having an umbrella function over the other cognitive processes of attention, memory, and reasoning. Components of executive function include anticipation and goal selection, organization and planning, initiation, awareness and self-monitoring, and use of feedback to make adjustments to plans.

TABLE 5-6

NEUROANATOMICAL REGIONS ASSOCIATED WITH MEMORY PROCESSES

Memory Process	Neuroanatomy
Working memory	Prefrontal cortex
Declarative memory	Neocortex and medial–temporal/diencephalic brain regions
Semantic memory	All sensory association cortices
Procedural memory	Basal ganglia
Priming	Neocortex

TABLE 5-7

STAGES OF THE GLOBAL DETERIORATION SCALE USED IN DESCRIBING COGNITIVE DECLINE IN INDIVIDUALS WITH DEMENTIA

Stage	Label and Clinical Phase
1	No cognitive impairment; normal
2	Very mild cognitive decline; forgetfulness
3	Mild cognitive decline; early confusional
4	Moderate cognitive decline; late confusional
5	Moderately severe cognitive decline; early dementia
6	Severe cognitive decline; middle dementia
7	Very severe cognitive decline; late dementia

From Reisberg, B., Ferris, S., de Leon, M.J., & Crook, T. (1982). The global deterioration scale for assessment of primary degenerative dementia. *American Journal of Psychiatry, 139,* 1136–1139.

Dementia

Individuals suffering from dementia, of many types, will demonstrate communication difficulties grounded in their cognitive decline. The various disease processes noted earlier (e.g., Alzheimer's, Pick's disease, multiinfarct) result in dementia and the associated cognitive-communicative impairment. A popular scale for grossly rating cognitive decline following dementia diagnosis is the *Global Deterioration Scale* (Reisberg, Ferris, de Leon, & Crook, 1982); Table 5-7 presents the levels for this scale.

The earliest symptoms of AD are changes in personality (e.g., becoming defensive) and memory. Early impairments are reflected in a breakdown of episodic memories and executive functioning especially at the level of working memory. Working memory requires sustained attention and is a component of executive functioning (Sohlberg & Mateer, 2001). Individuals with dementia have difficulty holding on to what was just heard or seen to make these judgments and/or encode information into long-term memories (Bayles, 2006).

Santo Pietro and Ostuni (2003) present the characteristics of communication loss across the stages of Alzheimer's type dementia in regard to memory, understanding, speech and language skills, and social skills. The following is summarized from their work.

The communication deficits during the *early stage* of dementia are relatively mild and reflect the memory problems already mentioned. Individuals lose their orientation to time, their ability to retrieve recent memories, or their ability to use short-term memory to hold on to a short list or a phone number. Conversation may seem abrupt or they may become argumentative. This may be due to decreased abilities to comprehend more complex or rapidly presented information. They may lose their train of thought and have difficulties keeping up with conversation. Word retrieval is affected, but at this stage, they are often aware of errors and make attempts at self-correction.

Communication during the *middle stage* is quite affected and difficulties are immediately obvious. Orientation is impacted for both time and place; however, they still know who they are. Memory problems become more apparent in conversation with more egocentrism and less perspective taking, less questioning, less initiation, and rare self-correction. Auditory and reading comprehension is impacted although they retain the ability to read extra-linguistic cues (e.g., facial expressions). Individuals at this stage also retain the mechanics of reading such as in oral reading and demonstrate the ability to comprehend at the single word or the short phrase level in a meaningful context (Bourgeios & Hopper, 2005).

Communication is devastated in the *late stage* of Alzheimer's type dementia. All orientation is lost: person, place, and time. They cannot form new memories nor even recognize family members. Awareness of the rules of social engagement is lost as is a desire to communicate. In fact, at this stage, the patient may lose speech production and comprehension altogether and appear to be mute.

Primary progressive aphasia (PPA) is a subtype of frontotemporal dementia, labeled as such because of the areas of the brain that are degenerating. PPA differs from the clinical picture seen with Alzheimer's dementia, as it manifests itself in progressive decline of language abilities followed by a decline in cognition. The term aphasia applies because the initiating symptoms are in language. It differs from aphasia associated with stroke or other focal lesions due to its (1) insidious onset; (2) focal affect on the language-dominant hemisphere; (3) progressive worsening of symptoms; and (4) ultimate cognitive involvement. In addition to the progressive aphasia, progressive AOS has also been noted with certain individuals (Duffy, 2005). AOS is a motor speech disorder that will be discussed in the next section.

MOTOR SPEECH DISORDERS

A myriad of speech disorders are associated with lesions involving the motor centers and pathways of the central and peripheral nervous systems. Recall from Chapter 4 the many structures, tracts, and nerves responsible for planning and executing motor actions. Centrally, these include the premotor cortex, the anterior insular cortex, the precentral gyrus, the corticospinal and corticobulbar tracts, the basal ganglia, the cerebellum and associated tracts, the brainstem (i.e., cranial nerve motor nuclei), and the spinal cord (i.e., anterior horns). Peripherally, recall the motor component of the cervical spinal nerves and the cranial nerves involved with motor execution. These are the trigeminal (V), facial (VII), glossopharyngeal (IX), vagus (X), spinal accessory (XI), and hypoglossal (XII). Any neuropathology that affects these systems has the potential to result in a motor speech disorder; thus, stroke, tumor, degenerative disease, or TBI may result in a motor speech disorder.

Motor speech disorders are defined as "...speech disorders resulting from neurologic impairments affecting the motor planning, programming, neuromuscular control, or execution of speech" (Duffy, 2005, p. 6). There are two motor speech disorders: AOS and dysarthria. Duffy defines AOS as a "...motor speech disorder characterized by a disturbance in motor planning or programming of sequential movement for volitional speech production" (p. 5) and dysarthria as a "...speech disorder characterized by disturbances in speech muscle control due to paralysis, paresis, weakness, slowness, incoordination, and/or altered muscle tone" (p. 5). These same motor problems resulting in speech difficulties are often also manifested in other parts of the body. For example, an individual with uncoordinated speech may also show uncoordinated body movements. Thus, individuals with these disorders *look* like they have motor problems.

Apraxia of Speech

AOS is rarely found in isolation; rather, it is typically concomitant with aphasia. This makes sense when one thinks of the lesion sites associated with AOS. Lesions resulting in this motor speech disorder are always in the language-dominant hemisphere but not necessarily localized to one particular region. Nonetheless, AOS is most often seen following lesions to the third frontal convolution, or Broca's area, with the anterior insular cortex often implicated as well (Miller, 2002). This is consistent with the speech description of those with nonfluent aphasia described earlier in this chapter. Second, the supplementary motor area is important for planning and programming of volitional movements (Duffy, 2005). Other areas of lesion have also been implicated in AOS such as subcortical lesions involving the basal ganglia or regions of the parietal lobe including the somatosensory cortex and the supramarginal gyrus (Square-Storer & Apeldoorn, 1991). These areas are responsible for the integration of sensory information, a prerequisite for skilled motor activity (Duffy, 2005).

The process of motor planning and programming can be looked at as a sort of bridge between language formulation and motor execution (Halpern, 2000). A problem in language formulation is aphasia; a problem in motor execution is dysarthria; a problem with the bridge is AOS. This bridge seems to require a "... transformation of the abstract phonemes to a neural code that is compatible with the operations of the motor system" (Duffy, 2005, p. 309). This transformation is responsible for "... connecting the inner language processes into the endless number of speech utterances" (Halpern, 2000, p. 218). A breakdown in this motor process results in interesting speech symptoms.

Individuals with AOS have speech output that reflects a concentrated effort to sequentially and volitionally produce phonemes for intelligible speech. Wertz, LaPointe, and Rosenbek (1984) describe this speech as consisting of "islands" of fluent, intelligible speech interrupted by periods of effortful, off-target groping for the speech sounds. These islands of fluent speech are usually automatic phrases that are produced without thinking. For example, a client may be struggling to say a target word when all of a sudden he says "gosh, this is just so hard!" perfectly clear. However, when asked to repeat that utterance, he is unable to do so without hesitation and effort.

Speech output secondary to AOS can be described in regard to articulatory disturbance and prosodic disturbance. Symptoms evident in articulation include inconsistent *trial and error* responding, increased difficulty with increased utterance length and complexity, and frequent speech sound substitutions. Symptoms resulting in the disrupted prosodic contours of speech include slow speech rate, hesitations, and difficulty initiating speech (known as *articulatory groping*).

Dysarthria

Dysarthria is actually a syndrome or a collection of motor speech symptoms reflective of the disturbed motor system. Darley, Aronson, and Brown (1975) completed a seminal study and subsequently published a now classic text categorizing and describing six types of dysarthria that are very specifically related to site of lesion (a seventh type was described years later). It is important to note that it is the site of lesion rather than the etiology of the lesion that determines the type of dysarthria. For example, a brainstem stroke, ALS, or an acoustic neuroma can all result in symptoms associated with flaccid dysarthria. The original six types of dysarthria are flaccid, spastic, ataxic, hypokinetic, hyperkinetic, and mixed. The seventh type, a relatively mild dysarthria, is named for its lesion site—unilateral upper motor neuron (UUMN) dysarthria. Unlike AOS, dysarthria reflects impairment in the ability to execute motor movement for speech production. Also unlike AOS, dysarthria often affects all speech processes—respiration, phonation, resonation, articulation, and prosody—whereas AOS primarily impacts articulation and prosody. Speech characteristics associated with the disrupted processes for dysarthria are highlighted in Table 5-8. Each of the subtypes of dysarthria, along with its correlated lesion site, is described next.

UUMN dysarthria results from lesions to the UMNs and is the mildest of the dysarthrias. More specifically, the lesion involves disruption to the tracts carrying

TABLE 5-8

SPEECH SYMPTOMS COMMONLY ASSOCIATED WITH THE DYSARTHRIA TYPES

Dysarthria Type	Speech Symptoms
Unilateral upper motor neuron	Imprecise articulation
Spastic	Strained-strangled phonation Hypernasal resonance Slow, imprecise articulation
Flaccid	Short breath groups Breathy phonation Reduced loudness Inhalatory stridor Hypernasal resonance Nasal air emission Imprecise articulation
Ataxic	Loudness and pitch variations Normal resonance Irregular articulatory breakdowns
Hypokinetic	Breathy phonation Reduced loudness Monotone vocal quality Normal resonance Imprecise articulation Rapid speech rate
Hyperkinetic (dystonia)	Intermittent strained phonation Phonatory arrests Normal resonation Intermittent, slow, articulatory distortions
Hyperkinetic (chorea)	Abrupt phonatory arrests Normal resonation Intermittent, quick, articulatory distortions

neural information to the brainstem and spinal cord. Symptoms of UUMN are seen contralateral to the site of lesion and are manifested in lower facial weakness and tongue weakness. For this reason, articulation is most often impacted. However, lesions to UMNs may also result in damage to tracts that are important for posture, muscle tone, and reflexes (Duffy, 2005). Because of the site of lesion, these individuals often present with aphasia and/or AOS. In fact, interventions for those communication disorders are a priority over a mild dysarthria.

Spastic dysarthria results when bilateral lesions to the UMNs occur. Bilateral lesions result in significant dysarthria and are also called **pseudobulbar palsy**. This is because the lesion occurs above the level of the brainstem (i.e., the bulbar region). These bilateral lesions result in lack of inhibitory neural information reaching the cell bodies that give rise to the LMNs in the brainstem and spinal cord. This, in turn, results in muscle weakness, too much muscle tone (i.e., *hypertonia*) with limited range of movement, and exaggerated reflexes. The pathology involved is often bilateral strokes or TBI, but other etiologies (e.g., degenerative disease) account for some cases.

Lesions affecting the LMNs result in *flaccid dysarthria*. Recall that LMNs include motor neuron cell bodies (located in the brainstem or the spinal cord), the peripheral nerves (cranial nerves or spinal nerves), the neuromuscular junction, and, end with the muscle fibers innervated. Lesions occurring anywhere along the LMN can result in flaccid dysarthria; thus, etiologies vary. These include, but are not limited to, brainstem stroke, TBI or other induced trauma (e.g., surgeries), ALS, myasthenia gravis (a disorder of the neuromuscular junction), and muscular dystrophies. In contrast to spastic dysarthria, there is decreased muscle tone (i.e., *hypotonia*), muscle weakness, and atrophy of the affected muscles. The extent and severity of speech systems affected are contingent on site of lesion. If a lesion occurs peripherally, closer to the innervation of the targeted muscle, then the symptoms will reflect that interruption. For example, if the recurrent laryngeal branch of the vagus nerve is damaged during thoracic surgery, symptoms will be specific to the phonatory system. Alternatively, symptoms are more pervasive and severe when a lesion occurs higher up (i.e., at or near the brainstem), thus impacting multiple cranial nerves. In this case, all speech systems will likely be affected.

Ataxic dysarthria results from damage to the cerebellum and/or the tracts associated with it. Degenerative disease, stroke, TBI, and tumor are the most common causes of lesion. Recall that the cerebellum is responsible for coordinating movement through the control of range, force, direction, and timing of movements. When this is disrupted, movements become uncoordinated and lack synergy. In fact, the resulting dysarthria is often described as "drunken speech." This lack of coordination crosses all speech systems, especially impacting the prosodic features of speech.

Hypokinetic dysarthria is caused by damage to the basal ganglia system, specifically involving the substantia nigra. This is the dysarthria associated with the degenerative disorder of Parkinson's disease (PD). The name refers to the decreased (hypo) movement (kinetic), or bradykinesia, seen in PD. Additional motor symptoms include muscle rigidity, resting tremor, and difficulty initiating movement. It is common to see individuals with PD presenting with stooped posture, decreased facial expression (i.e., masked facies), and a shuffle in their walk (i.e., festinating gait). Most speech processes are affected with notable symptoms in phonation and articulation.

Hyperkinetic dysarthria is classified into two types of dysarthria that are both a result of involuntary movements but named for the speed of these movements. Dysarthria associated with slow, writhing movement is called slow hyperkinetic dysarthria such as with dystonia. These uncontrolled movements slowly build to a peak and are sustained before subsiding. Quick hyperkinetic dysarthria is associated with chorea. In contrast to dystonic movement patterns, choreic movements are fast, only briefly sustained if at all, and unpredictable. Pathologies affecting the basal ganglia and associated circuitry in the cerebral hemispheres are responsible for hyperkinetic dysarthrias. These pathologies include congenital cerebral palsy of the athetoid type resulting in dystonia and degenerative Huntington's disease resulting in chorea. However, often times the pathology underlying these disruptive movement disorders is unknown (Duffy, 2005).

Mixed dysarthrias, as the name implies, result from a combination of two or more of the above types. This most often occurs with degenerative disorders such as amyotrophic lateral sclerosis (ALS) or multiple sclerosis (MS) or when trauma affects multiple locales of the nervous system such as with traumatic brain injury (TBI) or multiple strokes. The speech systems affected will vary dependent on the combination of dysarthria types.

Swallowing Disorders

Swallowing impairments are referred to as **dysphagia**. Dysphagia has multiple etiologies; here, the focus is on swallowing difficulties due to acquired neurologic disorders. It is appropriate that a discussion of dysphagia follows motor speech disorders, especially dysarthria, because these disorders often co-occur. This is due to the impact of the associated pathology on the motor system and the resultant affects on the muscles across the different stages of the swallow. The pathologies resulting in **neurogenic dysphagia** are similar to those mentioned earlier and include stroke, TBI, tumors, and degenerative diseases (Corbin-Lewis, Liss, & Sciortino, 2005). Unlike the dysarthrias, a clear correlation between lesion site and expected symptoms does not exist for neurogenic dysphagia. Instead, the swallowing impairment is described based on the disrupted stage(s) of the swallow (these stages were described in Chapter 4).

Lesions resulting in decreased or disordered movement of the facial, labial, and lingual musculature results in *oral preparatory* and *oral stage* impairments. Lesions involving the LMNs of the facial, trigeminal, and hypoglossal cranial nerves will obviously result in problems at these stages of swallow. However, lesions to higher cortical centers, such as the UMNs, the cerebellum and its tracts, or the basal ganglia and their tracts, can also result in problems in these stages. Pathologies associated with these lesions are consistent with that already mentioned. Notable symptoms include drooling, reduced mastication and bolus formation, pocketing of food, and difficulty propelling the bolus posteriorly to initiate the swallow. Oral transit delay can result in food and drink passing inadvertently into the hypopharynx, entering the laryngeal vestibule, and possibly penetrating the vocal folds (see Chapter 8) with resultant aspiration. Aspiration is defined as food, drink, or saliva that enters the airway (i.e., trachea) below the level of the true vocal folds.

The *pharyngeal stage* is highly automatized and requires rapid integration of multiple movements for a safe swallow to occur. The velum elevates to close the nasopharyngeal port at the same time as the larynx moves up and forward and the epiglottis moves down and back. A lesion impacting the movements required for this stage of the swallow is of priority concern as the result can be aspiration. Pathologies affecting this stage are those that result in large, multiple, or diffuse nervous system lesions such as multiple strokes, TBI, and degenerative diseases (Corbin-Lewis et al., 2005). Symptoms associated with problems in this stage include a delayed trigger of the swallow reflex and food and drink getting hung up (called *residue*) in the val-

leculae and pyriform sinuses. The individual with problems in this stage will often cough or choke or, more seriously, not feel anything penetrate the airway. When the later happens, it is referred to as **silent aspiration**.

The *esophageal stage* of the swallow requires intact function of the upper esophageal sphincter to allow the bolus to enter and proper motility of the skeletal and smooth muscle of the esophagus to propel food to the stomach. Problems with this stage are primarily under the purview of the gastroenterologist. Texts devoted to swallowing disorders review the various disorders that influence esophageal function (e.g., Corbin-Lewis et al., 2005; Crary & Groher, 2003; Logemann, 1998).

Dysphagia can also be the result of limited cognition due to neuropathology. Swallowing concerns are especially prevalent in the later stages of dementia. Although these individuals may have adequate function across stages of the swallow, their cognitive deficits impact remembering to chew and remembering to swallow! This can even be a problem earlier in the course of the disease, as they may not even remember to eat. All of this can result in malnutrition and dehydration for the individual which, in turn, impacts cognitive functioning as evidenced by increased confusion and lethargy.

A stagnate bolus of food in the oral cavity impacts a safe swallow. If chewing is not adequate, a bolus too large for safe passage into the esophagus may enter the airway and result in aspiration and/or penetration—an episode of choking. Likewise, holding a masticated bolus in the oral cavity for a prolonged period of time increases the risk of aspiration or penetration as well. Imagine someone laying down for their afternoon nap following lunch or a snack. As you can imagine, mealtime assistance with reminders to chew and swallow as well as follow-up oral hygiene is absolutely critical for these individuals.

Individuals with end-stage dementia pose unique challenges in regard to dysphagia management. At this stage, individuals may refuse food by turning away, gagging, or spitting food out. The choice to provide nutrition and hydration support through tube feeding or going with a **palliative care** approach needs to be decided upon. At this time, the speech–language pathologist serves an important role in educating staff and family regarding options and outcomes. Although it may sound unkind to withhold nutritional support, persons with advanced dementia on tube feedings have been found to not fare any better than those without tube feedings in regard to aspiration risk (Finucane, Christmas, & Travis, 1999).

Alternatively, palliative care refers to providing food and/or drink that are accepted by the individual such as using ice chips on the lips for comfort.

Summary

This chapter presented the many communication disorders that result from neurologic disturbance. The neuropathologies that can result in communication breakdowns are also many and varied including cardiovascular incidents, trauma, and disease. The resultant communication disorders can be in language (e.g., aphasia), cognition (e.g., disorders secondary to right hemisphere damage, TBI, or dementia), speech (e.g., AOS, dysarthria), or any combination. Key to this discussion of the various neurogenic communication disorders is understanding the neurological substrates associated with the various disorders. Referring back to Chapter 4 of this part will greatly assist you in connecting neuropathology to neuroanatomy and physiology. Conversely, understanding various neurological disorders assists in meaningful application of the detailed information presented in Chapter 4.

Clinical Teaser—Follow-Up

At the beginning of this part, you were asked to note any terms or concepts in the case study that were unfamiliar to you. As you read Chapter 4, you were to pay particular attention to the anatomy and physiology pertinent to this case. Now we return to the case for further discussion.

Following the format of Chapter 5, we can interpret this case regarding etiology, neuropathology, and resulting communication disorder(s). Sisi suffered an ischemic stroke affecting the frontal branch of the middle cerebral artery. Based on site of lesion and symptoms, brain areas damaged included the left precentral gyrus (Brodmann area 4), the third frontal convolution (Brodmann areas 44, 45), and the anterior insular cortex. The lesion may have extended into subcortical white matter as well. Information from the speech–language evaluation leads to the conclusion that Sisi evidences unilateral upper motor neuron dysarthria and nonfluent aphasia. More information is required to determine if apraxia of speech (AOS) is present. What information from Chapters 4 and 5 assisted you in drawing these conclusions? What information do you need to (1) further classify this aphasia as a particular syndrome and (2) determine if AOS is present? Lastly, would you expect swallowing ability to be affected and if so, which stage(s)?

PART 2 SUMMARY

Part 2 (Chapters 4 and 5) presented information critical to understand the basic functions of the nervous system and what can go wrong with it to result in a communication disorder. The understanding of the nervous system and its pathologies prepares the reader for the subsequent chapters of this book. The brain is the overseer of body function via the conversion of thought to action and sensation to integration in general and for speech production specifically. Thus, muscles of the speech and swallowing mechanism—respiratory, phonatory, resonatory, and articulatory—all receive innervation via spinal and cranial nerves which, in turn, receive neural commands from higher cortical centers and pathways. Also, sensory receptors send neural information, via spinal and cranial nerves, to the central nervous system. This sensory feedback includes auditory information and both conscious and unconscious information regarding muscle position. Thus, it can be appreciated that the nervous system allows for a continuous feed forward and feedback mechanism for speech and swallowing through messages sent to muscle for movement and messages received at the brain for thought and response. Damage can occur to the nervous system in a number of ways: by disease or by injury such as stroke or traumatic brain injury. This damage may, in turn, result in disorders of communication. The communication disorder is a result of where damage occurs in the nervous system and can take the form of an acquired language disorder (e.g., aphasia), a motor speech disorder (e.g., dysarthria or apraxia of speech), or a cognitive-communicative disorder. There are different types of aphasia (e.g., Broca's aphasia) and different types of dysarthria (e.g., flaccid dysarthria) depending on lesion site. There are also different manifestations of cognitive-communication disorders which are variably described based on lesion site (e.g., right hemisphere damage), type of injury (e.g., traumatic brain injury) or disease (e.g., dementia). This part concludes with a brief description of the impact of neurological damage on swallowing function across the stages of the swallow as well as the impact dementia has on eating and swallowing.

PART 2 REVIEW QUESTIONS

1. Describe the components of the fully developed central nervous system using neurodevelopmental (i.e., "-encephalon") terminology.

2. Name two gyri and sulci associated with each of the four lobes of the cerebrum: frontal, parietal, temporal, and occipital.

3. Describe the flow of cerebrospinal fluid beginning with the lateral ventricles and ending with the dural sinuses.

4. How do glial cells differ from neurons? Name four types of glial cells and describe each one's function.

5. List the steps for an action potential beginning with a stimulus to the presynaptic neuron, resulting in depolarization.

6. Define IPSP and EPSP. What is the difference between the two?

7. What communication disorder is most likely to result from a lesion to the following areas of the central nervous system: brainstem, Brodmann area 22, hippocampus, orbital gyri, and cerebellum?

8. What communication disorder is most likely to result from the following medical etiologies: right hemisphere stroke; left hemisphere stroke; amyotrophic lateral sclerosis, Alzheimer's dementia; Parkinson's disease; and encephalitis?

9. Differentiate nonfluent aphasia from fluent aphasia.

10. Name the three cognitive functions that are especially vulnerable to traumatic brain injury.

11. Contrast declarative with nondeclarative memory.

12. Name three symptoms of middle stage Alzheimer's type dementia that can impact communication.

13. Describe several ways in which dysarthria differs from apraxia of speech.

14. List the seven types of dysarthria and indicate the probable site of lesion for each type.

PART 3

Anatomy, Physiology, and Pathology of the Respiratory System

CHAPTER 6

Anatomy and Physiology of the Respiratory System

Knowledge Outcomes for ASHA Certification for Chapter 6
- Demonstrate knowledge of the biological basis of the basic human communication processes (III-B)
- Demonstrate knowledge of the neurological basis of the basic human communication processes (III-B)

Learning Objectives
- You will be able to describe the framework that supports the respiratory system.
- You will be able to describe the lungs and their linkage to the thoracic cavity.
- You will be able to discuss the muscles that mediate inspiration and expiration.
- You will be able to define the basic concepts involved in respiration, including but not limited to airflow, Boyle's law, elastic recoil, gravity, pressure, torque, and volume.
- You will be able to explain the mechanics of quiet, vegetative breathing.
- You will be able to discuss the differences in respiratory mechanics between quiet, vegetative breathing and breathing to support vocal activity.

AFFIX AND PART-WORD BOX

TERM	MEANING	EXAMPLE
brachial	pertaining to the arm and shoulder	**brachial** nerve
cardiac	pertaining to the heart	**cardiac** impression
chondro-	pertaining to cartilage	**chondro**-osseous juncture
-clavius	pertaining to the clavicle	sub**clavius**
-cleido-	pertaining to the clavicle	sterno**cleido**mastoid
costal	pertaining to the ribs	**costal** pleura
costarum	pertaining to the ribs	levator **costarum** brevis
crico-	pertaining to the cricoid cartilage	**crico**tracheal ligament
dorsi	pertaining to the back	latissimus **dorsi**
glottic	pertaining to the glottis, the variable-sized opening between the vocal folds	sub**glottic** pressure
ilio-	pertaining to the ilium	lateral **ilio**costalis
inter-	between	**inter**vertebral disc
intra-	within or inside of	**intra**tracheal membrane
lumbo-	pertaining to the lumbar region of the vertebral column	quadratus **lumbo**rum

TERM	MEANING	EXAMPLE
odontoid	shaped like a tooth	**odontoid** process
osseo-	pertaining to bone	chondro-**osseo**us juncture
parietal	pertaining to the wall of a cavity	**parietal** pleura
pectoral	pertaining to the chest	**pectoral**is major
pelvic	pertaining to the pelvis	**pelvic** girdle
peri-	around or surrounding	**peri**cardium
phrenic	pertaining to the diaphragm	**phrenic** nerve
pulmo-	pertaining to the lungs	alveoli **pulmo**ni
sacral	pertaining to the sacrum	**sacral** foramina
serratus	having a sawtooth or jagged appearance	**serratus** anterior
spiro-	pertaining to the process of breathing	**spiro**meter
sterno-	pertaining to the sternum	**sterno**cleidomastoid
sub-	below or inferior to	**sub**clavius
tracheal	pertaining to the trachea	intra**tracheal** membrane
vertebro-	pertaining to the vertebral or spinal column	**vertebro**sternal

Clinical Teaser

Richard is a 35-year-old teacher who comes to your speech and language clinic complaining of an inability to produce a strong, clear voice. It seems that every time he attempts to speak, he just does not seem to have enough breath to speak in a clear voice for any more than a few seconds at a time. He suspects he has asthma, but denies that there is a family history of the disorder. Richard claims to be healthy otherwise. When you ask him, he admits that he has been smoking for approximately 10 years—perhaps, a pack to a pack and a half each day. He also relates to you that his condition seems to be worse after his three-times-weekly exercises. Finally, through further inquiry, you learn that Richard has had chronic gastroesophageal reflux disease for well over 15 years. You note that he presents a pronounced stridor upon inhalation.

Being well versed in the anatomy and physiology of the respiratory system, you suspect that a number of things could be causing the problem. Immediately coming to mind are asthma, emphysema, neuropathology, and paradoxical vocal fold movement (PVFM) disorder. You suggest to your client that he get a complete medical work up from his personal physician.

Your client does indeed follow up with your suggestion. His primary care physician conducts a general health check-up. All medical signs do not appear to support a diagnosis of asthma. Because of Richard's history of cigarette smoking,

the doctor suspects that perhaps he is in the initial stages of emphysema. The doctor refers the patient to a pulmonary specialist for further evaluation.

The pulmonary specialist conducts a thorough assessment of Richard, including respiratory measures (e.g., vital capacity [VC], flow-volume loop testing) and endoscopy. An endoscopic examination reveals no subglottic inflammation typically seen in asthma patients. In fact, all testing seems to reveal normal structure and function of the respiratory system. Not able to provide a definitive diagnosis, the pulmonary specialist refers Richard to an otolaryngologist.

Taking into consideration the information that has been obtained to this point, the otolaryngologist has Richard engage in vigorous exercise for 20 minutes before conducting an endoscopic examination. The doctor notices right away that Richard's stridor is more pronounced. The doctor begins the endoscopic exam, which immediately reveals an abnormal adduction of the vocal folds during inhalation with a small posterior, triangular glottal chink. Further testing supports a diagnosis of PVFM disorder.

Note any terms or concepts in the foregoing case study that are unfamiliar to you. As you read the first chapter of this part, pay particular attention to the anatomy and physiology pertinent to this case, then try to relate that information to the discussion of respiratory pathologies presented in Chapter 7.

Introduction

Now that you have a basic understanding of the nervous system—the battery that drives the entire speech and hearing mechanisms—it is time to take a closer look at the three systems that comprise the human vocal mechanism. These three are the respiratory, phonatory, and articulatory/resonance systems. The anatomy and physiology of the phonatory system will be discussed in Chapter 8, and the articulatory/resonance system will be presented in Chapter 10. Your attention is turned toward the respiratory system in this chapter.

As discussed in Chapter 4, the nervous system can be envisioned as the apparatus that overrides the entire vocal mechanism. In other words, each of the three systems that comprises the vocal mechanism is able to function and contribute to the process of speech production because of the influence of the nervous system (see Figure 6-1). The greatest contribution the nervous system makes to the vocal mechanism is through the innervation of voluntary muscles that comprise each of the systems of speech production. However, the nervous system may also influence the vocal mechanism through the autonomic nervous system.

The respiratory system can be thought of as the power source for speech production. It is through our expired air that energy is created to cause **phonation** of the vocal folds, thereby producing a **complex tone** that is further modified as it passes through the vocal tract. In other words, the respiratory system provides input to the phonatory system by way of expired air from the lungs. In turn, the phonatory system is responsible for producing the vocal tone (this will be discussed at length in Chapter 8), which is then modified through the processes of **articulation** and **resonance** (see Chapter 10) to produce speech

sounds such as consonants and vowels. The net result of these activities is speech production.

The remainder of this chapter will be devoted to a thorough discussion of the anatomy and physiology of the respiratory system. It is expected that upon reading this chapter, you will be well versed in the structure and mechanics of respiration.

Anatomy of the Respiratory System

In describing the anatomy of the respiratory system, it may be helpful to use the analogy of building a house. First, a foundation is laid and the house's framework is erected. Once the framework is in place, electricians and plumbers will install the electrical and plumbing systems. Then, carpenters will fill the wall, floor, and ceiling spaces with insulation. Finally, the inner and outer walls of the house will be constructed. In many instances, the builder may install appliances prior to completion of the house.

Take the framework first. In anatomy, the framework is the skeletal system. The skeletal system is composed of bones, cartilages, and connective tissue such as membranes, ligaments, and tendons. Nerves and blood vessels can be viewed as the electrical and plumbing systems. The house's insulation corresponds to muscles; that is, muscles are an integral part of the skeletal system in much the same way that insulation is an integral part of the house's framework. Finally, the mucous membranes that cover the muscles, nerves, and blood vessels are analogous to the walls of the house. Any organs that may be part of a particular system (e.g., the lungs as part of the respiratory system) can be thought of as the house's appliances.

Keeping this analogy in mind, the anatomy of the respiratory system will be presented in a logical order. First, the framework will be discussed (i.e., bones, cartilages, membranes, ligaments, and tendons). Then, muscles that are an important component of the system will be presented. Following the muscles, mucous membranes and organs will be described in detail. Finally, a brief discussion will be provided about the neural underpinnings of the respiratory system (structures of the circulatory system will not be discussed).

THE FRAMEWORK FOR THE RESPIRATORY SYSTEM

The framework of the respiratory system includes five structures: the vertebral (or spinal) column, the rib cage, the pectoral girdle, the pelvic girdle, and

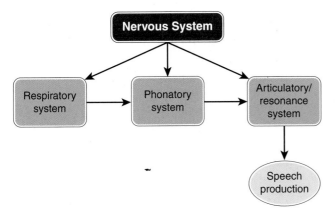

Figure 6-1 A schematic overview of the speech production mechanism.

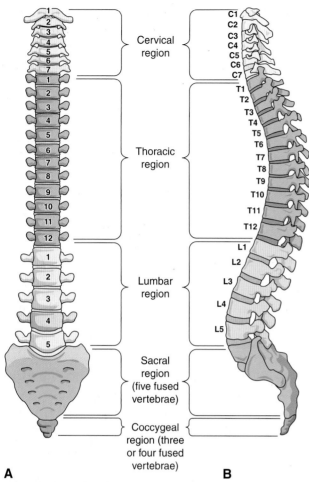

A   **B**

Figure 6-2   The human vertebral column with individual verte-brae numbered. **A**. Anterior view. **B**. Lateral view. (Reprinted with permission from Cohen, B.J., Taylor, J.J. (2009). *Memmler's the human body in health and disease* (11th ed.). Baltimore, MD: Wolters Kluwer Health.)

the trachea and bronchial tree. These five structures will be examined more closely in the paragraphs that follow.

The Vertebral (Spinal) Column

The vertebral—or spinal—column makes up the axis of the human body (see Figure 6-2). It is composed of 32 or 33 individual bones stacked upon each other vertically. An individual bone is referred to as a vertebra. In the upper regions of the vertebral column (i.e., the cervical, thoracic, and lumbar regions), the vertebrae for the most part do not actually make contact as they are stacked upon each other; instead, cartilaginous discs (called **intervertebral discs**) reside between adjacent vertebrae throughout most of the length of the vertebral column. These discs are non-existent in the fused vertebral structures known as the sacrum and coccyx, which are the lowermost regions of the vertebral column.

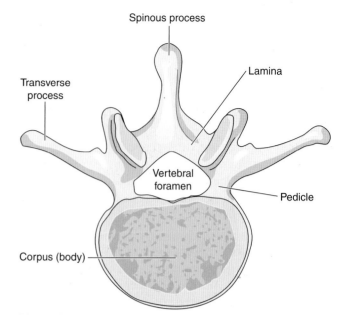

Figure 6-3   Landmarks on a typical human vertebra (superior view). (Reprinted with permission from Cohen, B.J., Taylor, J.J. (2009). *Memmler's the human body in health and disease* (11th ed.). Baltimore, MD: Wolters Kluwer Health.)

Figure 6-3 shows the landmarks of a typical vertebra. Anteriorly, a vertebra has a corpus or body. Proceeding posteriorly from the corpus are two legs or pedicles. The two pedicles are joined together by laminae that form the **neural arch**. The pedicles and neural arch create an inner chamber immediately posterior to the corpus. This chamber is called the vertebral foramen. When the majority of vertebrae are stacked vertically, this foramen becomes a passageway from the base of the skull to the lower back. The spinal cord resides within this passageway. At the juncture where each pedicle meets a lamina, a somewhat laterally directed process emerges, one on the right-hand side and one on the left. These are called **transverse processes**. Finally, proceeding posteriorly from the point where the two lamina meet is another process called the **spinous process**. When one runs a finger down the center of their back, they will feel bumps along its length. These are the spinous processes. The vertebrae are bound together by a series of anterior and posterior longitudinal ligaments, as well as several accessory ligaments, thereby forming the vertebral column.

In a typical adult, the vertebral column is approximately 72 to 75 cm in length. It is divided into regions and the individual vertebrae are coded according to their sequence in any given region. Proceeding at the base of the skull and moving toward the tailbone, these regions are the cervical, thoracic, lumbar, sacral, and coccygeal regions.

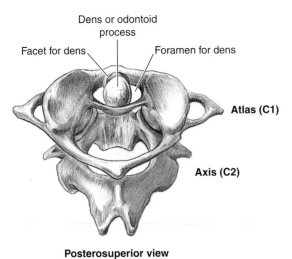

Dens or odontoid process

Facet for dens

Foramen for dens

Atlas (C1)

Axis (C2)

Posterosuperior view

Figure 6-4 Articulation of the atlas (C1) with the axis (C2). (Reprinted with permission from Anatomical Chart Company.)

The cervical region is found in the neck. It consists of seven vertebrae coded C1 through C7. C1 and C2 also have names. C1 is known as the atlas because it articulates with the skull. Similar to the mythological character of the same name, the atlas can be envisioned as holding the weight of the world (i.e., the skull) on its shoulders. C2 is also referred to as the axis because of its articulation with C1. The axis has a special process known as the **dens** or **odontoid process**, upon which the atlas rests and rotates (see Figure 6-4). This action allows us to turn our head from side to side. In addition to the landmarks mentioned earlier for a typical vertebra, the cervical vertebrae have a distinguishing characteristic. On the proximal end of the transverse processes are small holes called **transverse foramina** (C7 may or may not have these). The purpose of these foramina is to provide a passageway for some nerves and blood vessels as they pass through the neck region. Incidentally, an interesting fact about cervical vertebrae is that most mammals have the same number. This means that a giraffe and a human have the same number of cervical vertebrae, although obviously the giraffe's are much larger (as much as 8½ inches in length!).

The thoracic region of the vertebral column consists of 12 vertebrae coded T1 through T12. As one proceeds from T1 to T12, the individual vertebrae become larger. In addition to the typical landmarks, the thoracic vertebrae are unique in that they house the articular facets for the ribs. These facets can be found along the posterolateral aspects of the corpus and the transverse processes.

The lumbar region consists of five vertebrae that are very large in size by comparison to the other vertebrae. The large size is necessary to support the individual's weight. The lumbar vertebrae are coded L1 through L5. Other than their large size, the lumbar vertebrae have no uniquely distinguishing landmarks.

The sacral and coccygeal regions consist of a number of fused vertebrae. The sacrum is composed of five vertebrae whose discs have ossified. The overall shape of the sacrum is somewhat like a wedge. The sacrum contains four pairs of **sacral foramina**. These allow nerves and blood vessels to pass from the pelvic region into the lower extremities. The coccyx is the terminal region of the vertebral column and consists of three or four fused vertebrae. Collectively, the coccygeal vertebrae resemble a rattlesnake's rattle.

The Rib Cage and Sternum

The primary organs of respiration are the lungs. The two lungs are housed within the rib cage, also referred to as the thoracic cavity. The rib cage is composed of 12 pairs of ribs arranged vertically (see Figure 6-5). The uppermost ribs and the lowermost ribs are somewhat smaller than the ribs in the middle of the rib cage. This gives the rib cage a barrel-like appearance. Anatomists refer to the individual ribs by number along with a letter "R" to indicate "rib." For example, the first pair of ribs is labeled R1 and the last pair of ribs is labeled R12.

Figure 6-6 is an illustration of a typical rib. The key landmarks of a typical rib are the *shaft* (the length of the rib), *neck and head* (the posterior terminal end of the rib that articulates with thoracic vertebrae), and *costal groove* (a depression running along the length of the shaft on the undersurface of the rib, where blood vessels and nerves are housed). Finally, the *costal angle* (also known as the "angle of the rib") is the abrupt change in curvature of the rib as it is bent in two directions, causing it to appear twisted upon its axis.

Posteriorly, all 12 pairs of ribs articulate with the vertebral column. One would think that because there are 12 pairs of ribs and likewise 12 thoracic vertebrae, each rib would articulate with its corresponding vertebra. However, the articulations are not that simple. Table 6-1 summarizes the articulations of the ribs with the thoracic vertebrae. The posterior articulations are between the head of the ribs and the corpora (the plural of corpus) of the thoracic vertebrae, and between the neck of the ribs and the transverse processes of the thoracic vertebrae (with the exception of R11 and R12, which do not articulate with the transverse processes). The head of each rib is held in place by the articular capsule, radiate ligament, and interarticular ligament. The neck of each rib is held in place by the

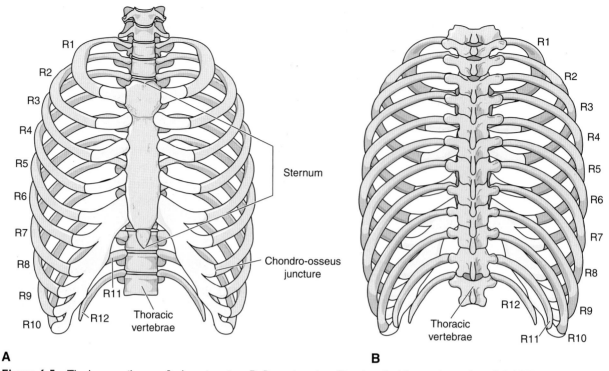

A   **B**

Figure 6-5 The human rib cage. **A**. Anterior view. **B**. Posterior view. (Reprinted with permission from LifeART image copyright © 2010. Lippincott Williams & Wilkins. All rights reserved.)

articular capsule, anterior costotransverse ligament, posterior costotransverse ligament, ligament of the neck of the rib, and ligament of the tubercle of the rib. The joints formed by these articulations are arthrodial or slightly gliding joints. Because of this arrangement, the lateral rib cage can rotate upward and outward or downward and inward, somewhat analogous to raising and lowering the handle on a water bucket. This increases and decreases the transverse volume of the thorax.

Unlike their posterior attachments, not all of the ribs have an anterior articulation. R1 through R10 articulate anteriorly with the **sternum**, more commonly known as the breastbone (see Figure 6-7). The sternum is an elongated bone that has three parts. From

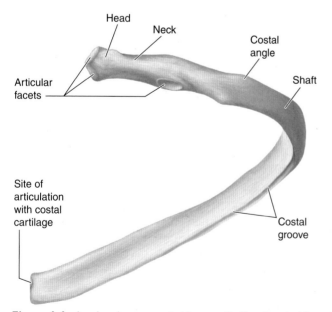

Figure 6-6 Landmarks on a typical human rib. (Reprinted with permission from Tank, P.W., Gest, T.R. (2008). *Lippincott Williams & Wilkins atlas of anatomy*. Baltimore, MD: Lippincott Williams & Wilkins.)

TABLE 6-1		
ARTICULATIONS OF THE RIBS WITH THE THORACIC VERTEBRAE		
Rib Number	**Articulates with the Corpus of**	**And the Transverse Process of**
1	T1	T1
2	T1 and T2	T2
3	T2 and T3	T3
4	T3 and T4	T4
5	T4 and T5	T5
6	T5 and T6	T6
7	T6 and T7	T7
8	T7 and T8	T8
9	T8 and T9	T9
10	T10	T10
11	T11	(None)
12	T12	(None)

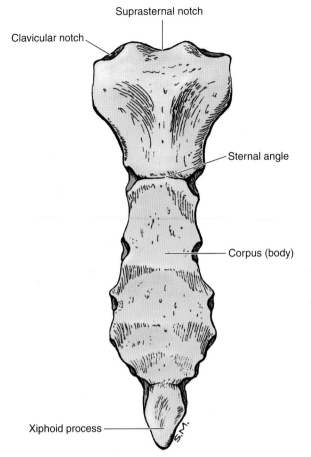

Figure 6-7   Landmarks on a human sternum. (Reprinted with permission from Agur, A.M., Dalley, A.F. (2008). *Grant's atlas of anatomy* (12th ed.). Baltimore, MD: Lippincott Williams & Wilkins.)

superior to inferior, these parts are the manubrium, corpus, and xiphoid (or ensiform) process. Landmarks on the manubrium include the suprasternal (or jugular) notch and the clavicular notches. The suprasternal notch is on the superior surface of the manubrium and can be felt by pressing down on the bone at the midline base of the neck. The clavicular notches are on the superior-lateral surfaces of the manubrium and are the point of articulation of the sternum with the clavicles (or collarbones). The corpus of the sternum is the anterior point of articulation for most of the ribs, as described more fully later. The xiphoid process does not have a direct articulation with any of the ribs. It is a delicate structure that should never be depressed during artificial resuscitation.

> ### *Why You Need to Know*
>
> *If pressure is placed directly upon the bony xiphoid process, it can break off of the body of the sternum. Being somewhat spearheaded in shape, the xiphoid process could be driven into the liver, resulting in a rupture of this vital organ that may prove fatal.*

The ribs themselves do not actually come in contact with the sternum; rather, the articulations between ribs and sternum are accomplished by a series of cartilages that extend from the anterior terminals of the ribs. R1 through R7 have direct articulations with the sternum, that is, each rib has its own cartilage that makes contact with the sternum. Because of this, R1 through R7 are referred to as **vertebrosternal** (or "true") ribs because they have direct articulations with the vertebral column and the sternum. R8 through R10 also have articulations with the sternum, but these attachments are more indirect. The cartilages for these ribs merge and join with the cartilage of R7 before making a single articulation with the sternum. Because of this, R8 through R10 are referred to as **vertebrochondral** or "false" ribs. Finally, R11 and R12 do not have an anterior attachment at all. Because their only articulation is with the vertebral column, they are referred to as **vertebral** or "floating" ribs. In terms of the specific location of the articulations for R1 through R10, R1 articulates with the lateral surface of the manubrium immediately inferior to the clavicular notch. R2's articulation is at the juncture between the manubrium and corpus of the sternum. Finally, the remaining ribs articulate with the sternum along the lateral edge of its corpus. All costal articulations with the sternum are held in place by a series of radiate sternocostal ligaments.

Two types of joints are formed by the articulations of the ribs with the sternum. The joint formed by the articulation of R1 with the manubrium is a synchondrosis, which means that the joint ossifies with age. The joints formed between R2 through R10 and the sternum are synovial, which allow a variety of movements. Considering the synovial action of the ribs' anterior articulations, the anterior rib cage can move upward and outward or downward and inward, similarly to raising and lowering the handle on an old water well pump. This action creates slight increases and decreases in the anteroposterior dimension of the thorax. It should be noted that this anterior action occurs simultaneously with the action of the lateral rib cage by virtue of the ribs' posterior articulations with the vertebral column.

The Pectoral Girdle

The pectoral girdle refers to the bony structure in the chest region that provides support for the upper extremities (see Figure 6-8). Two bones comprise the pectoral girdle: the **clavicle** and the **scapula**. The clavicle was mentioned briefly earlier. It is also known as the collarbone. There are two clavicles: each one articulates medially with the manubrium of the sternum at the

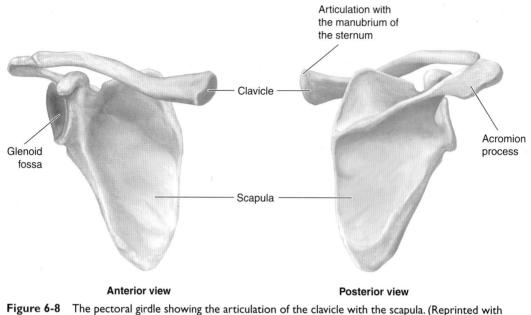

Anterior view   **Posterior view**

Figure 6-8   The pectoral girdle showing the articulation of the clavicle with the scapula. (Reprinted with permission from Tank, P.W., Gest, T.R. (2008). *Lippincott Williams & Wilkins atlas of anatomy.* Baltimore, MD: Lippincott Williams & Wilkins.)

clavicular notch. The lateral articulation of the clavicle is with the scapula (or shoulder blade), more specifically at the **acromion** which is its most lateral point. Therefore, each clavicle runs horizontally along the shoulder from the sternum to the scapula. The two scapulae are somewhat triangular in shape and lie dorsal to the upper seven or eight ribs. The scapulae are literally suspended in place by their articulations with the clavicles. Besides the acromion, each scapula has another important landmark—the **glenoid fossa**. The glenoid fossa is a crater-like depression in which the head of the humerus (the upper bone of the arm) rests. Being inquisitive, you no doubt wonder what the pectoral girdle has to do with respiration. The answer is that several muscles that play a part in respiration have their origin somewhere on the pectoral girdle. The same is true of the pelvic girdle.

The Pelvic Girdle

The pelvic girdle (see Figure 6-9) is to the lower extremities as the pectoral girdle is to the upper extremities. It consists of a pair of coxal bones. Each coxal bone has three parts: the **ilium**, the **ischium**, and the **pubis**. The pubis from each coxal bone merges anteriorly at the **pubic symphysis**. This joint is generally immovable but will "soften" in females during late pregnancy to allow the baby's head to pass through. The sacrum of the vertebral column articulates with the ilium posteriorly, forming the sacroiliac joint. The sacrum and coccyx together with the coxal bones is referred to as the bony pelvis. The **acetabulum**, a crater-like

depression along the lateral aspect of the ischium, is the point of articulation with the femur—the large, upper leg bone. Finally, running obliquely from the anterior superior iliac spine to the pubic symphysis on either side are the **inguinal ligaments**. These ligaments separate the contents of the lower abdomen from the lower extremities.

The Trachea and Bronchial Tree

The trachea (or windpipe) is a singular tube composed of a series of vertically arranged rings of cartilage that extends from the level of C6 to T5 (see Figure 6-10).

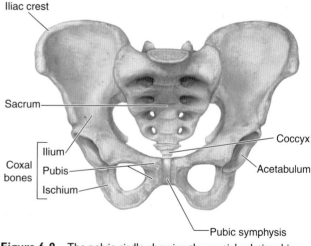

Figure 6-9   The pelvic girdle showing the spatial relationships of the coxal bones, sacrum, and coccyx. (Reprinted with permission from Tank, P.W., Gest, T.R. (2008). *Lippincott Williams & Wilkins atlas of anatomy.* Baltimore, MD: Lippincott Williams & Wilkins.)

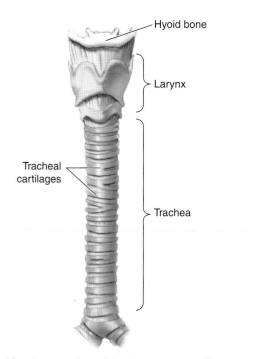

Figure 6-10   Anterior view of the human trachea. (Reprinted with permission from Premkumar, K. (2004). *The massage connection anatomy and physiology.* Baltimore, MD: Lippincott Williams & Wilkins.)

Its superior articulation is with the cricoid cartilage, which is the base of the larynx. This articulation is held together by the **cricotracheal ligament**. To articulate with the cricoid cartilage, the first tracheal ring must be large by comparison with the other tracheal rings. At its inferior terminal, the trachea bifurcates at the **carina**, forming two main stem bronchi—one bronchus proceeds to the left lung while the other proceeds to the right.

In all, the trachea is composed of approximately 16 to 20 horseshoe-shaped rings of hyaline cartilage. The rings are incomplete posteriorly; this posterior region is filled by fibrous tissue and smooth muscle fibers. The esophagus runs immediately behind and parallel to the trachea. The cartilaginous rings do not actually touch each other, as they are stacked vertically. A small space exists between adjacent rings. The spaces are filled with a fibroelastic membrane called the **intratracheal membrane**. This membrane is actually double layered. At each ring, the two layers separate. One layer covers the interior of the trachea, while the other covers the outside. Between the rings, the two layers come together to form a single unit. Superficial to the inner layer of the intratracheal membrane (i.e., inside the trachea) is a mucous membrane consisting of pseudostratified ciliated, columnar epithelial cells. **Goblet cells** are also located here; their purpose is to secrete mucous. The cilia within the mucous mem-

brane continuously push the mucous (and any foreign material it may trap) upward toward the larynx. Finally, **phagocytic cells** assist by ingesting bacteria and other undesirable organisms to prevent infection. With the cartilaginous rings and intratracheal membrane taken together, the net result is a tube that is approximately 11 to 12 cm in length and 2 to 2½ cm in diameter.

> ### *Why You Need to Know*
>
> *The word "phagocytic" comes from the Greek term "phagein" which literally means to eat. Phagocytic cells ingest and destroy foreign matter such as microorganisms. As such, they could be considered the immune system's first line of defense against disease within the respiratory system.*

As mentioned earlier, the trachea terminates inferiorly by bifurcating into two main stem bronchi. The bronchi will divide two more times into lobar (or secondary) bronchi and then again into segmental (or tertiary) bronchi. The three generations of bronchi form what is known as the bronchial tree (see Figure 6-11). Only a part of the main stem bronchi lay outside the lungs. The main stem bronchi pierce the

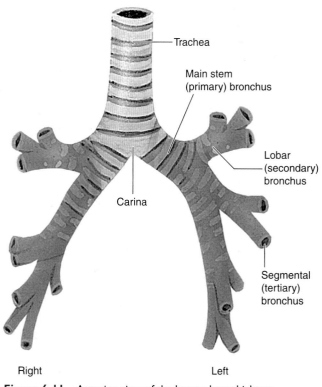

Figure 6-11   Anterior view of the human bronchial tree. (Reprinted with permission from Anatomical Chart Company.)

lung tissue at the **hilum** so that all further parts of the bronchial tree are housed entirely within the lungs.

The two main stem bronchi are approximately half the diameter of the trachea. The right bronchus is somewhat larger than the left bronchus in diameter, but it is also shorter in length. The two main stem bronchi are similar in structure to the trachea, except that they are not quite as cartilaginous and instead consist of more smooth muscle tissue. The right bronchus divides into three lobar bronchi, whereas the left bronchus divides into two.

Why You Need to Know

For people with the affliction, asthma is an immune system response to certain stimuli (e.g., cold air, physical exertion, allergens) that affects the bronchi. Spasms within the bronchi lead to inflammation of their internal membranes. The inflammation creates an obstruction that results in greater resistance to inspired air. This pathological condition will be discussed in greater detail in Chapter 7.

Each lobar bronchus supplies a specific lobe of the lungs. Being the astute student you are, you quickly deduce that the right lung has three lobes while the left lung has two. Within each lung, the lobes are further divided into smaller regions called segments. The lobar bronchi divide into the same number of segmental bronchi as there are segments in that lung (i.e., the three lobar bronchi of the right lung will further divide into 10 segmental bronchi, whereas the lobar bronchi of the left lung will divide into eight segmental bronchi).

The segmental bronchi will continue to divide approximately 20 times until the last generations are microscopic in size. As the bronchi continue to divide, there will be less and less cartilage and more and more smooth muscle. The last generation of bronchi gives way to the bronchioles, which in turn give way to the terminal bronchioles. Finally, the terminal bronchioles give way to the alveolar ducts, which open into the air sacs where the exchange of oxygen and carbon dioxide takes place at the **alveoli pulmoni**.

THE MUSCLES OF RESPIRATION

We turn our attention now to the muscles of respiration. A cycle of respiration has two phases: inspiration (i.e., breathing in) and expiration (i.e., breathing out). For each of these phases of respiration, there is a series of muscles whose action facilitates that particular phase. Therefore, for discussion purposes, the muscles of respiration are categorized as either muscles of inspiration or muscles of expiration. That said, it must be emphasized that sometimes there is not a clear dichotomy between muscles that are inspiratory and muscles that are expiratory. As you will see, a small number of muscles are involved in both inspiration and expiration. For example, a small number of muscles within the rib cage can be either inspiratory or expiratory in their function. Similarly, the muscles we typically classify as abdominal wall muscles (and therefore expiratory) are often active during inspiration.

In describing muscles—whether they are muscles of respiration, phonation, or articulation/resonance—the origin and insertion are usually highlighted as well as the action of the muscle. To act upon a body part, a muscle must have two attachments (usually to bone or cartilage). The point of attachment that remains relatively constant during muscle contraction is the origin and is usually the proximal structure. The insertion is usually the distal attachment and is associated with the body part that moves during contraction. In some cases, the action of a single muscle may be noteworthy because of its importance, but in most instances, it is the action of several muscles as a group that causes a particular body part to move. As the muscles are being discussed in the sections that follow, these characteristics will be described more fully. It should be noted that in the vast majority of cases muscles are paired, even though the discussion may refer to them in the singular case. If the discussion does not mention that a particular muscle is unpaired, you should assume that the muscle is paired.

The Muscles of Inspiration

The majority of muscles involved in respiration assist in regulating inspiration. These muscles are found throughout the thoracic region as well as the neck. To assist you in remembering the muscles, the muscles of inspiration have been organized into two groups: (1) primary muscles and (2) secondary muscles. The secondary muscles are subclassified according to their general location: (1) ventral thorax; (2) dorsal thorax; and (3) neck. The origins, insertions, and actions of the muscles of inspiration are summarized in Table 6-2.

Primary Muscles of Inspiration

Three muscles perform the greatest work during inspiration. They are the *diaphragm, external intercostals,* and *internal intercostals.* Of these, the diaphragm is unpaired, while the external and internal intercostals are paired.

TABLE 6-2

MUSCLES OF INSPIRATION WITH THEIR ORIGINS, INSERTIONS, AND ACTIONS

Muscle	Origin	Insertion	Action
Diaphragm	Sternal: xiphoid process Costal: inner aspect of R7–R12 Vertebral: lumbar vertebrae	Central tendon	The primary muscle of inhalation; increases the longitudinal volume of the thoracic cavity and compresses the abdominal viscera
External intercostals	Lower border of R1–R11	Upper surface of the rib immediately below	As each successive upper rib is anchored, the rib immediately below is elevated
Internal intercostals	Lower border of R1–R11	Upper surface of the rib immediately below	The portions of these muscles along the anterior rib cage (i.e., sternum) act similarly to the external intercostals
Lateral iliocostalis cervicis	Outer surfaces of R3–R6	C4–C6	Elevates R3–R6
Lateral iliocostalis thoracis	Upper edges of R7–R12	Lower edges of R1–R6	Works in concert with the lateral iliocostalis cervicis to stabilize the back of the rib cage wall
Latissimus dorsi	Spines of lower thoracic vertebrae, lumbar vertebrae, sacrum, and R10–R12	Upper humerus	With the humerus fixed, the fibers of this muscle that insert into R10–R12 will elevate them
Levator costarum brevis	Transverse processes of C7 and T1–11	Tubercle and angle of the rib immediately below	Elevates the posterior rib cage
Levator costarum longus	Fasciculi of lower four brevis muscles	Second rib below their origin	Elevates the lower posterior ribs
Pectoralis major	Medial clavicle and entire length of sternum	Greater tubercle of the humerus	With the humerus fixed, elevates the sternum and anterior ribs
Pectoralis minor	Anterior aspect of R2–R5	Coracoid process of the scapula	With the scapula fixed, elevates R2–R5
Scalenus anterior	Transverse processes of C3–C6	Inner border of upper surface of R1	Elevates R1
Scalenus medius	Transverse processes of C2–C7	Upper surface of R1	Elevates R1
Scalenus posterior	Posterior tubercles of C6–C7, and in some cases C5	Outer surface of R2	Elevates R2
Serratus anterior	R1–R8 and in some cases R9	Outer surface of the ribs and inner surface of the scapula	With the scapula fixed, elevates R1–R8 and in some cases R9
Serratus posterior superior	Spinous process of C7 and T1–T2 or in some cases T3	Lateral to the angle of R2–R5	Elevates R2–R5
Sternocleidomastoid	Sternum: anterior manubrium Clavicle: proximal (sternal) end	Two heads unite and attach to the mastoid process	With the head fixed, elevates the sternum and clavicle
Subclavius	Junction of R1 and its cartilage	Inferior surface of the clavicle, near the acromion of the scapula	With the clavicle fixed, elevates R1

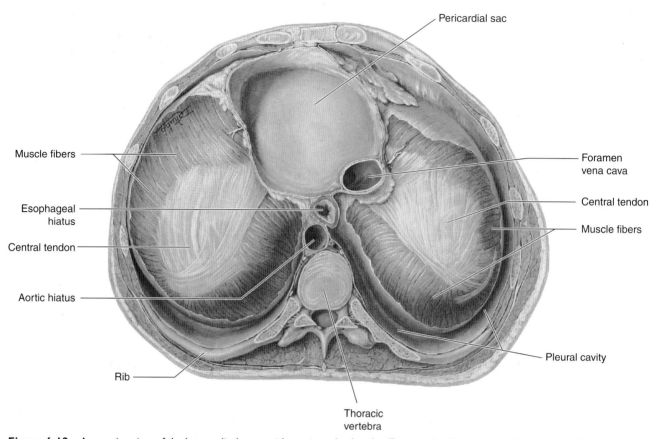

Figure 6-12 A superior view of the human diaphragm with pertinent landmarks. (Reprinted with permission from Agur, A.M., Dalley, A.F. (2008). *Grant's atlas of anatomy* (12th ed.). Baltimore, MD: Lippincott Williams & Wilkins.)

The Diaphragm

The diaphragm is the primary muscle of respiration, essentially being the workhorse of inspiration (see Figure 6-12). It is a single muscle that separates the thorax from the abdomen and is bi-domed, similarly to the humps on a camel. The dome on the right-hand side is situated a bit higher than the dome on the left because the liver occupies the upper right-hand quadrant of the abdomen. The diaphragm is among the largest muscles in the body. As it lies in place, it looks rather large and resembles an open umbrella. However, if you were to remove the diaphragm and spread it out flat on a table, you would note that it is relatively thin and broad.

The muscle fibers insert into a core of connective tissue called the **central tendon**, which is actually an aponeurosis that resembles a trifoliate leaf (somewhat like the maple leaf on a Canadian flag). Because the diaphragm separates the thorax from the abdomen, it is perforated with several openings to allow structures to pass from the thorax to the abdomen. Noteworthy are the (1) aortic hiatus, which allows the aorta to pass through to the abdomen; (2) foramen vena cava, which allows the vena cava to pass through

to the abdomen; and (3) the esophageal hiatus, which allows the esophagus to pass through on its way to the stomach.

The diaphragm has three points of origin: a sternal portion that attaches to the posterior surface of the xiphoid process; a costal portion that anchors onto the lowermost six ribs; and a lumbar portion that attaches to L1 through L3 by way of two legs called crura. Of these three attachments, the lumbar attachment is inflexible. Since the lumbar attachment is inferior to the body of the diaphragm, contraction will result in the diaphragm descending toward its lumbar attachments. In other words, during contraction, the diaphragm lowers toward the contents of the abdomen, thereby increasing the longitudinal (or vertical) volume of the thorax. Because of its costal and sternal attachments, contraction of the diaphragm will also pull down on the sternum and lower six ribs. In addition to these three points of origin, the diaphragm also has connections to the lungs (by way of the **visceral pleura**; a more thorough discussion of the pleurae can be found in the section that describes the lungs) and the fibrous layer of the **pericardium**.

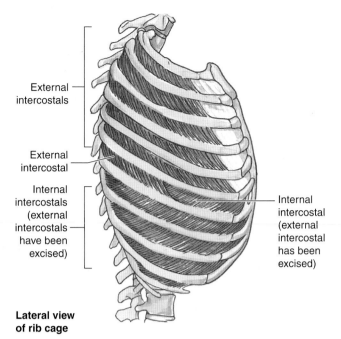

External
intercostals

External
intercostal

Internal
intercostals
(external
intercostals
have been
excised)

Internal
intercostal
(external
intercostal
has been
excised)

**Lateral view
of rib cage**

Figure 6-13   The internal and external intercostal muscles. (Reprinted with permission from Agur, A.M., Dalley, A.F. (2008). *Grant's atlas of anatomy* (12th ed.). Baltimore, MD: Lippincott Williams & Wilkins.)

The Intercostal Muscles

The external and internal intercostals also play a significant role in inspiration. As their name implies, the intercostal muscles can be found between the ribs (see Figure 6-13). The terms external and internal refer to their relative position to each other—the externals are superficial and the internals are deep. The 12 pairs of ribs have 11 spaces between them. Not surprisingly, there are 11 pairs of internal and external intercostal muscles. The fibers of the intercostal muscles are oriented obliquely (i.e., diagonally) although in opposite directions (essentially crisscrossing each other). This crisscrossing of the two muscles occurs throughout most of the distance between each adjacent pair of ribs. However, at the sternal and vertebral terminals, only one of the two muscles can be found. At the vertebral terminal, the external intercostals continue all the way to the vertebral column but the internal intercostals stop short of it. At the sternal terminal, the opposite is true. The internal intercostals proceed all the way to the sternum, but the external intercostals terminate approximately at the **chondro-osseous juncture** (the point where the rib ends and the cartilage that continues to the sternum begins). Any space that is not occupied by either the internal or external intercostal muscle is occupied by connective tissue.

The external intercostal muscles are stronger than the internal intercostals. The net action of the external intercostal muscles is to expand the rib cage by elevating the ribs. The origin for each external intercostal muscle is the rib immediately above, and the insertion is the rib immediately below. As each external intercostal muscle contracts, the lower rib to which it is attached elevates. The sum of the contraction of all 11 pairs of external intercostals then is an increase in the transverse volume of the thorax.

The internal intercostal muscles may actually have a dual purpose. Not only do they apparently assist in inspiration, but they are also thought to assist in forced expiration. The ventral fibers of the internal intercostals (i.e., from the sternum to approximately the chondro-osseous juncture) act in much the same way as the external intercostals. However, the greater length of the internal intercostals (i.e., from the chondro-osseous juncture to a few centimeters away from the vertebral column) has the opposite effect on the ribs. Along the lateral and posterior wall of the rib cage, the internal intercostal muscles *lower* the ribs.

The intercostal muscles are thought to have an additional function besides elevating and lowering the rib cage. Evidence seems to suggest that these muscles also keep the intercostal spaces rigid during respiration so that they do not bulge out during expiration or get drawn in during inspiration (Agur & Dalley, 2005). One might expect that by expanding the rib cage, the outward force that is placed on the ribs will generate an inward force on the intercostal spaces. Similarly, the inward force that is generated by contraction of the rib cage will generate an outward force on the intercostal spaces. The intercostal muscles serve to make the intercostal spaces rigid to prevent these forces from acting upon them.

Secondary Muscles of Inspiration

In all, 14 additional muscles can be considered muscles of inspiration, and any number of them may be called upon to assist when there is a greater demand for air intake. All of them are paired muscles. These secondary muscles include the *lateral iliocostalis cervicis, lateral iliocostalis thoracis, latissimus dorsi, levator costarum brevis, levator costarum longus, pectoralis major, pectoralis minor, scalenus anterior, scalenus medius, scalenus posterior, serratus anterior, serratus posterior superior, sternocleidomastoid,* and *subclavius.* In the following sections, these muscles have been subclassified according to their location: ventral thorax, dorsal thorax, and neck.

The Ventral Thorax

There are four pairs of muscles situated within the ventral thorax. These are the *pectoralis major, pectoralis minor, subclavius,* and *serratus anterior*

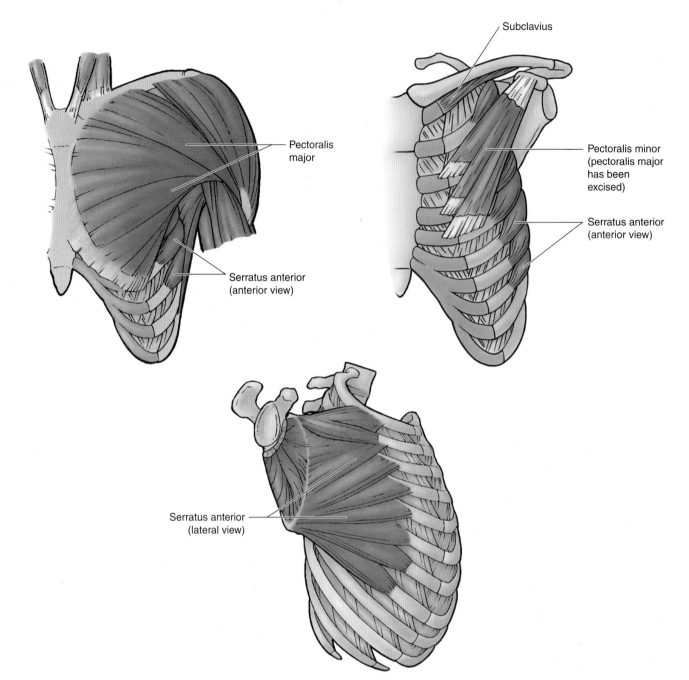

Figure 6-14 Muscles of the upper thorax, including the pectoralis major and minor, subclavius, and serratus anterior. (Reprinted with permission from Agur, A.M., Dalley, A.F. (2005). *Grant's atlas of anatomy* (11th ed.). Baltimore, MD: Lippincott Williams & Wilkins.)

(Figure 6-14 illustrates all four of these muscles). The primary purpose of these muscles is to assist in moving the arm and shoulder. However, they may play a minor role in respiration by assisting in deep inspiration, such as what would occur during vigorous exercise or yawning. The pectoralis major is a fan-shaped muscle that has three attachments: the clavicle, the sternum, and the humerus. The clavicular and sternal attachments are this muscle's origin while the humerus is the insertion. When the pectoralis major contracts and the humerus is in a fixed position, it will elevate the sternum and with it the anterior aspect of the ribs attached thereon.

The pectoralis minor is deep to the pectoralis major and runs from the anterior aspect of R2 through R5 to the scapula. When this muscle contracts and the scapula is in a fixed position, the net effect will be elevation of ribs 2 through 5.

The subclavius gets its name from the fact that it courses immediately below and parallel to the clavicle. Its origin is the chondro-osseous juncture of the first rib and its insertion is the inferior surface of the clavicle. When the clavicle is in a fixed position, contraction of this muscle will result in elevation of the first rib.

Finally, the serratus anterior is a sawtooth-shaped muscle (hence, the term "serratus") that has its origin on R1 through R8 (and in some cases R9) and its insertion on the inner surface of the scapula and outer surfaces of the ribs. When the scapula is in a fixed position and this muscle contracts, the first eight (and in some cases, the ninth) ribs will elevate.

The Dorsal Thorax

Six pairs of muscles comprise the dorsal region of the thorax. These are the *lateral iliocostalis cervicis, lateral iliocostalis thoracis, latissimus dorsi, levator costarum brevis, levator costarum longus,* and *serratus posterior superior.* The lateral iliocostalis cervicis originates on the outer surfaces of the third through sixth ribs and inserts into C4, C5, and C6. When it contracts, it elevates ribs 3 through 6. Its partner, the lateral iliocostalis thoracis, runs from the upper edges of R7 through R12 and terminates at the lower edges of the first six ribs. This muscle works in concert with the lateral iliocostalis cervicis by stabilizing the posterior rib cage wall. The lateral iliocostalis muscles can be seen in Figure 6-15.

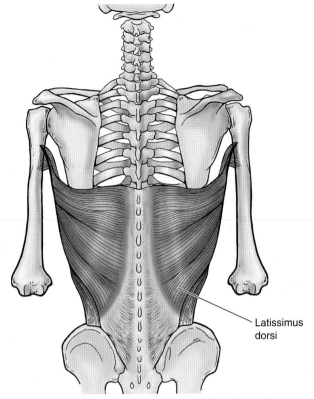

Figure 6-16 The latissimus dorsi muscle. (Modified with permission from Moore, K.L., Agur, A.M., Dalley, A.F. (2005). *Clinically oriented anatomy* (5th ed.). Baltimore, MD: Lippincott Williams & Wilkins.)

The latissimus dorsi muscle is wider medially than it is laterally (see Figure 6-16). It originates at the lower thoracic, lumbar, and sacral vertebrae and then inserts onto the upper aspect of the humerus. If the humerus is fixed in position and this muscle contracts, it will elevate the last three ribs.

The two sets of levator costarum muscles—the levator costarum brevis and the levator costarum longus (see Figure 6-17)—can be found along the posterior rib cage immediately lateral to the vertebral column. The terms "brevis" and "longus" refer to the relative length of the muscles. The brevis muscles are 12 in number; each rib receives a pair of brevis muscles. The origin of the brevis muscles is on the transverse processes of C7 through T11, with the insertion being the rib immediately below (i.e., the first pair of brevis muscles originate on the transverse processes of C7 and insert onto R1 and so on until the final pair of brevis muscles originates on the transverse processes of T11 and inserts onto R12). The longus muscles are confined to the last four pairs of ribs. Their origins are also on the transverse processes of the thoracic vertebrae, but their insertion is onto the second rib below (in essence making them approximately twice the length of the brevis muscles). With this in mind, the

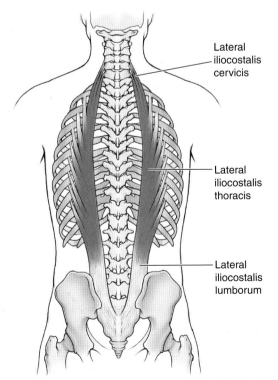

Figure 6-15 The lateral iliocostalis muscle. (Modified with permission from Moore, K.L., Agur, A.M., Dalley, A.F. (2009). *Clinically oriented anatomy* (6th ed.). Baltimore, MD: Lippincott Williams & Wilkins.)

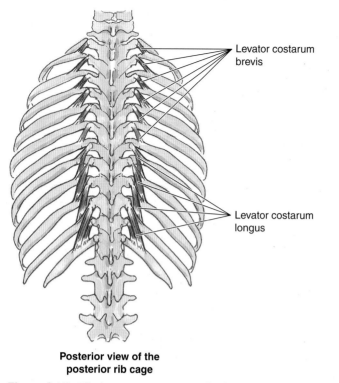

**Posterior view of the
posterior rib cage**

Figure 6-17 The levator costarum muscles (brevis and longus). (Modified with permission from Moore, K.L., Agur, A.M., Dalley, A.F. (2009). *Clinically oriented anatomy* (6th ed.). Baltimore, MD: Lippincott Williams & Wilkins.)

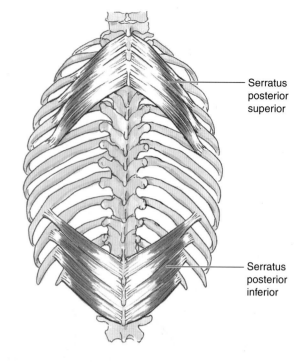

**Posterior view
of the rib cage**

Figure 6-18 The posterior serratus muscles (superior and inferior). (Modified with permission from Moore, K.L., Agur, A.M., Dalley, A.F. (2009). *Clinically oriented anatomy* (6th ed.). Baltimore, MD: Lippincott Williams & Wilkins.)

first pair of longus muscles originates on the transverse processes of T7 and inserts onto R9, whereas the last pair of longus muscles originates on the transverse processes of T10 and inserts onto R12. As their names imply, the levator costarum muscles elevate the posterior rib cage when they contract.

Finally, the serratus posterior superior is illustrated in Figure 6-18. The term "serratus" refers to the fact that this muscle has a jagged appearance as it inserts into the ribs. The serratus posterior superior originates on the spinous processes of C7 through T3 and then inserts lateral to the angle of R2 through R5. When it contracts, it elevates ribs 2 through 5.

The Neck Muscles

Four pairs of muscles in the neck region may contribute to inspiration. These are the *scalenus anterior, scalenus medius, scalenus posterior,* and *sternocleidomastoid.* All of these muscles are illustrated in Figure 6-19. As a whole, these four neck muscles serve to elevate the first two ribs, sternum, and clavicle. The net effect of this action is a slight increase in the anteroposterior dimension of the rib cage, such as would be needed for deep inhalation during strenuous exercise or yawning.

The three scalenes are among the deepest muscles in the neck. They originate on the transverse processes

and posterior tubercles of most of the cervical vertebrae and then insert either onto R1 (the scalenus anterior and medius) or R2 (the scalenus posterior). Contraction of the scalenus anterior and scalenus medius will result in elevation of the first rib, whereas contraction of the scalenus posterior will result in elevation of the second rib.

The sternocleidomastoid is an interesting muscle not only in its architecture but also in its action. It has three attachments, as its name implies: the sternum, the clavicle, and the **mastoid process** (the rounded part of the base of the skull immediately posterior to the ear). The primary purpose of this muscle is to allow us to turn our head from side to side. It accomplishes this action because of how it is situated. The mastoid process is behind the axis of the body (i.e., the vertebral column), but the sternum and clavicle are anterior to the axis. With the sternum and clavicle anchored, the sternocleidomastoid will pull upon the mastoid process, thereby turning the head to one side. However, the head turns to the side that is opposite to the muscle that is contracting. That is, when the sternocleidomastoid on the right side of the neck contracts, it turns the head to the left, and vice versa. If the mastoid process is anchored, the sternocleidomastoid will slightly elevate the sternum and clavicle.

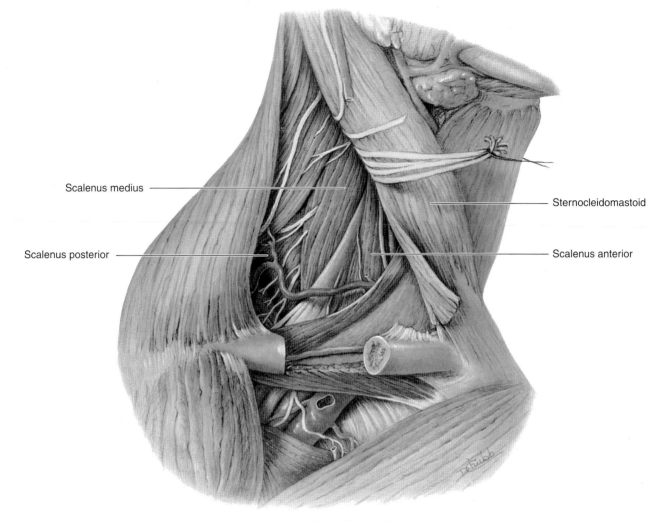

Scalenus medius

Sternocleidomastoid

Scalenus posterior

Scalenus anterior

Lateral view of the neck

Figure 6-19   Muscles of the neck, including the sternocleidomastoid and scalenus muscles (anterior, medius, and posterior). (Reprinted with permission from Agur, A.M., Dalley, A.F. (2008). *Grant's atlas of anatomy* (12th ed.). Baltimore, MD: Lippincott Williams & Wilkins.)

As a unified, coordinated whole, the muscles of inspiration serve to increase the longitudinal, transverse, and anteroposterior volumes of the thoracic cavity. Having the lungs contained within, expansion of lung tissue will also occur in any of these three dimensions that are at work. A more thorough discussion of these mechanics is reserved for the section on Physiology of the Respiratory System.

The Muscles of Expiration

The muscles of expiration are generally located in the abdomen and are categorized into two groups: primary muscles and secondary muscles. The primary muscles are found within the wall of the abdomen and hence they are referred to as abdominal wall muscles. All of the secondary muscles of expiration (with the exception of the quadratus lumborum) can be found within the thorax. The quadratus lumborum is a deep abdominal muscle. Table 6-3 summarizes the origins, insertions, and actions of the muscles of expiration.

Primary Muscles of Expiration

Four pairs of muscles within the abdominal wall play a part in expiration. These are the *external oblique, internal oblique, rectus abdominus,* and *transversus abdominus.* Removal of the epidermis of the abdomen will reveal the external oblique and rectus abdominus along with a network of connective tissue that binds the muscles together. The connective tissue includes the lumbodorsal fascia posteriorly, the inguinal ligament inferiorly, and the abdominal aponeurosis anteriorly. Of particular note is the latter. The abdominal aponeurosis forms the **linea alba** (literally, "white line") at the midline of the belly, coursing from the xiphoid process to the pubic symphysis.

TABLE 6-3

MUSCLES OF EXPIRATION WITH THEIR ORIGINS, INSERTIONS, AND ACTIONS

Muscle	Origin	Insertion	Action
External oblique	Posterior surfaces and lower borders of R5–R12	Anterior half of iliac crest and abdominal aponeurosis	Pulls the lower ribs downward and compresses the anterior and lateral walls of the abdomen
Internal intercostals	Lower border of R1–R11	Upper surface of the rib immediately below	The portions of these muscles along the sides and back of the rib cage pull down on the ribs
Internal oblique	Lateral half of inguinal ligament and anterior iliac crest	Linea alba and the cartilages of R10–R12 and in some cases R9	Pulls the lower ribs downward and compresses the anterior and lateral walls of the abdomen
Lateral iliocostalis lumborum	Lumbodorsal fascia, lumbar vertebrae, and posterior surface of the coxal bone	Lower edges of R7–R12	Depresses the lower six ribs
Lateral iliocostalis thoracis	Upper edges of R7–R12	Lower edges of R1–R6	Works in concert with the lateral iliocostalis lumborum to stabilize the back of the rib cage wall
Latissimus dorsi	Spines of lower thoracic vertebrae, lumbar vertebrae, sacrum, and R10–R12	Upper humerus	Contraction of this muscle as a whole compresses the lower portion of the rib cage wall
Quadratus lumborum	Iliac crest and iliolumbar ligament	Transverse processes of L1–L4; lower border of R12	Pulls down on R12
Rectus abdominus	Crest of the pubis	Cartilages of R5–R7 and xiphoid process	Pulls down on the sternum and lower ribs and compresses the anterior abdominal wall
Serratus posterior inferior	Spinous process of T11–T12 and L1–L3	Inferior border of R8–R12	Depresses R8–R12
Subcostals	Same course as the internal intercostals	Same as the internal intercostals but may traverse more than one rib	Pull down on the ribs to which they are inserted
Transversus abdominus	Inner surfaces of R6–R12, diaphragm, and transversus thoracis	Deepest layer of the abdominal aponeurosis and the pubis	Compresses the anterior and lateral walls of the abdomen
Transversus thoracis	Posterior surface of sternum, xiphoid process, and R5–R7	Lower borders and inner surfaces of R2–R6	Pull downward on R2–R6

With the linea alba positioned vertically in the middle of the abdomen, the muscles of the abdominal wall are all paired with one on each side of midline.

Upon dissection of the epidermis and connective tissue, the external oblique and rectus abdominus are the first muscles in view. The external oblique is the largest and strongest of all the abdominal wall muscles (see Figure 6-20). It is broad and thin, originating on the posterior surfaces of the lower eight ribs

and terminating at the anterior aspect of the iliac crest as well as the abdominal aponeurosis. As its name implies, the fibers of the external oblique run in a diagonal direction. When this muscle contracts, it pulls the lower ribs downward and also compresses the anterior and lateral walls of the abdomen.

To be able to view the internal oblique, the external oblique and rectus abdominus must be removed. The fibers of the internal oblique also course in a diagonal

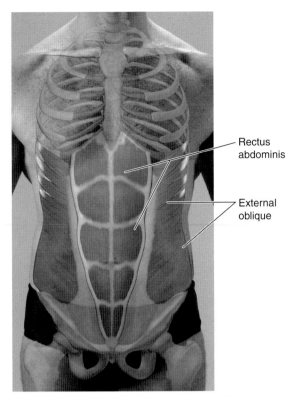

Figure 6-20 labels: Rectus abdominis / External oblique

Figure 6-20 The external oblique and rectus abdominus muscles. (Modified with permission from Agur, A.M., Dalley, A.F. (2008). *Grant's atlas of anatomy* (12th ed.). Baltimore, MD: Lippincott Williams & Wilkins.)

rior two-thirds of the iliac crest, whereas the insertion is the linea alba and the 10th through 12th ribs (and in some people, the 9th). Contraction of this muscle will pull downward on the lower ribs and compress the anterior and lateral walls of the abdomen.

The rectus abdominus is immediately lateral to the linea alba and runs parallel to it. Along its length, the rectus abdominus is compartmentalized by a series of tendinous inscriptions, giving this muscle the "washboard effect" when it is well developed. The fibers of the rectus abdominus course vertically from the pubis to the xiphoid process and R5 through R7 (see Figure 6-20). When the rectus abdominus contracts, it pulls down on the sternum and ribs 5 through 7. This muscle also assists in compressing the anterior abdominal wall.

Once the internal oblique is dissected, the deepest abdominal wall muscle can be seen—the transversus abdominus (see Figure 6-21). Fibers of this muscle run horizontally from the inner surfaces of R6 through R12, the diaphragm, and the transversus thoracis to the pubis and abdominal aponeurosis. Contraction of the transversus abdominus causes a compression of the anterior and lateral walls of the abdomen.

It should be noted that the primary purpose of the abdominal wall muscles is to allow an individual to bend his or her body. If both muscles in each pair contract, the body will bend forward. If contraction is unilateral (i.e., only one of the two muscles in each pair contracts), the body will bend in the opposite direction. In terms of expiration, if the vertebral column is

direction, although the direction is opposite that of the external oblique (see Figure 6-21 and compare with Figure 6-20). The origin of the internal oblique is the lateral half of the inguinal ligament and the ante-

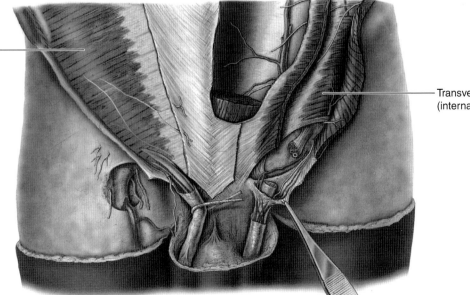

Internal oblique (external oblique excised)

Transversus abdominus (internal oblique excised)

Lower abdomen

Figure 6-21 The internal oblique and transversus abdominus muscles. (Reprinted with permission from Agur, A.M., Dalley, A.F. (2008). *Grant's atlas of anatomy* (12th ed.). Baltimore, MD: Lippincott Williams & Wilkins.)

kept rigid, contraction of these muscles will depress the ribs, thereby decreasing thoracic volume while at the same time generating increased intra-abdominal pressure by compressing the anterior and lateral abdominal walls.

Secondary Muscles of Expiration

There are eight pairs of secondary muscles of expiration. They include the *internal intercostals, lateral iliocostalis lumborum, lateral iliocostalis thoracis, latissimus dorsi, quadratus lumborum, serratus posterior inferior, subcostals,* and *transversus thoracis.* All of these muscles are found in the thorax except the quadratus lumborum, which is found deep within the abdomen.

You may recall that the internal intercostals, lateral iliocostalis, and latissimus dorsi were all described earlier in the section that described the muscles of inspiration (refer back to Figures 6-13, 6-15, and 6-16, respectively). These muscles play a dual role in respiration. You learned earlier that the portions of the internal intercostals that abut the sternum function similarly to the external intercostals, that is, they perform an inspiratory function. However, when the lateral and posterior portions of the internal intercostals contract, they depress the rib cage, which is an expiratory function. Similarly, the latissimus dorsi plays an inspiratory role when only the costal portion of this muscle contracts, but it plays an expiratory role when the entire body of the muscle contracts. When the whole muscle contracts, the latissimus dorsi compresses the lower portion of the rib cage. Finally, the lateral iliocostalis is a muscle that has three parts: cervicis, thoracis, and lumborum. The cervicis and thoracis bundles are involved in inspiration, whereas the lumborum and thoracis bundles are involved in expiration. The lateral iliocostalis lumborum originates at the lumbodorsal fascia, lumbar vertebrae, and posterior surface of the coxal bone and inserts into the lower edges of ribs 7 through 12. When it contracts, it depresses the lower six ribs. The lateral iliocostalis thoracis works with the lumborum bundle by simply stabilizing the back of the rib cage (which it also does with the lateral iliocostalis cervicis during inspiration).

The remaining three pairs of expiratory muscles within the thorax—the serratus posterior inferior, subcostals, and transversus thoracis—all serve to depress a number of the ribs. The serratus posterior inferior begins on the spinous processes of T11 through L3 and inserts into the inferior border of R8 through R12 (see Figure 6-18). When this muscle contracts, it pulls down on ribs 8 through 12. The subcostal muscles (see Figure 6-22) can be seen running in an oblique

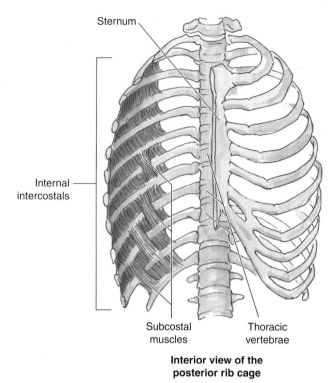

Figure 6-22   The subcostal muscles. (Reprinted with permission from Agur, A.M., Dalley, A.F. (2008). *Grant's atlas of anatomy* (12th ed.). Baltimore, MD: Lippincott Williams & Wilkins.)

direction on the internal surface of the lower ribs near their angles, in relative proximity to the vertebral column. The specific ribs into which they insert differ from person to person. Contraction of these muscles will pull down on the ribs to which they are attached. Finally, the transversus thoracis muscles resemble the legs of a spider as they extend from the posterior surface of the sternum, xiphoid process, and R5-R7 to the posterior surfaces of R2 through R6 (see Figure 6-23). When this muscle contracts, it pulls downward on ribs 2 through 6.

The final secondary muscle of expiration is the quadratus lumborum (see Figure 6-24). To see this muscle from the ventral side of the body, the abdominal contents (e.g., intestines, stomach, liver) must be removed. The point of origin for this muscle is the iliac crest and iliolumbar ligament. Its insertion is the transverse processes of L1–L4 and the lower border of the 12th rib. Its action is thought to be to anchor R12 during forced expiration.

NEURAL INNERVATION OF THE MUSCLES OF RESPIRATION

In Chapter 4, you were introduced to the human nervous system. A thorough discussion of the nervous system was provided there, and therefore will not be provided here. However, it is important that you

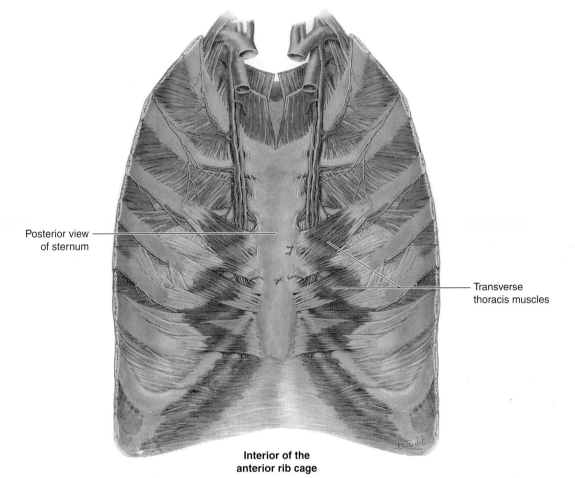

Posterior view of sternum

Transverse thoracis muscles

Interior of the anterior rib cage

Figure 6-23   The transversus thoracis muscles. (Modified with permission from Agur, A.M., Dalley, A.F. (2008). *Grant's atlas of anatomy* (12th ed.). Baltimore, MD: Lippincott Williams & Wilkins.)

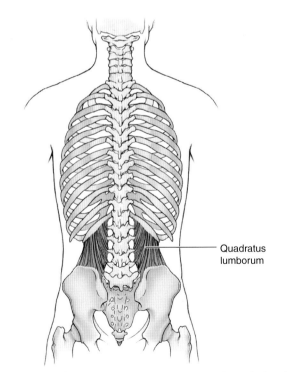

Quadratus lumborum

Figure 6-24   The quadratus lumborum muscle. (Modified with permission from Moore, K.L., Agur, A.M., Dalley, A.F. (2009). *Clinically oriented anatomy* (6th ed.). Baltimore, MD: Lippincott Williams & Wilkins.)

understand the neural innervation of the many of the important muscles of respiration because in many cases, pathology of the respiratory system may be a result of nerve damage (see Chapter 7 for a more thorough discussion of the impact of neurological impairment on breathing).

Table 6-4 provides a summary of most of the muscles of inspiration and expiration and their neural connections. In all, 23 spinal nerves (8 cervical, 12 thoracic, and 3 lumbar) are involved in the motor innervation of the muscles of respiration. In addition, the sternocleidomastoid is innervated in part by a cranial nerve.

As was mentioned earlier in this chapter, the diaphragm is the primary muscle of respiration, accounting for the longitudinal dimension of thoracic cavity expansion. The diaphragm is innervated by the **phrenic nerve**, which arises from the third through fifth cervical spinal nerves. Two branches of the phrenic nerve pass through the neck in proximity to the scalenus anterior muscle and carotid artery on their way to the thoracic cavity. The left phrenic nerve proceeds directly to the diaphragm to innervate it, but the right phrenic nerve passes through the

TABLE 6-4

NEURAL INNERVATION OF SELECTED MUSCLES OF RESPIRATION

Muscle	Innervation
Diaphragm	C3–C5 (phrenic nerve)
External intercostals	T1–T11 (intercostal nerves)
External oblique	T7–T12
Internal intercostals	T1–T11 (intercostal nerves)
Internal oblique	T7–L1
Latissimus dorsi	C6–C8
Levator costarum muscles	C8–T11
Pectoralis major	C5–C8
Pectoralis minor	C5–C8
Quadratus lumborum	T12–L3
Rectus abdominus	T7–T12
Scalenus muscles	C2–C8
Serratus anterior	C5–C7; T2 and T3
Serratus posterior inferior	T9–T12
Serratus posterior superior	T2 and T3
Sternocleidomastoid	Spinal accessory (cranial nerve XI); C1–C5
Subclavius	C5 and C6
Subcostal	T1–T11 (intercostal nerves)
Transversus abdominus	T7–L1
Transversus thoracis	T2–T6

foramen vena cava at the level of T10 and then rises to meet the diaphragm. In addition to innervating the diaphragm, the phrenic nerves also provide sensory innervation to the **mediastinum, pleurae**, liver, and gall bladder.

> ### Why You Need to Know
>
> *Damage to the phrenic nerves will result in paralysis of the diaphragm. Because the diaphragm is responsible for mediating longitudinal expansion of the thorax—and hence accounts in part for tidal volume—an individual with paralysis of the diaphragm will require a ventilator to assist in respiration. The good news is that since the diaphragm receives bilateral innervation, it would be difficult (although not impossible) to completely paralyze it. That would require a pathological condition that is more central rather than peripheral. Paralysis and its effect on the breathing mechanism will be discussed in more detail in Chapter 7.*

Secondary to the diaphragm, the intercostal muscles play a significant role in the inspiratory process.

Both sets of intercostals muscles (i.e., external and internal) are innervated by the intercostal nerves, which are formed by the anterior (i.e., ventral) rami of spinal nerves T1 through T11. Each intercostal muscle receives its own intercostal nerve. However, the thoracic spinal nerves innervate more than just the intercostal muscles.

The remaining muscles of inspiration are innervated by various combinations of cervical and/or thoracic spinal nerves. The pectoralis major and minor are innervated by C5 through C8. The subclavius receives its innervation from cervical spinal nerves 5 and 6. The three pairs of scalenus muscles are innervated by C2 through C8. The levator costarum muscles (brevis and longus) receive innervation from C8 as well as thoracic spinal nerves 1 through 11. The serratus anterior receives innervation from cervical (C5–C7) and thoracic (T2 and T3) spinal nerves. The serratus posterior superior is innervated by T2 and T3. Finally, the sternocleidomastoid is the only muscle that receives innervation from a cranial nerve (the spinal accessory nerve—cranial nerve XI). However, it also receives motor commands from cervical spinal nerves 1 through 5.

The muscles of expiration within the abdominal wall are all innervated by spinal nerves T7 through T12; the internal oblique and transversus abdominus are innervated by the first lumbar spinal nerve (L1) as well. The quadratus lumborum is innervated by T12 in addition to L1–L3. The subcostals are innervated by the intercostal nerves (T1 through T11). The latissimus dorsi (which is also classified as a muscle of inspiration) is innervated by cervical spinal nerves 6 through 8. The serratus posterior inferior is innervated by T9 through T12. Finally, the transversus thoracis receives its innervation from thoracic spinal nerves 2 through 6.

THE LUNGS AND PLEURAE

The two lungs consist of spongy, porous tissue and are housed within the rib cage, one on the right-hand side and the other on the left (see Figure 6-25A). Between the two lungs, posterior to the sternum, and anterior to the vertebral column is the mediastinum, which contains all of the thoracic viscera except the lungs (see Figure 6-25B). These viscera include the heart and pericardium, aorta, vena cava, phrenic nerves, esophagus, trachea, main stem bronchi, lymph nodes of the central thorax, and lesser blood vessels and nerves. The mediastinum is encapsulated by loose connective tissue.

A comparison between the two lungs reveals that the right lung is larger than the left, but it is also

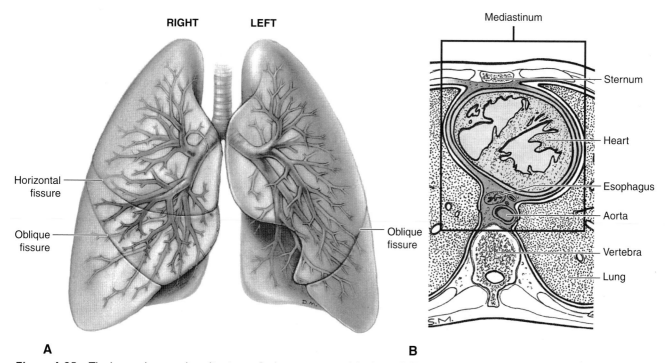

RIGHT   **LEFT**

Horizontal fissure

Oblique fissure

Oblique fissure

Mediastinum

Sternum

Heart

Esophagus

Aorta

Vertebra

Lung

A

B

Figure 6-25 The human lungs and mediastinum. **A**. Anterior view of the lungs. **B**. Transverse section through the lungs and mediastinum. (Reprinted with permission from Agur, A.M., Dalley, A.F. (2008). *Grant's atlas of anatomy* (12th ed.). Baltimore, MD: Lippincott Williams & Wilkins.)

shorter in part because of the liver below it. The left lung is smaller because the heart occupies some of the space of the left lung, in a concavity called the **cardiac impression**. Both lungs are divided into lobes: the right lung has three lobes separated by the oblique and horizontal fissures, whereas the left lung has two lobes separated by the oblique fissure. You may recall from the discussion of the bronchial tree that each lobe receives its own lobar or secondary bronchus. Although the bronchial tree has considerable smooth muscle tissue within it (especially as the tree divides further and further), lung tissue has very few smooth muscle fibers. This means that the action of the lungs is passive; that is, the lungs must rely on outside forces to act upon them to make them expand and contract during respiration. The interior volume of an average adult male's lungs is approximately 5 liters (5000 cc); in an average adult female, the volume is approximately 4 liters (4000 cc). That is, for an adult female, the capacity of air for each lung would be equivalent to a 2-liter bottle of your favorite soft drink.

In adults, there are approximately 300 million alveoli pulmoni—small pits or depressions within the air sacs of the lungs. At birth, there are approximately 25 million alveoli. That number increases to the adult number of 300 million by age 8 years, and remains at that number throughout life. The alveoli pulmoni consist of Type I and II cells as well as phagocytic cells. Type I

cells are epithelial cells arranged in a single layer. Type II cells are responsible for producing pulmonary surfactant, a somewhat soapy substance that breaks up surface tension within the alveoli during respiration. Phagocytic cells in the lungs assist in eliminating any bacteria or other organisms that have found their way to the alveoli. The alveoli pulmoni are engorged with an elaborate system of capillaries where carbon dioxide is released from the bloodstream so that it can be exhaled, and oxygen is taken up by the bloodstream so it can be distributed throughout the body.

Why You Need to Know

A baby born prematurely tends to have underdeveloped lungs. For example, Type II cells may not be fully developed, leading to a reduction in the production of pulmonary surfactant resulting in an increase in surface tension within the alveoli. The baby may show signs of respiratory distress and may be placed on a ventilator until the lungs develop more fully to allow her to breathe independently. Similarly, underdevelopment of phagocytic cells may leave the baby susceptible to infectious processes such bacterial or viral pneumonia.

Each lung is somewhat triangular in shape, with the apex extending into the root of the neck and the base making contact with the diaphragm. Each lung is enclosed within a double-layered membrane called the pleurae. The pleurae that surround each lung are independent of each other. This is a protective mechanism; if the pleura of one lung is compromised, the other lung will not be affected. The pleurae not only line the lungs but also line the inner surface of the rib cage, superior surface of the diaphragm, and mediastinum. The outer layer of each pleura lines the inner surface of the ribs and hence is referred to as the **costal** (or **parietal**) **pleura**. The inner layer covers the diaphragm and is known as the visceral pleura. The thoracic visceral pleura continues beyond the diaphragm and is continuous with the visceral lining of the abdomen. A potential space exists between the two pleurae; this space is referred to as the pleural cavity or intrapleural space and contains a serous fluid that allows the two layers to glide upon each other without friction during respiration.

The two layers of the pleurae adhere to each other and are airtight. This vacuum is known as **pleural linkage** and essentially binds the lungs to the interior of the rib cage and to the superior surface of the diaphragm. Approximately 75% of the surface of the lungs is in contact with the interior wall of the rib cage. The remaining 25% is in direct contact with the superior surface of the diaphragm as well as indirectly with the abdominal wall muscles. This means that the diaphragm must exhibit greater movement than the rib cage to effect comparable changes in lung volume.

Because of pleural linkage, whenever the rib cage and/or diaphragm are displaced, the lungs will also displace proportionately. Analogous to Mary and her little lamb (i.e., the rib cage and the diaphragm are Mary and the lungs are her little lamb), wherever Mary goes, the lamb is sure to follow. This is a very important part of the physiology of breathing.

Physiology of the Respiratory System

In the first half of this chapter, the physiology of respiration was alluded to during the discussion of various anatomical structures. In this section of the chapter, a more thorough and integrated discussion of respiratory physiology will be presented. With a firm understanding of the anatomical structures of respiration, you should have little difficulty comprehending how the process of respiration takes place. The clinician in training must be able to describe respiratory physiology as it relates to normal, quiet breathing (referred to as vegetative breathing), and then be able to describe the changes that take place when respiration is used for the purpose of vocal activity. Before discussing the actual mechanics though, you need to understand some basic concepts that are related to breathing.

BASIC CONCEPTS

Volume, Pressure, and Airflow

To understand the mechanics of inspiration, you must understand some very basic concepts. Two of these are volume and pressure. These two concepts are integrally related to each other. According to **Boyle's law**, assuming temperature is kept at a constant, volume and pressure will be inversely related to each other. In other words, as the value of one increases, the value of the other decreases proportionately. This very simple law of physics applies to gases, and of course, the air we breathe is a gas. Figure 6-26 illustrates the relationship. Assume we have two containers, one being larger than the other. Assume also that each container is filled with the very same number of air molecules. Because one container is larger than the other, its interior volume is also larger. The air molecules in the larger container "spread out" to fill the interior volume of that container. For the smaller container, the air molecules are more compacted because they do not have as much interior space to occupy as the larger container. Because the air molecules in the smaller container are compacted, they exert a greater amount of pressure within the container as compared with the larger container where the molecules are not quite as compacted. If there was a way to further reduce the interior volume of the container, the air pressure within would continue to increase as its volume gets

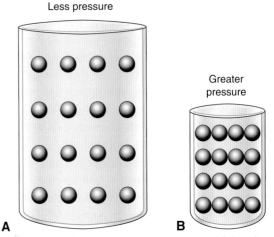

Figure 6-26   A schematic representation of Boyle's law. As volume decreases (as depicted when going from container A to container B), air molecules are more compacted, resulting in greater pressure within the container.

smaller and smaller. The inverse is also true: if you make the container larger and larger, its interior volume will also get larger and larger and along with it, the pressure within will continue to decrease.

Now let us move from the containers to the human lungs. The lungs are also containers of air, and their interior volume can be manipulated. Recall from the discussion of anatomy that the lungs consist of relatively few smooth muscle fibers, so they must be manipulated by external forces. As the lungs expand, their interior volume increases. As the lungs contract, their interior volume decreases. Taking Boyle's law into consideration, as the lungs expand, the air pressure within the alveoli decreases because the air molecules "spread out" to occupy the increased volume. Conversely, as the lungs contract, the air pressure within the alveoli increases because the air molecules become more compacted.

To understand the process of inspiration, one must also understand fluid mechanics. The term "fluid" is used to denote any gas or liquid. One of the principles of fluid mechanics states that a fluid will always flow from areas of greater pressure to areas of lesser pressure. Of course, this implies that there are two areas (referred to as gradients) of pressure. Recall from the discussion immediately above that one gradient of pressure is within the lungs. This is referred to as **pulmonary pressure**. The other gradient of pressure is the air outside the body—what we commonly refer to as **atmospheric pressure**. If pulmonary pressure is equal to atmospheric pressure, there will be no flow of air from one gradient of pressure to the other. However, if either of these pressures changes relative to the other, air will flow from the gradient of greater pressure to the gradient of lesser pressure.

Understanding these basic concepts, you are well equipped to comprehend how inspiration takes place. Before a breath is taken, when the lungs are at **resting volume**, pulmonary pressure and atmospheric pressure are essentially equivalent. Expansion of the lungs causes their interior volume to increase, thereby resulting in a decrease in pulmonary pressure relative to atmospheric pressure. Because fluids always flow from gradients of greater pressure to gradients of lesser pressure, the air outside the body will enter the respiratory passageway and fill the lungs until pulmonary pressure once again is equal to atmospheric pressure, at which time airflow will cease. The individual has just "taken a breath," that is, inspired air.

Notice that humans inspire air by creating negative pressure within the lungs. Because of this, humans are referred to as negative pressure breathers. Some animals are positive pressure breathers. For example, a frog generates positive pressure by puffing its cheeks in and out like a piston. A frog has no diaphragm, so it cannot generate negative pressure in its lungs.

Passive Forces

When the thorax expands during inspiration, several physical phenomena are set into motion. These are referred to as passive forces and include *elastic recoil, torque, intra-abdominal pressure*, and *gravity*. Newton's Third Law of Motion comes into play here. It states that for every action, there is an opposite and equal reaction. Elastic recoil, torque, and intra-abdominal pressure are all forces that conform to this basic law. First, because the lungs are composed of elastic tissue, they have the ability to be "stretched" during inspiration. Expansion of lung tissue creates a certain force, and there is an opposite and equal force that acts upon the lungs to collapse them. This is elastic recoil. Second, rib cage expansion is accomplished by rotation of the ribs upon their longitudinal axes. The force that is generated by this rotation is known as torque. Once again, when the ribs rotate upon their axes, an opposite and equal force exists in opposition to the torque that is created. Third, when the diaphragm contracts, it descends toward the abdomen. Think of the diaphragm as acting somewhat like a piston. As it descends, it applies downward pressure on the abdominal contents, creating what is referred to as intra-abdominal pressure. Intra-abdominal pressure exerts itself proportionately on the inferior surface of the diaphragm, attempting to force the diaphragm back to its resting position.

In part, these three phenomena account for the expiratory phase of respiration along with gravity. Gravity assists the expiratory phase by acting upon the ribs. As the ribs are elevated during inspiration, gravity pulls on them to lower them back to their resting position. The net effect of these four passive forces is contraction of the rib cage, which subsequently results in expiration. In some cases, these passive forces are all that is needed to mediate expiration. In other cases, expiration is more active (i.e., it requires contraction of certain muscles).

Lung Volumes and Capacities

Obviously, the lungs are not always completely filled with air, neither are they ever completely empty. In fact, at rest when an individual is between breaths, the lungs are about 40% full of air. An individual cannot force out all the air in his lungs, neither does he typically breathe in as deeply as he possibly can during quiet vegetative breathing. As such, the lungs have certain volumes. A lung volume is a discreet unit that is independent of all other volumes. In other words, volumes do not overlap. **Tidal volume (TV)** is the air that is normally exchanged during a complete respiratory cycle (i.e., an inspiration followed by an expiration). In a typical adult male, TV is approximately 600 cubic centimeters (cc) or milliliters (ml) and in adult females TV is approximately 450 cc.

The lungs have volumes that extend beyond a normal tidal inspiration and a normal tidal expiration. These are referred to as **inspiratory reserve volume (IRV)** and **expiratory reserve volume (ERV)**, respectively. A typical adult has an IRV of approximately 2500 cc and an ERV of approximately 1000 cc. You can reach your IRV by taking a normal tidal inspiration, stopping, and then gulping in as much additional air as you can. IRV will be the amount of additional air you gulped in. By the same token, you can access your ERV by taking a normal tidal expiration, stopping, and then forcing out all the air you can. The additional air you forced out (before you started wheezing and coughing!) is ERV.

Even upon forcing out as much air as possible, some air will remain in the lungs. This is known as **residual volume (RV)** and remains in the lungs to keep them from collapsing. RV is approximately 1100 cc in a typical adult. Finally, air fills structures within the respiratory passageway outside the lungs—the oral and nasal cavities, larynx, trachea, and bronchi. These are referred to as dead air spaces, and they contain approximately 150 cc of air. Incidentally, upon inspiration, the first 150 cc of air to enter the lungs will come from the dead air spaces. Conversely, the final 150 cc of air released from the lungs upon expiration will fill these dead air spaces.

Although lung volumes are discreet, independent units, lung capacities are not. Lung capacities are formed by the combination of lung volumes. Humans only use a portion of their total lung volume during vegetative breathing and vocal activity. When there is a greater demand for air (e.g., when exercising or when engaging in vocal activity), we have the ability to call upon our IRV and/or ERV. In other words, healthy lungs have the *capacity* to meet our every demand for air. Lung capacities include **inspiratory capacity (IC), functional residual capacity (FRC), vital capacity (VC),** and **total lung capacity (TLC)**. IC can be expressed as TV + IRV. In other words, an individual's IC is the amount of air he or she can maximally inhale from a resting expiratory level. FRC is equal to ERV + RV; that is, FRC is the amount of air in the lungs at a resting expiratory level. The formula for VC is IRV + TV + ERV.

It is the amount of air a person can maximally and forcibly exhale upon taking a deep inspiration. Finally, TLC is the combination of all lung volumes (IRV + TV + ERV + RV).

Why You Need to Know

All lung capacities are important from a clinical standpoint, but VC is very likely of greatest clinical interest to a speech–language pathologist because it includes TV, IRV, and ERV—all of the volumes that may come into play during vocal activity. One can determine by using a mathematical formula the expected VC for a given individual. For adult males, expected VC can be determined by multiplying the person's age by 0.112, subtracting that number from 27.63, and then multiplying the result by that individual's height (in centimeters, or cm). For adult females, one would multiply the individual's age by 0.101, subtract that number from 21.78, and then multiply the result by the individual's height (in cm). VC is typically used as a general indicator of an individual's ability to provide breath support for vocal activity. In some cases, persons with voice disorders or neuromotor problems will exhibit a diminished ability to provide adequate breath support for speech. In these cases, VC may be considerably less than what the clinician may expect. An instrument called a **spirometer** *is used to measure VC, and norms exist to give the clinician an idea as to how much VC a person should be able to generate. Although beyond the scope of this textbook to discuss, there are other instruments that we use to study respiration. These include, but are not limited to, the* **pneumotachometer** *and* **plethysmograph**. *A more thorough discussion of instrumentation and its use in studying respiratory physiology can be found in Hixon, Weismer, and Hoit (2008).*

Lung volumes and capacities can vary considerably from person to person. An individual's size, gender, and age often influence his or her lung volumes and capacities. For example, VC tends to change with age. It first increases gradually up until a person reaches the age of 20 years, levels off until age 25 years, and then decreases at the rate of approximately 100 cc each year thereafter. Similarly, a person's position (e.g., lying down vs. standing up) and posture will also affect measurements of lung volume and capacity. In the supine position, for example, resting lung volume drops from 40% to about 20% because of the effect of gravity. The strength of the muscles that assist in mediating respiration will also have an effect on these measures. Finally, disease processes may also affect lung volumes and capacities (a more thorough discussion of some of these disease processes can be found in Chapter 7).

Breathing and the Exchange of Air

A typical human takes approximately 12 breaths per minute when engaging in quiet, vegetative breathing. Of course, for more strenuous activity, the number of breaths taken per minute will increase—in some cases, quite dramatically. In the section immediately above, it was mentioned that TV is approximately 600 cc (or ml) for an adult male and 450 cc for an adult female. In other words, with each breath, a typical male exchanges approximately 600 cc and an adult female exchanges approximately 450 cc of air. Considering an average of 12 breaths per minute, a typical male exchanges approximately 7.2 liters of air per minute (12 breaths per minute times 600 cc equals 7200 cc or 7.2 liters). This is known as the individual's **minute volume**. A person's **maximum minute volume** is the amount of air that person can maximally exchange each minute (assuming he or she does not hyperventilate during the process!). Maximum minute volumes range from approximately 150 to 170 liters, which indicates that humans only use a fraction of their VC during quiet breathing.

> ### Figure This Out
>
> *What would a typical adult female's minute volume be if she took 12 breaths per minute with an average TV of 450 cc?*

The human body must have oxygen to function properly. The air we breathe actually contains relatively little oxygen—only about 20% of atmospheric air is oxygen; the remaining 80% is nitrogen, carbon dioxide (0.04%), and other elements and compounds. Although only one-fifth of air is oxygen, it is still more than enough to sustain life. In fact, only 20% of the oxygen humans inspire is actually consumed by the body! Expired air is composed of approximately 16% oxygen, 4% carbon dioxide, and 75% nitrogen. Note that the carbon dioxide we breathe out is 100 times greater than the carbon dioxide we breathe in. With more than 6 billion people on earth breathing, we generate a lot of carbon dioxide. Of course, plants use carbon dioxide like humans use oxygen.

Let us do some more math. If a person has a respiratory rate of 16 breaths per minute with TV measured at 500 cc per breath, the total amount of oxygen consumed by that individual in a minute is 320 cc (minute volume = 8000 cc of air; 8000 cc of air × 20% oxygen = 1600 cc of oxygen; 1600 cc of oxygen × 20% actually consumed = 320 cc). If you do your math right, you will realize that approximately 4% of inspired air is actually consumable oxygen (20% of 20% is 4%).

> ### Figure This Out
>
> *How much oxygen would a person consume per minute if he has a TV of 550 cc and a respiratory rate of 14 breaths per minute?*

> ### Why You Need to Know
>
> *Emphysema, a disease that adversely affects the alveoli and elasticity of the lungs, can dramatically alter blood oxygen levels. Consumable oxygen may be well below 4% of inspired air in individuals who present with this disease. Emphysema will be discussed in greater detail in Chapter 7.*

THE PROCESS OF VEGETATIVE BREATHING

Inspiration

Now that you understand the basic concepts involved in respiration, a question that may come to mind is "How do the lungs expand so that pulmonary pressure will decrease resulting in the sequence of events that creates inspiration?" Your knowledge of respiratory muscles now comes into play. Recall from the discussion of anatomy that certain muscles are responsible for inspiration. These muscles are summarized in Table 6-2. The action of all these muscles will result in expansion of the thoracic cavity in three dimensions—longitudinal, transverse, and anteroposterior—although all three dimensions may not be acted upon at any given time.

Vegetative breathing is primarily an automatic function (i.e., you do not have to consciously think about taking a breath) that is regulated by the lower brain center for breathing housed within the medulla oblongata. This center does two things: (1) regulates the levels of oxygen and carbon dioxide in the arterial blood and (2) controls the rhythmic pattern of breathing. Whenever the medulla senses that there is too much carbon dioxide and not enough oxygen in the blood, it sends neural signals to the nerves that control respiratory muscle activity. The appropriate muscles that enable us to yawn contract. A yawn is simply a reflexive behavior mediated by the lower brain center for breathing.

The diaphragm is responsible primarily for longitudinal expansion of the thoracic cavity. As this muscle contracts, it descends toward the abdomen. Because of its attachments, the diaphragm not only expands the thoracic cavity in the vertical dimension (i.e., longitudinally), but it also pulls down on the lower rib cage and distends the abdominal wall outward. This generates negative pressure within the thorax. When a person is standing or sitting in an upright position, muscles in the chest wall and abdominal wall contract to prevent the rib cage from being "sucked" inward by the negative force being generated by the diaphragm. The counteraction of the abdominal wall muscles also exerts an upward force on the diaphragm, which assists the diaphragm in lifting the rib cage. Although the diaphragm remains in a contracted (i.e., lowered) position, its body is spread out superiorly and laterally by the intra-abdominal pressure exerted upon it by contraction of the abdominal wall muscles. Because the diaphragm has attachments to the lower ribs, the net effect will be an expansion of the lower rib cage. In this way, not only does the diaphragm mediate longitudinal expansion of the thorax but also assists in transverse expansion. When an individual is lying in the supine (i.e., "belly up") position, gravity will exert an inward force on the diaphragm so that the abdominal muscles do not need to contract.

The external intercostal muscles are second only to the diaphragm in terms of their importance to vegetative breathing. During shallow breathing, the external intercostals may not even be called upon; their contribution to inspiration becomes more pronounced when you take a deeper than normal breath (e.g., yawning or sighing). Recall that the external intercostals course from each rib to the rib immediately below. As these muscles contract, they pull up on the rib below. The articulations the ribs have with the thoracic vertebrae and sternum allow the ribs to rotate on their longitudinal axes. The ribs evert, resulting in greater lateral thoracic volume.

During quiet, vegetative breathing, there may be measurable upward and forward movement of the sternum, as the anterior ribs are acted upon by the internal intercostal muscles. This movement will create a slight increase in the anteroposterior dimension of the thoracic cavity. Contraction of the neck muscles will also generate a slight increase in the anteroposterior dimension of the thorax, but these muscles are usually not involved in the process unless vegetative breathing becomes strenuous. For example, as an individual engages in heavy aerobic exercise, the demand for more oxygen may cause the individual to contract the neck muscles as he or she strains to get more air into the lungs.

The majority of muscles involved in inspiration are relegated to a secondary role. The remaining inspiratory muscles of the thorax (as well as the neck muscles just mentioned) typically do not play a role in inspiration unless there is a greater demand for oxygen by the body or if an individual wants to generate considerable vocal volume (i.e., yell or scream). Under these scenarios, the secondary muscles contract to further expand the transverse and anteroposterior volumes of the thoracic cavity.

It should be noted that intrapleural pressure (the pressure within the potential space between the costal and visceral pleurae) is always negative throughout respiration. At rest (i.e., between breaths), intrapleural pressure is approximately -6 cm H_2O. During inspiration, the contraction of the diaphragm pulls on the visceral pleura. This generates even more negative intrapleural pressure (from -6 cm H_2O to approximately -10 cm H_2O). Boyle's law plays a role here. Expansion of the rib cage and descent of the diaphragm increases the volume within the intrapleural space, which causes the drop in pressure. Upon expiration, contraction of the rib cage and elevation of the diaphragm generates greater (i.e., more positive) intrapleural pressure, although overall the pressure is still negative.

What does this mean in terms of inspiring air? As was mentioned briefly in the section on anatomy, not only are the lungs made of elastic tissue, they also act as a unit with the diaphragm and rib cage because of pleural linkage (remember Mary and her little lamb). The visceral and costal pleurae act like two compressed plates of glass with liquid between them, meaning that they glide upon each other but do not separate. Longitudinal and transverse expansion of the lungs creates greater volume within the alveoli pulmoni. The greater volume in the alveoli results in lower pulmonary pressure by comparison to atmospheric pressure (pulmonary pressure is approximately -2 cm H_2O relative to atmospheric pressure). Air will flow from outside the body to within the lungs to equalize the drop in pressure. Once the pressure is equalized, airflow ceases and you are at the end of the inspiratory phase of the respiratory cycle (i.e., pulmonary pressure is 0 cm H_2O relative to atmospheric pressure).

Why You Need to Know

Under certain pathological conditions such as asthma or chronic bronchitis, the individual may contract the neck muscles in an attempt to create greater lung volume to compensate for reduced tidal inspiration due to the obstruction within the bronchi. These pathological conditions will be discussed in Chapter 7.

Expiration

Once air gets into the lungs, how do we get it out? Does it require additional muscle activity? From the discussion about respiratory anatomy, you know that there are certain muscles that are classified as muscles of expiration. However, for quiet, vegetative breathing, the action of these muscles is typically negligible. In fact, the expiratory muscles (especially the abdominal wall muscles) actually assist in the process of *inspiration*. What then serves as the impetus for expiration?

For the most part, passive forces act upon the thorax to contract it. As was mentioned earlier, these passive forces include elastic recoil, torque, intra-abdominal pressure, and gravity. As the muscles of inspiration relax, these forces act upon the thorax to compress it. As the thorax compresses back to its resting position, the alveoli within the lungs are compressed as well. Compression of the alveoli results in an increase in pulmonary pressure relative to atmospheric pressure (i.e., pulmonary pressure is now $+2$ cm H_2O relative to atmospheric pressure). With pulmonary pressure being greater than atmospheric pressure, air will flow from the lungs to outside the body. The lungs deflate until they reach their resting volume, which is also the point at which pulmonary pressure once again equals atmospheric pressure (i.e., the pressure differential is 0 cm H_2O).

With these passive forces at work, what prevents the thorax from compressing before we have a chance to use the oxygen from the air? The answer is the inspiratory muscles (especially the external intercostals) and the abdominal wall muscles. Upon inspiration, the diaphragm almost immediately relaxes. However, the external intercostals and the abdominal wall muscles remain active throughout inspiration. This prevents the rib cage from contracting prematurely. Interestingly enough, when the external intercostal muscles start to relax, the internal intercostal muscles may contract, exerting a downward and inward force on the ribs to assist in deflating the thorax. Once the thorax has returned to its resting state, another cycle of respiration begins.

The Respiratory Cycle

During quiet, vegetative breathing, the inspiratory phase is active. In other words, muscles are always involved in the process. Muscles of inspiration are needed to initiate the inspiratory phase. Other than the possible contraction of the internal intercostals, the expiratory phase is usually passive. Newton's Third Law of Motion acts upon the thorax to initiate expiration by generating the passive forces of elastic recoil, torque, and intra-abdominal pressure. Gravity also plays a role in the expiratory process.

If one were to time a typical cycle of respiration during quiet, vegetative breathing, it would be evident that the timing of the inspiratory and expiratory phases is almost equivalent. The inspiratory phase accounts for approximately 40% of the respiratory cycle, whereas the expiratory phase accounts for 60% of the cycle. As an example, if a complete cycle of respiration takes 2 seconds to complete, inspiration will account for 800 msec (0.8 seconds) of the cycle, while expiration will account for the remaining 1200 msec (1.2 seconds).

When the thorax is at rest (i.e., when a person is between breaths), the air in the lungs occupies approximately 40% of VC. This is referred to as resting lung volume. The TV that is created during quiet, vegetative breathing accounts for an additional 10% of VC. This means that on average, only 50% of VC is used during quiet, vegetative breathing. When we yawn, we go into IRV. For example, inspiration during a vigorous yawn can occupy as much as 90% or more of VC. You can imagine that an activity like physical exercise will also cause us to utilize more of our IRV and thus VC.

THE PROCESS OF BREATHING FOR VOCAL ACTIVITY

When an individual uses the breath stream for vocal activity, the respiratory system undergoes distinct physiological changes. These changes affect both the mechanics and timing of the respiratory cycle. The primary difference between vegetative breathing and using the breath stream for vocal activity is the introduction of the phonatory system into the equation. The vocal folds remain abducted (i.e., separated) during vegetative breathing, but they adduct (i.e., come together) during vocal activity. The phonatory system will be described more fully in Chapter 8. In this section, we will describe respiratory physiology as it relates to vocal activity. More specifically, we will discuss what happens when we engage in two vocal activities—continuous, steady phonation and conversational speech.

Continuous Phonation

Continuous, steady phonation is defined as the sustaining of phonation with little variation in pitch or intensity. An example of this would be sustaining a vowel sound or a single musical note. The speaker inspires air and then continuously phonates until he or she runs out of breath.

During vocal activity, expired air is used to generate vocal fold vibration. Because inspired air is not involved in phonation, the mechanics of inspiration do not change considerably from what one would observe during quiet, vegetative breathing. The same phenomena that explain vegetative inspiration still apply. To inspire air, the individual simply contracts the diaphragm, external intercostal muscles, and possibly some secondary muscles of inspiration. The internal intercostals and abdominal wall muscles contract to stiffen the rib cage so that the intercostal spaces are not sucked in by the negative pressure. The net result of this muscle activity is expansion of the thorax. Because of pleural linkage, the lungs expand as well. Pulmonary pressure decreases relative to atmospheric pressure because of the increased volume within the alveoli. Air enters the lungs to equalize the drop in pressure.

Although the basic inspiratory mechanics are the same for continuous vocal activity as they are for vegetative breathing, an observable difference is that IRV will likely be called into play during continuous vocal activity. In other words, the speaker will take a deeper breath than he or she normally would during vegetative breathing. If the speaker is asked to sustain continuous phonation until he or she runs out of breath, then ERV will also be accessed. This will necessitate a change in expiratory mechanics as well.

Take note of Figure 6-27. The upper part of the figure shows the changes in lung volume that occur during continuous vocal activity. Point "A" represents the

peak of the volume trace. Here, the speaker has taken a deep breath, essentially going into IRV. Then, there is a gradual decrease in lung volume throughout the vocal activity until it "bottoms out" (point "B"). The speaker is below resting lung volume; in other words, the speaker has accessed ERV. Now note the trace below the volume trace. This second trace represents pulmonary pressure. You can see that although lung volume diminishes over time throughout continuous vocal activity, pulmonary pressure remains relatively constant. Pulmonary pressure is what we use to set the vocal folds into vibration (except at the vocal folds, it is referred to as **subglottic pressure**). At a normal loudness level, it only takes approximately 5 to 8 cm H_2O of subglottic pressure to maintain vocal fold vibration.

In terms of inspiration, accessing IRV means that more air is introduced into the alveoli. The speaker is in a condition of high lung volume (point "A" in Figure 6-27). High lung volume means greater pulmonary pressure. Greater pulmonary pressure means greater relaxation pressure (remember that for every action, there is an opposite and equal reaction). To counter the increased relaxation pressure, we must put a brake on the expiratory forces (referred to as the **checking mechanism**) that act to make the rib cage collapse (Hixon, Mead, & Goldman, 1976). This is accomplished by the chest wall inspiratory muscles (i.e., the external intercostals primarily, but other muscles may also be active). Refer back to Figure 6-27. Note the muscles that are involved in inspiration (from the beginning of the graph to point "A"). The diaphragm and external intercostals contract simultaneously, but the diaphragm relaxes almost immediately. The external intercostals remain active beyond relaxation of the diaphragm. This is done to counter the increased relaxation pressure at high lung volume as the speaker begins to phonate on expired air. Note also that the abdominal wall muscles (e.g., the external obliques and rectus abdominus) are also active during inspiration. These muscles contract to counter the negative force on the intercostal spaces.

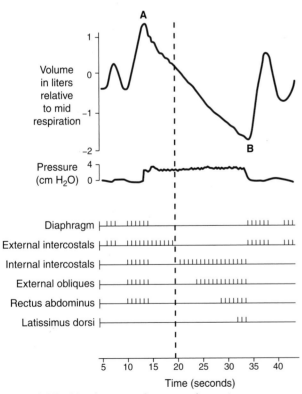

Figure 6-27 Muscle activity during steady, continuous phonation.

Why You Need to Know

Any neuromuscular disease or disorder that affects the braking mechanism of the external intercostal muscles will have a concomitant effect on phonation time, that is, an individual's ability to maintain vocal fold vibration beyond a few seconds. The individual may not be able to speak but a few words before running out of breath. Neuromuscular pathologies will be discussed in greater detail in Chapter 7.

At the point of the vertical dotted line in Figure 6-27, when the external intercostal muscles relax, the speaker is approaching resting lung volume (i.e., is in mid lung volume), but phonation continues uninterrupted. As the speaker continues to phonate, expiratory rib cage muscles (i.e., internal intercostals) contract to maintain the steady (5 to 8 cm H_2O) subglottic pressure to sustain vocal activity. The speaker continues to phonate and begins to tap into ERV. At this point, the speaker is below resting lung volume, and pulmonary pressure is negative in relation to atmospheric pressure (i.e., the speaker is at low lung volume). However, subglottic pressure for phonation remains a steady 5 to 8 cm H_2O. To be able to do this, the speaker has to apply even greater muscular pressure on the breathing mechanism. At this point, the abdominal wall muscles (especially the external obliques and rectus abdominus) become active. By contracting these muscles, greater intra-abdominal pressure is exerted upon the diaphragm, which in turn exerts greater pressure on the lungs. As the speaker continues more and more into ERV, expiratory thoracic muscles (e.g., latissimus dorsi) and additional abdominal muscles become active until the speaker runs out of breath (point "B" in Figure 6-27).

It should be noted that muscle activity during vocal activity is not an all-or-none event. In other words, it is not a matter of the inspiratory muscles contracting first, then relaxing, and then finally the expiratory muscles contracting. Breathing for vocal activity requires a coordinated and overlapping effort between all of the muscles of inspiration and expiration. This way, rib cage wall and abdominal wall volume will decrease at a constant rate throughout phonation. Lung volume will also decrease at a relatively constant rate throughout phonation, providing the steady and constant pulmonary pressure that is necessary to initiate and maintain vocal fold vibration.

Conversational Speech

The physiological changes that occur during conversational speech are even more remarkable than for continuous, steady phonation. In the latter case, vocal pitch and intensity remain somewhat constant throughout phonation. In the case of conversational speech, we vary our vocal pitch, intensity, and quality quite a bit. Changes in vocal pitch and intensity are what allow us to vary our lexical stress and intonation. For example, in some contexts, lexical stress allows us to differentiate the meaning of words (say

the word "record" with stress on the first syllable and then with stress on the second syllable). Similarly, intonation also plays a part in conveying the meaning of our utterances (e.g., say the sentence "We are going to the store tonight" first with a rising intonation at the end of the sentence and then with a falling intonation). Nine of the 24 consonant sounds in English are produced without vocal fold vibration. Therefore, in conversational speech, there are intermittent periods where vocal fold vibration is either "on" or "off."

Another difference between continuous, steady phonation and conversational speech is that we do not typically utilize a large portion of IRV or ERV for conversational speech. We tend to take quick, rapid inspirations (going slightly into IRV) and then speak until we go a little into ERV. We could use all of IRV and ERV to speak, but it would cause a disruption in our ability to produce conversational speech in a smooth, uninterrupted manner.

Because of these changes, respiratory physiology is once again altered somewhat. Volume and pressure change considerably throughout our conversational speech. For conversational speech, lung volume is primarily a mid-range event. Remember that VC at resting lung volume is approximately 40%. Normal tidal inspiration adds another 10% to VC, meaning that we only use about 50% of our VC for vegetative breathing. During conversational speech at a normal intensity level, inspiration accounts for approximately 60% of VC; in other words, we utilize only a small portion of our IRV. We then speak on expired air and continue until we are relatively close to resting lung volume. In some cases, we might even go into ERV a bit (to about 30% to 35% VC). In these cases, the checking mechanism during high lung volume and the active contraction of muscles of expiration during low lung volume will not likely come into play to the degree they would during steady, continuous phonation. We do not typically go well into IRV unless we want to increase our vocal intensity (such as in yelling or screaming), and we do not go too far into ERV unless we continue to speak until we run out of breath (such as might occur when we are excited or when we are trying to hold the floor during conversation).

For such activities like singing, reading loudly, or yelling, we do go more into our IRV and may use more of our ERV. According to Hixon (1973), our inspiration accounts for approximately 80% of VC when we read loudly and as much as 85% to 90% when we yell or sing classically. At the end of expiration, we are usually around 35% VC. In other words, for vocal activity produced at greater intensity, we typically use between 45% and 55% of our VC. Naturally, if we go more and more into our ERV, we will utilize more and more of our VC.

What are the physiological mechanisms during conversational speech? In essence, we tend to "charge" the respiratory system during conversational speech by taking quick inspirations intermittently throughout our speech. Slight upward and downward variations in pulmonary (and hence, subglottic) pressure override our expiratory breath stream and allow us to alter our vocal pitch, intensity, and quality. We generate slight increases in pulmonary pressure to mediate lexical stress and slight decreases in pulmonary pressure at the end of breath groups where pitch and intensity tend to level off.

Once again, the same basic mechanics apply for inspiration during conversational speech as they do for vegetative breathing and steady, continuous phonation. The difference, of course, is whether we require as much braking activity by the external intercostals at high lung volume or more active participation of the expiratory abdominal and chest wall muscles at low lung volume. The greatest change in physiology involves the expiratory phase.

The expiratory phase is mediated by the expiratory abdominal and chest wall muscles. These muscles are typically not involved in inspiration during conversational speech. This allows these muscles to be at the ready to drive expiration as soon as the inspiratory phase has ended. When the abdominal wall muscles contract, they generate greater intra-abdominal pressure that exerts itself upon the diaphragm. This results in three actions. First, it increases the diaphragm's radius of curvature and elongates its principal muscle fibers. This allows the diaphragm to produce quick, powerful inspirations so that there are minimal disruptions to running speech. Second, upward force on the diaphragm generates an upward force on the rib cage, which elevates it. This in turn stretches the fibers of the expiratory rib cage muscles to allow them to produce quick expiratory pulses for varying lexical stress and vocal intensity. Finally, inward incursion of the abdominal wall muscles prevents an outward excursion of the abdomen when the diaphragm acts upon the rib cage to elevate it. If this did not take place, there would be a reduction in the expiratory chest wall muscles' ability to generate the expiratory pulses necessary to effect changes in intensity, stress, and intonation. That is, if the expiratory chest wall muscles contracted without opposition from the abdominal wall muscles, the inward pressure generated by the expiratory chest wall muscles would simply dissipate by outward excursion of the abdomen.

The abdominal muscles then mechanically "tune" the breathing mechanism for inspiration and expiration during conversational speech.

The Respiratory Cycle

It should be clear to you that dramatic changes occur to the respiratory cycle during vocal activity. First and probably most obvious are the mechanical changes that take place, especially during the expiratory phase. Perhaps not quite as obvious are the changes that occur to the timing of respiration. As you learned earlier in this chapter, during quiet, vegetative breathing, inspiration accounts for approximately 40% of the respiratory cycle, while expiration accounts for the remaining 60%. During vocal activity, the ratio between inspiration and expiration changes dramatically to approximately 10% and 90%, respectively. This makes sense when one considers what is going on physiologically during vocal activity. Because the vocal folds adduct for phonation, they create an obstacle to the expired air so that it takes longer for the expiratory phase to be completed. To a lesser degree, the checking mechanism of the external intercostal muscles during expiration also causes the expiratory phase to be prolonged. In addition, we tend to utilize more of our VC during vocal activity than what we do during quiet, vegetative breathing. We use varying amounts of our inspiratory and expiratory reserve volumes during vocal activity. These volumes are not utilized as much during tidal breathing.

Summary

This chapter provided a thorough description and discussion of the anatomy and physiology of the respiratory system. The respiratory system is the power source for vocal activity. Without adequate breath support, humans would not be able to generate a vocal tone, that is, they would not have a voice. Indeed, there are many pathological conditions that may result in poor breath support for speech, and as expected, individuals exhibiting any of these pathologies will also have voice problems. Some of these pathologies will be discussed in Chapter 7. Then, in Chapter 8, a thorough discussion of the phonatory system will be presented. Through a discussion of the phonatory system, you should gain a greater appreciation for the important role respiration plays in the process of speech production.

CHAPTER 7

Pathologies Associated with the Respiratory System

Knowledge Outcomes for ASHA Certification for Chapter 7

- Demonstrate knowledge of the biological basis of the basic human communication processes (III-B)
- Demonstrate knowledge of the neurological basis of the basic human communication processes (III-B)
- Demonstrate knowledge of the etiologies of voice and resonance disorders (III-C)
- Demonstrate knowledge of the etiologies of swallowing disorders (III-C)
- Demonstrate knowledge of the characteristics of swallowing disorders (III-C)

Learning Objectives

- You will be able to list and briefly describe the medical etiologies associated with respiratory pathologies.
- You will be able to explain the impact of respiratory pathologies on speech breathing and voice production.
- You will be able to explain the impact of respiratory pathologies on swallowing.

AFFIX AND PART-WORD BOX

TERM	MEANING	EXAMPLE
chemo-	responding to chemicals	**chemo**receptor
de-	decrease	**de**saturation
hyper-	increased or excessive	**hyper**inflation
hypo-	decreased or reduced	**hypo**xemia
-itis	infection	bronch**itis**
mechano-	responding to movement	**mechano**receptor
-ologist	specialist	pulmon**ologist**
oro-	pertaining to the oral cavity	**oro**pharynx
-osis	state of disease	tubercul**osis**
pneumo-	pertaining to the lungs	**pneumo**nia
sclera-/sclero-	scar, plaque	multiple **sclero**sis
-sia	abnormal or pathological state	dyskine**sia**

Introduction

Breathing is not only our life force, it is our "speech force" because the breath serves as the very foundation of each and every vocal utterance. A number of pathologies can disrupt this force and result in disrupted speech production. A brief review of the respiratory anatomy and physiology will set the stage to discuss these pathologies.

Breathing is a twofold process of **ventilation** and **respiration**. Ventilation refers to the movement of air in and out of the lungs via the upper airway beginning at our nostrils and mouth opening and continuing through the oral and nasal cavities posteriorly to the pharyngeal regions: **nasopharynx, oropharynx**, and **hypopharynx**. As the air travels through these passages lined with mucous membranes—especially those of the nasal cavity—it is warmed, moistened, and freed from unwanted debris. Indeed, consider breathing in the cold winter weather where it is a necessity to warm the air by breathing through your nose. Take even a modest breath through your mouth in near zero temperatures and you will find yourself coughing. The breath stream continues inferiorly through the larynx and the trachea prior to following the branching of the bronchi. The bronchi and their multiple generations (see Chapter 6) distribute the air to the right and left lung segments. Finally, the air reaches the bronchioles and alveoli where the process of respiration actually takes place, that is, the vital exchange of oxygen (O_2) for carbon dioxide (CO_2). The CO_2 is expired and that completes one breath cycle. Any disruption in this system can result in respiratory pathology that can have ramifications for speech production.

Respiratory Pathologies

There are a number of pathologies that can affect respiratory function through obstruction, an interrupted neural supply, a disrupted respiratory process, or a musculoskeletal disorder. A list of such pathologies (modified from Hixon & Hoit, 2005; Kersten, 1989) can be found in Table 7-1.

Some of these pathologies are specific to respiration, while others affect multiple body systems. For example, **emphysema, tuberculosis**, and **pneumothorax** primarily affect lung function. Emphysema is a chronic condition associated with smoking and other environmental toxins. Its pathology is characterized by an enlargement of the alveoli and

TABLE 7-1
RESPIRATORY PATHOLOGIES

1. Obstructions
    - i. Allergies
        - (a) Hay fever
        - (b) Asthma
    - ii. Diseases
        - (a) Cystic fibrosis
        - (b) Interstitial fibrosis
        - (c) Pulmonary fibrosis
        - (d) Tuberculosis
        - (e) Chronic obstructive pulmonary disease
            1. Chronic bronchitis
            2. Emphysema
        - (f) Congestive heart failure
            1. Pulmonary edema
            2. Adult respiratory distress syndrome
        - (g) Pneumonia
        - (h) Lung cancer
        - (i) Pulmonary embolism
2. Musculoskeletal pathologies
    - i. Muscular dystrophy
    - ii. Scoliosis
    - iii. Kyphosis
3. Neurological etiologies
    - i. Myasthenia gravis
    - ii. Amyotrophic lateral sclerosis
    - iii. Postpolio syndrome
    - iv. Multiple sclerosis
    - v. Parkinson's disease
    - vi. Dystonia
    - vii. Tremor
    - viii. Stroke
    - ix. Spinal cord injury
4. Trauma
    - i. Pneumothorax
    - ii. Laryngeal trauma

a resultant decrease of elasticity with consequential decreased efficiency of blood–oxygen exchange. For the patient, this results in effortful breathing, shortness of breath, and associated fatigue. Tuberculosis is a bacterial infectious disease with symptoms including a bad cough, a fever, and chest pain. Pneumothorax refers to a collection of air or gas in the pleural cavity resulting in a collapsed lung due to trauma or disease. Symptoms of pneumothorax also include shortness of breath, chest pain, and fatigue in addition to a rapid heart rate. In fact, a caveat is in order in that any disorder that affects lung function can and often does impact cardiac function. There is a reason the entire system is referred to as the cardiopulmonary system. Pulmonary blood circulation refers to the blood vessels that receive deoxygenated blood from the right side of the heart, circulate it through the lungs to become oxygenated, and return the blood to the heart's left side (Kersten, 1989). An example of the impact of less efficient oxygen exchange is chronic emphysema. Individuals have enlarged hearts due to the extra effort required by the heart to pump oxygenated blood to muscles and organs. Alternatively, many of the disorders listed in Table 7-1 impact systems beyond the cardiopulmonary. Such is the case with congenital disorders such as **muscular dystrophy (MD)**, an inherited disease of progressive muscle deterioration and weakness, and neurological disorders such as **multiple sclerosis (MS)**, a disease of the central nervous system affecting the myelin covering of the axons. Also, some disorders may be only temporary or transient in nature with proper medical treatment, such as those associated with allergies such as **asthma** and **hay fever** or infections of the lungs such as **pneumonia** or tuberculosis. Other disorders progressively worsen with respiratory function decreasing over time such as with **amyotrophic lateral sclerosis (ALS)** (also known as Lou Gehrig's disease).

Speech–language pathologists (SLPs) become involved when respiratory function impacts speech breathing beyond the acute phase. Thus, individuals with chronic breathing problems may benefit from evaluation and intervention for speech breathing. You will recall from Chapter 6 that our respiratory system is extremely flexible, generating positive and negative pressures for inspiration and expiration, respectively, that go well beyond that needed for conversational speech. Because of this excess "reserve," individuals with significantly reduced respiratory capacity can often speak intelligibly at adequate intensities, although those same individuals may not have long utterances or be able to speak loudly or shout with as much success. When lung volume and capacities become too small for functional speech, then the patient becomes ventilator dependent and collaborative work with the respiratory therapist begins and/or efforts switch to the use of augmentative and alternative communication systems.

This chapter now turns to a brief description of some of the respiratory pathologies an SLP may encounter in his or her practice. As mentioned earlier, a number of disorders resulting in respiratory difficulties can be medically managed without a referral for speech therapy services. However, it should be understood that whenever the breath stream is compromised, speech production is also likely compromised. The extent to which SLPs intervene is presented in great detail in Hixon and Hoit's (2005) comprehensive

text on evaluation and management of individuals who have speech breathing disorders.

AIRWAY OBSTRUCTION

A number of respiratory difficulties are secondary to obstructions in the upper and lower airways that hinder the flow of air and gas exchange at the alveoli. Selected respiratory disturbances will be discussed as they relate to the power supply for speech production.

Asthma and Paradoxical Vocal Fold Movement

Asthma and **paradoxical vocal fold movement (PVFM)** can be mistaken for one another, as they both are a function of airway obstruction and both result in sudden difficulty breathing. However, there are a number of differences that distinguish the two. A hallmark symptom of PVFM is difficulty *breathing in* air (Hixon & Hoit, 2005), whereas asthma is better described as difficulty *breathing out*. Further, PVFM is an upper airway obstruction that occurs secondary to sudden adductor spasms of the vocal folds that interfere with normal breathing (Mathers-Schmidt, 2001). In contrast, asthma is a lower airway obstruction due to constriction of both large and small pulmonary passages (e.g., bronchi, bronchioles). In asthma, there is abnormal sensitivity of smooth muscle surrounding the bronchioles causing them to close and trapping air inside the lungs (Goodman, 2003). In addition, an "asthma attack" brings about inflammation of the bronchial lining and the production of mucus as depicted in Figure 7-1A. Abnormal "noise" when breathing is heard with both disorders, but again, there are differences. Asthma is associated with wheezing and a concomitant patient complaint of tightness in the chest; this wheezing emanates from the pulmonary passages. The sound associated with PVFM is **inhalatory stridor**. Stridor is caused by the creation of air turbulence during inspiration through the adducted vocal folds; thus, the sound emanates from the larynx. Further, when the vocal folds fully adduct during breathing, **dyspnea** or complete cessation of breathing can occur.

There are varying views espoused in the literature concerning the etiologies of PVFM. It has been considered an organic disorder similar to asthma in that it may be brought on by a response to environmental allergens and/or strenuous exercise. Alternatively, it may be a functional disorder with a psychological component (see Chapter 9, for a discussion of organic versus functional voice disorders). Mathers-Schmidt

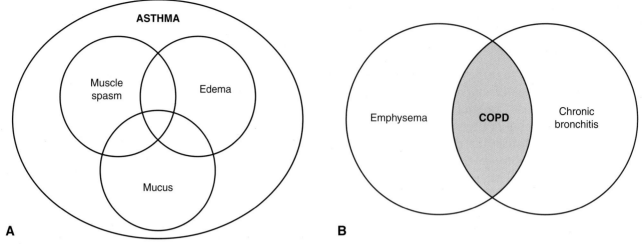

Figure 7-1   Airway obstruction. **A**. The triad of symptoms secondary to an asthma attack. **B**. The combination of emphysema and chronic bronchitis results in chronic obstructive pulmonary disease (COPD). (From Kersten, L. (1989). *Comprehensive respiratory nursing: A decision making approach.* Philadelphia, PA: W.B. Saunders.)

(2001) blends the two views and considers PVFM a complex, heterogeneous laryngeal disorder. The American Speech-Language-Hearing Association (n.d.) concurs by including the following as possible triggers for PVFM:

- Shouting/coughing.
- Physical exercise.
- Acid reflux.
- Cold air breathing.
- Smoke and air pollution.
- Psychosocial issues.
- Neurological issues.

It should be noted that an individual can present with both PVFM and asthma. When obstruction occurs to the lower airway, accessory muscles of respiration come into play to assist the primary muscles in moving air in and out of the lungs.

Chronic Obstructive Pulmonary Disease

Chronic obstructive pulmonary disease (COPD) is a general and nonspecific term that refers to **chronic bronchitis** and emphysema as illustrated in Figure 7-1B. Chronic bronchitis is the continuous over production of mucus due to the structural changes of the bronchi because of environmental pollutants and allergens such as smoking (see Why You Need to Know Box). Emphysema results in the breaking down of the walls of the air sacs resulting in clumps of alveoli and decreased surface area for gas exchange (see Figure 7-2). Furthermore, the alveoli become thick walled and lose their elastic-

ity. COPD then impacts both ventilation and respiration. Through medical treatment, ventilation is maintained by medication administered through inhalers and **nebulizer** treatments. Respiration is managed but cannot be improved by the use of oxygen support. You may have seen individuals carrying or pulling oxygen tanks attached to tubing inserted into their nose by way of **nasal cannulae**; most likely, these individuals have COPD (although lung cancer may also be the culprit). In addition, individuals with advanced emphysema are termed "pink puffers" by medical personnel, as they have a ruddy complexion and are short of breath (the "puffing"), often breathing through pursed lips.

Individuals with COPD are able to speak conversationally but may use shorter **breath groups** or get fatigued more easily with speech. A breath group is simply the quantity of speech, as measured by number of syllables or words, produced in a single breath. As you can imagine, as lung volume decreases, breath group length also decreases. Along with the reduced phrase length, expect the reduced lung volumes and capacities to also result in lower **subglottic pressure** and reduced vocal intensity all while requiring increased respiratory effort on the part of the speaker (Seikel, King, & Drumright, 2005). The fatiguing effect of speaking is related to decreased oxygen in the blood stream. Hixon and Hoit (2005) provide a clinical example of managing speech breathing to decrease fatigue in an individual with moderate emphysema. In clients at risk for **desaturation** during speaking activities, monitoring of oxygen saturation (SpO_2) levels and/or end-tidal breathing partial pressure of carbon dioxide (PCO_2) is done under the direction of a pulmonolo-

Figure 7-2 An illustration of airway obstruction in chronic bronchitis and the breakdown of alveolar walls in emphysema (chronic obstructive pulmonary disease [COPD]) compared with normal respiratory function. (Modified with permission from Nettina, S.M. (2009). *Lippincott manual of nursing practice* (9th ed.). Philadelphia: Lippincott Williams & Wilkins.)

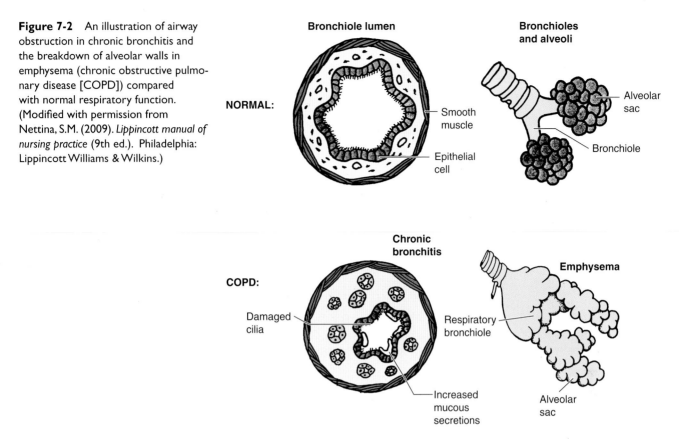

gist and with the assistance of a respiratory therapist (Hixon & Hoit, 2005). Hixon and Hoit suggest using a **pulse oximeter** to monitor oxygen saturation (SpO_2) to assist in determining the type of speaking behavior that causes desaturation and teach strategies to reduce this (e.g., incorporating nonspeech breaths between speech breaths).

> ### Why You Need to Know
>
> *Smoking is clearly linked to lung disease attributing to 438,000 deaths in the United States each year. The majority of these deaths are a result of COPD (chronic bronchitis and emphysema) and lung cancer (Centers for Disease Control, 2005). Although prevalence rates have declined in young adults 18 to 24 years of age in the United States, smoking is still the most prevalent in this age group (American Lung Association, 2007). Furthermore, adult males and females who smoke lose an average of 13.2 and 14.5 years of life, respectively, as compared with nonsmokers.*

Congestive Heart Failure

The weakening of the heart's ability to efficiently and adequately pump blood leads to **congestive heart failure (CHF)**. This, in turn, causes decreased circulation of blood with fluid buildup in the lungs as well as other tissues. Congestion refers to this buildup of fluid and concomitant swelling (i.e., edema). Causes are many and include years of uncontrolled high blood pressure and coronary artery disease. Individuals with CHF have chronic shortness of breath and persistent coughing up of phlegm. Most typically, the left ventricle or chamber of the heart fails and blood backs up into tissues (e.g., the swelling seen in the lower extremities) and organs. Lung congestion, or **pulmonary edema**, occurs with this left-sided heart failure. This fluid then fills the alveoli and prevents gas exchange or respiration from occurring. Speech is impacted due to decreased lung volume and decreased ability to generate and sustain the subglottic pressures necessary for continuous speech with adequate loudness. In addition, patients with CHF present with a wet or gurgly sounding voice and persistent coughing; this makes it hard to determine at bedside if they are at risk for aspiration of food and drink because these symptoms mimic those that indicate swallowing problems.

MUSCULOSKELETAL CONDITIONS

Conditions affecting voluntary skeletal muscle include the various forms of muscular dystrophy (MD). Muscular dystrophies are inherited genetic diseases resulting in degeneration of skeletal muscle

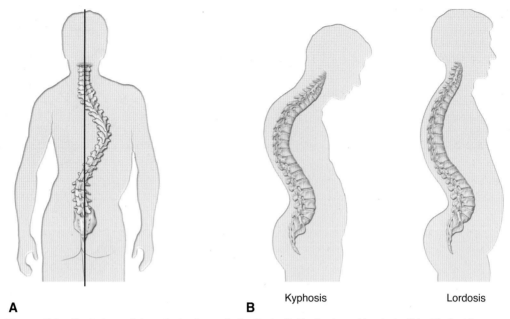

A   **B**

Kyphosis   Lordosis

Figure 7-3   Deviations of the spinal column. **A**. Scoliosis. **B**. Kyphosis and lordosis. (Modified with permission from *Stedman's medical terminology* (2010). Baltimore: Lippincott Williams & Wilkins.)

and associated progressive muscle weakness. The types of MD vary in terms of age of onset, distribution of affected muscle groups, rate of progression, and extent of muscle weakness (National Institute of Neurological Disorders and Stroke, n.d.). Although involvement of the muscles of respiration are not a required characteristic of the disease, it is often the case that MD results in such severely weakened respiratory muscles that the patient's breathing becomes **ventilator** dependent.

Individuals with MD may present with a variety of respiratory issues affecting speech breathing. The progressive muscle weakness leads to reduced lung capacities and decreased ability to generate adequate subglottic pressures for phonation (Seikel et al., 2005). Furthermore, Seikel and colleagues indicate that the reduced range of motion seen in individuals with MD, as well as other dysarthrias of the flaccid type, can result in reduced breath groups, impaired prosody, and reduced vocal intensity.

Spinal column deformities, when severe, also hinder breathing abilities. **Scoliosis** (also termed **kyphoscoliosis**) refers to a lateral (i.e., sideways) spinal curvature that is a deviation from the normal vertical line of the spine or vertebral column. Figure 7-3A illustrates a right thoracic scoliosis, as the spinal deviation is to the right at the thoracic region of the vertebral column. According to the National Scoliosis Foundation (n.d.a), scoliosis is found in 2%–3% of the US population, affecting infants to adults with an average age of onset between 10 and 15 years. If the lateral curvature is severe, the ribcage may press against the lungs and heart and compromise cardiopulmonary function.

The vertebral column is aligned in the center of our back and has two areas of normal anterior curvature at the cervical and lumbar regions. These curves are important to maintain an erect posture and provide for maximal mechanical efficiency for breathing. Thus, structural deformities of the vertebral column will limit the natural and efficient expansion and recoil of the ribcage. **Lordosis** refers to abnormally large anterior curvatures of the vertebral column. All of us have a little bit of what may be referred to as "swayback." Typically, an underlying disease is at the root of a serious lordosis such as with MD (National Scoliosis Foundation, n.d.c). **Kyphosis** (or "round back") is the opposite of lordosis. It is an abnormal increase in the posterior curvature of the vertebral column (National Scoliosis Foundation, n.d.b). This is most often seen in the thoracic vertebral region where we have a certain degree of natural rounding. Figure 7-3B shows these spinal curvatures via a lateral view. You might be familiar with **Dowagers hump**, often associated with aging women. This hump is a type of kyphosis due to a collapse of the vertebrae in the upper thoracic region because of low bone density or **osteoporosis**. The key to minimizing or avoiding this is prevention through consuming adequate levels of calcium and vitamin D and performing weight-bearing exercises.

NEUROLOGICAL PATHOLOGIES

Neurological traumas and diseases are numerous as you read about in Chapter 5. Those disorders of the nervous system that result in dysarthria likely have a respiratory component. Neurological damage impacting ventilation and respiration can be widespread from the central nervous system to the peripheral nervous system. In the central nervous system, the upper motor neurons (UMNs), the control circuitry of the cerebellum and basal ganglia, the medullary respiratory center, the brainstem cranial nerve nuclei, and the anterior horns of the spinal cord are all involved in breathing. In the peripheral nervous system, the lower motor neurons (LMNs), the neuromuscular junction, and the muscles of inspiration and expiration are all involved. You are referred back to Chapter 5 on neurological pathologies for a discussion of the various dysarthrias associated with the neuropathologies mentioned in this chapter. Here, the focus will be on

select pathologies that have a significant respiratory component involved with management and treatment. These include spinal cord injuries and progressive neurological diseases.

Prior to a discussion of certain neurological pathologies, a review of the central nervous system control of respiration is in order. As presented in Chapter 4, central control of respiration is both conscious and unconscious in nature. Voluntary control over breathing is evidenced in simple activities such as taking a big breath, holding the breath, and breathing faster or slower, and in more complex activities such as breathing for speech production. Voluntary neural mechanisms for breathing include frontal lobe motor cortices (e.g., premotor cortex, motor strip), parietal lobe somatosensory areas, the basal ganglia, thalamus, and cerebellum. In addition, breathing changes associated with emotions are mediated by the limbic lobe (see Figure 7-4). Next time you become emotional,

Figure 7-4   The brainstem respiratory center with input from higher brain regions, the vascular system, and the lungs and output to the muscles of respiration. (Modified with permission from Premkumar, K. (2004). *The massage connection anatomy and physiology.* Baltimore: Lippincott Williams & Wilkins.)

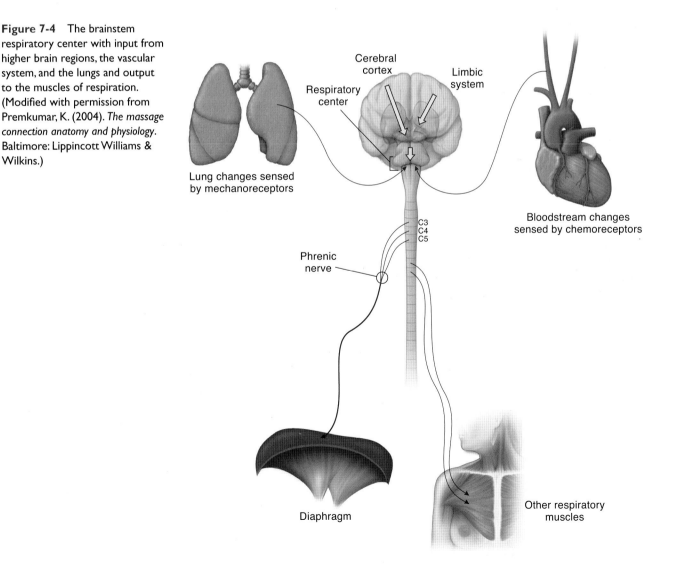

take special note of the effect on your breathing. In fact, you may not even be able to generate and control the breath to speak in emotionally charged situations. Although volitional and emotional breathing occurs, our breath is primarily involuntarily controlled as dictated by blood chemistry.

Importantly, minute changes in blood chemistry sensed by **peripheral chemoreceptors** in the blood stream and carbon dioxide levels in cerebrospinal fluid by **central chemoreceptors** at the level of the medulla indirectly control breathing. The **medullary rhythmicity center** with separate inspiratory and expiratory centers controls automatic breathing. In the pons, the **apneustic area** promotes inspiration and the **pneumotaxic area** inhibits inspiration; together these areas provide input to the medulla to regulate respiratory coordination. These critical brainstem respiratory centers may be suppressed through trauma, or "narcotized" by drugs or alcohol (see Why You Need to Know box).

> ### Why You Need to Know
>
> *Excessive drinking by college students can result in pulmonary aspiration and/or respiratory failure and death. This excessive drinking is often referred to as "binge drinking" roughly defined as five or more drinks in two hours for men or four or more drinks in two hours for women. As the body is unable to metabolically keep up with the alcohol, the effects are ultimately revealed in decreased heart rate, breath rate, and gag reflex. In turn, the decreased gag reflex may result in pulmonary aspiration of vomit, potentially fatal due to its asphyxiation of the lungs. In addition, both cardio and pulmonary effects are seen when blood alcohol levels (from 0.35 to 0.40) suppress the medullary respiratory center. Hence, never let a drunk friend "sleep it off;" instead stay with your friend and call for help if breathing rate is reduced (i.e., eight breaths or less per minute; recall that a normal quiet breathing rate is around 12 breaths per minute), if they are unconscious or semiconscious and do not rouse to a shout or pinch, if their skin is cold or clammy and has a bluish complexion, or if they are vomiting without waking! ANY of these signs warrant getting help. Of course, you want to avoid this situation by urging friends, family, and yourself to drink in moderation if at all.*

Select cranial nerves and a number of spinal nerve pairs are also involved in ventilation. Cranial nerves IX (glossopharyngeal), X (vagus), XI (spinal accessory), and XII (hypoglossal) innervate muscles and mucosa involved with the upper airway structures of the velopharyngeal port, the pharynx, the larynx, and the accessory neck muscles for breathing. Twenty-three spinal nerve pairs (i.e., 8 cervical, 12 thoracic, and the upper 3 lumbar pairs) are involved with innervating both the primary and accessory muscles of respiration. You are encouraged to refer back to Chapter 6 to review the neural innervation for the muscles presented there. The motor commands that are sent out from the brainstem and spinal cord are mediated by the afferent input not only from the chemoreceptors but also from the **mechanoreceptors** located in the pulmonary apparatus itself (e.g., alveoli) and those located in the chest wall responding to muscle stretch (Hixon & Hoit, 2005). Damage to any of these nerves can have a detrimental effect on respiration.

Spinal Cord Injury

Trauma involving the spinal cord at almost any level can impact breathing with trauma at the cervical level being the most severe (see Figure 7-5). For example, Christopher Reeve, the well-known actor and advocate for spinal cord research, suffered a high cervical spinal cord injury (SCI) (C1-C2) during an equestrian race resulting in quadriplegia and the need for ventilator supported breathing for the remainder of his life. According to the National Spinal Cord Injury Statistical Center (n.d.), spinal cord injuries have a variety of causes with sports-related injuries accounting for approximately 9% of cases. The leading cause of spinal cord injuries is motor vehicle accidents (approximately 48%) followed by falls (approximately 23%). Similar to traumatic brain injury (TBI), spinal cord injuries are most prevalent in young adult men.

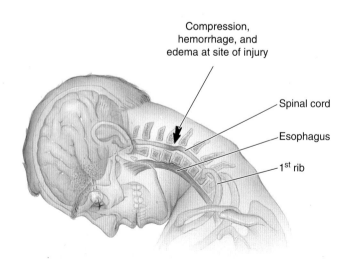

Figure 7-5   An illustration of cervical spinal cord injury. (Modified with permission from Anatomical Chart Company.)

Trauma to the spinal cord is often secondary to fractured vertebrae due to displaced bone and/or discs that compress the cord itself (Young, 2003), although one can suffer vertebral fracture without SCI. When the spinal cord is involved both tissue gray and white matter of the CNS can be impacted as well as spinal nerves of the PNS carrying afferent and efferent neural information to and from the spinal cord, respectively. Thus, SCI disrupts sensory, motor, and autonomic nervous system functions. The body location and extent of the disruption is dependent on the level and severity of the injury.

One way to classify SCI is "complete" or "incomplete" in regard to the amount of remaining function below the level of injury. The level of injury refers to the spinal cord segments and vertebrae and their corresponding numbers: cervical (1–8), thoracic (1–12), lumbar (1–5), and sacral (1–5). Complete SCI refers to no function below the level of the injury, that is, no sensation or voluntary movement on either side of the body below the level of injury. An incomplete SCI is defined as some function present below the level of injury. In addition, symptoms can also be secondary to autonomic nervous system disruption. These symptoms can include disruption of bowel and bladder control, blood pressure regulation, and body temperature regulation. More specifically to the interest of the SLP is weakness or paralysis of respiratory muscles for speech breathing and for swallow safety. For example, if the injury results in weakened or paralyzed intercostal and abdominal muscles, the patient will not be able to produce a productive cough and will be at increased risk for aspiration and pneumonia. An SCI above C4 may require a ventilator for breathing.

Hixon and Hoit (2005) present two case examples of clients with SCI. Here, a brief summary of each case is presented to give you a glimpse at the type of interventions that can be done to assist individuals with SCI to gain improved speech function. A young woman with a C6 injury as a result of a fall was quadriplegic with limited residual function in her arms and hands. Although she could speak, her breath support for speech was severely limited due to weakened muscles of respiration. Her voice lacked intensity, she spoke in short breath groups, and became fatigued with speaking. Due to the level of her injury, innervation to the diaphragm was spared (recall that the diaphragm is innervated by the phrenic nerve that arises at C3–C5, above her level of injury). Following the SLP's evaluation and consultation with the **pulmonologist**, an elastic wrap-around binder was used to position the abdominal wall inward and support the body trunk.

This treatment resulted in longer breath group productions and improved vocal intensity. A second client was described as a young adult male who suffered a C2 level SCI following a motor vehicle accident. Due to the level of SCI, he was left with paralysis of the diaphragm, muscles of the rib cage, and muscles of the abdomen. As expected, he required a ventilator to breath. After extensive medical consultation and testing, he was determined to be a candidate for a phrenic nerve pacer (see Figure 7-6). A phrenic nerve pacer acts as a respiratory neural prosthesis that electrically stimulates the phrenic nerves for diaphragm contraction and resultant inspiration (Hoit & Shea, 1996). The pacer, along with abdominal binding and behavioral treatment, resulted in such good speech production that he often sounded like a normal speaker (Hixon & Hoit, 2005).

> ### *Why You Need to Know*
> *A phrenic nerve pacer, also called a diaphragmatic pacer, is an electrode that is placed in the cervical region behind the phrenic nerve with a radiofrequency receiver that communicates with an external radiofrequency transmitter. The patient is introduced to the pacer gradually and stimulation is adjusted according to ventilation needs. Potential candidates for this type of pacer include individuals with SCI, ALS, and MS, whereas individuals with COPD would not be candidates (Hoit & Shea, 1996).*

Progressive Neurological Diseases

The diseases that result in degeneration of certain aspects of the nervous system vary widely in rate of symptom progression. Some diseases progress slowly such as Parkinson's disease (PD), some diseases progress rapidly such as amyotrophic lateral sclerosis (ALS) and some are widely variable in progression rate such as multiple sclerosis (MS). Entire texts are devoted to the speech and swallowing disorders and management associated with these diseases (e.g., Yorkston, Miller, & Strand, 2003). Here, a brief overview of selected diseases is presented along with a description of each disease's potential impact on breathing.

Freidreich's Ataxia

Freidreich's ataxia (FA) is a hereditary spinocerebellar degenerative disorder named for the German physician who first described its symptoms in 1863. It is an autosomal recessive genetic disease meaning that the

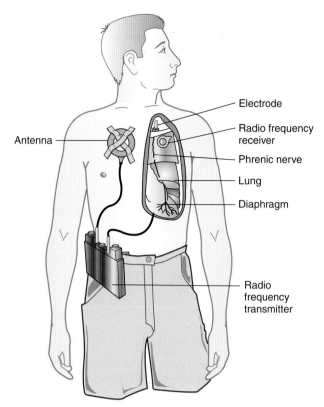

Figure 7-6 An implanted phrenic nerve pacer. (From a Google image search of "phrenic nerve pacer.")

affected individual must inherit two affected genes, one from each parent. For this reason, there may be no apparent family history as each parent would be "silent carriers." Signs and symptoms associated with this type of ataxia include a progressive loss of balance and coordination beginning with a poor gait and progressing to include the trunk and upper extremities. Initial symptoms typically occur between 5 and 15 years of age; however, rate of progression varies widely across individuals (Muscular Dystrophy Association, n.d.). In addition, muscles atrophy over time and individuals may develop scoliosis. FA also affects the heart and can result in congestion as described previously; these symptoms are managed medically. As the disease progresses, speech and swallowing are also affected by decreased muscle coordination and timing of movements. Respiratory effects with ataxic dysarthria in general include reduced coordination between speech processes and within the process of respiration itself. For example, decreased ability to coordinate inspiration and expiration with resulting inappropriate timing and explosive expiratory bursts may occur (Seikel et al., 2005). Thus, respiratory control is an apt target for intervention along with targeting improved timing of tongue, jaw, and lip movement.

Multiple Sclerosis

Multiple sclerosis (MS) is a progressive disease that results in multiple lesions of the oligodendroglia comprising the myelin in the central nervous system. Thus, disrupted myelin can occur in the brain, spinal cord, or optic nerves. Sclerosis refers to the scar tissue that is left to replace patches of destroyed myelin, producing lesions known as MS plaques. As mentioned earlier, the progression is highly variable across individuals with the most common pattern involving remission and relapse. Relapsing-remitting MS is typified by nearly full remissions following an exacerbation of symptoms with a period of stability or incomplete remissions with a chronic progression of symptoms. MS is usually diagnosed in young adults between the ages of 18 and 40 years and is more common among woman than men. Life expectancy is not affected for 85% of those diagnosed with MS (Yorkston, Miller, & Strand, 1995). Table 7-2 lists the various types of MS based on progression of the disease.

Given the varied lesion sites associated with MS, symptoms may also be varied. Motor, sensory, and visual systems may be impacted with symptoms of unilateral vision loss, sensory loss, and/or motor weakness and spasticity (Johnson & Jacobson, 2007). When dysarthria is present, it is the mixed type, most often a spastic–ataxic type with respiratory and phonatory symptoms prominent (Darley, Aronson, & Brown, 1975; Duffy, 2005). More specific to respiration, Chiara, Martin, and Sapienza (2007) state that the dysfunctional neural control of expiratory muscles in particular results in reduced subglottic pressure for adequate speech production. This, in turn, leads to phonatory problems. The additional difficulty in coordinating respiratory and phonatory function may also result in reduced breath groups. Nonspeech respiratory characteristics can include decreased vital

TABLE 7-2	
MULTIPLE SCLEROSIS SUBTYPES BASED ON PROGRESSION CHARACTERISTICS	
Subtype	**Course of Disease**
Benign	One or few episodes
Relapsing–remitting	Deterioration followed by near complete recovery
Remitting–progressive	Gradual accumulation of deficits
Progressing	Sudden onset and continuous progression without remission

capacity and, more rarely, the need for ventilatory support (Darley, Brown, & Goldstein, 1972).

Parkinson's Disease

Parkinson's disease (PD) is also a progressive disorder of the central nervous system. In the case of PD, the basal ganglia are involved; more specifically, the dopamine producing neurons of the substantia nigra degenerate. This results in the characteristic symptoms of bradykinesia, rigidity, and resting tremor. Individuals with PD often present with a masked-like face, a stooped posture, and a "pill-rolling" movement of the hands. As can be seen in Figure 7-7, the trunk flexion of an individual with PD is one problem that compromises the respiratory system. The onset of PD is typically in the sixth or seventh decade of life and its rate of progression varies.

Individuals with PD have a decreased ability to automatically execute learned motor plans. This includes the ease at which they can utilize the respiratory system for efficient and effective speech production. Duffy (2005) notes that the primary speech issues for individuals with PD center on phonation, articulation, and prosody. Specific respiratory symptoms that are reflected in speech breathing difficulties include decreased vital capacity, decreased chest wall excursion, decreased respiratory muscle strength, irregular breathing patterns, and increased breathing rate. These symptoms may be due to an "... alteration in the agonistic/antagonistic relationship between respiratory muscles during breathing" (Duffy, 2005, p. 198). Furthermore, individuals with PD evidence a bowing of the vocal folds which further hinders the ability of the respiratory and laryngeal systems to collaborate for loud, clear speech production. The interaction between these two systems is exemplified well in the Lee Silverman Voice Treatment program, or LSVT (see Why You Need to Know box).

> ### *Why You Need to Know*
> *The Academy of Neurologic Communicative Disorders and Sciences (ANCDS) has taken the lead in providing systematic reviews of treatment and presenting practice guidelines in the various areas of neurologic communication disorders. One such review was a paper on behavioral management of respiratory/phonatory dysfunction in dysarthria (Yorkston, Spencer, & Duffy, 2003). Among studies reviewed were those by Ramig and colleagues, who investigated the effects of Lee Silverman Voice Treatment (LSVT) with individuals with Parkinson's disease. LSVT focuses on the voice through effortful and repetitive exercises at the respiratory and phonatory levels to increase loudness, and in so doing, improve speech quality. The ANCDS concluded that evidence supporting LSVT is good for immediate posttreatment improvement and has some evidence that supports long-term maintenance of treatment effects (Yorkston et al., 2003).*

Amyotrophic Lateral Sclerosis

As mentioned in Chapter 5, ALS is a progressive disease of the motor neurons (refer back to Figure 5-1) that results in both UMN and LMN symptoms. Early symptoms may be manifested in limb weakness or in weakness of the muscles of the head and neck resulting in speech and swallowing problems (i.e., bulbar symptoms). Onset of the disease is in adulthood and life expectancy ranges on average from 1 to 5 years postdiagnosis. However, a quarter of individuals diagnosed with ALS survive for more than 12 years (Bromberg, 1999). Death is usually due to respiratory failure (Duffy, 2005).

Consistent with involvement of upper and lower motor neurons, a mixed dysarthria of the spastic-flaccid type is common in individuals with ALS. Those speech characteristics most indicative of respiratory involvement include decreased loudness, reduced breath groups, and decreased use of prosody manifested in

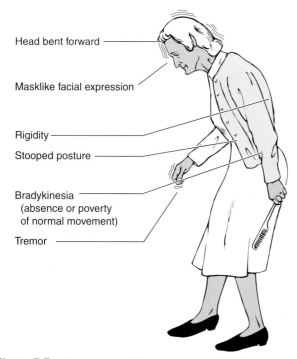

Head bent forward

Masklike facial expression

Rigidity

Stooped posture

Bradykinesia
(absence or poverty
of normal movement)

Tremor

Figure 7-7   A woman exhibiting symptoms of Parkinson's disease. (Modified with permission from LifeART image copyright © 2010 Lippincott Williams & Wilkins. All rights reserved.)

monoloudness and monopitch. In addition, individuals with ALS may exhibit decreased ability to generate sub-glottic pressure sufficient for coughing (Duffy, 2005). Shortness of breath and decreased vital capacity while in the supine position, as well as weakness of the dia-phragm, inspiratory and expiratory chest wall muscles, and abdominal muscles can all be expected (Hixon & Hoit, 2005).

Tracheotomy and Mechanical Ventilation

Individuals with a variety of respiratory pathologies resulting in airway obstruction and/or muscle weak-ness may depend on artificial airways and/or venti-lators to meet their respiratory needs. Many of the etiologies associated with these patient groups have already been discussed in this or previous chapters; these include stroke, TBI, SCI, laryngeal or chest trauma, and pulmonary, cardiopulmonary, and neu-rodegenerative diseases. Most typically, these patients present in intensive care units (ICUs) either in the **acute** stage of trauma or, alternatively, at end stages of progressive disease.

Tracheotomy often follows oral/nasal **endotra-cheal** intubation (see Figure 7-8). A tracheotomy refers to the surgical incision (see Figure 7-9) made around the second or third tracheal rings, whereas a tracheo-stomy refers to the opening made by the incision. This opening is also referred to as the **stoma**. Furthermore, a tracheostomy tube is a short artificial airway that is inserted into the trachea through the stoma during

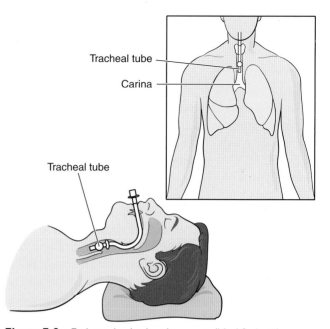

Figure 7-8   Endotracheal tube placement. (Modified with permission from LifeART image copyright © 2010 Lippincott Williams & Wilkins. All rights reserved.)

the surgery (also see Figure 7-9). This tube allows for a direct airway into the lower respiratory passages, bypassing upper airway obstruction due to trauma, disease, or surgery. Notice in Figure 7-10 that the tra-cheostomy tube is inserted below the subglottic space directly into the trachea, and thus it is below the true vocal folds. This has important implications for voic-ing possibilities.

A tracheostomy tube has multiple components. As pictured in Figure 7-11, the outer most tube is referred to as the outer cannula and the innermost tube is the inner cannula. The obturator is necessary for

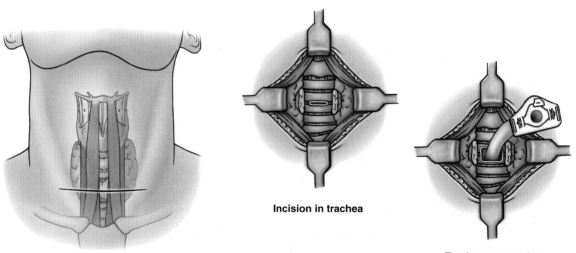

Tracheotomy

Incision in trachea

Tracheostomy tube inserted in tracheal opening (stoma)

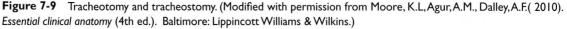

Figure 7-9   Tracheotomy and tracheostomy. (Modified with permission from Moore, K.L, Agur, A.M., Dalley, A.F.(2010). *Essential clinical anatomy* (4th ed.). Baltimore: Lippincott Williams & Wilkins.)

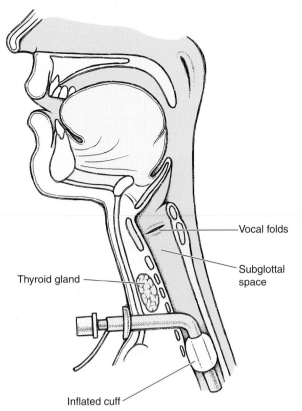

Figure 7-10 Sagittal view of the placement of a tracheostomy tube. (Modified with permission from *Stedman's medical dictionary* (2005) (28th ed.). Baltimore: Lippincott Williams & Wilkins.)

condition, a deflated cuffed tracheostomy tube acts in the same way as an uncuffed tube.

There are different options when it comes to speaking with a tracheostomy tube in place. For example, one can deflate a cuffed tracheostomy tube or simply wear an uncuffed tube. When either an uncuffed or deflated cuffed tube is worn and the stoma is occluded, expired airflow is directed superiorly through the larynx. This allows the air to pass between the adducted vocal folds and through the oral and nasal cavities, thereby allowing for speech to occur. The stoma can be occluded either manually with a finger or by using a speaking valve (see Figure 7-12). This is a one-way valve that is fitted on the stoma end of the tracheostomy tube that allows the patient to breathe in through the valve, but on expiration the pressure of expired air closes the valve so that air is redirected to the upper airway similar to manual occlusion (see the Why You Need to Know box for a discussion of various speaking valves). The speaking valve then allows the patient to speak on expired air without having to manually occlude the stoma.

When it comes to deflating a cuffed tube or using an uncuffed tube, a caveat is in order. There may be contraindications regarding cuff deflation. For instance, the patient may be at risk for aspiration due to excessive oropharyngeal and tracheal secretions. Therefore, working closely with nursing staff and obtaining medical clearance prior to targeting voice and speech production is imperative. Similarly, decisions must be made regarding the necessity and advantage of placing a tracheostomy tube over the more short-term endotracheal intubation. Many texts offer in-depth discussion of these matters for the SLP (e.g., Johnson & Jacobson, 2007).

tube insertion. A tracheostomy tube can be cuffed or uncuffed. For a cuffed tube, a small balloon (or cuff) surrounds the outer cannula. This cuff can be inflated or deflated. When the cuff is inflated, expired air cannot travel up to the larynx but instead is directed back out of the stoma. When the cuff is deflated, expired air is free to travel around the cannula and up through the larynx as long as the stoma is occluded. In this

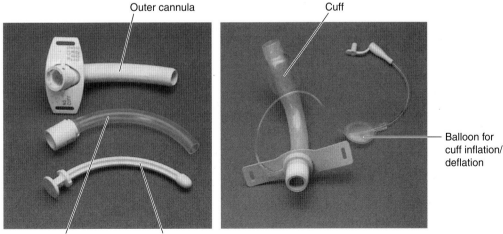

Figure 7-11 Components of a tracheostomy tube. (Modified with permission from Pillitteri, A. (2009). *Maternal and child health nursing: Care of the childbearing and childrearing family* (6th ed.). Philadelphia: Lippincott Williams & Wilkins.)

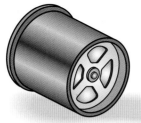

Figure 7-12 An example of a speaking valve (Aqua PMV 007; Passy-Muir Inc., Irvine, CA). (From Passy-Muir Web site product catalog (http://www.passy-muir.com/products/pmvs/pmv007.aspx).)

Why You Need to Know

A number of considerations must be given prior to the placement of a speaking valve for a tracheostomy and/or ventilator-dependent patient. Often times, an SLP is consulted early in the process for consideration of a speaking valve. The preplacement evaluation of the patient is conducted ideally with collaboration among team members—the SLP, the respiratory therapist, and the nursing staff under the direction of the pulmonologist. Areas the SLP will be directly responsible for include an in-depth oral motor examination, evaluation of cognitive and motivational status for speaking, and adequate alertness throughout most of the day to support verbal communication (Johnson & Jacobson, 2007). In addition, the SLP should be knowledgeable regarding the various types of speaking valves that are available as well as manufacturer support. Fortunately, professional meetings such as the annual convention of the American Speech-Language-Hearing Association provide extensive opportunities to view and learn about tracheostomy tubes and the various speaking valves available through demonstration and interaction directly with manufacturers' representatives.

Patients may require mechanical ventilation—or a breathing machine—for breath support due to **hypoxemia, hypercapnia**, or both. Hypoxemia refers

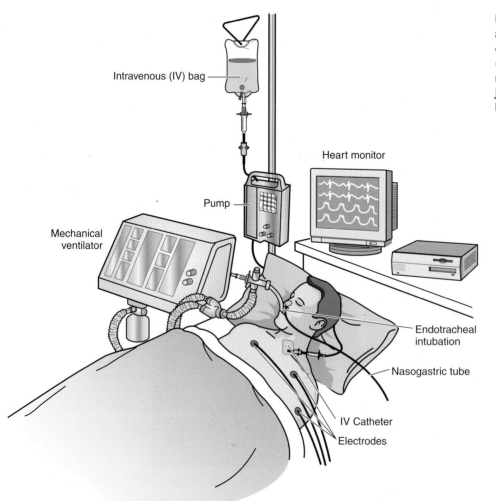

Figure 7-13 A patient in an intensive care unit on mechanical ventilation for breathing. (From http://www.medem.com/medem/images/jamaarchives/JAMA_Practice_HealthCare_lev20.)

Intravenous (IV) bag

Heart monitor

Pump

Mechanical ventilator

Endotracheal intubation

Nasogastric tube

IV Catheter

Electrodes

to low pulmonary artery oxygen levels and hypercapnia refers to elevated blood carbon dioxide levels. Ventilators are set according to air pressure, air volume, and respiratory rate. A number of factors play into these settings such as disease state and medical status of the patient. Regardless, it is the physician, most typically a pulmonologist, who determines the settings and works with a team of professionals to carry out the orders and keep the physician informed. This team includes a respiratory therapist, a nurse, and, often, an SLP. Although mechanical ventilation is common in intensive care and acute settings, sometimes it is necessary over the long term and therefore is also seen in home health settings and long-term care settings. Indeed, some individuals function remarkably well for a number of years with portable ventilators. It should also be noted that a number of less invasive means are available to assist a patient with the work of breathing if full ventilator support is not needed (e.g., a full facial mask that delivers positive pressure to the patient's airway). Figure 7-13 illustrates a patient on a ventilator; the pictured scene is typical of the number of tubes and machines utilized in an ICU.

SLPs may work with patients as they are weaned from ventilators and tracheostomy tubes to spontaneously breathe on their own. A speaking valve may be a good intermediate step for this weaning process as the patient goes from full breathing through a tracheostomy tube to the complete occlusion of the tube through capping it (Johnson & Jacobson, 2007).

Summary

This chapter provided an introduction to a number of respiratory pathologies that can affect speech breathing and the potential role of the SLP. When disease or trauma disrupts one's ability to breathe, the power source for voice and indeed all of speech is curtailed. Difficulties range from total inability to use the breath for speech as in intubated patients to primary impact on the ability to coordinate and control the airstream for the most efficient use for speech as seen in patients with ataxic dysarthria. Because respiration serves as the very foundation of speech, understanding the various pathologies and their impact on the air supply equips the speech–language professional to target respiratory management in a team setting to achieve the best outcome possible for speech.

Clinical Teaser—Follow-Up

Your study of Chapter 7 should have informed you of a number of factors that support the physician's diagnosis of PVFM disorder. In thinking about respiratory pathologies, PVFM disorder is a result of airway obstruction, where the vocal folds themselves get in the way of inspiration. This was noted in the case description regarding inhalatory stridor. Recall that stridor is caused by the creation of air turbulence during inspiration through adducted vocal folds. Indeed, a hallmark symptom of this disorder is difficulty breathing in. Another clue that this may be a case of PVFM disorder is the close association of symptoms to physical exercise. Other triggers for PVFM include smoking and acid reflux, both exhibited by this patient. Although the diagnosis of PVFM disorder is accurate, the physician would likely take the opportunity to educate Richard regarding what he is doing to his lungs through his smoking behavior and the possible outcome of chronic bronchitis and emphysema. Quality of life is often diminished when one is forced to live with COPD. This could turn out to be a real issue for Richard if he does not defeat his smoking habit.

PART 3 SUMMARY

Part 3 (Chapters 6 and 7) presented information regarding respiratory anatomy, physiology, and pathology. The understanding of the respiratory system and its pathologies prepares you to build on this foundational knowledge for speech production as we move to the upstream speech systems of phonation, articulation, and resonance. Respiration serves as the power supply for speech production. Air pressures, volumes, and flows are generated in the pulmonary apparatus by active (i.e., muscles) and passive (e.g., elastic recoil of the lungs) forces. The movement of air in and out of the lungs through the process of ventilation is critical for the life-sustaining process of respiration but also quite literally gives us air to speak on. Thus, pathologies that affect ventilation for respiration also affect our power supply for speech. These pathologies are many and varied, resulting from diverse etiologies such as airway obstruction, musculoskeletal deformities, and neurologic disease. Some of these pathologies are transient in nature and are resolved with acute medical intervention (e.g., asthma); others are persistent and move into chronic and oftentimes progressive stages such as chronic obstructive pulmonary disease, muscular dystrophy, and amyotrophic lateral sclerosis. Chapter 7 concluded with an introduction to the breath support systems of tracheostomy and mechanical ventilation. The speech–language pathologist needs to be aware of the impact these diseases and support systems have on breathing for speech production to effectively intervene with these patients given a team approach (e.g., doctors, respiratory therapists).

PART 3 REVIEW QUESTIONS

1. Describe the support framework for the respiratory system in as much detail as possible.
2. How does the exchange of oxygen and carbon dioxide take place within the lungs?
3. What is the difference between lung volume and lung capacity? List and describe as many of the volumes and capacities as you can. As far as breath support for speech or other vocal activity is concerned, which lung capacity is probably most relevant, and why?
4. How do the inspiratory and expiratory phases of respiration change from vegetative to vocal function?
5. Explain how passive forces act during respiration.
6. Describe how inspiration takes place, using such terms as pulmonary pressure, atmospheric pressure, and Boyle's law.
7. What are the neural underpinnings of the respiratory system? How might neurological pathology affect breathing?
8. Contrast ventilation with respiration and indicate one respiratory pathology that compromises each.
9. How do the respiratory symptoms associated with paradoxical vocal fold movement disorder differ from symptoms associated with asthma?
10. Why do individuals with chronic obstructive pulmonary disease speak on shorter breath groups?
11. Why do individuals with congestive heart failure speak with decreased loudness?
12. Name two musculoskeletal conditions that may impact breathing for speech.

13. Why would an individual with a spinal cord injury at C1/C2 be a better candidate for a phrenic nerve pacer than an individual with a spinal cord injury at C6/C7?

14. Providing therapy on the timing of the respiratory cycle and coordination of the structures involved with ventilation is appropriate for an individual with what type of progressive neurological disease?

15. Individuals with pathologies affecting the respiratory system often have increased risk for aspiration. Why?

16. What impact could an uncuffed or deflated cuffed tracheostomy tube have on swallow safety?

PART 4

Anatomy, Physiology, and Pathology of the Phonatory System

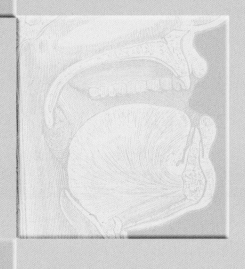

CHAPTER 8

Anatomy and Physiology of the Phonatory System

Knowledge Outcomes for ASHA Certification for Chapter 8

- Demonstrate knowledge of the biological basis of the basic human communication processes (III-B)
- Demonstrate knowledge of the neurological basis of the basic human communication processes (III-B)

Learning Objectives

- You will be able to discuss the framework that supports the phonatory system.
- You will be able to list and describe the muscles that mediate phonatory activity.
- You will be able to define the basic concepts involved in phonation, including but not limited to airflow, Bernoulli effect, fundamental frequency, harmonics, octaves, and subglottic pressure.
- You will be able to describe the mechanics of phonation in terms of the Myoelastic Aerodynamic Theory and the Cover–Body Model.

AFFIX AND PART-WORD BOX

TERM	MEANING	EXAMPLE
ary-	pertaining to the arytenoid cartilages	**ary**epiglottic folds
cerato-	horns	**cerato**cricoid ligaments
crico-	pertaining to the cricoid cartilage	**crico**tracheal membrane
genio-	pertaining to the chin	**genio**hyoid muscles
glosso-	pertaining to the tongue	**glosso**epiglottic folds
hyo-	pertaining to the hyoid bone	**hyo**thyroid membrane
infra-	below	**infra**hyoid muscles
inter-	between	**inter**arytenoid muscles
musculo-	pertaining to muscles	**musculo**cartilaginous
myo-	pertaining to muscles	**myo**elastic aerodynamic theory
para-	beside; to the side of	**para**median position
pars	part of a larger anatomical structure	**pars** oblique
stylo-	pertaining to the styloid process	**stylo**hyoid ligament
sub-	below	**sub**glottic pressure
supra-	above	**supra**hyoid muscles
thyro-	pertaining to the thyroid cartilage	**thyro**arytenoid muscles

Clinical Teaser

Destiny is a typical 15-year-old sophomore in high school. She has many friends and is a very sociable person. She is active in extracurricular school activities, especially cheerleading and singing in the school choir. She has a younger sister and an elder brother at home. Because of all the activities she and her siblings are into, home life is a bit chaotic. The entire family is quite vocal and there is a lot of yelling among Destiny and her siblings. Destiny loves being the center of attention; however, she constantly has to vie for her parents' attention along with her brother and sister. It seems like the child who is loudest is usually the one noticed by mom and dad.

Over the past several months, Destiny has noticed that her voice fatigues very rapidly over the course of a typical day. She also notices that her vocal pitch is much lower than it normally is. She has been struggling with the vocal aspect of her cheerleading and also notices that while she sings she has trouble hitting the high notes. Her voice quality is very hoarse and there is a certain degree of breathiness in her voice as well. Although it is sometimes painful for Destiny to cheerlead and sing, she continues to do so.

Destiny's parents have also noticed the deterioration of her voice over the last couple of months. They are concerned that Destiny's voice is worsening. They call their primary care physician who examines Destiny and then recommends her to an otorhinolaryngologist, or ENT doctor. The ENT conducts a more thorough examination of Destiny's voice. She uses a fiberoptic endoscope with stroboscopy to observe the anatomy and physiology of Destiny's vocal folds as she phonates. Based on the examination, the ENT diagnoses Destiny with bilateral vocal nodules, approximately 1.5 mm in size, on the juncture of the anterior one-third of the length of the vocal folds. The ENT refers Destiny to your clinic and recommends that she receive voice therapy.

Note any terms or concepts in the foregoing case study that are unfamiliar to you. As you read the first chapter of this part, pay particular attention to the anatomy and physiology pertinent to this case. We will return to this case at the conclusion of this part.

Introduction

In Chapter 4, you learned that the nervous system is the control center for speech production in much the same way the CPU is the control unit for a computer. The respiratory, phonatory, and articulatory/resonance systems then can be thought of as the computer's peripherals, although these peripherals have quite different functions than the peripherals you'd see with a computer. You learned in Chapter 6 that the respiratory system is the power source for speech production. In this chapter, your attention will be turned toward the phonatory system—the motor or generator for speech production. The phonatory system is responsible for the creation of the vocal tone. In other words, it is the system by which humans generate voice. An acoustic signal is produced by vibration of the vocal folds. This signal is then modified and transformed as it passes through the vocal tract on the way out the lips. The process of modification and transformation is accomplished by the articulatory/resonance system, which will be the focus of Chapter 10. For now, you will learn to appreciate the beauty and sophistication of the human vocal mechanism.

Anatomy of the Phonatory System

In Chapter 6, a house building analogy was used to describe the anatomy of the respiratory system. To a lesser extent, the same analogy can be used to describe the anatomy of the phonatory system. Recall that the house building analogy involved the construction of a foundation and framework (i.e., bones, cartilages, and connective tissue); installation of insulation (i.e., muscles); erection of walls (i.e., mucous membranes); and installation of the electrical system (i.e., the nervous system).

In the sections that follow then, the anatomy of the phonatory system will be presented according to this analogy. The foundation and framework (i.e., bones, cartilages, and connective tissue) will be discussed first. Then, muscles that are important to the function of the phonatory system will be presented (i.e., the insulation). Following the muscles, mucous membranes (i.e., the walls) will be described. Finally, the neural underpinnings (i.e., the electrical system) of the phonatory system will be presented.

THE FRAMEWORK FOR THE PHONATORY SYSTEM

The foundation or framework of the phonatory system includes the **hyoid** bone and the **larynx**. The hyoid bone can be thought of as the superior boundary of the phonatory system. The larynx is a **musculocartilaginous** structure that resides inferiorly to the hyoid bone and is attached to it by membranes. The trachea is immediately inferior to the larynx and is also attached to it by a membrane or ligament (the trachea was described more fully in Chapter 6 as part of the respiratory system). Figure 8-1 provides an illustration of the phonatory system.

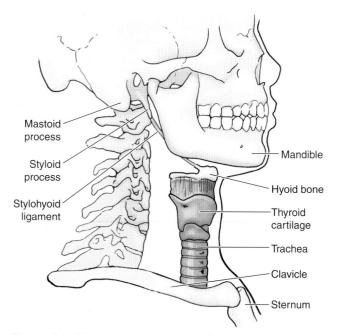

Figure 8-1 The phonatory system, including the larynx, hyoid bone, and other associated structures. (Modified with permission from Moore, K.L., Dalley, A.F., Agur, A.M. (2009). *Clinically oriented anatomy* (6th ed.). Baltimore, MD: Lippicott Williams & Wilkins.)

The Hyoid Bone

The hyoid bone can be seen in Figure 8-1 and is further illustrated in greater detail in Figure 8-2. It is located in the upper region of the neck approximately at the level of the third cervical vertebra (C3) and is immediately superior to the larynx. Upon inspection, the hyoid is somewhat horseshoe or U shaped, with the open end facing posteriorly (i.e., toward the esophagus). An interesting fact about the hyoid bone is that it does not articulate with any other bone, but rather it is suspended in place by the **stylohyoid ligaments** coming from the **styloid processes** of the temporal bones of the skull.

Technically, although the hyoid bone and larynx are connected, the hyoid is not considered an integral component of the larynx. Rather, the hyoid is considered part of the tongue complex, serving as the point of attachment for several tongue muscles coming from above. Not only do muscles make attachments to the hyoid bone from above, but muscles also make attachments to the hyoid from below. As such, the hyoid bone is literally suspended in place by a total of 22 or 23 pairs of muscles. Many of these muscles will be presented later in this chapter.

As illustrated in Figure 8-2, the hyoid bone consists of a corpus (i.e., body), two greater cornua (i.e., horns), and two lesser cornua. The corpus has a convex anterior surface and a concave posterior surface. Projecting posteriorly and somewhat superiorly are

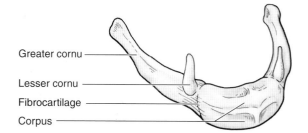

Right anterolateral view of hyoid bone

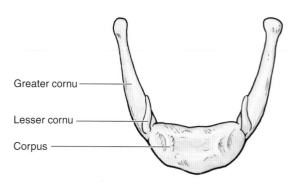

Anterosuperior view of hyoid bone

Figure 8-2 Anterolateral and anterosuperior views of the hyoid bone, with selected landmarks. (Modified with permission from Moore, K.L., Dalley, A.F., Agur, A.M. (2009). *Clinically oriented anatomy* (6th ed.). Baltimore, MD: Lippicott Williams & Wilkins.)

the two greater cornua, each one attached to a lateral border of the corpus. The lesser cornua rise superiorly from the juncture of the corpus and greater cornua. They resemble "devil's horns." Both the greater and lesser cornua, as well as the corpus of the hyoid, are the point of origin or insertion of muscles.

> ### Why You Need to Know
>
> *The hyoid bone is variable from specimen to specimen. For example, in some instances, one or both lesser cornua may be absent. This does not create a problem for the person who has this condition. The muscles will simply attach to an alternate structure.*

The Larynx

The human larynx is a complex musculocartilaginous structure found in the anterior region of the neck (see Figures 8-1, 8-3, and 8-4) approximately from the level of the third cervical vertebra (C3) to C6. For most people (especially males), the larynx can be located quite readily by the prominent bulge extending outward in the neck, commonly referred to as the Adam's apple. In reality, the Adam's apple is a landmark on the largest of all the cartilages composing the larynx.

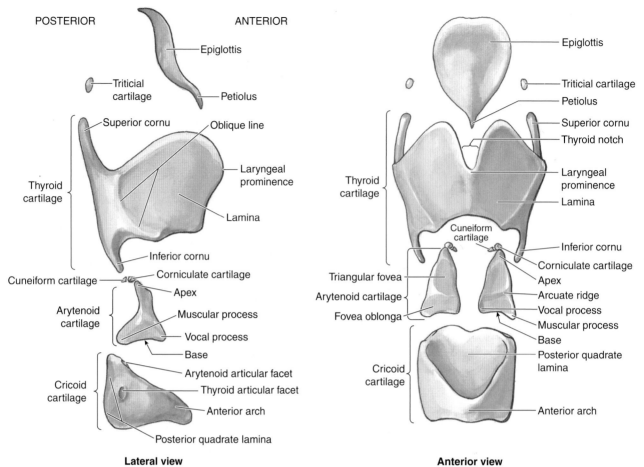

Figure 8-3 The cartilages of the larynx with selected landmarks. (Modified with permission from Agur, A.M., Dalley, A.F. (2008). *Grant's atlas of anatomy* (12th ed.). Baltimore, MD: Lippincott Williams & Wilkins.)

As seen in Figure 8-3, the larynx is composed of a total of nine cartilages along with their connecting membranes and ligaments. Although there are nine cartilages in total, only six have distinct names as three of the cartilages are paired. The three unpaired cartilages are the **thyroid, cricoid**, and **epiglottis**. The three paired cartilages are the **arytenoids, cuneiforms**, and **corniculates**. The thyroid, cricoid, and arytenoids are all classified as hyaline cartilage, which has a tendency to ossify with advanced age. The remaining cartilages (i.e., epiglottis, cuneiforms, and corniculates) are classified as elastic cartilage. In the following paragraphs, a more thorough description will be provided for each cartilage, along with the connecting membranes that are noteworthy.

Thyroid Cartilage

The thyroid cartilage is further illustrated in Figure 8-4. It is the largest of all the laryngeal cartilages. The thyroid is formed by two quadrilateral-shaped plates of cartilage called the **thyroid laminae**. The two laminae are fused together at midline anteriorly, forming the **thyroid angle**. In adult males, this angle is approximately 90 degrees; in adult females, the angle is approximately 120 degrees. The fusion of the two laminae is not complete. Instead, the two laminae separate superiorly forming the **thyroid notch**. Immediately below the thyroid notch is the point where the thyroid cartilage projects most anteriorly. This point of projection is called the **thyroid prominence** or the Adam's apple. The manner in which the two laminae fuse anteriorly means that the thyroid cartilage is similar in shape to the hyoid bone with an open posterior. On each thyroid lamina, there may be a prominent ridge running obliquely along the surface. This ridge is referred to as the **oblique line**, and actually may be a tendon for the sternothyroid and thyrohyoid muscles that attach to the larynx at this point.

An examination of Figure 8-4 (A, B, and D) reveals two pair of cornua projecting superiorly and inferiorly (one pair of each is found at the posterior terminus of each thyroid lamina). By comparison, the two **superior cornua** are longer yet more slender than the two **inferior cornua**. The superior cornua project superiorly, posteriorly, and somewhat medially (i.e., they take an upward, backward, and slightly inward

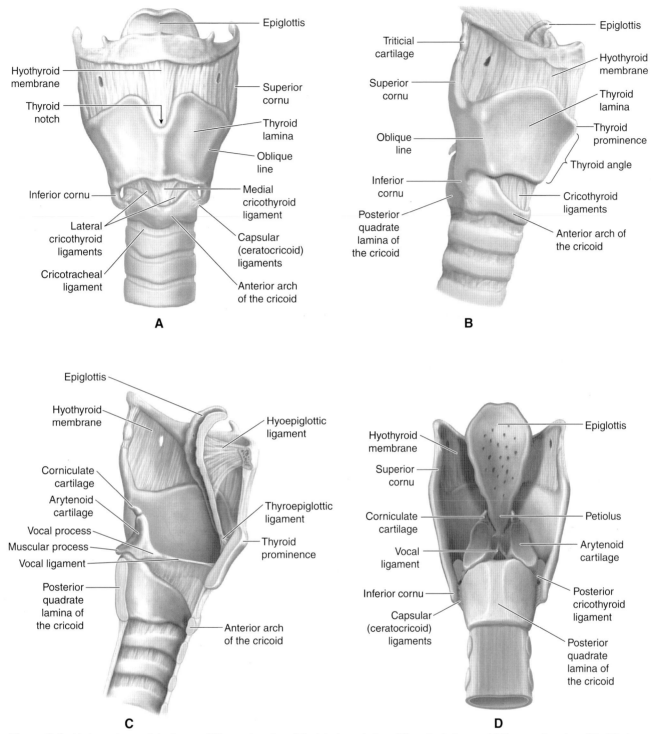

Figure 8-4 Various views of the larynx: (**A**) anterior view, (**B**) right lateral view, (**C**) sagittal view, and (**D**) posterior view. (Modified with permission from Tank, P.W., Gest, T.R. (2008). *Lippincott Williams & Wilkins atlas of anatomy.* Baltimore, MD: Lippincott Williams & Wilkins.)

direction). The superior cornua articulate indirectly with the greater cornua of the hyoid bone by way of the **lateral hyothyroid ligaments** (in fact, the entire superior surface of the thyroid cartilage articulates with the inferior surface of the hyoid bone by way of the **hyothyroid membrane**; the lateral hyothyroid ligaments are simply a thickening of the hyothyroid

membrane where the superior cornua of the thyroid cartilage articulate with the greater cornua of the hyoid). The inferior cornua of the thyroid cartilage articulate directly with the cricoid cartilage and are held in place by the **capsular ligaments**, which are actually composed of a series of ligaments: the anterior, posterior, and lateral ceratocricoid ligaments. The union of the thyroid and cricoid cartilages forms the bilateral **cricothyroid joints**. These joints will be described in more detail later in this section on anatomy as well as in the section on physiology.

> ### Why You Need to Know
>
> *The thyroid cartilage is variable from specimen to specimen. For example, in about one-third of the population, there are small foramens in the region of the superior cornua where blood vessels may pass as they enter the interior of the larynx (Zemlin, Simmon, & Hammel, 1984). For about 5% of the population, one of the superior cornua may be missing. Although the thyroid cartilage has a symmetric shape for most people, there may be a few cases where the cartilage exhibits asymmetry.*

Cricoid Cartilage

Greater detail for the cricoid cartilage is provided in Figures 8-3 and 8-4. This cartilage serves as the lowermost border or base of the larynx and articulates with the first cartilaginous ring of the trachea by way of the **cricotracheal ligament**. The cricoid is smaller than the thyroid cartilage, but it is also more stout. The cricoid is composed of two parts: an **anterior arch** and a **posterior quadrate lamina**. The two parts are continuous so that the cricoid cartilage is a circular ring, similar to a signet ring. The anterior arch lies immediately below the angle of the thyroid where the two thyroid laminae meet. The posterior quadrate lamina is somewhat broad so that it occupies a portion of the open space in the posterior region of the thyroid cartilage.

There are three landmarks of note on the cricoid cartilage. The first landmark is a pair of oval articular facets along the lateral margin of the cricoid where the anterior arch ends and the posterior quadrate lamina begins. These facets are the point of articulation of the cricoid cartilage with the inferior cornua of the thyroid cartilage, forming the cricothyroid joints mentioned earlier. The second landmark is a vertically oriented ridge along the midline of the posterior quadrate lamina with two shallow depressions on either side of the ridge. The ridge is the point of insertion of some fibers from the esophagus, whereas the shallow depressions are the point of insertion for the posterior cricoarytenoid (PCA) muscles. Finally, the third landmark is a pair of articular facets along the superior surface of the posterior quadrate lamina that serve as the point of articulation of the cricoid cartilage with the two arytenoid cartilages.

Epiglottis

The epiglottis is further illustrated in Figures 8-3 and 8-4. It somewhat resembles a leaf, with a broad body tapering into a short, slender stalk. The broad portion is referred to as the corpus, and the stalk is called the **petiolus**. The anterior, or lingual, surface of the corpus is convex and its surface is relatively smooth. The posterior surface of the corpus is concave and appears pitted.

The epiglottis has a vertical orientation. Superiorly, the corpus lies immediately posterior to the root of the tongue and the corpus of the hyoid bone. As illustrated in Figure 8-5, the anterior surface of the corpus is continuous with the root of the tongue by way of a single medial and two lateral **glossoepiglottic folds**. The medial glossoepiglottic fold is separated from the two lateral glossoepiglottic folds by two pits called **valleculae**. The corpus of the epiglottis is anchored to the interior surface of the corpus of the hyoid bone by the **hyoepiglottic ligament** (see Figure 8-4C). Adipose tissue forming a fat pad lies between the epiglottis and hyoid bone. Inferiorly, the petiolus extends just behind the thyroid notch and is anchored there by the **thyroepiglottic ligament** (see Figure 8-4C).

Arytenoid Cartilages

Greater detail for the arytenoid cartilages is provided in Figure 8-6. The two arytenoids lie on the posterior sloping border of the posterior quadrate lamina of the cricoid cartilage, forming the **cricoarytenoid joints**. The arytenoids resemble a three-sided pyramid with an apex and a base. The three sides include the medial surface, posterior surface, and anterolateral surface. The medial surfaces of the arytenoids face each other. The posterior surfaces are on the same plane as the posterior quadrate lamina of the cricoid. The medial and posterior surfaces of each arytenoid are at a 90-degree angle. The anterolateral surface then proceeds from the medial surface to the posterior surface.

The medial surface of each arytenoid is nondescript. The posterior surface houses some important muscles that will be discussed in detail later. The anterolateral surface of each arytenoid is the most detailed of the three surfaces. The anterolateral surfaces have several landmarks including the **triangular fovea, arcuate ridge**, and **fovea oblonga**. The two foveae are depressions on the anterolateral surface; the triangular fovea is found toward the apex of the arytenoid and the fovea oblonga lies along the base. The arcuate ridge separates the triangular fovea from the fovea oblonga. Each of these three landmarks serves as a point of attachment for muscles.

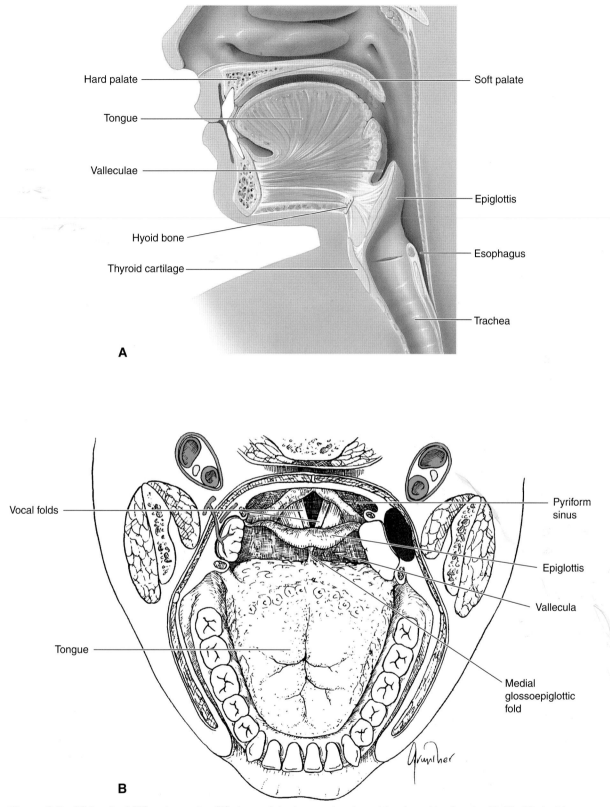

Figure 8-5   Mid-sagittal (**A**) and superior (**B**) views of the laryngeal region with selected landmarks. (**A**: Modified with permission from Anatomical Chart Company; **B**: Modified with permission from Snell, R. (2004). *Clinical anatomy* (7th ed.). Philadelphia, PA: Lippincott, Williams & Wilkins.)

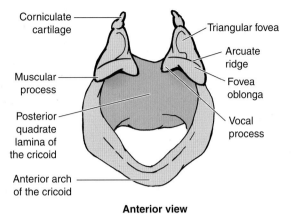

Anterior view

Figure 8-6 Relationship of the arytenoid cartilages to the cricoid cartilage. (Modified with permission from Oatis, C.A. (2008). *Kinesiology* (2nd ed.). Baltimore, MD: Lippincott Williams & Wilkins.)

In addition to the three landmarks of the anterolateral surface, there are other noteworthy landmarks on the arytenoid cartilages. Along the base of each arytenoid where the anterolateral surface meets the posterior surface is a prominent, laterally directed landmark known as the **muscular process**. Similarly, along the base where the anterolateral and medial surfaces meet is an anteriorly directed landmark called the **vocal process**. These two processes serve as a point of attachment for some very important muscles that will be presented later.

Cuneiform and Corniculate Cartilages

To understand the paired cuneiform and corniculate cartilages, you must know that two folds of tissue run along the interior of the larynx from the lateral borders of the corpus of the epiglottis to the arytenoid cartilages. These folds are referred to as the **aryepiglottic folds** (see Figure 8-7). Both the cuneiform and corniculate cartilages are embedded within the aryepiglottic folds, thereby providing a measure of stability to the folds. The corniculate cartilages rest atop the apexes

of the arytenoids, and the cuneiform cartilages are found immediately anterolateral to the corniculates. Because they are embedded within the aryepiglottic folds, you would not be able to see these cartilages but instead would see little bumps in the posterior region of the aryepiglottic folds. The two medial bumps are the **corniculate tubercles** and the two lateral bumps are the **cuneiform tubercles** (see Figure 8-7).

Laryngeal Joints

Two pairs of joints are formed by articulation of the arytenoid and thyroid cartilages with the cricoid cartilage. The joints formed by articulation of the arytenoid cartilages with the cricoid cartilage are the *cricoarytenoid* joints. Bilateral articulation of the thyroid cartilage with the cricoid cartilage creates the *cricothyroid* joints.

The cricoarytenoid joints are formed by the articulation of the **arytenoid articular facets** located on the base of the muscular process of each arytenoid cartilage with the **cricoid articular facets** located on the lateral sloping border of the posterior quadrate lamina of the cricoid cartilage. The arytenoid articular facets are concave, whereas the cricoid articular facets are convex. These articulations result in saddle joints that allow for rocking and some limited gliding movement. A series of ligaments hold these joints in place. For each joint, a **posterior cricoarytenoid ligament** limits the amount of forward movement of the arytenoid cartilage upon the cricoid, whereas an **anterior cricoarytenoid ligament** limits the amount of backward movement. As you will learn in more detail later, the lateral and posterior cricoarytenoid muscles (LCAs and PCAs, respectively) and the interarytenoid (IA) muscles (i.e., oblique and transverse arytenoids) act upon this joint by moving the arytenoid cartilages backward, forward, laterally, and medially upon the posterior quadrate lamina of the cricoid.

The cricothyroid joints are created by articulation of the inferior cornua of the thyroid cartilage with the cricoid cartilage in the region, where its anterior arch ends and posterior quadrate lamina begins. On each side, the **ceratocricoid ligaments** (anterior, lateral, and posterior) loosely hold the joints in place. The cricothyroid joints are pivot joints, allowing the cricoid and/or thyroid cartilages to pivot upon the axes created by these joints. This is accomplished by contraction of the cricothyroid, thyroarytenoid, and superior thyroarytenoid muscles that act upon this joint.

The Laryngeal Membranes

An intricate series of membranes binds the various cartilages of the larynx into a singular unit. Some of these membranes have one of their attachments to a laryngeal

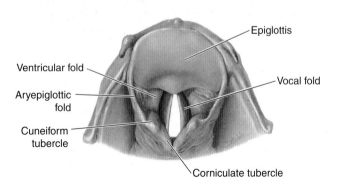

Figure 8-7 The aryepiglottic folds with corniculate and cuneiform tubercles. (Modified with permission from Agur, A.M., Dalley, A.F. (2008). *Grant's atlas of anatomy* (12th ed.). Baltimore, MD: Lippincott Williams & Wilkins.)

cartilage, but the other attachment is to a structure outside the larynx. These are referred to as **extrinsic** membranes. Conversely, there are other membranes whose attachments are found entirely within the cartilaginous confines of the larynx. These are called **intrinsic** membranes. Incidentally, the muscles that will be discussed later are also classified as either extrinsic or intrinsic for the same reason as the membranes discussed here.

Extrinsic Laryngeal Membranes

Three major membranes anchor the larynx in place superiorly and inferiorly. As was mentioned earlier, immediately superior to the larynx is the hyoid bone and immediately inferior is the trachea. The extrinsic membranes then bind the larynx to the hyoid bone and trachea. All three of these membranes were mentioned previously, but for the sake of enhancing your learning, they bear mentioning again. The three extrinsic membranes are the hyothyroid, hyoepiglottic, and cricotracheal. The prefix and root of each of these words indicates where the membrane is located.

As its name indicates, the hyothyroid membrane occupies the space between the inferior border of the hyoid bone and the superior surface of the thyroid cartilage (refer back to Figure 8-4). This membrane is somewhat thicker in its mid-region and also posteriorly where it bridges the space between the greater cornua of the hyoid and the superior cornua of the thyroid cartilage. In these regions, the hyothyroid membrane is referred to as the medial and lateral hyothyroid ligaments. In many cases, small cartilages called the tritricial cartilages are embedded within the lateral hyothyroid ligaments. The tritricial cartilages were not mentioned as components of the larynx because they reside outside the cartilaginous confines of that structure.

As you have probably already discerned, the hyoepiglottic membrane binds the epiglottis to the hyoid bone. More specifically, it is an unpaired, elastic ligament found midline that connects the lingual surface of the corpus of the epiglottis to the upper, posterior surface of the corpus of the hyoid bone. Recall from a previous section that the epiglottis is bound in place by two ligaments. The hyoepiglottic membrane is one of them. The other—the thyroepiglottic ligament—is not classified as an extrinsic membrane because it resides completely within the larynx (attaching the petiolus of the epiglottis to the thyroid cartilage).

The cricotracheal membrane binds the cricoid cartilage (i.e., the base of the larynx) to the first tracheal ring. Because of the size of the cricoid cartilage, the first tracheal ring tends to be larger than all of the other tracheal rings. The membrane courses from the inferior border of the cricoid to the superior border of the first tracheal ring, thereby providing an inferior anchor for the larynx.

Intrinsic Laryngeal Membranes

The intrinsic laryngeal membranes are more complex and are not quite as distinct as the extrinsic membranes. Figure 8-8 provides a schematic diagram of the organization of the intrinsic membranes, while Figure 8-9 provides an illustration of these membranes according to posterior and sagittal views of the larynx. Almost all of the intrinsic laryngeal membranes are a part of a single, continuous layer of fibroelastic tissue called the **elastic membrane**. Nearly the entire interior of the larynx is lined by this membrane. The elastic membrane is divided into two components: the upper portion is referred to as the **quadrangular membrane** and the lower portion is known as the **conus elasticus**.

Figure 8-8 A schematic representation of the elastic membrane.

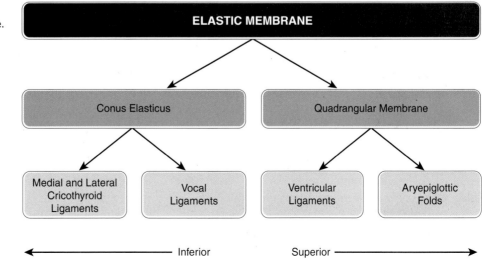

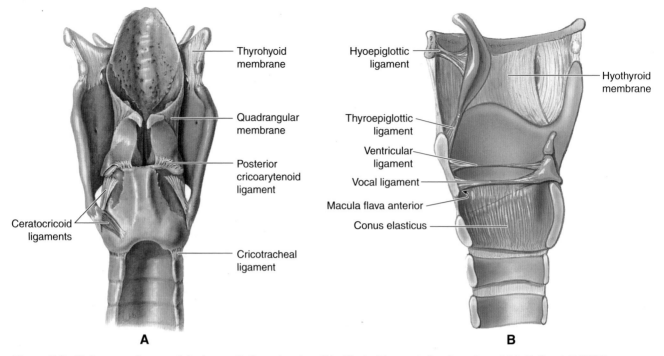

Figure 8-9 Various membranes of the larynx. **A**. Posterior view. (Modified with permission from Agur, A.M., Dalley, A.F. (2008). *Grant's atlas of anatomy* (12th ed.). Baltimore, MD: Lippincott Williams & Wilkins.) **B**. Right sagittal view. (Modified with permission from Anatomical Chart Company.)

The quadrangular membrane is actually a paired membrane that originates superiorly along the lateral borders of the epiglottis, then continuing around the adjacent interior walls of the thyroid cartilage until they terminate at the corniculate cartilages and medial surfaces of the arytenoid cartilages. This superior portion of the quadrangular membrane is known as the aryepiglottic folds. As was mentioned in a previous section of this chapter, embedded within the aryepiglottic folds posteriorly are the corniculate and cuneiform cartilages. There may be muscle fibers within the aryepiglottic folds, but they tend to be poorly developed. From the aryepiglottic folds, the quadrangular membrane continues inferiorly until it terminates as a pair of thickened ligaments called the **ventricular ligaments**. The ventricular ligaments course from the angle of the thyroid immediately below the epiglottic attachment to the triangular foveae of the arytenoid cartilages. Recall that the triangular foveae are found on the anterolateral surfaces of the arytenoids in proximity to their apexes. Because of this arrangement, the two ventricular ligaments approximate each other anteriorly (i.e., at their thyroid attachment) but separate as they proceed posteriorly to the arytenoids. The ventricular ligaments serve as the point of attachment for the **ventricular folds**, more commonly referred to as the "false folds."

The purpose of the conus elasticus is to bind the thyroid, cricoid, and arytenoid cartilages. Inferiorly, this membrane starts as the medial and lateral **cricothy-**

roid ligaments. The medial cricothyroid ligament can be found at midline, running from the superior border of the arch of the cricoid to the inferior border of the thyroid cartilage at the thyroid angle. The two lateral cricothyroid ligaments begin at the superior lateral margins of the cricoid cartilage, then proceed into the interior of the larynx, terminating immediately below the ventricular ligaments from the quadrangular membrane. At this superior margin, the lateral cricothyroid ligaments attach themselves anteriorly to the thyroid cartilage just behind and below the thyroid notch in a region called the **macula flava anterior**. They then proceed posteriorly to the vocal processes at the base of the arytenoids. This superior margin of the conus elasticus is known as the **vocal ligaments**. The vocal ligaments are the anchor for the true vocal folds.

Note that both the ventricular ligaments and vocal ligaments originate at the inner aspect of the thyroid cartilage and then proceed back to the arytenoids. Both sets of ligaments converge at this anterior attachment but separate as they move posteriorly. Although the course of the ventricular and vocal ligaments is parallel, the ventricular ligaments are superior to the vocal ligaments, terminating closer to the apices of the arytenoids as opposed to their bases. Subsequently, the ventricular folds are superior to the true vocal folds.

In summary, if you were to label the elastic membrane from its superior margin to its inferior margin, the landmarks would include the aryepiglottic folds, ventricular ligaments, vocal ligaments, and finally the medial and lateral cricothyroid ligaments. The first two landmarks are part of the quadrangular membrane and the remaining landmarks are part of the conus elasticus.

THE MUSCLES OF THE PHONATORY SYSTEM

The muscles of the phonatory system are classified similarly to the laryngeal membranes. That is, muscles are classified as either extrinsic or intrinsic. Extrinsic muscles have either their origins or insertions on a laryngeal cartilage, but the other attachment is to a structure outside the larynx. Intrinsic muscles have their origins and insertions within the cartilaginous confines of the larynx. An intrinsic muscle may reside between two different laryngeal cartilages (e.g., between the cricoid and arytenoid cartilages) or between the two partners of a pair (e.g., from the left arytenoid to the right arytenoid).

With the extrinsic muscles, in most cases, one of the attachments is to the hyoid bone. Some of the muscles come from anatomical structures superior to the hyoid and then insert somewhere along the superior margin of the hyoid. Others come from structures inferior to the hyoid and then rise to attach to some point along the inferior margin of the hyoid. These muscles are referred to as **suprahyoid** and **infrahyoid** muscles, respectively. A small number of extrinsic muscles come from structures below the hyoid bone but do not insert onto the hyoid. Although these could be considered infrahyoid muscles, they are not typically classified in that manner because they do not make an attachment to the hyoid. These few muscles will simply be classified as miscellaneous extrinsic muscles.

Although the extrinsic membranes were presented before the intrinsic membranes, the intrinsic muscles will be described first in this section. As far as the physiology of the larynx is concerned, the intrinsic muscles play a greater role than the extrinsic muscles, and for this reason, the intrinsic muscles will be discussed first.

It should be noted that all laryngeal muscles—intrinsic and extrinsic muscles alike—are paired. Although Table 8-1 provides the actions of the

TABLE 8-1

ORIGINS, INSERTIONS, AND ACTIONS OF THE INTRINSIC LARYNGEAL MUSCLES

Muscle	Origin	Insertion	Action
Cricothyroid	Anterolateral arch of the cricoid	Pars oblique into the anteroinferior cornu of thyroid; pars recta into the inner aspect of the lower margin of the thyroid lamina	With thyroid anchored, elevates cricoid; with cricoid anchored, depresses thyroid; increases the distance between the thyroid and arytenoid cartilages to increase vocal fold tension
Lateral cricoarytenoid	Anterolateral arch of the cricoid	Muscular process and anterior surface of the arytenoid	Adducts the vocal folds
Oblique arytenoid	Posterior muscular process and posterolateral surface of arytenoid	Near the apex of the opposite arytenoid	Approximates the arytenoids for medial compression
Posterior cricoarytenoid	Shallow depression of posterior cricoid lamina	Posterosuperior surface of the muscular process of the arytenoid	Abducts the vocal folds by pulling the arytenoids backward and outward
Superior thyroarytenoid	Upper limit of thyroid notch	Muscular process of arytenoid	Tilts thyroid back to relax vocal folds; pulls muscular processes forward to aid in medial compression
Thyroarytenoid: muscularis	Angle of thyroid; posterior surface	Fovea oblonga and base of arytenoids	Primarily serves as a regulator of longitudinal tension, but can also act as a vocal fold adductor
Thyroarytenoid: vocalis	Angle of thyroid; posterior surface	Latero-inferior aspect of the vocal process of the arytenoid	
Transverse arytenoid	Lateral margin and posterior surface of one arytenoid	Lateral margin and posterior surface of the other arytenoid	Approximates the arytenoids for medial compression

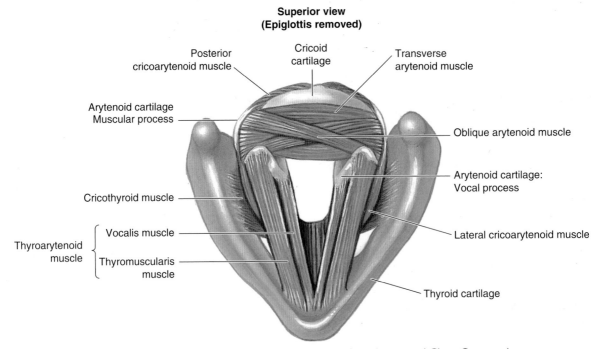

**Superior view
(Epiglottis removed)**

Figure 8-10   The thyroarytenoid muscles. (Modified with permission from Anatomical Chart Company.)

laryngeal muscles, only a brief anatomical description of each muscle will be provided in this section. Muscle action will be discussed more fully in physiology section of this chapter.

Intrinsic Laryngeal Muscles

A brief summary of the origin, insertion, and action of each intrinsic laryngeal muscle is provided in Table 8-1. The intrinsic muscles include the *thyroarytenoids, posterior cricoarytenoids (PCAs), lateral cricoarytenoids, oblique arytenoids, transverse arytenoids,* and *cricothyroids.* The name of each of these muscles is a direct hint as to its origin and insertion.

Thyroarytenoid Muscles

The thyroarytenoid muscles course from the inner aspect of the angle of the thyroid cartilage back to the vocal processes and foveae oblonga along the bases of the arytenoids (see Figure 8-10). In essence, the thyroarytenoids make up the bulk of the vocal folds. These muscles have two parts—a medial bundle (i.e., thyrovocalis) that flanks the vocal ligament and a lateral bundle (i.e., the thyromuscularis) that serves as the body of the muscle. During **abduction**, both portions of the thyroarytenoids appear straight, but upon **adduction**, the thyromuscularis presents a somewhat twisted appearance. Because the vocal folds are composed primarily of muscle tissue, they have the ability to contract. The interesting thing about the thyroarytenoids is the dual

function they play in phonation. The primary purpose of thyroarytenoid contraction is to increase vocal fold tension, but this muscle is also involved in decreasing vocal fold tension (this will be discussed in greater detail in the section Modifications of Vocal Pitch). To a lesser degree, the thyroarytenoids may also play a part in their own adduction.

According to Hirano (1974, 1981), the thyroarytenoids consist of five layers of tissue (these layers are summarized in Figure 8-11). The epithelial layer (composed of squamous cells) is the most superficial of all the layers and assists in maintaining the shape of the vocal folds. The superficial layer of the lamina propria is soft and

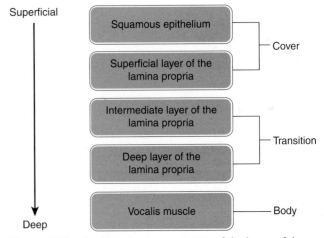

Figure 8-11   A schematic representation of the layers of the thyroarytenoid muscles.

somewhat gelatinous in its consistency. This layer is responsible for the **mucosal wave** that can be viewed when the vocal folds vibrate. The intermediate layer of the lamina propria is soft and rubbery due to the elastic fibers that are found there. The fourth layer, the deep layer of the lamina propria, is collagenous in consistency, giving it an appearance similar to cotton fibers. Finally, the vocalis muscle is composed of stiff, rubbery fibers. As Figure 8-11 indicates, the epithelial layer and superficial layer of the lamina propria are collectively referred to as the cover of the thyroarytenoid muscles. The intermediate and deep layers of the lamina propria are referred to as the transition. Finally, the vocalis muscle is considered to be the main body of the thyroarytenoids.

Vocal fold length varies greatly from individual to individual. However, on average, vocal fold length in adult males is in the range of 17 to 24 mm. For adult females, the range is between 13 and 17 mm. Naturally, the vocal folds of children are even shorter but become longer as they mature until they reach the adult size for their gender.

Why You Need to Know

In approximately half of the world's population, there may be an additional muscle called the superior thyroarytenoid. This muscle originates at the superior-most limit of the thyroid notch and proceeds posteriorly to insert onto the muscular process of the arytenoids. Upon contraction, the superior thyroarytenoids tilt the thyroid cartilage back, thereby shortening the distance between the thyroid cartilage and the arytenoid cartilages. This in turn creates a shortening of the vocal folds, which relaxes them.

Posterior Cricoarytenoid Muscles

The posterior cricoarytenoid muscles (referred to as the PCA muscles) are illustrated in Figure 8-12. These muscles originate at the shallow depressions immediately lateral to the vertical ridge on the posterior quadrate lamina of the cricoid cartilage. They then insert onto the muscular processes of the arytenoids. Because the origins of the PCAs are posterior and inferior to their insertions, contraction will cause the muscular processes of the arytenoids to rotate posterolaterally. Because the vocal folds are attached to the vocal processes and foveae oblonga of the arytenoids, the net action is abduction of the vocal folds. In fact, the PCA is the only abductor muscle in the larynx.

Lateral Cricoarytenoid Muscles

The origin of each LCA is the arch of the cricoid cartilage in proximity to where the arch ends and the posterior quadrate lamina begins (see Figure 8-12). The insertion is the muscular process of each arytenoid cartilage. In this case, the point of origin is anterior and inferior to the point of insertion, so contraction of the LCA will have just the opposite effect of the PCA. In other words, the LCA is an adductor muscle; its purpose is to assist in bringing the vocal folds to midline. To a lesser degree, the LCA also assists in relaxing the vocal folds.

Oblique and Transverse Arytenoid Muscles

The oblique and transverse arytenoid muscles originate on one of the two arytenoid cartilages and then inserts onto the other. Because these two muscles are confined to the arytenoid cartilages, coursing from one to the other, they are collectively referred to as the **interarytenoid (IA) muscles** (see Figure 8-12). The origin of each oblique arytenoid muscle is the posterior surface of the muscular process. The muscle then proceeds along the posterior surface to the opposite arytenoid cartilage near its apex. This arrangement gives the oblique arytenoids an "X" appearance. You would be able to see the "X" formed by these muscles because they are superficial to the transverse arytenoid muscles.

The transverse arytenoid muscles originate at the lateral aspect of the posterior surface of one arytenoid cartilage and then course horizontally across the posterior surface of the two arytenoids to the lateral aspect of the opposite arytenoid cartilage. Some of the deeper fibers continue around to the anterolateral surface to intermingle with fibers of the thyroarytenoid muscles. When the oblique and transverse arytenoid muscles contract, they cause the two arytenoid cartilages to approximate each other. Because the vocal folds are attached to the vocal processes and foveae oblonga, the net action is adduction of the vocal folds. Therefore, the IA muscles are classified as adductor muscles, along with the LCA described earlier.

Cricothyroid Muscles

As their name implies, the cricothyroid muscles run between the cricoid and thyroid cartilages (see Figure 8-13). The muscles are actually composed of two bundles, the **pars recta** and **pars oblique**. Both bundles have their origin at the anterior arch of the cricoid, somewhat lateral to midline. The pars oblique bundle has its insertion along the anterior aspect of the inferior cornua of the thyroid cartilage. The pars recta bundle inserts into the inner aspect of the inferior margin of the thyroid lamina.

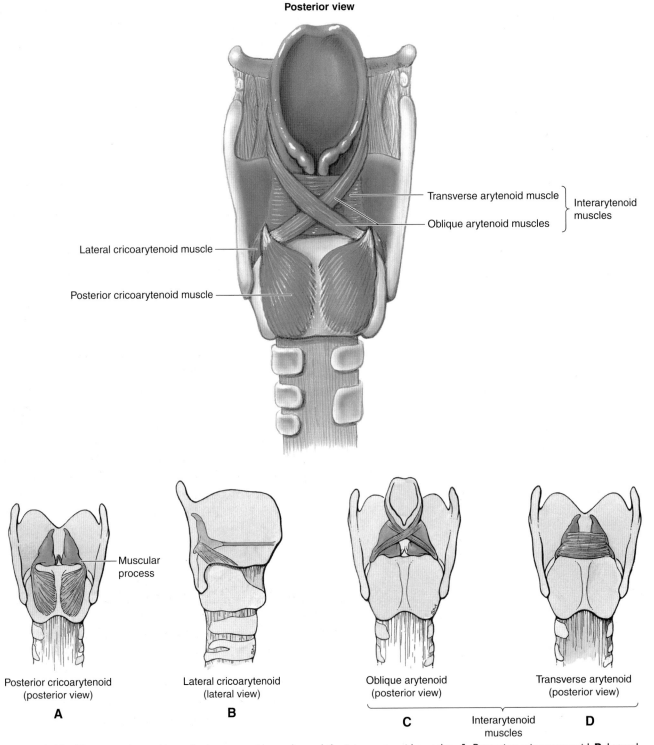

Posterior view

Transverse arytenoid muscle ⎤
Oblique arytenoid muscles ⎦ Interarytenoid muscles

Lateral cricoarytenoid muscle

Posterior cricoarytenoid muscle

Muscular process

Posterior cricoarytenoid (posterior view)
A

Lateral cricoarytenoid (lateral view)
B

Oblique arytenoid (posterior view)
C

Transverse arytenoid (posterior view)
D

Interarytenoid muscles

Figure 8-12 The posterior and lateral cricoarytenoid muscles and the interarytenoid muscles. **A.** Posterior cricoarytenoid. **B.** Lateral cricoarytenoid. **C.** Oblique arytenoid. **D.** Transverse arytenoid. (*Top*: Modified with permission from Anatomical Chart Company; **A–D**: Modified with permission from Agur, A.M., Dalley, A.F. (2008). *Grant's atlas of anatomy* (12th ed.). Baltimore, MD: Lippincott Williams & Wilkins.)

There is a space between the anterior arch of the cricoid and the thyroid cartilage. The relationship between these two cartilages is similar to the visor on the helmet of a suit of armor. When the cricothyroid muscles contract, the thyroid tilts downward and forward and/or the cricoid tilts upward, somewhat simi-larly to lowering the visor on the helmet. This changes the angle between the thyroid and cricoid cartilages and increases the distance between the interior aspect of the thyroid cartilage and the arytenoid cartilages. Because the vocal folds course between these two points, contraction of the cricothyroid muscles results

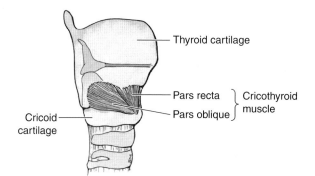

Thyroid cartilage

Pars recta ⎫
Pars oblique ⎬ Cricothyroid muscle

Cricoid cartilage

Figure 8-13 The cricothyroid muscle. (Modified with permission from Agur, A.M., Dalley, A.F. (2008). *Grant's atlas of anatomy* (12th ed.). Baltimore, MD: Lippincott Williams & Wilkins.)

in a lengthening of the vocal folds, thereby increasing their tension. As such, the cricothyroid muscles are classified as tensor muscles.

Extrinsic Laryngeal Muscles

The extrinsic laryngeal muscles are subclassified as either suprahyoid or infrahyoid muscles. Suprahyoid muscles have one of their attachments superior to the hyoid bone; infrahyoid muscles have one of their attachments inferior to the hyoid bone. Upon contraction, the net action of suprahyoid muscles is an elevation of the hyoid bone, and subsequently the larynx because the hyoid and larynx are coupled by the hyothyroid membrane. The net effect of contraction of the infrahyoids (and the miscellaneous muscles mentioned later) is to depress or lower the hyoid bone

and larynx. The importance of these actions will be discussed more fully in the section on physiology.

Suprahyoid Muscles

The suprahyoid muscles include the *digastricus, stylohyoid, mylohyoid, geniohyoid, hyoglossus,* and *genioglossus*. Table 8-2 provides a summary of the origins, insertions, and actions of these muscles. Four of these muscles originate in the region of the mandible (i.e., the jaw). From superficial to deep, these include the digastricus (anterior body), mylohyoid, geniohyoid, and genioglossus. Superficial refers to muscles that are closer to the surface of the skin. Deep then refers to muscles that are farther away from the surface of the skin, or closer to the base of the tongue inside the oral cavity in this case.

As its name indicates, the digastricus has two bellies—an anterior one and a posterior one (see Figure 8-14). The anterior belly has its origin inside the lower border of the mandible. It then courses downward and backward until it joins with the posterior belly in an **intermediate tendon** that penetrates the stylohyoid muscle before inserting onto the lesser cornua of the hyoid bone. The posterior belly originates at the **mastoid process**, which is the rounded base of the skull immediately behind the ear, then courses downward and forward to meet the anterior belly at the intermediate tendon. If the hyoid bone is anchored, contraction of the digastricus will assist in depressing the mandible (i.e., opening the mouth). With the mandible fixed, contraction will assist in elevating the hyoid bone and larynx.

TABLE 8-2			
ORIGINS, INSERTIONS, AND ACTIONS OF THE SUPRAHYOID EXTRINSIC LARYNGEAL MUSCLES			
Muscle	**Origin**	**Insertion**	**Action**
Digastricus: anterior belly	Inside lower border of mandible	Lesser cornua of hyoid bone	Elevates the hyoid bone or depresses the mandible
Digastricus: posterior belly	Mastoid process of temporal bone	Lesser cornua of hyoid bone	
Genioglossus	Mental symphysis of mandible	Lower fibers to hyoid; upper fibers to inferior tongue	Primarily an extrinsic tongue muscle; it may also help position larynx
Geniohyoid	Lower part of mental symphysis of mandible	Anterior corpus of hyoid	With the mandible anchored, pulls the hyoid bone up and forward
Hyoglossus	Corpus and greater cornua of hyoid	Posterolateral surface of tongue	Primarily an extrinsic tongue muscle; it may help position larynx
Mylohyoid	Inner surface of body of mandible	Midline raphe; posterior fibers to hyoid corpus	Elevates the hyoid bone or depresses the mandible
Stylohyoid	Styloid process of temporal bone	Junction of hyoid corpus and greater cornua	Elevates the hyoid bone up and back

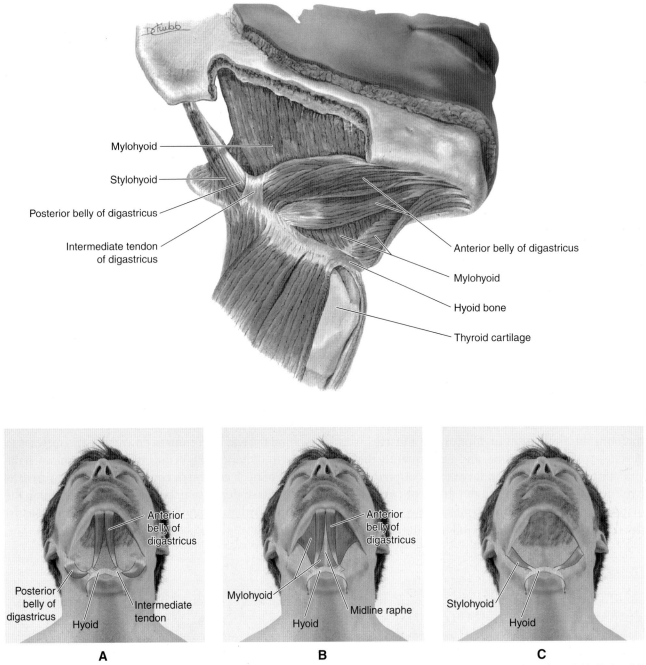

Figure 8-14 Suprahyoid muscles: **A.** digastricus, **B.** mylohyoid, and **C.** stylohyoid. (*Top*: Modified with permission from Agur, A.M., Dalley, A.F. (2008). *Grant's atlas of anatomy* (12th ed.). Baltimore, MD: Lippincott Williams & Wilkins; **A–C**: Modified with permission from Cael, C. (2009). *Functional anatomy: Musculoskeletal anatomy, kinesiology, and palpation for manual therapists.* Baltimore, MD: Lippincott Williams & Wilkins.)

The stylohyoid muscle passes from the styloid process at the base of the skull to the junction of the corpus and greater cornua of the hyoid bone (see Figure 8-14). Upon contraction, this muscle will draw the hyoid bone and larynx upward and backward.

The mylohyoid muscle is also illustrated in Figure 8-14. It forms essentially the muscular floor of the oral cavity. Its origin is the **mylohyoid line** that runs along the inner surface of the corpus of the mandible. Fibers from each side of the mandible course downward and medially until the two sides meet at the **midline raphe**.

The posterior-most fibers along the midline raphe insert onto the corpus of the hyoid bone. When this muscle contracts, it will either elevate the hyoid bone and larynx or depress the mandible, depending upon which anatomical structure is anchored and which is not.

The geniohyoid muscle originates at the lower portion of the **mental symphysis** of the mandible (i.e., inside the chin) and then courses inferiorly to insert onto the anterior surface of the corpus of the hyoid bone (see Figure 8-15). Contraction of this muscle will result in elevation of the hyoid bone in a forward direction.

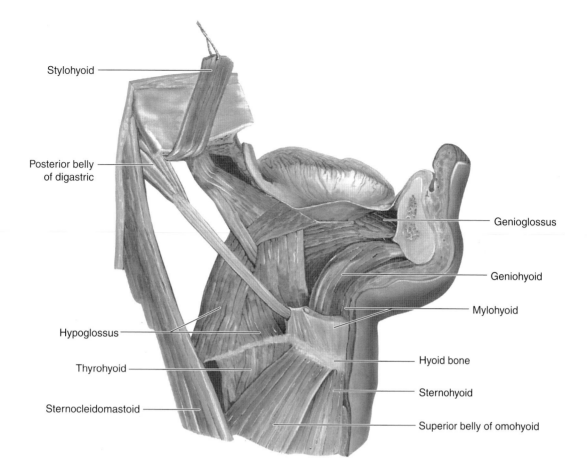

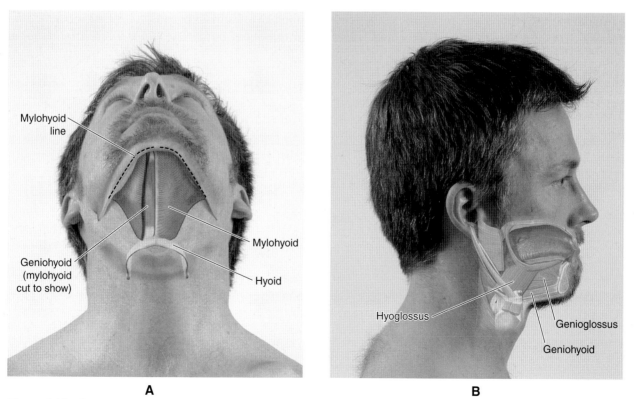

Figure 8-15   Suprahyoid muscles: **A.** geniohyoid, **B.** genioglossus, geniohyoid, and hyoglossus. (*Top*: Modified with permission from Agur, A.M., & Dalley, A.F. (2008). Grant's atlas of anatomy (12th ed.). Baltimore, MD: Lippincott Williams & Wilkins; **A, B**: Modified with permission from Cael, C. (2009). *Functional anatomy: Musculoskeletal anatomy, kinesiology, and palpation for manual therapists.* Baltimore, MD: Lippincott Williams & Wilkins.)

The hyoglossus muscle is also illustrated in Figure 8-15. It is a muscle primarily associated with the tongue, but it does have an indirect action upon the larynx by way of the hyoid bone. Its origin is the corpus and greater cornua of the hyoid bone, and its insertion is along the sides and back of the tongue. This muscle is thought to influence positioning of the larynx in relation to tongue activity.

The course of the genioglossus muscle is from the inner aspect of the mental symphysis of the mandible to the tongue and hyoid bone (see Figure 8-15). As the genioglossus runs in a posterior direction, upper fibers insert into the inferior regions of the tongue, whereas lower fibers insert onto the corpus of the hyoid bone. Although this muscle is primarily associated with the tongue, it may play a part in positioning the larynx in much the same way as the hyoglossus muscle.

Infrahyoid Muscles

The extrinsic infrahyoid muscles are summarized in Table 8-3 according to their origins, insertions, and actions. The infrahyoids include the *thyrohyoid, sternohyoid,* and *omohyoid* muscles. The thyrohyoid muscles course from the oblique lines of the thyroid cartilages to the lower margin of the greater cornua of the hyoid bone (see Figure 8-16, top drawing and drawing C). Upon contraction, the thyrohyoid muscles will either depress the hyoid bone or elevate the thyroid cartilage, depending on which of these two structures is anchored.

As can be seen in Figure 8-16 (top drawing and drawing A), the sternohyoid muscles originate along the posterior aspect of the manubrium of the sternum as well as the medial aspect of the clavicle, then course vertically to insert into the inferior border of the corpus of the hyoid bone. Contraction of these muscles results in depression (i.e., lowering) of the hyoid bone.

Similar to the digastricus muscles, the omohyoid muscles consist of two bodies joined by intermediate tendons (see Figure 8-16, top drawing and drawing B). The inferior bellies of the omohyoid muscles have their origins along the superior borders of the scapulae. The fibers then course almost completely horizontally until they join fibers of the superior bellies at the intermediate tendons. The intermediate tendons are held in place by tendinous slips that anchor onto the sternum and first rib. From the intermediate tendons, fibers of the superior bellies course vertically and somewhat medially to insert into the inferior margin of the greater cornua of the hyoid bone. Although the omohyoid muscles assist in preventing the neck region from collapsing during deep inhalation, they may also assist in depressing the hyoid bone.

Miscellaneous Extrinsic Muscles

Two muscles act upon the larynx in much the same way as the infrahyoid muscles, yet they are not classified as infrahyoid because they have no attachment to the hyoid bone. These are the *sternothyroid* and

TABLE 8-3

ORIGINS, INSERTIONS, AND ACTIONS OF THE INFRAHYOID AND MISCELLANEOUS EXTRINSIC LARYNGEAL MUSCLES

Muscle	Origin	Insertion	Action
Inferior pharyngeal constrictor[a]	Lower portion of tube which originates at the base of the skull	Eventually becomes continuous with the esophagus	Provides resonance characteristics for speech; may pull down on the posterior quadrate lamina of the cricoid
Omohyoid: inferior belly	Upper border of scapula	Intermediate tendon	Prevents the neck region from collapsing during deep inhalation; may assist in depressing the hyoid bone
Omohyoid: superior belly	Intermediate tendon	Lower border of greater cornua of hyoid	
Sternohyoid	Posterior manubrium of sternum and medial clavicle	Lower border of corpus of hyoid	Depresses the hyoid bone; anchors the hyoid when the mandible is opened against resistance
Sternothyroid	Posterior manubrium of sternum and first costal cartilage	Oblique line of thyroid lamina	Depresses the thyroid cartilage
Thyrohyoid	Oblique line of the thyroid lamina	Lower border of greater cornua of hyoid bone	Depresses the hyoid bone or elevates the thyroid cartilage

[a]The lower portion of this muscle has some fibers inserting into the posterior thyroid and cricoid cartilages.

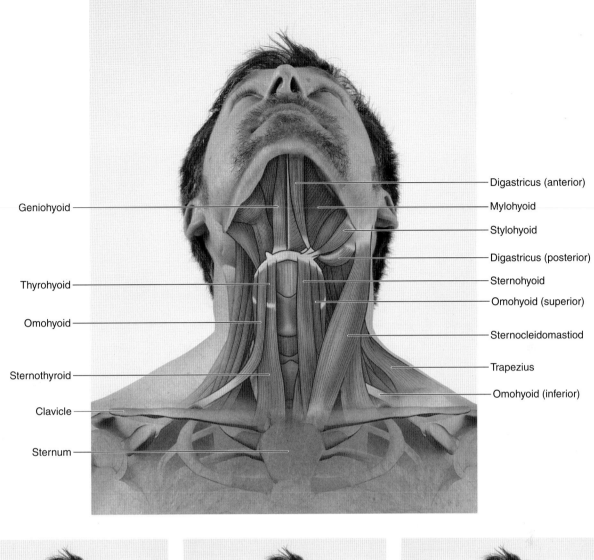

Geniohyoid

Thyrohyoid

Omohyoid

Sternothyroid

Clavicle

Sternum

Digastricus (anterior)

Mylohyoid

Stylohyoid

Digastricus (posterior)

Sternohyoid

Omohyoid (superior)

Sternocleidomastiod

Trapezius

Omohyoid (inferior)

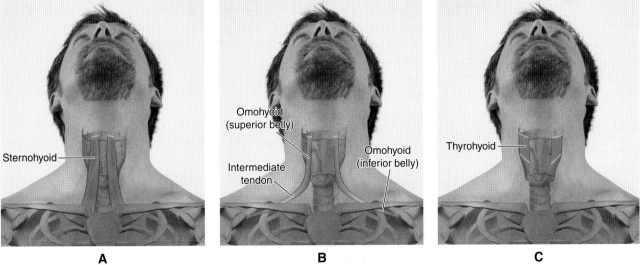

Sternohyoid

Omohyoid
(superior belly)

Intermediate
tendon

Omohyoid
(inferior belly)

Thyrohyoid

A   **B**   **C**

Figure 8-16   Infrahyoid muscles: **A.** sternohyoid, **B.** omohyoid, and **C.** thyrohyoid. (Modified with permission from Cael, C. (2009). *Functional anatomy: Musculoskeletal anatomy, kinesiology, and palpation for manual therapists.* Baltimore, MD: Lippincott Williams & Wilkins.)

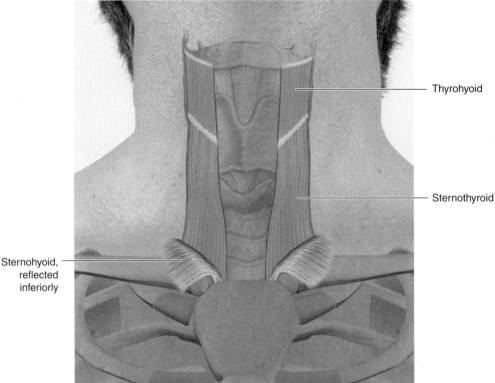

Thyrohyoid

Sternothyroid

Sternohyoid, reflected inferiorly

Figure 8-17 Infrahyoid muscles: sternothyroid. (Modified with permission from Cael, C. (2009). *Functional anatomy: Musculoskeletal anatomy, kinesiology, and palpation for manual therapists*. Baltimore, MD: Lippincott Williams & Wilkins.)

inferior pharyngeal constrictor muscles (see Figures 8-17 and 8-18, respectively). Table 8-3 provides summary information relating to the origin, insertion, and action of these two muscles.

The sternothyroid muscles originate along the posterior aspect of the manubrium of the sternum and the cartilage of the first rib. Their fibers then travel vertically to insert into the lower border of the oblique line of the thyroid cartilage. With the sternum and first rib anchored, contraction of these muscles will result in bilateral depression of the thyroid cartilage.

The inferior pharyngeal constrictor muscles make up the lower part of the **pharynx** and are actually formed by a number of individual muscles that intermingle (these muscles will be discussed in more detail in Chapter 10). Some of the fibers of these muscles insert into the vertical ridge located at midline on the posterior quadrate lamina of the cricoid cartilage as well as the posterior borders of the thyroid cartilage. The action of these muscles assists in mediating the resonant characteristics of the vocal tone.

MUCOUS MEMBRANE

The entire laryngeal cavity is lined by a mucous membrane that is continuous with the mucous membrane found within the pharynx above and trachea below.

This membrane is tight and closely adheres to the epiglottis, aryepiglottic folds, and vocal folds, but it tends to be loose elsewhere within the larynx. The mucous membrane on the regions of the vocal folds that approximate during phonation is composed of squamous epithelium. The mucous membrane that lines the interior of the cricoid cartilage (referred to as the subglottic space) is ciliated, similarly to the mucous membrane of the trachea immediately below.

Why You Need to Know

Orlikoff and Kahane (1996) describe a laryngeal feedback system. Mechanoreceptors can be found throughout the joints, membranes, and muscles of the larynx. These specialized receptor cells are thought to allow the brain to determine and maintain the status of the larynx, making reflexive adjustments as necessary. To date, relatively little is known about the specifics of this feedback system.

NEURAL INNERVATION OF THE MUSCLES OF PHONATION

Table 8-4 provides a summary of the neural innervation of select intrinsic and extrinsic muscles of the phonatory system. Four cranial nerves are involved in

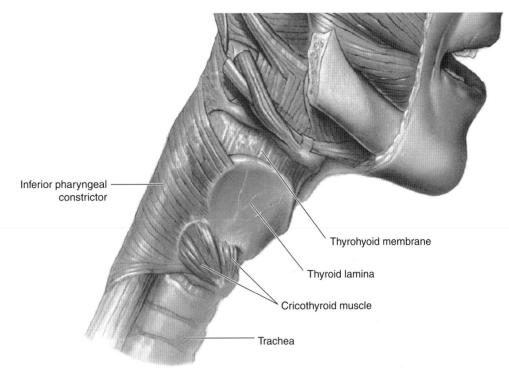

Inferior pharyngeal constrictor

Thyrohyoid membrane

Thyroid lamina

Cricothyroid muscle

Trachea

Figure 8-18 Infrahyoid muscles: inferior pharyngeal constrictor. (Modified with permission from Agur, A.M., Dalley, A.F. (2008). *Grant's atlas of anatomy* (12th ed.). Baltimore, MD: Lippincott Williams & Wilkins.)

TABLE 8-4

NEURAL INNERVATION OF THE EXTRINSIC AND INTRINSIC LARYNGEAL MUSCLES

Muscle	Innervation
Extrinsic Muscles	
Digastricus (anterior belly)	Trigeminal (cranial nerve V), mylohyoid branch
Digastricus (posterior belly)	Facial (cranial nerve VII), digastric branch
Genioglossus	Hypoglossal (cranial nerve XII)
Geniohyoid	Hypoglossal (cranial nerve XII), geniohyoid branch
Hyoglossus	Hypoglossal (cranial nerve XII)
Inferior pharyngeal constrictor	Vagus (cranial nerve X); possibly spinal accessory (cranial nerve XI)
Mylohyoid	Trigeminal (cranial nerve V), mylohyoid branch
Omohyoid	Hypoglossal (cranial nerve XII) with C1–C3
Sternohyoid	Hypoglossal (cranial nerve XII) with C1–C3
Sternothyroid	Hypoglossal (cranial nerve XII) with C1–C3
Stylohyoid	Facial (cranial nerve VII), stylohyoid branch
Thyrohyoid	Hypoglossal (cranial nerve XII) with C1.and C2
Intrinsic Muscles	
Cricothyroid	Vagus (cranial nerve X), superior laryngeal nerve
Lateral cricoarytenoid	Vagus (cranial nerve X), recurrent laryngeal nerve
Oblique arytenoid	Vagus (cranial nerve X), recurrent laryngeal nerve
Posterior cricoarytenoid	Vagus (cranial nerve X), recurrent laryngeal nerve
Superior thyroarytenoid	Vagus (cranial nerve X), recurrent laryngeal nerve
Thyroarytenoid	Vagus (cranial nerve X), recurrent laryngeal nerve
Transverse arytenoid	Vagus (cranial nerve X), recurrent laryngeal nerve

the process of phonation. These include the facial (VII), hypoglossal (XII), trigeminal (V), and vagus (X). Cranial nerves V, VII, and XII innervate the extrinsic muscles, whereas cranial nerve X innervates the intrinsics.

Innervation of the Intrinsic Muscles

All of the intrinsic laryngeal muscles receive their motor innervation from one of two branches of the vagus nerve (cranial nerve X). All intrinsic laryngeal muscles except the cricothyroids are innervated by the **recurrent laryngeal nerve**. The cricothyroid muscles are innervated by the **superior laryngeal nerve**.

The recurrent laryngeal nerve gets its name from the fact that it takes the "scenic route" on its way to the intrinsic muscles of the larynx (see Figure 8-19). The left recurrent laryngeal nerve passes under and around the aorta on its way to the larynx, whereas the right recurrent laryngeal nerve passes under and around the subclavian artery. Because the aorta is inferior to the subclavian artery, the left recurrent laryngeal nerve is a bit longer than the right recurrent laryngeal nerve. However, there is no discernible effect on the timing of neural impulses to the muscles these two nerves serve. By comparison with the recurrent laryngeal nerves, the superior laryngeal nerves take a more direct route on their way to the cricothyroid muscles.

Innervation of the Extrinsic Muscles

The suprahyoid muscles receive their innervation from either the facial (VII), hypoglossal (XII), or trigeminal (V) cranial nerve. The anterior belly of the digastricus and the mylohyoid muscles receive their motor supply from branches of the trigeminal nerve. The posterior belly of the digastricus and the stylohyoid muscles are innervated by branches of the facial nerve. The geniohyoid, genioglossus, and hyoglossus muscles all receive innervation from branches of the hypoglossal nerve.

The three infrahyoid muscles are innervated by branches of the hypoglossal nerve along with branches coming from various spinal nerves. The sternohyoid and omohyoid muscles are innervated by a branch of the hypoglossal nerve whose fibers intermingle with fibers from spinal nerves C1 through C3. The thyrohyoid muscles are innervated by branches from the hypoglossal nerve that interdigitate with fibers from spinal nerves C1 and C2.

Finally, the inferior pharyngeal constrictor is innervated by the vagus nerve (cranial nerve X), with possible contribution from the spinal accessory nerve (XI). The sternothyroid muscle is innervated by the hypoglossal nerve (XII) with contributions from C1, C2, and C3.

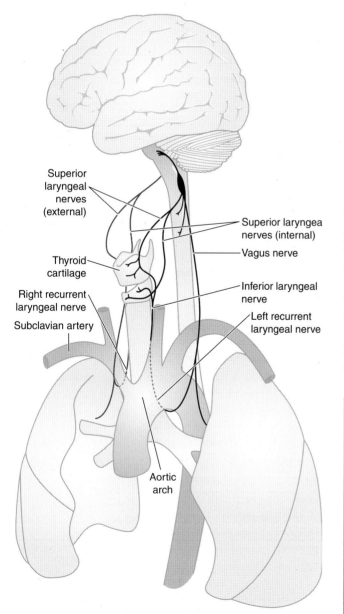

Superior laryngeal nerves (external)

Thyroid cartilage

Right recurrent laryngeal nerve

Subclavian artery

Superior laryngea nerves (internal)

Vagus nerve

Inferior laryngeal nerve

Left recurrent laryngeal nerve

Aortic arch

Figure 8-19 The superior and recurrent laryngeal nerves.

Why You Need to Know

In rare instances, the laryngeal branches of the vagus nerve may be severed or damaged during neck surgery or because of an accident. This can result in severe voice problems for the patient. Depending on the extent of damage, the patient may not have a voice at all, or the voice may sound dull and monotonous due to the patient experiencing problems in regulating pitch. The patient's voice may be whispery with diminished intensity. A more thorough discussion of the effects of vagus nerve damage on voice will be presented in Chapter 9.

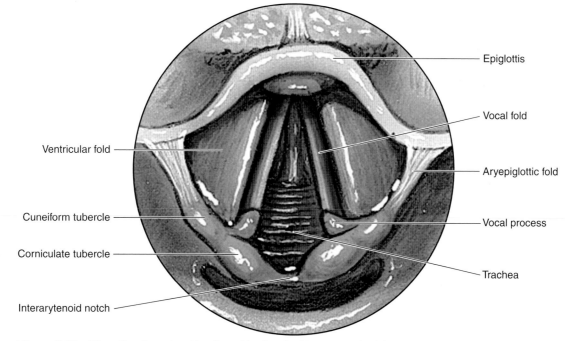

Epiglottis

Vocal fold

Aryepiglottic fold

Ventricular fold

Vocal process

Cuneiform tubercle

Corniculate tubercle

Trachea

Interarytenoid notch

Figure 8-20   The aditus laryngis with selected landmarks (the ventricular folds are superior to the true vocal folds). (Modified with permission from Anatomical Chart Company.)

THE LARYNGEAL CAVITY

Now that the larynx is complete with all the cartilages, connective tissue, and muscles, you will note that the interior of the larynx is a tube with several spaces residing within. If you were to look into the laryngeal cavity, you would see the two ventricular folds and the two true vocal folds extending into the space. The ventricular folds are superior to the true vocal folds (see Figure 8-20). The "shelves" formed by the ventricular folds and true vocal folds serve to divide the laryngeal cavity into several regions.

Figure 8-21 provides a schematic organization of these regions. Starting at the very top of the larynx

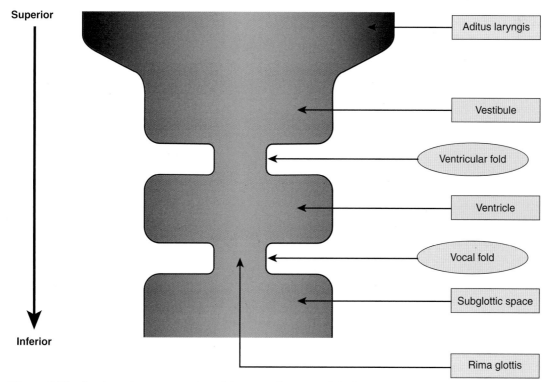

Superior

Inferior

Aditus laryngis

Vestibule

Ventricular fold

Ventricle

Vocal fold

Subglottic space

Rima glottis

Figure 8-21   A schematic representation of the internal cavities of the larynx.

and making your way down, these include the **aditus laryngis, vestibule, ventricle**, and **subglottic space**. The aditus laryngis is the entryway into the laryngeal cavity. It is bounded by the epiglottis anteriorly, the aryepiglottic folds laterally, and the arytenoid cartilages posteriorly. Immediately below the aditus laryngis and immediately above the ventricular folds is an open area called the vestibule. Between the ventricular folds and true vocal folds is a space that runs horizontally along the length of the two sets of folds. This space is called the ventricle. Finally, immediately inferior to the true vocal folds is a space corresponding to the interior of the cricoid cartilage. This space is referred to as the subglottic space.

Although not really a space, there is a variable-sized opening between the two true vocal folds known as the **rima glottis**, or simply the glottis. Variable-sized means that the width of the glottis can change depending on what the vocal folds are doing. When the vocal folds fully adduct, there is zero glottis—no opening between the vocal folds. During normal quiet vegetative breathing, the vocal folds are in a somewhat half-open position known as the **paramedian position**. In this case, the glottis is open but not quite as wide as it has the potential to be (for adult males, with the vocal folds in the paramedian position, the glottis is approximately 8 mm at its widest point). When a person yawns or starts to breathe heavily due to strenuous exercise, the vocal folds abduct even more, beyond their paramedian position. In this scenario,

the glottis is at maximum width (for adult males, as much as 16 to 18 mm at its widest point).

The glottis is divided into two parts. The first part is referred to as the membranous glottis and the second is the cartilaginous glottis. The membranous glottis corresponds to the portions of the vocal folds that are attached to the vocal ligaments (which are membranous). This makes up approximately 60% of the length of the glottis (approximately 15 mm in adult males and 12 mm in adult females). The remaining 40% of the length (i.e., the cartilaginous glottis) corresponds to the vocal processes and foveae oblonga of the arytenoid cartilages (approximately 10 mm in adult males and 8 mm in adult females). The entire length of the glottis then is approximately 25 mm in adult males and 20 mm in adult females.

Laryngeal Regions

The laryngeal cavity is typically divided into three regions: the supraglottic, glottic, and subglottic regions. The supraglottic region involves all laryngeal structures above the level of the vocal folds (since the vocal folds form the glottis). This would include the aditus laryngis (i.e., epiglottis, aryepiglottic folds, and arytenoid cartilages), vestibule, ventricular folds, and ventricle. As illustrated in Figure 8-22, the pyriform sinuses are posterolateral to the aditus laryngis. These sinuses are formed by the space between the superior cornua of the thyroid and the arytenoid cartilages.

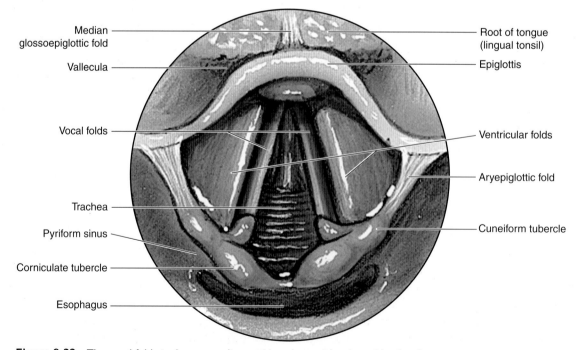

Median glossoepiglottic fold

Vallecula

Vocal folds

Trachea

Pyriform sinus

Corniculate tubercle

Esophagus

Root of tongue (lingual tonsil)

Epiglottis

Ventricular folds

Aryepiglottic fold

Cuneiform tubercle

Figure 8-22 The vocal folds in the paramedian position along with selected landmarks.

> **Why You Need to Know**
>
> *For persons with swallowing disorders, food or drink may pocket within the pyriform sinuses because the patient does not have the ability to propel the food past the larynx and into the esophagus. The patient may choke or aspirate on the food or drink.*

> **Why You Need to Know**
>
> *The Valsalva maneuver is also used by cardiologists to assess the condition of the heart, and may also be used by persons experiencing tachycardia to slow down their heart rate and/or lower their blood pressure. Otolaryngologists (ENTs) also know the utility of a different form of the Valsalva maneuver as a means of actively adjusting middle ear pressure (see Chapter 12).*

The vocal folds and the glottis that is formed by their abduction make up the glottic region. Finally, the space below the vocal folds is known as the subglottic space, and it corresponds to the subglottic region. The mucous membrane that lines the interior of the subglottic space is composed of ciliated epithelial cells. The hairlike projections rising from the mucous membrane continually beat toward the vocal folds. This helps move mucous and inhaled debris (e.g., dust particles) toward the vocal folds where it can be forcibly cleared by a reflexive cough.

Physiology of the Phonatory System

The primary structure of the phonatory system, the larynx, serves a couple of biological or primary functions. First, it acts as a protective mechanism for the lower respiratory passageway. The larynx prevents foreign objects from getting into the trachea, bronchi, and lungs. If by chance a foreign object did find its way into the larynx, contact with the vocal folds would generate a cough reflex to expel the foreign matter. This is especially true during the process of swallowing. When swallowed food or drink (referred to as a **bolus**) approaches the larynx, the epiglottis and aryepiglottic folds constrict the aditus laryngis so that the bolus cannot enter the larynx. The bolus then passes over the larynx posteriorly and into the esophagus. Anyone who has ever accidentally aspirated swallowed water can certainly recall the violent coughing that results!

The second biological function of the larynx is to serve as a valve during thoracic fixation (also known as the **Valsalva maneuver**). During this procedure, expired air is trapped beneath the adducted vocal folds, generating increased abdominal and/or thoracic pressure. The increased pressure is used by a person attempting to lift a heavy object, or by a person who may be straining to empty their bladder or rectum, or by a female giving birth.

The nonbiological or secondary purpose of the larynx is to serve as the sound source for the human voice. It accomplishes this by offering variable resistance to airflow coming from the lungs as expired air. As expired air is forced through the adducted vocal folds, it sets them into vibration. The vibration of the vocal folds is the sound source for voice. It is this particular function of the larynx to which the remainder of this chapter will be dedicated. Before entering into a thorough discussion of how the vocal mechanism works, you should be familiar with several basic concepts related to voice production.

BASIC CONCEPTS

Pure Tones and Complex Tones

Sound is produced by a variable disturbance of the pressure between molecules within a medium; in most cases, the medium is air. When an object is set into motion, it is said to vibrate (one complete back and forth vibration is called a cycle). The disturbance of air molecules transfers energy, referred to as acoustic energy. The acoustic energy travels from the source of the pressure disturbance from air molecule to air molecule in a **longitudinal wave** to the hearing mechanism of an animal or human where it is perceived.

If you have ever undergone an audiological evaluation or screening, you are no doubt familiar with the beeping tones to which you were to respond. These tones are referred to as **pure tones;** that is, each tone presented is a single, individual, discrete **frequency**. Frequency is the number of completed cycles of vibration that occur in one second (hence, cycles per second or cps). For example, an object (such as a tuning fork) that produces a 512 cps pure tone is completing 512 back and forth vibrations of its tines in one second. In other words, the vibrating tines of the tuning fork generate 512 pressure disturbances per second. Not only does a sound have frequency but it also has **intensity**. Intensity is the magnitude of energy carried along the sound wave and is measured in a unit known as the decibel (dB).

Frequency and intensity are physical measures, that is, they are constant and do not change because of humans' perceptions. In speech science, we use the measure of **Hertz (Hz)** to represent the number of cycles per second, so an object vibrating at 1000 cps is measured as 1000 Hz. Humans, however, perceive frequency as **pitch**. Pitch is the psychological perception of frequency and can change depending on people's perceptions. A sound that is perceived as low in pitch has a source that is vibrating at a slower rate than the source of a perceived high-pitched sound. Similarly, intensity is a physical measure of sound pressure level that has a perceptual correlate—**loudness**.

There are relatively few things in our world that produce pure tones. Most sounds are **complex tones**. Complex tones are sounds resulting from two or more pure tones blended together. Through a process known as **Fourier analysis**, a complex tone can be analyzed into its pure tone components along with their individual intensities. The vocal tone (i.e., the sound created by vibration of the vocal folds) is a complex tone that is composed of many frequencies; in other words, it includes a wide range of frequencies. The lowest frequency in this complex tone is referred to as the **fundamental frequency** (abbreviated F_0). Although the vocal tone is a complex tone with a range of frequencies, we usually refer to it in terms of its fundamental frequency instead of its range. The average adult male has a fundamental frequency of approximately 125 Hz, the average adult female has a fundamental frequency exceeding 200 Hz, and children (regardless of gender) have a fundamental frequency exceeding 300 Hz.

The vocal tone is said to be rich in **harmonics**. Harmonics are created by many different modes of vibration of the vocal folds. Fundamental frequency is created by vibration of the entire length of the vocal folds. However, not only does the entire length of the vocal folds vibrate, but sections along the vocal fold length also vibrate, literally creating "vibrations within vibrations." For example, the two halves of each vocal fold also vibrate, and the frequency of vibration of each of these halves is two times the fundamental. The relationship between frequency and length is an inverse one. As length gets shorter and shorter, frequency gets higher and higher. Therefore, since there are two equal halves instead of a whole, each half vibrates at twice the rate as the entire length. This is the second harmonic (the first harmonic is associated with the entire length of the vocal folds, i.e., the fundamental frequency). Not only does each half of the vocal fold vibrate, but each third, fourth, fifth, sixth, seventh, eighth, etc., also vibrates at a different mode that is a multiple of the fundamental frequency. These would be the third, fourth, fifth, sixth, seventh, eighth, etc., harmonics. As an example, if the fundamental frequency is 100 Hz, the harmonics are 100 Hz (first), 200 Hz (second), 300 Hz (third), 400 Hz (fourth), 500 Hz (fifth), 600 Hz (sixth), 700 Hz (seventh), 800 Hz (eighth), and so on. The human vocal tone on average can extend into as many as 20 or more harmonics although not all of them would likely be perceived. With each successive harmonic, vocal intensity tends to diminish at a rate of approximately 12 dB per **octave** until the higher-frequency harmonics are literally imperceptible.

In music, you might recognize the term octave as a series of eight musical notes. In speech science, an octave is defined as a successive doubling of frequency, usually in reference to the fundamental frequency. In the example above, the first octave would be 100–200 Hz (200 Hz represents a doubling of the fundamental frequency of 100 Hz). The second octave would be 201–400 Hz (400 Hz being a doubling of 200 Hz), the third octave would be 401–800 Hz (800 Hz being a doubling of 400 Hz), and the fourth octave would be 801–1600 Hz (1600 Hz being a doubling of 800 Hz). Although the vocal folds can generate a large number of harmonics (and therefore, octaves), vocal intensity diminishes at the rate of 12 dB per octave. Because the highest frequencies are practically imperceptible, the average human being has an *effective* vocal range of approximately two to two and a half octaves. By comparison, some humans have slightly greater vocal ranges. Although this is not confirmed scientifically, a quick search of the Internet reveals that singer Rob Halford (from the heavy metal band Judas Priest) is reported to have a vocal range of approximately four octaves. Mariah Carey (no introduction needed!) and Annie Haslam (from the 1970s progressive rock band Renaissance) are each reported to have a vocal range of five octaves. Trained, professional singers may have a naturally wider vocal range than most humans, but they also learn how to extend their vocal range to some degree.

Subglottic Pressure

Vocal fold vibration requires a coordinated effort between release of the expired air stream from the lungs and adduction of the vocal folds. As the expired air comes up from the lungs and approaches the larynx, the vocal folds adduct. Adduction of the vocal folds creates an obstruction to the expired air so that it becomes trapped below the vocal folds within the subglottic space. As the expired air continues to build below the vocal folds, it generates a certain amount of pressure against the inferior surfaces of the vocal folds. This is known as **subglottic pressure**. As you shall see in the sections that follow, subglottic pressure is a crucial component in vocal fold mechanics.

Longitudinal Tension and Medial Compression

The larynx is capable of making two primary adjustments that regulate the vocal tone. These are **longitudinal tension** and **medial compression**. Longitudinal tension refers to the amount of tension that is generated by changes in the length of the vocal folds. Anyone who has ever played with a rubber band knows that as the rubber band is stretched (i.e., as its length is increased), its tension increases. The same holds true for the vocal folds. Conversely, you could accurately assume that as the vocal folds are shortened, their tension decreases. As the vocal folds lengthen and shorten, other changes are also occurring. Vocal fold lengthening also results in a decrease in their cross-sectional area or mass. By the same token, shortening of the vocal folds results in increased cross-sectional area or mass. The relationship between cross-sectional area and tension is an inverse one. As cross-sectional area increases, tension decreases, resulting in a lower frequency vocal tone. As cross-sectional area decreases, tension increases; the net result is a higher frequency vocal tone. As you can no doubt deduce, changes in vocal fold tension and mass have direct effects on the frequencies that are produced when the vocal folds vibrate. Keep in mind that although changes in cross-sectional area and tension are what are responsible for changes in vocal tone frequency, the two are mediated by changes in vocal fold length. Other than serving as the mechanism for regulating cross-sectional area and tension, vocal fold length has essentially a negligible role in vocal tone frequency. For the most part, vocal fold length is a means toward an end.

Medial compression refers to the pressure that is generated by adduction of the vocal folds. In other words, medial compression could be thought of as the "force of adduction." Humans have the ability to regulate the amount of compression between the vocal folds from a very light contact to an excessive amount of compression. As medial compression increases, the vocal folds offer greater and greater resistance to subglottic pressure. The amount of subglottic pressure that would be needed to overcome the resistance of the vocal folds when the vocal folds are making a light contact with each other is much less than the subglottic pressure that would be needed when the vocal folds are adducted very tightly. Regardless of the amount of medial compression, at some point, subglottic pressure will overcome the resistance of the vocal folds. If there is minimal medial compression, then minimal subglottic pressure will accumulate before the vocal folds' resistance is overcome. Because so little subglottic pressure is generated, a relatively small puff of air will pass through the open vocal folds. Conversely, when there is maximum medial compression, maximum subglottic pressure will be necessary to overcome the resistance of the vocal folds. At the time the vocal folds are overcome, the massive subglottic pressure that had built up will be released as a relatively large puff of air. Essentially, the size of the puffs of air is associated with vocal intensity. Small puffs of air (generated by minimal medial compression) will result in a relatively low intensity vocal tone; large puffs of air will result in a vocal tone having greater intensity.

THE PROCESS OF PHONATION

Myoelastic Aerodynamic Theory of Phonation

Despite the advances of modern science, to this date it is still not completely clear as to how the vocal folds vibrate. Several theories have been posited over the years in an attempt to describe the process of phonation. Perhaps the most widely accepted theory of phonation is the **Myoelastic Aerodynamic Theory** (van den Berg, 1958). As its name indicates, this theory is concerned with principles of muscle tissue elasticity and aerodynamics. One would think that with all of the tools of modern science at our disposal, this theory would be a relatively recent one, but the theory was actually proposed by two 19th century scientists—Helmholtz and Müller—and was further refined by van den Berg in the 1950s.

Central to this theory are the concepts subglottic pressure, elasticity, and **Bernoulli effect**. Subglottic pressure was defined earlier as the force of air upon the inferior surfaces of the vocal folds when the vocal folds are adducted and expired air is trapped below them. Being composed of muscle tissue, the vocal folds have a certain elasticity; that is, they can be manipulated by external forces as well as internal mechanics. Finally, the Bernoulli effect states that when a gas or liquid flows through or around a constriction, velocity of the gas or fluid increases. The abrupt increase in velocity in turn results in a drop in pressure within the gas or fluid relative to the walls of the constriction through which it passes. The net result is a vacuum between the walls of the constriction. If you have ever been on a freeway passing a tractor-trailer and gotten the sensation that you are being "sucked" toward the bigger vehicle, it was the Bernoulli effect that caused that sensation. The differential in air velocity between the two vehicles created a vacuum. Lower air pressure was generated by the tractor-trailer (which was creating greater air velocity) and higher air pressure was generated by your car (which was creating less air velocity). Air flows from regions of higher to lower pressure, and hence your car was actually drawn toward the larger vehicle. It is also interesting to note that the Bernoulli effect is integral to the mechanics of flight. The contour of an airplane wing is designed in such a way that as air passes over and under the wing, velocity of air movement over the wing is greater than under the wing. This creates a drop in pressure above the wing by comparison with the pressure below it. Air below the wing creates "lift" as it attempts to equalize the drop in pressure above the wing.

According to the Myoelastic Aerodynamic Theory, when the vocal folds are adducted, they create resistance to expired air coming from the lungs. Air pressure (in the form of subglottic pressure) then builds within the subglottic space. At some point, subglottic pressure will overcome the resistance of the vocal folds. Because of their elasticity, subglottic pressure will force the vocal folds to separate creating a small glottis. As soon as this occurs, subglottic pressure is released immediately as airflow. The increase in velocity of the air as it passes through the glottis creates a drop in pressure of the air relative to the medial borders of the vocal folds. The vocal folds are literally brought back together by the vacuum that is created by the increased velocity (i.e., the Bernoulli effect), as well as by the recoil pressure that is created by their inherent elasticity. This entire sequence of events (buildup of subglottic pressure; subglottic pressure overcoming the resistance of the vocal folds; increase in velocity creating a vacuum that brings the vocal folds back together again) results in one cycle of vibration. For a vocal tone with a fundamental frequency of 100 Hz, this entire cycle takes only 1/100 of a second to complete. To look at it another way, there would be 100 cycles of glottis open/glottis closed per second! At such a fast rate, subglottic air does not flow through the glottis continuously but rather, small puffs or bursts of air pass through the glottis very similarly to Native American smoke signals.

By the description immediately above, it should be clear that also inherent to vocal fold vibration are the laws of fluid mechanics. You will recall from Chapter 6 that when there is a difference in pressure between two gradients, gases and liquids will always flow from regions of greater pressure to regions of lesser pressure. When the vocal folds adduct for phonation, expired air is trapped below the vocal folds, creating subglottic pressure. By the time the vocal folds are forced open, subglottic pressure is greater than the atmospheric pressure above the vocal folds (referred to as supraglottic pressure). As the vocal folds open, subglottic pressure is released and flows upward through the glottis and vocal tract to equalize the drop in supraglottic pressure.

Cover–Body Model

In recent decades, advances in computer-assisted modeling and imaging techniques such as **videostroboscopy** have allowed scientists to get a better look at how the vocal folds vibrate. Among the pioneers in this area are Titze (1994, 2006) and Hirano et al. (e.g., Hirano, Kakita, Kawasaki, Gould, & Lambiase, 1981; Hirano, Yoshida, & Tanaka, 1991). As a result of his studies involving computer-assisted modeling, Titze (2006) proposed a modification to the Myoelastic Aerodynamic Theory commonly referred to as the Cover–Body Model.

Titze's studies on vocal fold vibration (referred to as oscillations) lead him to believe that the Bernoulli effect alone could not account for how the vocal folds maintain their vibratory mechanics once phonation is initiated. That is, he discovered that the vocal folds have the ability to continue oscillating even during brief periods when there is no energy source. The Bernoulli effect cannot account for this. Instead, Titze found that the inherent structure of the vocal folds plays a big part in their ability to maintain vibration.

To understand how this happens, you should realize that the entire masses of the vocal folds do not vibrate as a whole once subglottic pressure overcomes their resistance. In other words, the vocal folds do not separate from each other *en masse*. Rather, the vocal folds vibrate in a wavelike fashion from bottom to top. Figure 8-23 illustrates this concept. As you can see in Figure 8-23A, the vocal folds adduct as expired air comes up from the lungs, thereby generating subglottic pressure. At some point (see Figure 8-23B), subglottic pressure overcomes the resistance of the vocal folds, and the lower parts of the vocal folds are forced laterally by the pressure. At this point, the lower parts of the vocal folds are wider apart than the upper parts, and this creates convergent airflow. The air continues upward and forces the upper parts of the vocal folds to move laterally (see Figure 8-23C). At the same time this is happening, the lower parts return to midline. Now the upper parts of the vocal folds are wider apart than the lower parts. This creates divergent airflow. As illustrated in Figure 8-23D,

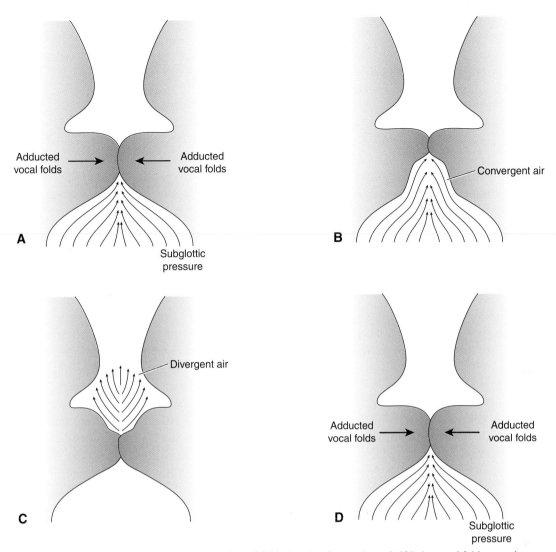

Figure 8-23   A schematic representation of vocal fold vibration (coronal view): (**A**) the vocal folds are adducted and subglottic pressure exerts a force upon their lower surfaces; (**B**) the lower portions of the vocal folds separate creating convergent air; (**C**) the upper portions of the vocal folds separate as the lower portions return to midline, thereby creating divergent air; and (**D**) the upper portions of the vocal folds return to midline. This cycle repeats itself (**A–B–C–D**), creating oscillations of the vocal folds.

the upper parts of the vocal folds return to midline and subglottic pressure once again exerts a force upon their inferior surfaces. This process repeats itself over and over again.

The vocal folds can be thought of as a mass-spring system. According to Titze (1994, 2006), the body (i.e., thyroarytenoid muscle proper) is one mass, whereas the cover (i.e., epithelium and superficial layer of the lamina propria) is composed of many masses from the bottom of the vocal folds to the top. All of the masses (cover and body together) are connected by virtual springs, but their movements are independent of one other. This allows the masses within the cover to be displaced in a wavelike fashion from bottom to top, thereby creating regions of convergent and divergent airflow through the glottis. This is referred to as a vertical phase difference. Air pressure during regions of convergent airflow is greater than during regions of divergent airflow. Titze contends that it is the asymmetry in pressures between convergent and divergent airflow (i.e., the vertical phase difference) that sustains the vocal folds' oscillatory ability and not the Bernoulli effect per se.

Why You Need to Know

A short section in this textbook cannot do justice to the beauty of vocal fold vibration as described by Titze. For a more fascinating and in-depth look at vocal fold mechanics, you are encouraged to read Titze's works—Principles of Voice Production (1994) and The Myoelastic Aerodynamic Theory of Phonation (2006).

The Mechanics of Phonation

The Process

It is clear that phonation occurs when the vocal folds are nearly or fully adducted. They cannot vibrate if they are overly abducted. This begs the question: How do humans adduct the vocal folds so that they can phonate? Conversely, how do humans abduct the vocal folds so that they will stop phonating?

In a single word, the answer is muscles. In two words: intrinsic muscles. Recall from the discussion of the anatomy of phonatory muscles that some of them were classified as adductors, and one of them was classified as an abductor. The adductors are the LCA and the transverse and oblique arytenoids (collectively referred to as the interarytenoids, or IAs). The lone abductors are the PCAs.

As expired air passes from the lungs through the bronchi and up to the trachea, the LCA and IA muscles contract. Contraction of the IA muscles literally squeezes the two arytenoid cartilages together (i.e., adducts them). Because the vocal folds are attached to the arytenoids at the vocal processes and foveae oblonga, they too will be adducted. Simultaneous with IA contraction is LCA contraction. LCA contraction causes the muscular processes of the arytenoids to rotate medially, thereby pulling the vocal ligaments downward and toward midline. Keep in mind that the PCA ligaments restrict the amount of forward and downward movement of the arytenoid cartilages when the LCA contracts. In summary, the net action of the adductor muscles is to bring the arytenoid cartilages forward, medially, and downward. This action causes the vocal folds to adduct. The adductor muscles can be contracted in varying degrees, which means that humans have the ability to adjust the amount of medial compression between the vocal folds.

Now that the vocal folds are adducted, they have the capacity for phonation. As discussed earlier, the Myoelastic Aerodynamic Theory of phonation and Cover-Body Model describe how this process takes place. It should be noted, however, that during phonation, the arytenoids remain adducted by the IA and LCA muscles throughout the entire process. Vibration of the vocal folds is *not* the result of continuous adduction and abduction of the arytenoid cartilages. For the most part, the arytenoid cartilages remain adducted during phonation. Vibration is the result of subglottic pressure overcoming the resistance of the vocal folds, and then the vocal folds' natural recoil and a vertical phase difference bringing them back together again.

> ### Why You Need to Know
> As the vocal folds vibrate, a wave is created that travels from their medial borders to their lateral margins near to where the vocal folds are overlapped by the ventricular folds. This is referred to as the mucosal wave (Berke & Gerratt, 1993; Hirano et al., 1981). The first two layers of the vocal folds (i.e., the epithelial layer and the superficial layer of the lamina propria) slide over the remaining three layers as the vocal folds vibrate. The mucosal wave is used as a diagnostic tool. An absent or abnormal mucosal wave may signal a pathological condition.

There does not need to be complete, absolute adduction of the vocal folds to effect phonation. By the same token, not a lot of subglottic pressure is necessary to set the vocal folds into vibration. As little as 2 to 3 cm H_2O is all the subglottic pressure that is needed to set the vocal folds into vibration. For conversational speech at approximately 60-dB intensity, subglottic pressure averages between 7 and 10 cm H_2O. It increases to approximately 15 to 20 cm H_2O for loud speech, and even higher for high-intensity vocal activity such as yelling or screaming.

How do we abduct the vocal folds, and under what conditions do they abduct? Abduction of the vocal folds is the result of a single pair of muscles—the PCAs. Contraction of the PCA muscles causes the muscular processes of the arytenoids to rock upward and backward. This separates the arytenoid cartilages, thereby also abducting the vocal folds. Keep in mind that the anterior cricoarytenoid ligaments restrict the amount of backward movement of the arytenoids. Obviously, abduction of the vocal folds is necessary for the individual to breathe, but the vocal folds also abduct periodically during vocal activity. The English language consists of approximately 41 speech sounds—24 consonants, 14 pure vowels, and three diphthongs. The vast majority of these sounds are classified as **voiced** sounds, that is, they require vocal fold vibration. All of the pure vowels and diphthongs are voiced, as well as most of the consonants. Only nine consonant sounds are **unvoiced** (/p, t, k, f, s, ʃ, Θ, h, tʃ/). During speech, whenever a voiced sound is encountered, the vocal folds adduct so that they can vibrate. They will remain adducted as long as there is a continuous stream of voiced speech sounds. As soon as an unvoiced speech sound is encountered, the vocal folds abduct so that vocal fold vibration ceases. Upon encountering the next voiced sound, the vocal folds adduct again to phonate. You should immediately gain an appreciation for how rapidly the vocal folds must respond to the demands of the sound system of a language!

Phases of Phonation

The process of phonation is divided into two phases—the **prephonation phase** and the **attack phase**. The first phase is defined as the period of time during which the vocal folds move from the paramedian position to a nearly adducted or fully adducted position. The timing between the prephonation phase and expiration of air is crucial. Mistiming between respiration and prephonation will likely result in aberrations of the attack phase.

The attack phase begins at the moment the vocal folds are adducted and continues through the first cycles of vibration. If timing between expiration and prephonation is optimal, the expired air will reach the vocal folds at the same time the attack phase begins. This is referred to as a **simultaneous attack**. By comparison, if air is released from the lungs before the vocal folds have adducted, there will be a certain quantity of air wastage through the glottis before the vocal folds begin vibrating. This is called a **breathy attack**, and the person who exhibits this attack will have a breathy quality to their voice. On the opposite end of the spectrum, if the vocal folds are adducted before air is released from the lungs and medial compression is considerable, the person will exhibit a **glottal attack**. The voice will sound very explosive upon initiation of phonation.

> ### *Why You Need to Know*
> *As will be discussed in Chapter 9, mistiming between the prephonatory and attack phases of phonation can result in a voice disorder due to hypofunction or hyperfunction of the phonatory system. More times than not, these types of voice disorders tend to be functional in nature, that is, there appears to be no known physical or neurological etiology for the problem.*

MODIFICATION OF VOCAL TONE FREQUENCY AND INTENSITY

Humans have the ability to modify their voices. They can change their vocal pitch for the purpose of regulating **prosody** during speech or for the purpose of singing. Likewise, humans can vary the loudness of their voice from a barely audible whisper to a yell or scream. How do humans make these modifications to their voices? As was explained in an earlier section of this chapter, changes in vocal pitch are mediated by adjustments in longitudinal tension. Changes in vocal loudness are mediated by adjustments in medial compression. In the paragraphs that follow, the mechanics of vocal pitch and intensity will be discussed more fully.

Modifications of Vocal Pitch

Humans have the ability to change their vocal pitch from a very low-pitched guttural sound (called **glottal fry**) to a very high-pitched (i.e., **falsetto**) sound. During conversational speech, vocal pitch constantly varies due to the changes in **intonation** that occur in running speech. Very seldom, however, will an individual use their highest and lowest vocal pitches during speech. Most humans tend to speak toward the lower end of their pitch range, about one-fourth of the way from the bottom of their pitch range to the top. This is referred to as the person's **habitual pitch**. During singing and other vocal activity, a wider pitch range is typically used than during speech.

When the vocal folds are abducted, they are already close to their maximum length. During adduction then, the vocal folds shorten somewhat as they come to midline. The adjustments that occur to the vocal folds to create higher and lower pitches are accomplished relative to this basic mechanic. With that said, your attention is now turned toward the regulation of higher and lower vocal pitches, which is generally accomplished through changes in longitudinal tension.

Regulation of Higher Pitch

From their habitual pitch level, humans have the ability to create a range of higher pitches all the way to falsetto. If one were to gradually increase his or her pitch from habitual to falsetto, the first pitches would be mediated by intrinsic muscle activity. As the individual proceeds to the highest pitches (nearing falsetto), the limits of the intrinsic muscles would be reached so that certain extrinsic muscles would have to be called upon.

Initially, higher pitch is mediated by the cricothyroid muscles, with possibly some additional contraction of the thyroarytenoids and PCAs. The prevailing thought is that the cricothyroid muscles "load" the vocal folds for higher pitch by stretching them. Fine-tuning is accomplished by the vocal folds (i.e., the thyroarytenoids) themselves. The exact action the cricothyroids have on the pitch-changing mechanism continues to be debated to this day. Some scientists believe that contraction of the cricothyroid muscles elevates the anterior arch of the cricoid toward the thyroid cartilage immediately above while the thyroid cartilage remains essentially immobile. Others believe that contraction of the cricothyroid muscles causes the thyroid cartilage to tilt forward by decreasing the distance between its inferior border and the arch of the cricoid (in this case, the cricoid cartilage remains essentially immobile). Regardless of which cartilage is actually acted upon, the result is the same (recall the helmet visor analogy presented earlier). Action of the cricothyroid muscles creates greater distance between the interior of the thyroid angle and the vocal processes of the arytenoid cartilages. Because the vocal folds are attached to these two points, an increase in distance between these two points will result in a lengthening of the vocal folds. As the vocal folds lengthen, their cross-sectional area or mass will decrease (i.e., the vocal folds will get thinner) and their tension will increase. The net effect is an increase in pitch. Fine adjustments are made to the higher pitches by contraction of the muscle tissue within the vocal folds (i.e., the vocalis portion of the thyroarytenoid muscles). The PCAs play a minor role in this mechanic by preventing the arytenoid cartilages from tilting forward as the anterior structures are displaced. Anterior movement of the arytenoids is also limited by the PCA ligaments.

As pitch continues to increase toward falsetto, the intrinsic muscles will finally reach their limit. The vocal folds will be stretched maximally so that additional muscle action will have to play a role in the highest pitches. This muscle action comes from some of the extrinsic laryngeal muscles—more specifically, the suprahyoid muscles. The primary purpose of the extrinsic muscles is to provide support to, and maintain the position of, the larynx. Secondary to this, the suprahyoid muscles elevate the hyoid bone and larynx, while the infrahyoid muscles have the opposite effect. In terms of the production of the highest pitches, it is thought that when the suprahyoid muscles contract and the hyoid bone and larynx subsequently elevate, the result is increased tension of the conus elasticus, of which the vocal ligaments are a part. Indeed, if you were to look at your neck in a mirror during production of your highest pitches, you would very likely see the thyroid prominence (i.e., Adam's apple) move upward due to action of the suprahyoid muscles. Action of the suprahyoid muscles takes place *in addition* to the action of the intrinsic muscles. The final product is generation of the highest pitches in the human vocal range.

Regulation of Lower Pitch

You would be correct in assuming that if stretching of the vocal folds results in higher pitch, relaxing them will result in lower pitch. When the vocal folds are shortened, it results in an increase in their cross-sectional area with a concomitant decrease in tension. These factors result in lower pitch. Recall from the discussion above that vocal fold lengthening is accomplished by increasing the distance between the interior of the thyroid angle (i.e., the anterior attachments of the vocal folds) and the vocal processes of the arytenoid cartilages (i.e., the posterior attachments). Shortening of the vocal folds then requires that the distance between the anterior and posterior attachments be decreased. This is accomplished by contraction of the thyroarytenoid muscles themselves without supplemental contraction of any other intrinsic muscles. When the thyroarytenoids contract unopposed, they literally pull the thyroid cartilage back (the arytenoid cartilages remain stable during this action), thereby shortening the distance between the thyroid angle and vocal processes. The vocal folds basically "bunch up" on themselves. For 50% of the population that has them, the superior thyroarytenoid muscles perform the same function as the thyroarytenoids.

When you want to transition to your lowest pitches (i.e., glottal fry), additional muscle activity will be necessary. At this point, the vocal folds have been shortened as much as possible by intrinsic muscle activity so that the infrahyoid muscles must be called upon to assist in reaching glottal fry. The infrahyoid muscles depress the hyoid bone and larynx when they contract (this can be seen by viewing yourself in the mirror while producing very low pitches). Depression of these structures results in a lessening of tension on the conus elasticus, and subsequently the vocal ligaments. As is the case with the highest pitches, the lowest pitches are produced by the *combined* action of the appropriate intrinsic and extrinsic muscles.

Vocal Registers

As vocal pitch is varied from the lowest to the highest frequencies, physiological changes occur to the vocal folds. These are referred to as voice or vocal registers. Hollien (1972, 1974) identified three vocal registers during speech production: (1) the **pulse register** that is associated with the lowest frequencies in the vocal pitch range; (2) the **modal register** that is associated with the mid-frequencies of the vocal pitch range; and (3) the **loft register** that is associated with the highest frequencies in the vocal pitch range.

In the pulse register, there are low frequency irregularly timed bursts of air through the glottis. The vocal folds are compressed tightly and appear to be short, thick, and somewhat compliant. In some cases, the ventricular folds may descend and nearly touch the vocal folds. The bulk of the vocal folds move very little if at all; only the glottal margins appear to move in a floppy fashion. The infrahyoid muscles also contract to reduce tension on the vocal ligament. The result is a "bubbling" of air through the glottis. This bubbling sound contains very low frequencies, usually in the range of 50 Hz or less, and has been described as similar to the sound of popcorn popping or bacon frying.

In the modal register (which is where conversation speech occurs), the vocal folds have an upper and lower edge along the glottal margin and are still somewhat compliant. When air passes through the glottis, almost the entire vocal fold vibrates, starting with the inferior region and then spreading to the superior region. As pitch rises in the modal register, the vocal folds become longer and stiffer, and thus become less compliant. At the highest pitches within the modal register, the glottal margin appears as a single edge. The modal register accounts for the production of frequencies in the range of four to six octaves above the pulse register (roughly between 50 and 3200 Hz, but this range varies widely from individual to individual). Not only is a wide range of frequencies possible in the modal register, but also a wide range of intensities is also possible (approximately 40 to 110 dB). However, keep in mind that the highest frequencies will likely be imperceptible because of the 12 dB per octave loss of energy.

In the loft register, the vocal folds become so stiff and tense that only their medial-most borders vibrate and the vertical phase difference (mentioned earlier) is lost. There is only a single edge to the glottal margin. Because of the maximum tension that is produced, the anterior and posterior regions of the vocal folds barely move, thereby reducing the effective vibrating area of the vocal folds so that very high frequencies are produced. The suprahyoid muscles also contract to place even greater tension on the vocal ligament. The vocal folds vibrate similarly to strings in this case. Frequencies in the loft register typically exceed 1000 Hz.

Modifications of Vocal Loudness

Vocal intensity or loudness is a direct function of changes in the amount of subglottic pressure. Minimum levels of subglottic pressure will result in a voice that has reduced intensity. Conversely, maximum levels of subglottic pressure will create a voice having greater intensity. As was mentioned earlier in this section of the chapter, when the vocal folds vibrate, they release puffs of air through the glottis. The number of puffs of air that pass through the glottis per second is related to the frequency of vibration. The size of the puffs, on the other hand, is related to vocal intensity. The laryngeal

adjustment responsible for regulating pitch is longitudinal tension. The laryngeal adjustment that regulates vocal intensity is medial compression.

The more tightly the vocal folds are adducted during phonation, the more resistance they offer to subglottic pressure. Under a condition of minimum medial compression, minimum subglottic pressure will be necessary to overcome the resistance of the adducted vocal folds. Because so little subglottic pressure has built up by the time the vocal folds are blown apart, relatively tiny puffs of air will pass through the glottis. The net result is a voice having minimal intensity.

On the other hand, under a condition of maximum medial compression, the requirement for sufficient subglottic pressure to overcome the resistance of the vocal folds will be considerable. A very high level of subglottic pressure must be sustained to overcome the medial compression created by the adducted vocal folds. When this resistance is finally overcome, relatively large puffs of air will pass through the glottis. The net result is a voice having maximum intensity.

Another way to increase vocal intensity is to push more air through the glottis. The force of this action not only creates more pressure below the vocal folds when they are closed but also faster airflow through the glottis when the vocal folds separate. The faster airflow creates a greater drop in pressure between the vocal folds, which in turn draws the vocal folds back toward the midline faster and with greater force. When the vocal folds meet at midline, they become compressed with greater force due to inertia. This leads to a longer "closed phase" during phonation, which in turn leads to the opportunity for greater subglottic pressure to build up prior to the vocal folds being blown apart once again. To illustrate this, compare the phonatory cycle during conversational speech to the phonatory cycle during speech marked by increased vocal intensity. During conversational speech, vocal intensity is such that the vocal folds are open during 50% of the phonatory cycle, closing during 37% of the cycle, and closed during 13% of the cycle. By comparison, during loud speech, the open phase accounts for 33% of the phonatory cycle, the closing phase accounts for 37% of the cycle, and the closed phase accounts for the remaining 30%. In summary, airflow appears to be used for intensity changes at low frequencies, while maximum medial compression (mediated by muscle contraction) appears to be the mechanism by which greater intensity is generated at higher frequencies.

A general rule of thumb is that vocal intensity will rise on the magnitude of approximately 8 to 12 dB with each successive doubling of subglottic pressure. As was stated earlier, subglottic pressure for conversational speech at 60 dB is approximately 7 to 10 cm H_2O. To increase the intensity of speech to approximately 68 to 72 dB, subglottic pressure would have to double to approximately 14 to 20 cm H_2O. A yell or scream at 110 dB would require subglottic pressure on the magnitude of approximately 112 to 640 cm H_2O.

In the anatomy section of this chapter, you learned that three muscles are classified as vocal fold adductors. These are the LCAs and interarytenoids (i.e., the oblique and transverse arytenoids). Humans have the ability to adjust the contraction of these muscles, thereby mediating medial compression.

The Relationship Between Vocal Tone Frequency and Intensity

For the most part, vocal intensity is regulated by medial compression and its effect on subglottic pressure, while changes in vocal pitch are a result of adjustments to longitudinal tension of the vocal folds. However, there are instances where adjustments to medial compression may affect longitudinal tension as well. Anyone who has ever raised the intensity of their voice in an abrupt and dramatic fashion has probably noted that their pitch increased as well. This may be due to one or both of two factors: (1) at greater vocal intensity, reflexive tensing of the vocal folds may occur, and increased tension results in higher pitch; (2) with greater vocal intensity, increased subglottic pressure causes the vocal folds to adduct more quickly, and the quicker timing of adduction results in an increase in pitch.

Vocal pitch and intensity are used to mark the **suprasegmental** aspects of speech production such as intonation and stress. Intonation is mediated primarily by variations in vocal pitch, whereas stress is mediated by both pitch and intensity. This is accomplished very rapidly throughout the stream of speech—on average, about one-tenth of a second. In that very brief period of time, stress is generated by increases in subglottic pressure on the magnitude of about 2 cm H_2O along with slight increases in vocal pitch. Increases in subglottic pressure are accomplished by contraction of the muscles involved in medial compression (i.e., the lateral cricoarytenoids and IAs) as well as the internal intercostal muscles acting upon the rib cage. Increases in pitch are accomplished by generating greater tension on the vocal folds through action of the cricothyroids and thyroarytenoids (vocalis portion).

Intonation, of course, would involve only the pitch-change mechanism. For example, for a rising intonation pattern (typically seen in questions that require a "yes" or "no" response, such as "Are we going to the store?"), there is approximately a 50-Hz increase in the fundamental frequency of the vocal tone (Netsell, 1973). We have a natural tendency to lower our pitch at the end of a breath group. This means that when we encounter an utterance that has a rising intonation, we must work against this natural tendency by contracting the cricothyroid muscles.

Physiology of Other Forms of Vocal Activity

The foregoing discussion examined the physiology of phonation primarily in reference to typical speech activity. For other forms of vocal activity such as speaking or singing in falsetto or whispering, the physiology of phonation is a bit different. This final section of the chapter will briefly describe the phonatory physiology of falsetto and whisper.

Physiology of Falsetto

Recall that falsetto involves the production of frequencies at the uppermost end of the vocal pitch range. Not only is the rate of phonation affected, but the actual manner of phonation changes as well. Although there tends to be some degree of overlap between the upper end of an individual's modal register and the lower end of the loft register (where falsetto resides), there are laryngeal adjustments made that are particular to falsetto. During the production of falsetto, only the free medial borders of the vocal folds make contact and vibrate. The bulk of the vocal folds remain relatively firm and stationary. The appearance of the vocal folds is long, very stiff, and bowed. This results in a shorter effective vibrating area of the glottis, and hence higher frequency vibration. The suprahyoid muscles also assist the process by creating greater tension on the vocal ligament when they contract. Increased tension also results in higher frequency vibration. The vertical phase difference is not at play during falsetto.

Physiology of Whisper

A whisper is not voiced; that is, the vocal folds do not vibrate during this form of vocal activity. During normal phonation, the arytenoid cartilages come together medially and the two vocal folds are parallel to each other along their entire length. During whisper, however, the arytenoid cartilages do not come into contact with each other medially. Instead, they are slightly abducted with their vocal processes converging medially (i.e., the arytenoids are "toed in"). This is accomplished by contraction of the lateral cricoarytenoids with little to no contribution from the IAs (Monoson & Zemlin, 1984; Solomon, McCall,

Trosset, & Gray, 1989). Such a configuration creates an opening in the cartilaginous region of the vocal folds, referred to as a **glottal chink**. If you were to look at the length of the vocal folds from their adduction anteriorly to their abduction posteriorly, it would resemble an inverted "Y." As the person whispers, air passes through the glottal chink at a relatively rapid rate, creating turbulence (the rate of airflow during the normal production of vowel sounds is approximately 100 cc per second; for whisper, it is double this). The turbulence of air as it passes through the glottal chink is essentially what is perceived as the whisper.

Summary

This chapter provided a thorough description and discussion of the anatomy and physiology of the phonatory system. The phonatory system can be considered the motor or generator for vocal activity. Phonation is accomplished by vibration of the vocal folds and is mediated by intrinsic laryngeal muscle activity. Phonation also involves changes in frequency and intensity of the vocal tone. Changes in frequency are mediated by adjustments to longitudinal tension, while changes in intensity are primarily the result of adjustments to medial compression. Longitudinal tension involves activity of intrinsic and extrinsic laryngeal muscles. Medial compression is accomplished by intrinsic muscle activity, and more specifically by contraction of the vocal fold adductors. Basic principles of voice production (e.g., complex tones, fundamental frequency, and harmonics) and other forms of vocal activity (e.g., falsetto and whisper) were also discussed. The following chapter (Chapter 9) will assist you in understanding how aberrations in phonatory anatomy and/or physiology can result in disorders of voice. Then, Chapter 10 will show you how the vocal tone is shaped and molded into the acoustic phenomenon we recognize as human speech.

CHAPTER 9

Pathologies Associated with the Phonatory System

CHARLES L. MADISON

Knowledge Outcomes for ASHA Certification for Chapter 9
- Demonstrate knowledge of the biological basis of the basic communication processes (III-B)
- Demonstrate knowledge of the etiologies of voice and resonance disorders (III-C)

Learning Objectives
- You will be able to define normal and disordered voices.
- You will be able to explain the physiology of phonation (e.g., the Myoelastic Aerodynamic Theory of phonation).
- You will be able to explain how to clinically evaluate parameters of voice.
- You will be able to describe some of the common voice disorders.
- You will be able to explain clinical perspectives relevant to management of voice disorders.

AFFIX AND PART-WORD BOX

TERM	MEANING	EXAMPLE
a-	without; absence of	**a**phonia
dys-	abnormal; impaired	**dys**phonia
myo-	pertaining to muscles	**Myo**elastic Aerodynamic Theory
-phonia	sound; voice	dys**phonia**
presby-	pertaining to advanced age	**presby**laryngis
puber-	pertaining to puberty	**puber**phonia
segment	pertaining to phonemes (speech sounds)	supra**segment**al
supra-	above; overriding	**supra**glottic

Introduction

In this chapter, an introduction to **voice disorders** will be presented by building on the anatomical and physiological foundation offered in Chapter 8. The goal is to relate clinically relevant voice parameters to the structure and function (i.e., anatomy and physiology) of the larynx in a way that will make sense when the speech–language clinician, as a voice therapist, is faced with the responsibility of evaluating and offering remedial options to clients with voice concerns. Clinicians learn the anatomy of speech production for the purpose of relating structure to function as required to appropriately understand what they are hearing and how best to manage voice production for the most positive communication outcome. However, there are clearly challenges to effective evaluation and management of voice disorders. Deem and Miller (2000) noted four such challenges.

- There is no direct relationship between the perception of a voice disorder and the presence of pathology.
- Social acceptance of voice problems creates a significant challenge for the voice therapist.
- The patient's level of motivation to restore vocal health will be related to the importance of the voice in his or her profession.
- Terms used to describe voice disorders are often misunderstood among professionals (p. 3).

In this chapter, these challenges will be addressed, although not completely resolved, as the principles of voice production, voice perspective, and voice parameters are discussed. The goal is to present an introduction to voice that relates anatomy and physiology to normal voice, exceptional voice, and voice disorders in a clinically relevant way.

Voice Production

Respiration, phonation, articulation, and resonance are the underlying physiological processes of speech production. These processes are represented schematically in Figure 9-1 where air from the lungs causes vibration of the vocal folds (represented by the tuning fork) and thus a basic laryngeal tone (represented by the sine wave). Here, a simple tube represents the supraglottic resonators, and the repeating waveform at the right is a resulting vowel. The vowel wave could be that of any vowel, as the resonators serve to modify the basic laryngeal tone (i.e., fundamental) into the desired production.

As related to voice and voice disorders, the emphasis in this chapter will be on phonation as driven by respiration. Voice is the acoustic or audible result of the phonatory process or **phonation**. Sound is audible vibration, and phonation is the physiological process that results in vocal fold vibration and thus voice. Phonation and respiration are inexorably linked in oral human communication. For vocal fold vibration to occur, a driving force is necessary. In phonation, the force is the air provided and controlled by the subglottic respiratory mechanism. Movement of air is required. The phonatory process begins with closure of the **glottis**, that is, the vocal folds moving to midline. Subglottic air pressure increases to the point that it exceeds the resistance of the vocal folds. The vocal folds are blown apart and air is released. Based on the mass and elasticity of the vocal folds and the aerodynamic factors associated with air moving rapidly through a narrow orifice, the vocal folds return to a closed position and the process begins all over again (recall the discussion in Chapter 8 about the **Myoelastic Aerodynamic Theory** and Cover–Body Model).

This physical process of voice generation is the heart of the Myoelastic Aerodynamic Theory of phonation. Objects—including vocal folds—vibrate as a function of their physical properties, mass, and elasticity. For example, some guitar strings are larger (i.e., bigger in circumference) than others and thus have more mass. The larger thicker strings produce a lower pitched vibration than do the smaller thinner strings, and all strings produce a higher pitched vibration when made shorter and more taut by placing one's fingers on the frets. Analogous adjustments can be made by human producers of voice. Although we do not adjust the length of the vocal folds by using our fingers, we are able to vary their length by adjusting the relationship of the cricoid and thyroid cartilages, and we are able to vary the relative thickness/thinness of the vocal folds as well. It is the cricothyroid muscles that are primarily responsible for this adjustment. Interestingly, the cricothyroids are the only intrinsic muscles of the larynx that are not innervated by the recurrent laryngeal branch of the vagus nerve. The superior laryngeal branch of the vagus nerve serves the cricothyroid muscles, and thus insult to the superior branch might be suspected when a patient is unable to control vocal pitch.

The ability to make these changes in the mass and elasticity of the vocal folds affords us the opportunity to make incredible changes in the fundamental frequency perceived as pitch. The difference between the vibratory energy source for a guitar and the human

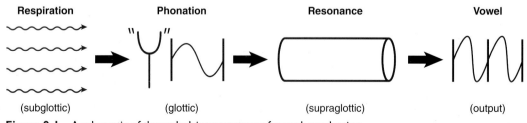

Respiration   **Phonation**   **Resonance**   **Vowel**

(subglottic)   (glottic)   (supraglottic)   (output)

Figure 9-1   A schematic of the underlying processes of speech production.

voice producing mechanism is acknowledged. We do not pluck or strum the vocal folds. Instead, we force subglottic air past them to generate vibration. Thus, we must recognize the importance of the physical properties of the air movement (aerodynamics) in phonation. Once the physiological process of phonation is understood, normal voices, exceptional voices, and disordered voices can be understood, appreciated, and managed. Voices that are appropriate for one's age and gender, do not call undue or negative attention to the speaker, or do not interfere with communication are considered normal. Some voices are considered exceptional because of their unique quality or the masterful control exhibited by the speaker or singer. Such voices are easily recognized and appreciated. They are exceptional in that they bring positive attention to the speaker or singer. By contrast, disordered voices are ones that bring negative attention to the speaker and/or interfere with communication. However, American society seems to have a liberal tolerance for voice differences, and thus noticeable voice differences may not be viewed as disordered. Deem and Miller (2000) noted that this circumstance may have an effect on patient motivation. Regardless of whether voices are considered normal, exceptional or disordered, the basic laryngeal anatomy is the same as are the physiological processes that result in phonation and the physical principles that underlie them. Our understanding of voice normalcy, exceptionality, or disorder is enhanced by our knowledge of the anatomy and physiology and the physical principles of vocal fold vibration.

Perspectives

Several common pathologies of voice are summarized in Table 9-1. Voice disorders can be viewed from several different perspectives, as speech–language pathologists seek to better understand them and effectively evaluate and treat them. In the discussion that follows, voice disorders will be discussed from the perspectives of the causes, prevalence, duration, and life span, then followed by an introduction to voice that focuses on the parameters that define it as normal, exceptional, or disordered.

ETIOLOGY

Voice disorders are frequently discussed from an etiological perspective, a perspective intended to help the clinician better understand the cause or causes of the problem. Voice disorders are categorized as being

psychogenic (i.e., functional) or **organic** in origin. Psychogenic voice disorders can be further differentiated as being subsequent to or a symptom of personality and adjustment disorders; for example, stress, anxiety, or mental health conditions. Psychogenic voice disorders can also be associated with personality type and/or faulty voice habits. In fact, faulty voice habits are most likely to be a factor in psychogenic voice disorders. Vocal abuse, in one form or another, is the leading cause of voice disorders. By contrast, organic voice disorders are viewed as a consequence of mass lesions or neurogenic conditions.

A voice disorder is organic if it is caused by structural (i.e., anatomic) or physiologic disease, either a disease of the larynx itself or by remote systemic illness which alters laryngeal structure or function (Aronson, 1990). Aronson goes on to identify congenital disorders, inflammation, tumors, endocrine disorders, trauma, and neurologic disease as organic etiological categories with voice consequences. Interestingly, psychogenic etiologies can result in organic pathologies, thus somewhat blurring the psychogenic–organic etiological dichotomy. For example, vocal abuse is accepted as the etiological basis for the development of **vocal nodules**. The nodules—clearly mass lesions—are generally agreed upon to be a consequence of vocal abuse, which must be addressed clinically to alleviate the voice disorder. Although organic in nature, vocal nodules (see Figure 9-2A), **polyps** (see Figure 9-2B), and contact ulcers (see Figure 9-2C) are often discussed as secondary pathologies consequent to abusive behavior, and thus are typically classified as being psychogenic in origin.

However, alternative causal factors suggest that both psychogenic and organic causes can result in the same pathology. Contact ulcers can result from abusive behaviors, but they can also result from gastroesophageal reflux disease. Pannbacker (1992) noted the difficulty in making a distinction between psychogenic and organic voice problems. In essence, there are frequently psychogenic elements associated with organic etiologies and psychogenic etiologies that result in organic factors. Pannbacker's thesis is that voice disorder etiologies can be viewed on a continuum ranging from psychogenic on one end to organic on the other.

PREVALENCE

Another perspective from which to view voice disorders is that of prevalence. Some voice problems occur much more frequently than others. Six percent of school-aged children have been found to present with

TABLE 9-1

COMMON VOCAL PATHOLOGIES

	Location	Size	Etiology	Description	Vocal Symptoms	Management
Carcinoma of the larynx (squamous cell, renal cell, melanoma, sarcoma)	Variable	Small (6 mm) to obstructive	• Unknown • Inhalation of suspected carcinogens	Variable; not a well-defined tumor	• Breathiness • Low pitch • Intermittent aphonia • Diplophonia • Hoarseness	• Chemotherapy • Radiation • Surgery • Voice therapy as part of rehabilitation
Contact ulcers	Vocal processes, typically bilateral	Small to obstructive	• Adults 30+ years • Upper gastrointestinal disorders	Hyperemia leading to sessile lesion; raised ulcer with inflamed margins	• Pain in the posterior laryngeal area when processes move to close, e.g., swallowing • Breathiness • Low pitch • Intermittent aphonia	• Voice therapy • Medical • Surgery (not recommended)
Essential tremor of the vocal folds	N/A	N/A	• Adults 45+ years • Central nervous system disease, typically genetic	• Mild cases: vocal tremor noticeable on prolonged vowels • Most severe cases: vocal tremor noticeable on all vocal attempts	• Quavering intonation • Phonation breaks • Rhythmic tremor • Laryngospasms in severe cases	• Medication may result in some improvement • Voice therapy is of limited value
Granuloma	Vocal processes, usually bilateral	Small to obstructive	• Surgical intubation • Esophageal reflux	Pain associated with any laryngeal movement (see contact ulcers)	• Breathiness • Low pitch • Diplophonia • Mild dysphonia • Tension • Clunking	• Voice therapy • Reflux management • Surgery (not recommended)
Interchordal cysts	Surface of vocal folds, typically unilateral (if bilateral, unpaired)	6–12 mm	• Obstruction of duct	Fluid-filled sacs, usually sessile	• Breathiness • Low pitch • Diplophonia	• Voice therapy • Surgical
Nodules	Juncture of the anterior $\frac{1}{3}$ and posterior $\frac{2}{3}$, typically bilateral	Pinpoint to 6 mm	• Vocal abuse • Hemorrhagic/sudden onset • Thickened epithelium/chronic	• Early (<6 months): soft, pink, normal epithelium • Mature (6 months or longer): white to yellow, firm epithelium	• Breathiness • Tension (early) • Pitch breaks • Hard attack on initial vowels • Intermittent aphonia • Diplophonia	• Vocal counseling • Voice therapy • Surgery (not usually necessary)
Papilloma	Vocal folds and surrounding area	6+ mm	• Viral	Wart-like: raspberry shape and texture	• Breathiness • Low pitch • Tension • Aphonia • Hoarseness	• Chemotherapy • Surgery • Voice therapy

TABLE 9-1

COMMON VOCAL PATHOLOGIES (Continued)

	Location	Size	Etiology	Description	Vocal Symptoms	Management
Polyps (unilateral or bilateral)	Laryngeal mucosa	Small (6 mm) to obstructive	• Airborne irritants: smoking, inhalation of toxins, etc. • Medications • Idiopathic	• Polypoid degeneration: soft globular mass exhibiting mucoid degeneration • Pedunculated: with a peduncle or stalk • Sessile: having no peduncle, attached directly by a broad base	• Breathiness • Low pitch • Intermittent aphonia • Diplophonia • Hoarseness (wet or dry)	• Vocal counseling • Surgical management • Postoperative vocal rest • Postoperative voice therapy
Spastic dysphonia	Larynx	N/A	Adults 30+ years	Adductor (most common) or abductor spasms	• Erratic vocal fold spasms	• Voice therapy (guarded prognosis at best) • Counseling • Surgery
Vocal fold edema (laryngitis)	Arytenoids, vocal processes to the anterior commissure	Typically widespread	• Viral infection • Bacterial infection • Allergic reaction	Reddened, swollen arytenoids, vocal processes and/or vocal folds	• Breathiness • Intermittent to complete aphonia • Diplophonia • Hoarseness • Tension • Low pitch	• Controlled vocal use • Medical • Vocal hygiene counseling
Vocal fold paralysis (unilateral or bilateral; abductor or adductor type)	Relative to type and position of paralysis	N/A	• Recurrent laryngeal nerve damage caused by surgery, disease, or trauma	Vocal fold immobility or partial mobility	• Unilateral abductor: breathiness, low pitch, diplophonia • Unilateral adductor: breathiness, diplophonia, low pitch, possible aphonia • Bilateral abductor: breathiness, fair vocal quality, obstructed airway, mild dysphonia • Bilateral adductor: vulnerable airway, aphonia	• Voice therapy • Surgery

Adapted from Wilson, F.B. (1990). *A program of diagnosis and management for voice disorders.* Bellingham, WA: VTI Voice Tapes, Inc.

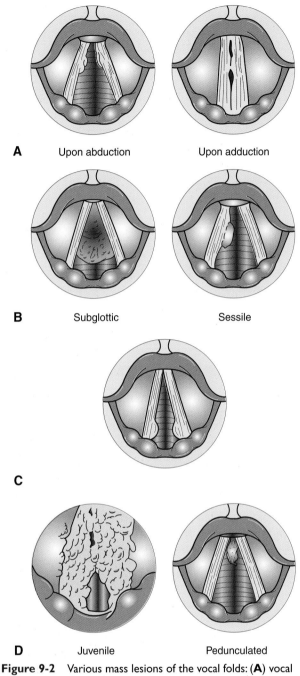

A   Upon abduction   Upon adduction

B   Subglottic   Sessile

C

D   Juvenile   Pedunculated

Figure 9-2 Various mass lesions of the vocal folds: (**A**) vocal nodules; (**B**) polyp; (**C**) contact ulcers; and (**D**) papilloma. (Reproduced with permission from CIBA Pharmaceutical Company, Summit, NJ; J. Harold Walton (Ed.), The larynx, W. Saunders, with illustrations by F.H. Netter, 1964.)

and management of them. Vocal nodules can be considered significant because of the frequency with which they occur. Comparatively, **papilloma** (see Figure 9-2D) is an example of a condition that affects voice, and occurs much less frequently than do vocal nodules, but it is no less important for the clinician to understand the anatomical and physiological consequences of these mass lesions and his or her role in the management of a child with papilloma.

DURATION

Some voice disorders present temporarily, usually as the consequence of abuse or some short-lived and treatable disease process. **Edema** of the vocal folds can result in a voice quality characterized by breathiness and tension, similar to vocal nodules, thus making it difficult to identify the cause of the **dysphonia** based on perceptual parameters alone. The anatomical nature of the edema on one hand or vocal nodules on the other is different and the physiological consequences of these conditions may be as well, but the resulting voice may be quite similar, ranging from mild breathiness and tension to **aphonia**. This is an example of the lack of direct relationship between how a voice sounds and the presence of a particular pathology. With respect to duration, the dysphonia associated with edema may last only a few hours or a day or so, but similar voice characteristics resulting from the presence of nodules may require months of vocal abuse management to eliminate.

Other voice disorders can last a very long time or be permanent. Spasmodic dysphonia is a progressive and often permanent condition. Although symptomatic relief is possible, in the vast majority of cases, patients must deal with the disorder for the rest of their lives. The loss of voice in the laryngectomee is clearly permanent. Once the larynx is removed, the patient will never phonate in the natural way as before the surgery. There are, of course, several alternative sound/phonation sources that will allow the laryngectomee to speak, but natural vocal fold phonation is permanently lost.

Why You Need to Know

We live in marvelous times! Until relatively recently, undergoing a laryngectomy or having unsalvageable trauma to the larynx meant the end of natural speech production. However, advances in the areas of bioengineering and organ transplantation may soon change the way speech–language pathologists conduct their business—especially in regard to persons with profound voice disorders. The first

chronically hoarse voices (Baynes, 1966), and 80% of that 6% were found to present with vocal nodules (Wilson, 1990). No other voice problem will approach the prevalence of the hoarseness associated with vocal nodules as a focus of concern for speech–language pathologists working in a school setting. Understanding the anatomical and physiological basis for the voice quality associated with nodules is important if the clinician is to deal effectively with the evaluation *attempts at laryngeal transplantation have proven to be successful for the most part. More incredible than this, though, is the recent advent of tissue engineering (i.e., creating complete organs from stem cells). Tissue engineering of the larynx has been accomplished successfully in animals. Just imagine how it will revolutionize the field of speech–language pathology if tissue engineering can be refined for use with humans!*

LIFE SPAN

Finally, viewing and understanding voice disorders across the life span also requires an understanding of the anatomical and physiological conditions that result in noticeable voice differences. Vocal nodules frequently result from the yelling and screaming that children do, and papilloma is typically found in preadolescent children when it does occur. The **presbylaryngis** of the elderly client results in voice characteristics for which there may be structural and physiological explanations—explanations inherent to the aging process and not typically associated with infancy, childhood, or even young adulthood. It should be noted, however, that following their review, Boone, McFarlane, von Berg, and Zraick (2010) concluded that the voice characteristics of the elderly are more a function of disease processes than of physiological deterioration.

In summary, regardless of perspective, when viewing voice disorders it is imperative to be able to relate structure and function of the voice producing mechanism to the affected parameters of voice. The voice clinician will always be better prepared to understand the disorder, to evaluate and monitor the voice, and to provide appropriate therapy and counsel if he/she is able to relate the perceptual consequences of the condition (i.e., the voice) to the structure and function of the mechanism.

Parameters of Voice

The psychological parameters of voice—pitch, loudness, quality, and flexibility—are the perceptual characteristics of voice that define it as either normal (i.e., pleasing to the ear, not calling undue or negative attention to the speaker, and not interfering with communication) or abnormal or disordered (i.e., dysphonic). Speech–language pathologists are faced with the responsibility of describing and documenting voices in terms of these parameters. When a clinician is able to do so effectively, the voice problem will be well understood, appropriate directions for therapy will be forthcoming, and treatment will likely be efficacious.

PITCH

In Chapter 8, pitch was defined as the psychological correlate of frequency. Pitch is primarily a function of the basic laryngeal tone, or **voice fundamental**—the frequency at which the vocal folds open and close (or release puffs of subglottic air) per second. Studies have documented the **habitual pitch** of the voice of various aged subjects. Thus, there is empirical evidence of habitual fundamental frequency as a function of age. As noted in Chapter 8, there is individual variation in vocal fold length from person to person as well as a significant difference in the length of the vocal folds between adult males and females. The difference in habitual pitch between males and females is evident in adults but not in children. In general, there is nearly an octave difference in habitual pitch between adult females and males, and females are able to achieve significantly higher frequencies at the upper end of their pitch range than are their male peers. Conversely, adult males are able to produce lower frequencies at the lower end of their pitch range than are adult females. These gender-related differences are explainable and understandable when you consider the anatomical variance between adult female and male speakers such as overall laryngeal size, degree of the thyroid angle, and vocal fold length and mass. Therefore, from a clinical perspective, normal pitch can be defined as a pitch that is appropriate for age and gender. Conversely, disordered pitch occurs when the speaker loses age or gender identity. For example, an adult female has lost age identity if she answers the phone and is asked if the caller can speak to her mother because the caller assumes from her voice that she's a child.

One of the most interesting, dramatic, and treatable disorders of pitch is **puberphonia**, a condition in which an inappropriately high pitch—often **falsetto**—is used by males in their late teens or early adulthood. Puberphonia has the capacity to affect gender identity and surely calls undue and negative attention to the speaker. Voices of somewhat high pitch, though not as dramatically so as puberphonia, can cause concern on the part of the speaker, and occasionally their employer, and may have implications for employment or promotions. It should be noted, however, that many therapists remain cautious about trying to dramatically effect pitch change in clients (puberphonia notwithstanding) for what might be termed "social" reasons. The concept that there is a habitual pitch that is best, and some might say healthiest, for each of us is discussed often in the literature. Our most natural pitch is referred to as **optimal pitch** and is thought to be the pitch at which our phonation producing mechanism is most efficient. The idea that there is a pitch that is most natural for the anatomical and physiological features of our larynx runs deep among voice therapists even when they disagree about how to establish optimal pitch and may be reluctant to facilitate change to optimal pitch as a therapeutic goal. It may be best to think of optimal pitch as the equivalent of habitual pitch for the vast majority of healthy nonabusive speakers.

Our discussion of pitch as a critical parameter of voice production would not be complete without consideration of **vocal registers**. The term vocal register refers to pitch ranges and to types of phonation, or ways in which the vocal folds function. Vocal registers are laryngeal events that can be identified on physical, acoustic, and perceptual bases and remind us of the incredible adaptability and flexibility of the laryngeal anatomy. These registers are ranges of vocal frequencies that overlap but are perceptually distinct. The vocal register that we use most is referred to as the **modal register** and is important because it is associated with the most common vibratory pattern of the vocal folds. Physiologically, when we phonate in our mid-range or normal voice, our vocal folds present an upper and lower edge that vibrates along their entire anteroposterior length. As pitch increases, the vocal folds are increasingly stretched and their thickness is decreased. In the modal register, the frequency range is one and a half octaves or more and a wide intensity range (40 to 110 dB) is possible. The quality of the modal register voice is considered rich, pleasing, and mellow. Normal vocal fold vibration is complex; as the puffs of air are released through the glottis, the thyroarytenoid muscle and the cover layers of the vocal folds vibrate differentially.

By contrast, in the **pulse register**, phonation is characterized by low frequency irregularly occurring bursts. The vocal folds are thick, short, and tightly compressed. The puffs of air may be individually perceived, and thus the phonation is referred to as **glottal** (or **vocal**) **fry**, sounding similar to the sound of bacon frying. In the pulse register, vocal intensity is limited and frequencies are in the range of 3 to 50 Hz. At the other end of the human phonation range, the highest frequencies are produced in the **loft register** or falsetto range. In this mode of phonation, the vocal folds stiffen to a single thin tense edge and only the free margins vibrate. The vibration is primarily in the area of the junction of the anterior and middle thirds of vocal fold length. Vocal fold movement is described as a simple opening and closing with no phase effects or **mucosal wave**. The resulting voice is high pitched with restricted intensity range and perhaps a breathy quality.

LOUDNESS

Loudness of voice is directly related to subglottic air pressure and is not a function of the mass and elasticity of the vocal folds as with pitch. To maintain a constant loudness level, one must be able to maintain constant air pressure below the glottis. The ability to maintain constant subglottic air pressure while constantly decreasing subglottic air volume is both a remarkable and achievable physiological ability for most people with a healthy respiratory and phonatory system. Controlled relaxation of the muscles of inspiration, including the diaphragm and intercostals, and support from the abdominal muscles is critical to the maintenance of constant subglottic air pressure.

Clinically, loudness is judged on the basis of its appropriateness for the social or environmental situation. For example, an individual having a personal one-to-one conversation with another person who brings attention to himself by speaking in a voice that is too loud for the situation may be perceived as having a voice loudness problem. Conversely, a teacher who is so soft spoken that students have difficulty hearing her lectures has a voice that is not loud enough for the demands of the classroom.

The ability to maintain loudness control may be compromised in neurological conditions or in patients with degenerative neurological diseases. More often however, vocal loudness that is inappropriate for the social or environmental situation is a function of hearing status. A person with a **sensorineural** hearing loss is likely to speak in a voice that is deemed too loud for the situation. Because of this person's inability to monitor the loudness of his own speech through the auditory system, he may speak in a voice that is louder than the situation requires. By contrast, a person experiencing a **conductive** hearing loss may speak in a soft voice—one considered not loud enough for the situation. The conductive hearing loss diminishes this person's perception of ambient noise, thus making his voice sound louder to himself than it really is. In this case, the speaker has a tendency to reduce the loudness of his voice to compensate for the increased loudness he perceives. Regardless of whether the impairment is sensorineural or conductive, hearing loss compromises a speaker's ability to monitor his voice and the parameter of vocal loudness is affected. It should be noted that in neither foregoing case is the anatomy or physiology of the voice producing mechanism affected. Anatomy and physiology are also not affected when diminished vocal loudness is attributable to psychological depression or to an excited (perhaps manic) psychological state, both of which are possible. Finally, it should be noted that vocal loudness may be attributable to environmental and cultural influences—for example, quiet soft spoken families or cultures verses louder, more verbally aggressive families or cultures. Again however, any noticeable differences in vocal loudness that can be attributable to environmental or cultural differences are not a function of anatomical or physiological factors.

QUALITY

Voice quality, similar to the parameter of pitch and unlike loudness, is very much a function of anatomical and/or physiological laryngeal factors. The primary problem of dealing clinically with voice quality is one of descriptive terminology. "Hoarse," "harsh," "breathy," "tense," "strident," and other terms have been used to describe voice quality. The clinician must ask the following questions: (1) Which terms are the most relevant when diagnosing dysphonia?

(2) Which terms assist the clinician in relating structure to function? And (3) Which terms help the clinician best plan for effective management? Wilson (1990) has suggested that a great deal can be understood and communicated about dysphonia by using the terms "breathiness" and "tension" as quality descriptors. Based on didactic and clinical experience, breathiness and tension are descriptive terms of voice quality that relate well to the Myoelastic Aerodynamic Theory of phonation, to the anatomical changes that affect voice production, and to the relevant management of dysphonia.

Breathiness relates directly to phonatory inefficiency. When the vocal folds are not vibrating in the normal way or cannot **adduct** appropriately, they become inefficient and more air escapes than under normal phonatory conditions. The excess air turbulence is perceived as a breathy voice quality. In **flaccid dysphonia**, for example, the vocal folds do not approximate normally (see Figure 9-3). The result is

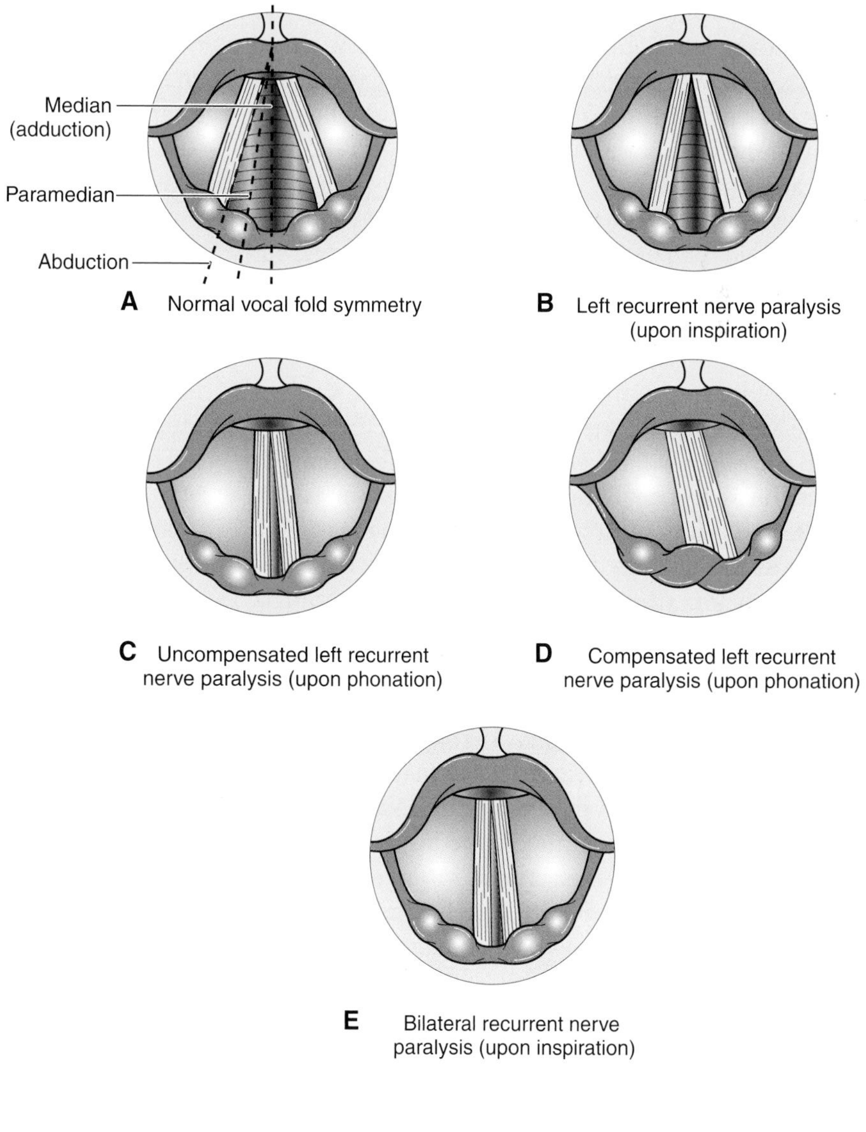

Figure 9-3 Normal vocal fold symmetry and vocal fold paralysis: (**A**) normal vocal fold symmetry; (**B–E**) various configurations of vocal fold paralysis. (Reproduced with permission from CIBA Pharmaceutical Company, Summit, NJ; J. Harold Walton (Ed.), The larynx, W. Saunders, with illustrations by F.H. Netter, 1964.)

Median (adduction)

Paramedian

Abduction

A   Normal vocal fold symmetry

B   Left recurrent nerve paralysis (upon inspiration)

C   Uncompensated left recurrent nerve paralysis (upon phonation)

D   Compensated left recurrent nerve paralysis (upon phonation)

E   Bilateral recurrent nerve paralysis (upon inspiration)

a breathy voice quality often described as weak, as it may be difficult for the speaker to produce a loud voice because of reduced ability to increase subglottic air pressure. Most frequently, a left vocal fold is flaccid and does not move to midline to approximate with the nonaffected fold, and thus there is no tension perceived in the voice.

At this point, it is important to remember that flaccid paralysis is associated with lower motor neuron and/or peripheral nerve damage. To illustrate this, consider the vagus nerve (cranial nerve X). The important branches of the vagus nerve for speech production are the pharyngeal branch, the superior branch of the laryngeal nerve (SLN), and the recurrent branch of the laryngeal nerve (RLN). Each of these branches is paired, which provides bilateral innervation to the velum and intrinsic muscles of the larynx. The pharyngeal branches of the vagus nerve provide motor innervation to the soft palate. The SLNs serve the cricothyroid muscles and the RLNs innervate all of the other intrinsic muscles of the larynx. Recall that the cricothyroid muscles are involved in the regulation of vocal pitch, while the other intrinsic laryngeal muscles mediate abduction and adduction of the vocal folds as well as vocal pitch and intensity. These three branches come off the vagus nerve in the following order (from superior to inferior): pharyngeal branch, SLN, and finally RLN.

The vagus nerve pathway is complex. Several features of voice can be affected depending on the extent of vagus nerve involvement. In general, the higher the damage to the vagus nerve, the more widespread (i.e., diffuse) the effect will be on the speech production mechanism. Conversely, the lower the damage to the vagus nerve, the less widespread (i.e., more focal) the effect will be. For example, if the damage is above the pharyngeal branch, not only will the velum be affected but the intrinsic muscles of the larynx on that side will also be affected because the SLN and RLN are below the level of the pharyngeal branch. The outcome of pharyngeal branch involvement likely will be **velopharyngeal incompetence** and hypernasality. Involvement of the RLN will be manifested in a diminished ability to abduct and adduct the vocal fold on the affected side; damage to the SLN will be manifested in a diminished ability to regulate vocal pitch, also on the affected side. On the other hand, involvement of the intrinsic laryngeal muscles without involvement of the velum means that vagus nerve damage must be below the pharyngeal branch but before either the SLN or RLN have branched off. Finally, when damage is even more peripheral—that is, on the pharyngeal branch, SLN, or RLN alone—

only the structures innervated by that specific branch will be affected.

Recurrent laryngeal nerve paralysis is more common on the left side than the right because of the longer pathway of the left recurrent laryngeal nerve. The more common flaccid paralysis of the left vocal fold can result from trauma, surgery, or heart disease although about one-third of the cases are idiopathic. Inability to adduct one or both vocal folds will result in a breathy voice quality. By contrast, in cases of excess tension in the voice, the vocal folds are extremely tense and may spasm tightly. This type of voice is described as **spasmodic dysphonia** and is considered the most extreme type of hypertensive dysphonia. Tension is the overwhelmingly predominant voice quality in cases of spasmodic dysphonia.

It is possible, and actually quite common, to have both breathiness and tension as voice quality characteristics. Two common examples are **edematous** vocal folds and vocal nodules. Edematous vocal folds occur commonly as a result of vocal abuse. Yelling at a ball game or talking over noise at a party or other public event can cause swelling of the vocal folds, thus changing their mass and elasticity and thereby changing their vibratory characteristics. The result is inefficiency that allows excessive air to escape, and thus breathiness. Our natural tendency is to increase laryngeal tension in an attempt to reduce breathiness. This same combination of breathiness and tension in voice quality is also common in cases of vocal nodules, the most common discrete lesion of the vocal folds. The nodules, also referred to as singer's, preacher's, or teacher's nodules, occur most often bilaterally on the free margins of the vocal folds at the junction of the anterior and middle thirds. The callous-like bumps on the folds cause them not to approximate in the normal way during phonation. Excessive air escapes, tension is increased to compensate for the breathiness, and the result is a breathy and tense voice quality.

SECONDARY CHARACTERISTICS

There are several secondary voice characteristics or features that are frequently present in association with a breathy and tense dysphonic voice. Glottal or vocal fry is a low-pitched sound that can be attributed to a paralyzed vocal fold or vocal polyp. From an anatomical and physiological perspective, it is important to understand that vocal fry can be the result of something that is vibrating in addition to the vocal folds. When this occurs, two pitches may be heard and this is referred to as **diplophonia**. The anatomical source of diplophonia is varied. It has been attributed to a difference in the vibratory pattern of the two vocal folds caused by paralysis of one fold or by a unilateral polyp, as noted earlier. Other sources for diplophonia include aryepiglottic and ventricular fold vibration occurring simultaneously with normal vocal fold vibration.

When coupled with breathiness and tension, vocal fry contributes to what is often referred to as hoarseness or a hoarse voice quality. However, it should also be recognized that vocal fry is used to describe a mode of vocal fold vibration—the pulse register—that is not associated with dysphonia but is simply a different vibratory pattern from that of typical phonation (i.e., the modal register) or falsetto (i.e., the loft register). Other secondary phonatory characteristics may include **pitch breaks** and **phonation breaks**. Pitch breaks are frequently associated with an abrupt shift from the typical (i.e., modal) register to the loft register (i.e., falsetto). Interestingly, when such pitch breaks are controlled musically, they are referred to as yodeling. Pitch breaks as secondary voice characteristic are likely associated with cricothyroid function and may be attributable to superior laryngeal nerve damage.

Phonation breaks or aphonic periods are associated with tense breathy voices, and are sometimes referred to as intermittent whisper. It appears that the vibratory pattern of the vocal folds is interrupted such that voice (i.e., audible phonation) is stopped briefly. This phenomenon is sometimes seen in cases of advanced or well-developed vocal nodules. In similar voices, a variation on the phonation break is delayed onset of phonation. In this case, the start of phonation is delayed at the beginning of an utterance and a brief period of aphonia or whispered speech is perceived prior to phonation beginning.

Other secondary features seen frequently in dysphonic patients include noisy inhalation and **inhalatory laryngeal stridor**. Both result from some degree of airway obstruction. Noisy inhalation and laryngeal stridor are audible features associated with several voice disorders. A paralyzed vocal fold could cause audible air turbulence during inhalation as could papilloma or other laryngeal obstruction. Secondary voice characteristics are important for the voice clinician to note because they are features that add to the overall impression of voice and are features that can be explained by the anatomy and physiology of the voice production mechanism. Secondary voice characteristics are closely associated with voice quality, as contrasted with pitch, loudness, and flexibility, and are important to document as part of the diagnostic and therapeutic process.

FLEXIBILITY

The final voice parameter that defines normal and abnormal voice is **flexibility**. As normal speakers, we expect, by both linguistic necessity and linguistic convention, to have a degree of variation in our vocal output. Speech that is void of pitch and loudness variation is monotonous, probably void of affect, and inconsistent with cultural expectations. Stress, pause, and **intonation** in language are linguistic necessities if one is to communicate effectively. These features in language can make a difference in meaning and when they do, they are referred to as **suprasegmental** phonemic elements. The rising intonation at the end of questions or the contrastive stress between the words *pro*duce and pro*duce* affect the speaker's meaning and perhaps the expectations for the listener. Even when pitch, loudness, and intonational features of voice do not affect meaning in specific ways, they are important to the communication of affect on the part of the speaker. Speech delivered in a monotonous, computer-like manner is void of emotional tone or affect. In general, as listeners we find such speech boring. The literal meaning of the message may be preserved but the importance, urgency, or mood is lost.

Flexibility in speech is not a function of specific anatomical structures or physiological processes but is secondary to those anatomical features and physiological processes that are important to the control of pitch and loudness. Clinically, a voice without appropriate flexibility can be described as lacking pitch and loudness variation and thus flat and dull. At the extreme, a computer- or robot-like voice is conspicuously monotonous and lacking in emotional color. Although clinically monotonous voices are not necessarily robot-like, they can bring negative attention to the speaker by the lack of conventional flexibility and affective communication. Cases where excessive flexibility is a voice liability are rare and are usually associated with personality issues ranging from over dramatic and excited to psychotic.

Clinical Perspectives

Students in speech–language pathology—beginning clinicians if you will—are encouraged to develop a clinical perspective or fundamental framework to guide their approach to evaluation and therapy. The proper perspective will help clinicians recognize their limitations, define their role, and guide their effectiveness. The following are some perspective suggestions for consideration when dealing with voice disorders.

PERSPECTIVE 1: MEDICAL CLEARANCE

With respect to voice disorders, it is important to keep in mind that medical clearance is critical. Because there is no direct relationship between voice characteristics and specific laryngeal pathology, the clinician cannot be certain of the cause of the voice disorder. Furthermore, it is outside the clinician's scope of practice to diagnose laryngeal pathologies. Speech–language pathologists must avoid treating clients until the etiology of the voice problem has been confirmed and it is agreed that voice therapy is indicated. Treating a dysphonic child, assuming the presence of vocal nodules when it is in fact papilloma that is present, is a critical error that must be avoided.

PERSPECTIVE 2: LISTENING

It might appear overly obvious or a trite admonition to emphasize listening as a clinical perspective when evaluating and treating voice disorders. After all, don't clinicians instinctively listen to their clients? Yes, but voice features can be subtle and confusing. Experience suggests that to be a good listener of voice parameters requires training and practice. Student clinicians are urged to take advantage of available recorded materials designed to help develop critical listening skills for primary and secondary vocal characteristics (e.g., Boone et al., 2010; Dworkin & Meleca, 1997; Wilson, 1990). Clinicians, as students or as practicing professionals, should never hesitate to consult colleagues about what they are hearing in the voices of clients. Listen, listen again, and discuss what you are hearing. Discussion of what is heard, confirmation of what is heard, and arrival at possible consensus can only be in the best interest of the client.

PERSPECTIVE 3: DOCUMENTATION

Documentation of voice characteristics and dysphonic qualities is critical to quality referral, appropriate diagnosis, and effective management and treatment. Careful description of pitch, loudness, quality, and flexibility is valuable to the physician to whom the client is referred and helps to build a respectful professional rapport. That same high quality professional description will always remain as the permanent record of your analysis of the voice at the time. When your perception has been confirmed by the perception of others, it is validated and thus respected. In addition, whenever possible, it is excellent practice to support your subjective perception of voice features with objective data.

It is acknowledged that in many settings, instrumentation for voice analysis is not available, but when available should be used to the extent possible to support perceptual judgments. Audio recordings serve as a relatively permanent documentation of the voice at a particular point in time. They serve as a source of comparison for future voice samples and can be used to garner the judgments of other professionals at any time. Computer programs for voice analysis are excellent sources of objective data, particularly on features related to pitch and flexibility. Voice fundamental, habitual pitch, and pitch range are examples of features of phonation that can be easily obtained with computer analysis. When computer analysis is not available, a pitch pipe or musical instrument like a piano can help the clinician establish a reasonable estimation of several pitch features. Loudness is highly subjective because it is a matter of appropriateness for the social situation. Computer programs provide some loudness documentation, but the information obtained is disassociated from the demands of the speaking situation. A simple sound level meter can be used in the communication environment, but that too is not likely to be accessible to clinicians in the public schools. The documentation of the quality of dysphonic voices is also highly subjective. Although there are features of computer analysis that relate to dysphonia, there is no substitute for the well-trained ear of the clinician. Again, audio recordings serve to preserve the voice sample for later analysis and comparison and provide a source of confirmation by others, thus validating the perceptions of the clinician.

> ### Why You Need to Know
>
> *Several instruments are used today to obtain objective data regarding the parameters of voice (i.e., pitch, intensity, and quality). One such computer-based instrument is the Computerized Speech Lab (CSL) by Kay Elemetrics. The CSL is a hardware/ software package that includes such analyses as nasometry, real-time pitch analysis, and spectography. One particular software program—the Multi-dimensional Voice Profile, or MDVP—can be used to objectively assess various parameters of vocal quality. Although it is beyond the scope of this textbook to provide a detailed discussion of instrumentation, you are encouraged to read about the advances that have been made in this particular area of speech–language pathology. Boone et al. (2010) provide a good primer in this area.*

PERSPECTIVE 4: EMPHASIS

When writing diagnostic reports, **SOAP notes**, and other therapy documentation, the clinician is urged to place appropriate emphasis on the most obvious and clinically relevant factors that characterize the voice. What stands out as most conspicuous in this voice? What is it about this voice that is within generally acceptable normal limits, and what is not? Of those features that appear not to be within normal limits, which, if any, are dominant? Reporting with appropriate emphasis and clearly relating the salient features of voice to the basic parameters of pitch, loudness, quality, and flexibility will clarify clinical communication while providing a clear record of the client's diagnosis and progress in therapy. Appropriate emphasis is particularly important in the summary and recommendation sections of reports, where other professionals are likely to first get the "big picture" of the case.

PERSPECTIVE 5: COMMUNICATION

In all of what we do clinically, there is no substitute for clear communication. Because voice cases almost always involve interdisciplinary interaction, the speech–language pathologist must be mindful of the limits of their role and the nature of their contribution. Although medical professionals are the most likely referral sources and referral recipients, school teachers, psychologists, and teachers of singing are also likely professionals to whom referrals are made and from whom referrals are received.

When communicating about voice disorders, the speech–language pathologist must be careful not to make a medical diagnosis or overstate the case in a way that might be construed as a medical diagnosis. The clinician should carefully describe the voice problem, support that description with as much objective and quantitative data as possible, identify the salient issues from the case history, and clearly pose any questions for which he or she hopes to receive answers. The clinician can go so far as to say that the nature of the dysphonia and the notable features of the history are consistent with the possible presence of vocal nodules, for example, but should present the case in a way so as not to positively confirm the presence of nodules. The following is an example of how the communication might be phrased:

Dr. ENT:

CL is a 6-year-old male who was evaluated on February 28, 2007 and who presented with a dysphonia characterized by tension and breathiness that is moderate in severity and is accompanied by phona-tion breaks and intermittent aphonia. The dysphonia appears to have increased in severity over the past six months as reported by CL's parents. They describe him as always having been an active child, prone to using a loud voice inside, and being among the most vocal in his play group outside. Yelling and screaming have increased since he has been involved in organized sports this year.

CL's voice and history are consistent with the possible presence of vocal nodules, but he has not had vocal fold visualization or a medical examination related to his voice problem. Please advise as to the appropriateness of therapy to help CL understand and reduce vocal abuse.

Respectfully,
Ima Therapist

Summary

The intent of this chapter was to provide you with an understanding of how the anatomy and/or physiology of the phonatory system relates to various common disorders of voice. Perhaps more so than any of the other systems involved in speech production (i.e., the respiratory and articulatory systems), there is a clear relationship between laryngeal anomalies and expected aberrations of voice. For example, increased mass on the vocal folds created by mass lesions such as vocal nodules, polyps, or papilloma will very likely result in a lower pitch than normal. Should the mass lesion invade the medial borders of the vocal folds, the vocal folds will not be able to approximate completely during phonation and the result will likely be manifested as a breathy voice quality. A differential in size or shape of bilateral lesions will likely cause the vocal folds to vibrate asynchronously, and the result will be a harsh voice quality. In cases of spasmodic dysphonia, the laryngeal mechanism may spasm so severely that the patient will exhibit a very labored vocal quality known as a "strain-strangled" voice. Having a good knowledge of the anatomy and physiology of the phonatory system will benefit the clinician greatly in assessing and treating voice disorders.

Clinical Teaser—Follow-Up

At the beginning of Chapter 8, we described Destiny, a 15-year-old high school student with diagnosed vocal nodules. Her history is clearly consistent with the medical diagnosis. Singing can be and cheering often is a factor in the history of young women with vocal nodules. The quality of her voice was described as hoarse with a degree of breathiness.

What is described as hoarseness (i.e., dysphonia) is very often a result of breathiness and tension, so the description of Destiny's voice is again quite consistent with the presence of nodules. In Destiny's case, her actual habitual pitch (as instrumentally confirmed) was not reported but is likely to be perceived as low because of her dysphonia. In fact, the entire history and description of her voice are consistent with vocal nodules with the exception of pain on phonation, which is less likely to be an associated symptom in vocal nodules and more likely to be reported in association with contact ulcers. It is important to keep in mind, however, that given the history and voice description, Destiny could have edematous vocal folds or, with the presence of pain on phonation, contact ulcers. Thus, the point is once again made that we cannot confirm pathology with vocal characteristics. Medical diagnosis and clearance to proceed with therapy are necessary.

The key to remediation of Destiny's voice problem is to reduce vocal abuse. It is most likely that singing and cheering are implicated as abusive activities, and it is also likely that cheering is the more deleterious of the two. Does this mean that Destiny can no longer participate in these activities? Should complete vocal rest (i.e., no voice use) for a period of time be recommended? The answer to both of these questions is no. In fact, complete and prolonged vocal rest can actually cause problems and will not solve the problem if—when voice use is resumed—vocal abuse continues.

From a management perspective, it is recommended that the clinician help Destiny to understand what vocal nodules are and what causes them. It is important for Destiny to take responsibility for her situation and the management of it. She is not at fault or to blame for having nodules, but she will need to be an active participant in her vocal remediation. She is likely to wonder, "Why me?" There is no explanation for why she has developed vocal nodules while her friends who participate in the same activities have not. Although she should not feel guilty, she will have to accept responsibility for change, something that may not be easy at her age. Understanding that she need not give up activities important to her may be a great boost to her motivation for change. Surgical removal of nodules is possible, but without change in vocal behavior (i.e., abuse reduction), nodules are likely to recur. Identification of abusive behaviors is recommended as a first step. Cheering and singing are likely to emerge at the top of a list of abusive behaviors for Destiny, but social vocal habits with friends, communication style at home, and other vocal habits (e.g., laughing, throat clearing, hard glottal attack) could also be factors contributing to her problem. Once a hierarchy is established, strategies can be explored to manage the abusive behaviors. For example, while cheering, Destiny might either lip-sync the cheers or speak them without yelling. During practice, she might refrain from vocalizing the cheers and instead concentrate on the physical aspects of cheerleading. Also, if Destiny were to "teach" others what she has learned about vocal abuse and its management, she might be able to help others avoid similar problems in the future. In that way, she could acknowledge her problem while helping others.

While singing, she might reduce vocal intensity, limit singing to only her modal register (i.e., mid-frequencies), limit the amount of participation, and avoid singing loudly with the car radio or in the shower. If singing is a very important activity for Destiny, she might consider getting a teacher of singing to aid in the development of healthy singing techniques. Elimination of vocal nodules will take time, but they will reduce in size and will eventually disappear through elimination of vocal abuse.

PART 4 SUMMARY

Part 4 (Chapters 8 and 9) provided you with a basic understanding of the anatomy and physiology of the phonatory system, along with some common pathologies associated with voice production. The primary structure of phonation—the larynx—is a musculocartilaginous structure that is supported by, and serves as a framework for, several muscle groups. The intrinsic laryngeal muscles are responsible for producing the vocal tone and for mediating the pitch and loudness of that tone. The extrinsic muscles are involved primarily in assisting pitch regulation. The process of vocal fold vibration was described according to the Myoelastic Aerodynamic and Cover-Body Theories of phonation. The result of phonation is a complex tone that is rich in harmonic structure. In Chapter 9, you were introduced to a number of pathologies associated with the phonatory system. A direct relationship was established between some common pathologies (e.g., mass lesions, vocal fold paralysis, spasmodic dysphonia) and the underlying anatomical and/or physiological anomalies associated with those pathologies. In addition, Chapter 9 offered several perspectives for diagnosing and remediating vocal pathologies.

PART 4 REVIEW QUESTIONS

1. Name all of the cartilages that comprise the larynx. Which of these cartilages are most important in the process of phonation?

2. Name the intrinsic and extrinsic membranes of the larynx and briefly describe each one's purpose.

3. Name the intrinsic laryngeal muscles and briefly describe how each of them contributes to phonation.

4. Describe how the extrinsic laryngeal muscles contribute to laryngeal physiology. What is the net effect of their contribution?

5. What are the contributions of the superior laryngeal nerve and recurrent laryngeal nerve to phonation?

6. From what cranial nerve do the superior and recurrent laryngeal nerves emerge? What other cranial nerves are involved in the process of phonation? Describe each one's contribution.

7. What are the underlying physiological processes of voice production? Explain their interdependence.

8. Briefly describe the Myoelastic Aerodynamic and Cover-Body Theories of phonation.

9. List and define the components of a complex tone.

10. Define medial compression and longitudinal tension. What is each one's contribution to voice production?

11. Describe the phases of phonation.

12. How are pitch and loudness of voice controlled?

13. What is dysphonia, and how does it relate to the parameter of voice quality?

14. Name three voice disorders presented in Chapter 9 and describe the effects they are likely to have on voice.

15. What is flexibility of voice, and in what ways is it important in conversation?

16. Why is medical clearance important in voice disorder management for the SLP?

PART 5

Anatomy, Physiology, and Pathology of the Articulatory/ Resonance System

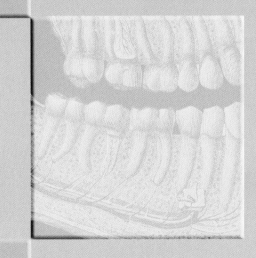

CHAPTER 10

Anatomy and Physiology of the Articulatory/Resonance System

Knowledge Outcomes for ASHA Certification for Chapter 10

- Demonstrate knowledge of the biological basis of the basic human communication processes (III-B)
- Demonstrate knowledge of the neurological basis of the basic human communication processes (III-B)
- Demonstrate knowledge of the acoustic basis of the basic human communication processes (III-B)

Learning Objectives

- You will be able to describe the framework that supports the articulatory/resonance system.
- You will be able to recall the major anatomical structures of articulation and resonance and their role in the process of speech production.
- You will be able to describe the muscles that mediate articulation and resonance.
- You will be able to discuss the basic concepts involved in speech production as described by Source-Filter Theory.

AFFIX AND PART-WORD BOX

TERM	MEANING	EXAMPLE
alae	wing-like processes	depressor **alae** nasi
alaeque	pertaining to a wing-like structure	levator labii superior **alaeque** nasi
bucco-	pertaining to the cheeks	**bucco**pharyngeus
cerato-	pertaining to a horn	**cerato**pharyngeus
chondro-	pertaining to cartilage	**chondro**pharyngeus
cranius	pertaining to the cranium	epi**cranius** frontalis
crico-	pertaining to the cricoid cartilage	**crico**pharyngeus
epi-	over or above	**epi**cranius frontalis
genio-	pertaining to the chin	**genio**glossus
glosso-	pertaining to the tongue	**glosso**pharyngeal
-glossus	pertaining to the tongue	palato**glossus**
hyo-	pertaining to the hyoid bone	**hyo**glossus
incisivus	pertaining to the incisor teeth	**incisivus** labii inferior
labii	pertaining to the lips	levator **labii** superior
mylo-	pertaining to the lower jaw	**mylo**pharyngeus

TERM	MEANING	EXAMPLE
nasi	pertaining to the nose	columella **nasi**
oculi	pertaining to the eye	orbicularis **oculi**
oris	pertaining to the mouth	orbicularis **oris**
palato-	pertaining to the palate, typically the velum	**palato**glossus
-pharygeus	pertaining to the pharynx	crico**pharyngeus**
pterygo-	pertaining to the pterygoid laminae	**pterygo**pharyngeus
salpingo-	pertaining to the Eustachian (auditory) tube	**salpingo**pharyngeus
stylo-	pertaining to the styloid process	**stylo**pharyngeus
thyro-	pertaining to the thyroid cartilage	**thyro**pharyngeus
veli palatini	pertaining to the velum	tensor **veli palatini**

Clinical Teaser

You are a speech–language pathologist working in a hospital setting. You are also a member of the local cleft palate team. On one particular day, you are asked to participate in an evaluation of Aidan, a 4-year-old boy who exhibits the features of Pierre Robin syndrome: micrognathia, cleft palate, and glossoptosis. Fortunately, these features are not pronounced to the degree that Aidan has been unable to thrive. However, unfortunately, Aidan's parents did not seek medical attention for their child's condition, so his orofacial anomaly has been left untreated. He has been brought to your hospital by authorities of Child Protective Services. Upon meeting Aidan for the first time, you observe that although he has little difficulty breathing, it is somewhat labored. You also note that he is generally malnourished. Because he has not received the proper medical intervention he needs, his development has been adversely affected.

The micrognathia, cleft palate, and glossoptosis are of primary concern to you. What would you expect to find when you perform a speech and language evaluation on this child? Would you expect articulation errors of any kind? If so, which speech sounds would he most likely produce in error? Would you expect any problems in terms of resonance? Would you suspect any other problems in terms of communication and/or swallowing? Assuming Aidan exhibits problems in these areas, what would your intervention strategy be?

Introduction

As presented in Chapters 6 and 8, the respiratory and phonatory systems work together to produce the human vocal tone. The respiratory system provides the air pressure that sets the adducted vocal folds into vibration. The vocal folds are housed within the larynx, which is part of the phonatory system. The phonatory system is not only responsible for producing the vocal tone but also has the ability to vary the intensity and frequency of the vocal tone. Once the vocal tone is generated, it passes through the vocal tract where it is shaped and molded into an acoustic signal we recognize as human speech. The anatomical structures within the vocal tract constitute the articulatory/resonance system.

In Chapter 8, the vocal tone* was described as a complex tone resembling a buzzing sound. The vocal tone itself would not be recognized as speech. It would therefore have to be transformed into an acoustic signal recognized as human speech. This process of transformation takes place by way of the articulatory/resonance system. You will note that the articulatory/resonance system has two components: **articulation** and **resonance**. These components will be described in more detail in the physiology section of this chapter, but for now it will be mentioned that these two components are not separate but rather act together simultaneously to shape the vocal tone into speech. To understand the processes of articulation and resonance, one must know the structures that comprise the vocal tract.

---

*You should not be mislead into thinking that the vocal tone is the only source of sound during speech production. In fact, in English, 9 of the 24 consonant sounds are produced without vocal fold vibration (and hence are referred to as "unvoiced" sounds). Sounds from the wide array of languages around the world come from a variety of sources and not just the vocal folds. We use the term "vocal tone" in this textbook to represent the acoustic signal that is generated by vocal fold vibration.

The remainder of this chapter will be devoted to a thorough discussion of the anatomy and physiology of the articulatory/resonance system. It is expected that upon reading this chapter, you will be well versed in the structure and mechanics of articulation and resonance, and how these processes work together to produce human speech. It should also be noted that many of the structures that make up the articulatory/resonance system are also involved in **deglutition**. Because speech–language pathologists work with persons having swallowing disorders, a discussion of the anatomy and physiology of the swallowing mechanism will also be presented in this chapter.

Anatomy of the Articulatory/ Resonance System

Three primary cavities form the vocal tract: pharyngeal, oral, and nasal (see Figure 10-1). The pharyngeal cavity extends from the base of the skull to the cricoid cartilage of the larynx. It has a vertical orientation. The oral cavity extends from the lips and teeth anteriorly to the **palatoglossal arches** posteriorly, and from the hard and soft palate superiorly to the tongue inferiorly. Its orientation is horizontal. Finally, the nasal cavity actually consists of two separate chambers. These chambers run horizontally from the nostrils anteri-orly to the uppermost portion of the pharynx posteriorly. Each of these three primary cavities consists of a number of anatomical structures and/or landmarks.

The oral cavity is composed of several anatomical structures and landmarks. These include the lips, teeth, alveolar ridge, hard palate, **velum**, tongue, and **mandible**. Each of these structures will be described in greater detail below. The nasal cavity includes the nose and two chambers separated at midline by the **nasal septum**. Within each chamber is a series of landmarks that will be discussed later. Finally, the pharyngeal cavity is rather unremarkable in terms of structures and landmarks but is composed of an intricate and complex network of muscles that will be discussed in a later section of this chapter.

The vocal tract then consists primarily of the following structures: lips, teeth, alveolar ridge, hard palate, velum, tongue, mandible, oral cavity, nasal cavity, and pharyngeal cavity. With the nasal and oral cavities being oriented horizontally and the pharyngeal cavity being oriented vertically, the vocal tract resembles a capital letter "F." In an adult male, the distance between the vocal folds and lips is approximately 17 cm. Five centimeters of this distance is the oral cavity, with the remaining 12 cm being the length of the pharynx.

Similar to many of the anatomical structures of the respiratory and phonatory systems, movement of the

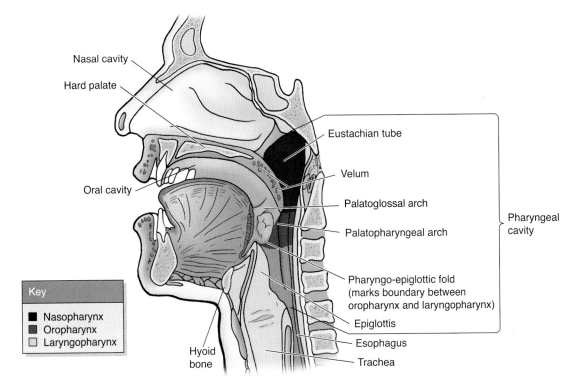

Figure 10-1 Sagittal view of the oral, nasal, and pharyngeal cavities. (Adapted with permission from Moore, K.L., Agur A.M., Dalley, A.F. (2009). *Clinically oriented anatomy* (6th ed.). Baltimore: Lippincott Williams & Wilkins.)

primary anatomical structures of the articulatory/resonance system are mediated by muscle activity. Therefore, this chapter will include a thorough discussion of the muscles that assist in articulation and resonance. Many of these muscles have their insertion or origin on bones of the skull. During the process of communication, facial expression may convey part of the message. Muscles are involved in facial expression, and many of these muscles also have attachments to the bones of the skull. Because of this, a discussion of the articulation/resonance system would not be complete without a description of the human skull. Once the human skull has been presented, the discussion will turn to the anatomical structures that make up the oral, nasal, and pharyngeal cavities.

THE SKULL

Figure 10-2 shows several views of the human skull. Upon first glance, the human skull appears to be a structure consisting of two parts: the skull proper and the jaw bone. However, in actuality, the skull is a complex structure that consists of 28 bones that articulate with each other similarly to a three-dimensional jigsaw puzzle. Some of these bones are paired and others are singular. All of them can be categorized into one of three groups: bones of the **cranium**, bones of the face, and miscellaneous bones. There are eight bones that comprise the cranium, the part of the skull that houses the brain. These include the unpaired *ethmoid, sphenoid, frontal*, and *occipital* and the paired *parietals* and *temporals*. The facial portion of the skull is that part that corresponds to the recognized human face. There are 14 bones that comprise the facial portion of the skull. These include the unpaired *mandible* and *vomer* and the paired *maxillae, nasals, palatines, lacrimals, zygomatics*, and *inferior nasal conchae*.

Finally, the miscellaneous bones are six in number and include a series of three tiny bones housed within each temporal bone of the cranium—the *malleus, incus*, and *stapes*—which are part of the hearing mechanism. These bones will be discussed at greater length in Chapter 12 and therefore will not be discussed in this chapter. Some anatomists include one additional bone under the miscellaneous category, resulting in a total of 29 bones for the skull. This is the hyoid bone which was discussed in detail in Chapter 8. Anatomists who include the hyoid bone as one of 29 do so because the hyoid is more intimately related to the tongue than to the larynx. However, because the hyoid does not articulate directly with any other bones of the skull, it is not included here as a part of the skull. Having been discussed in more detail in Chapter 8, the hyoid bone will not be described in detail here.

Gross anatomy of the skull will reveal several anatomical structures and landmarks. The orbits of the eye are prominent cavities where the eyeballs reside. Keeping to the analogy of a three-dimensional jigsaw puzzle, one will realize that the orbits are not composed of one bone but actually are composed of parts of several bones, among them the ethmoid, frontal, lacrimal, maxillary, palatine, sphenoid, and zygomatic bones. Similarly, within the nasal cavity is a vertical partition of bone. This partition is called the bony nasal septum, and it also is not a singular bone but actually composed of two bones: ethmoid (more specifically, the perpendicular plate) and vomer. Along the lateral walls of each chamber of the nasal cavity are three scrolls of bone known as the nasal conchae or **turbinates**. The two upper conchae (superior and medial) come from the ethmoid, whereas the lowermost scroll is an independent bone—the inferior nasal concha. The three nasal conchae form small chambers called meatuses. Returning to the exterior of the skull, one will note several landmarks: the **frons** (forehead), **occiput** (posteriormost point of the skull), and **vertex** (superior tip of the skull). Along the sides of the skull, where the facial part ends and the cranium begins, are depressions called **temporae**. These correspond to the temples when the soft tissue structures overlay the skull. Just lateral to and below each orbit is a prominent loop of bone called the zygomatic arch, more commonly referred to as the cheekbone. The zygomatic arch is not a singular bone but rather is created by parts of three bones: maxilla, temporal, and zygomatic.

If one were to remove the top of the skull by cutting around the circumference of the cranium, one would be holding the **calvaria** or skullcap. By then removing the brain from the cranium, one would note three major cavities within the floor of the cranium. These are the **anterior, medial**, and **posterior cranial fossae**.

On each side of the skull, immediately posterior to where the mandible articulates with the skull, is a small opening. This opening is the bony **external auditory meatus**. Immediately behind and projecting below each external auditory meatus is a rounded protuberance called the **mastoid process**. Medial to each external auditory meatus on the inferior surface of the skull is a sharp projection of bone known as the **styloid process**. At the base of the skull between and behind the styloid processes is a large hole. This hole is called the **foramen magnum**.

Finally, one will note that several jagged lines traverse the cranial part of the skull. These jagged lines

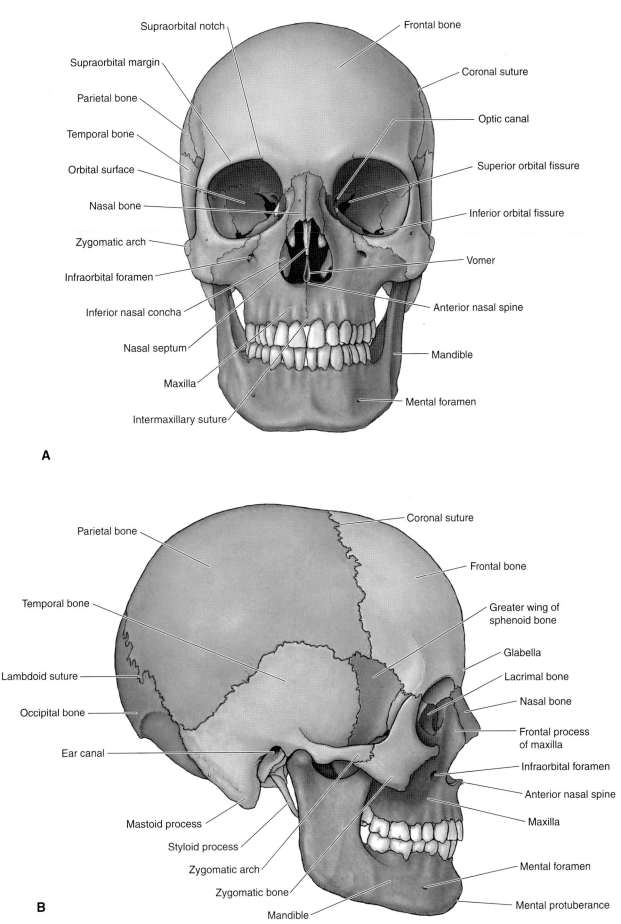

Figure 10-2   Various views of the human skull. **A**. Anterior view. **B**. Lateral view. (*continued*)

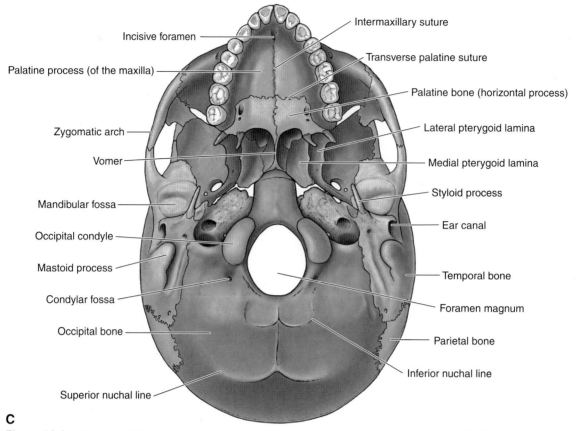

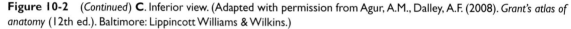

C

Figure 10-2 *(Continued)* **C**. Inferior view. (Adapted with permission from Agur, A.M., Dalley, A.F. (2008). *Grant's atlas of anatomy* (12th ed.). Baltimore: Lippincott Williams & Wilkins.)

are known as sutures. There are four prominent sutures: **coronal, sagittal, lambdoidal**, and **occipitomastoid**. The coronal and sagittal sutures are named in reference to the planes in which they course. The lambdoidal suture is named for the fact that it resembles the Greek letter lambda (λ). The occipitomastoid suture refers to the anatomical structures it joins together (i.e., the occipital bone and mastoid processes of the temporal bones).

Facial Bones

Maxillae

The paired maxillae are illustrated in Figure 10-3. These bones make up the greater portion of the central face just lateral to the nose and below the eyes and are second only to the mandible in size. The two maxillae fuse with each other at midline just below the nasal opening by way of the **intermaxillary suture**. This suture continues between the two upper central incisors and between the **palatine processes** of the maxillae. Immediately posterior to the upper central incisors is a small opening called the **incisive foramen**. In very early development, fine sutures that extend bilaterally from the incisive foramen to between the lateral incisors and canines form a triangular region referred to as the **premaxilla**. In some animals, this is a separate bone, but in

humans the sutures are usually completely fused and therefore the two halves of the premaxilla are counted as part of the palatine processes of the maxillae.

> ### *Why You Need to Know*
> *Sometimes in fetal development, the sutures of the maxillae fail to fuse properly, resulting in a condition known as cleft palate. The cleft may involve only the intermaxillary suture or may involve the sutures that define the premaxilla. Cleft palate will be discussed in greater detail in Chapter 11.*

Each maxilla has a corpus (i.e., body) and a number of processes. In all, each maxilla articulates with nine other bones. These include the ethmoid, frontal, inferior nasal concha, lacrimal, the opposite maxilla, nasal, palatine, vomer, and zygomatic. Of note is the frontal process that articulates with the frontal bone of the cranium and the zygomatic process that articulates with the zygomatic bone of the facial portion of the skull. Each maxilla also has an orbital process that creates much of the inferior **orbit** of the eye. Immediately below the orbit of the eye is a small opening called the **infraorbital foramen**. Each maxilla has a number of alveolar processes where the upper teeth are housed.

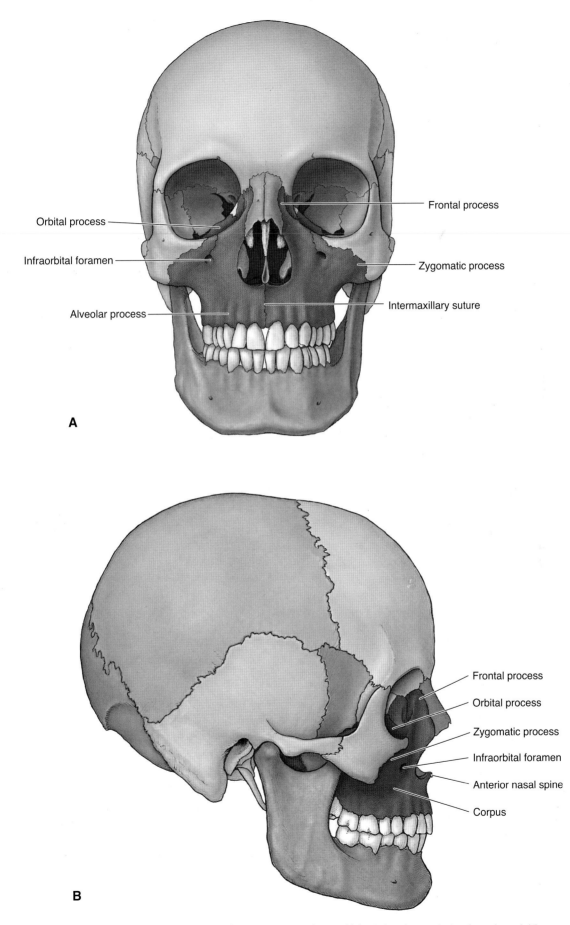

Figure 10-3 The maxillae. **A**. Anterior view. **B**. Lateral view. (Adapted with permission from Agur, A.M., Dalley, A.F. (2008). *Grant's atlas of anatomy* (12th ed.). Baltimore: Lippincott Williams & Wilkins.)

Of particular note is a somewhat vertically oriented ridge in the maxilla where the canine tooth resides (the third tooth from midline). Appropriately enough, this ridge is referred to as the canine eminence.

The palatine processes are noteworthy as they form the anterior three-fourths of the hard palate. The palatine process of each maxilla fuses with its partner to form most of the ceiling of the oral cavity and floor of the nasal cavity. On the nasal side of each palatine process is a small ridge called the nasal crest. The nasal crests from both maxillae form a horizontally directed groove where the perpendicularly directed vomer resides. The nasal crests continue in an anterior direction and terminate as the anterior nasal spine.

Upon close inspection of the maxillae, one will note that these bone are not solid but rather have a hollow interior. These are called the **maxillary paranasal sinuses**, and they are the largest of all the paranasal sinuses. The maxillary paranasal sinuses are present at birth.

Mandible

The mandible is more commonly referred to as the jaw bone and is illustrated in Figure 10-4. It is the largest of the facial bones of the skull. During embryonic development, the mandible starts as two halves joined together at the **mental symphysis** which courses vertically, starting between the two lower central incisors. The mandible consists of an anterior corpus and two posterior rami (the mandibular rami). In the region of the mental symphysis, the corpus extends outward forming the mental protuberance. The mental protuberance is bordered on each side by the mental tubercles. Along the superior margin of the corpus are dental alveoli for the lower teeth. Just lateral and somewhat superior to each mental tubercle is a small opening called the mental foramen. Also running from each mental tubercle somewhat posteriorly and superiorly is an indistinct ridge called the oblique line. On the inner (posterior) surface of the corpus is a more prominent ridge running horizontally from side to side. This ridge is known as the **mylohyoid line**.

The mandibular rami arise at an angle that is approximately 90 degrees to the corpus, although this angle may vary somewhat from person to person. On the superior border of the mandibular rami are two processes. The anterior process is called the **coronoid process** and the posterior process is referred to as the **condylar process**. The mandibular notch separates the coronoid process from the condylar process. The condylar process from each side articulates with the temporal bone of the skull to form the **temporomandibular joint (TMJ)**. This joint will be described in greater detail later.

Nasals

The paired nasal bones are illustrated in Figure 10-5. These bones form the bridge of the nose and lie medially to the frontal processes of the maxillae. Although they are rather small in size, they articulate with the frontal bone, **perpendicular plate of the ethmoid**, and maxillae as well as the **septal cartilage**. The two nasal bones are fused together at midline at the internasal suture. A nasal foramen may also exist in one or both bones.

Palatines

The paired palatine bones are somewhat "L" shaped and comprise the posterior one-fourth of the hard palate as well as a portion of the floor and lateral walls of the nasal cavity (see Figure 10-6). These bones also help form the inferior orbits of the eyes. Of particular note are the **horizontal processes** which form the posterior portion of the hard palate. The anterior border of each horizontal process is serrated to allow for a strong articulation with the palatine processes of the maxillae. The two horizontal processes when fused form a posterior nasal spine. The posterior border of the horizontal processes is free and forms the point of attachment for the velum. The palatine bones articulate with each other as well as the ethmoid, frontal, inferior nasal conchae, maxillae, and vomer.

Lacrimals

The lacrimal bones are the smallest bones of the facial portion of the skull (see Figure 10-7). They are so named because of their proximity to lacrimal (i.e., tear) glands. In addition to forming a small portion of the medial orbits of the eyes, these bones articulate with the ethmoid, frontal, inferior nasal conchae, and maxillae.

Zygomatics

The paired zygomatic bones are illustrated in Figure 10-8. They help form a portion of the lateral and inferior walls of the orbits of the eye. Each bone consists of a corpus and four processes: the frontosphenoidal; orbital; maxillary; and temporal, which describe their attachments to other bones (the frontal, maxillae, sphenoid, and temporal bones). Of particular note are the maxillary and temporal processes. Medially, the maxillary process of the zygomatic bone articulates with the zygomatic process of the maxilla. Laterally, the temporal process of the zygomatic bone articulates with the zygomatic process of the temporal bone. These articulations form the zygomatic arch, which is more commonly known as the cheekbone.

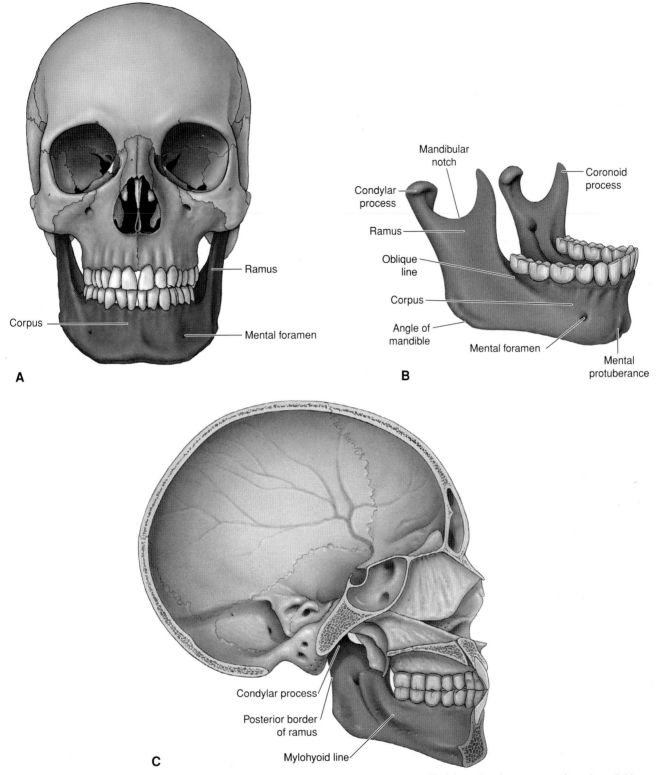

Figure 10-4   The mandible. **A**. Anterior view. **B**. Anterolateral view. **C**. Midsagittal view. (**A**: Adapted with permission from Agur, A.M., Dalley, A.F. (2008). *Grant's atlas of anatomy* (12th ed.). Baltimore: Lippincott Williams & Wilkins; **B** and **C**: Adapted with permission from Anatomical Chart Company.)

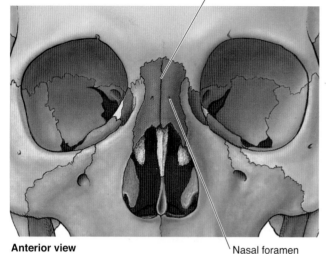

Internasal suture

Nasal foramen

Anterior view

Figure 10-5   The nasal bones. (Adapted with permission from Agur, A.M., Dalley, A.F. (2008). *Grant's atlas of anatomy* (12th ed.). Baltimore: Lippincott Williams & Wilkins.)

Inferior Nasal Conchae

The inferior nasal conchae are illustrated in Figure 10-9. One of these bones is found in each of the two chambers making up the nasal cavity, more specifically making up the lowermost part of its lateral wall. These bones articulate with the maxilla anteriorly and the palatine bones posteriorly. Along with the superior and medial nasal conchae (which are part of the ethmoid bone), the inferior nasal conchae are scrolls of thin bone that are also referred to sometimes as the turbinate bones.

Vomer

The vomer is a somewhat quadrilaterally shaped bone that comprises the lower half of the bony nasal septum (the upper half of the bony nasal septum comes from the perpendicular plate of the ethmoid bone). Illustrated in Figure 10-10, the vomer resides in the horizontally oriented groove created by the nasal crests of the maxillae. In addition to articulating with the maxillae, the vomer articulates with the palatine bones below and the perpendicular plate of the ethmoid and the rostrum of the sphenoid bone above. Its posterior border is free, but its anterior border articulates with the cartilaginous nasal septum.

Cranial Bones

Frontal

The frontal bone corresponds to the forehead region and the anterior portion of the top of the cranium. It is illustrated in Figure 10-11. The frontal bone consists of a squamous portion and an orbital portion. The squamous portion is the larger of the two and corresponds to the forehead and anteriormost part of the cranium. The orbital portion corresponds to the superior orbits of the eye and the eyebrow region. In infancy, there may be a **metopic suture** that divides the frontal bone into two halves.

Medially between the orbits of the eyes is a frontal spine. Superior to this spine, immediately between the two eyebrows is a region called the **glabella**. Lateral to the glabella are the supraorbital margins. These margins may be superimposed by either a supraorbital foramen or notch. Within the orbital surfaces are small depressions in the bone called lacrimal gland fossae. Tear glands are housed within these fossae. Finally, an opening exists between the orbital portions of the frontal bone and below the frontal spine. This opening is referred to as the ethmoidal notch. In an intact skull, this notch is occupied by the ethmoid bone.

In all, the frontal bone articulates with 12 bones: the singular ethmoid and sphenoid and the paired lacrimals, maxillae, nasals, parietals, and zygomatics. The posterior border of the squamous portion of the frontal bone articulates virtually along its entire length with the two parietal bones.

Similarly to the maxillae, the frontal bone is also hollow in its interior. Two cavities are separated by a thin bony septum, forming the paired **frontal paranasal sinuses**. These sinuses are virtually absent at birth. They start to develop during the first or second year of life but do not fully form until puberty.

Parietals

The parietal bones are illustrated in Figure 10-12. The two parietal bones articulate with each other at midline so that they form essentially the rounded roof of the cranium. The parietal bones are shaped somewhat like rectangles, meaning each one has four margins and angles. The frontal margin is that part of the parietal bone that articulates with the frontal bone. The sagittal margin is that part of the parietal bone that articulates with the other parietal bone. The occipital margin is the part of the parietal bone that articulates with the occipital bone, and, finally, the temporal margin is that part of the parietal bone that articulates with the temporal bone.

The articulation between the two parietals takes place along the sagittal suture. The articulation of the parietal bones with the frontal bone takes place along the coronal suture. The parietal bones also articulate with the occipital bone along the lambdoidal suture. The sagittal suture intersects the coronal suture anteriorly and the lambdoidal suture posteriorly.

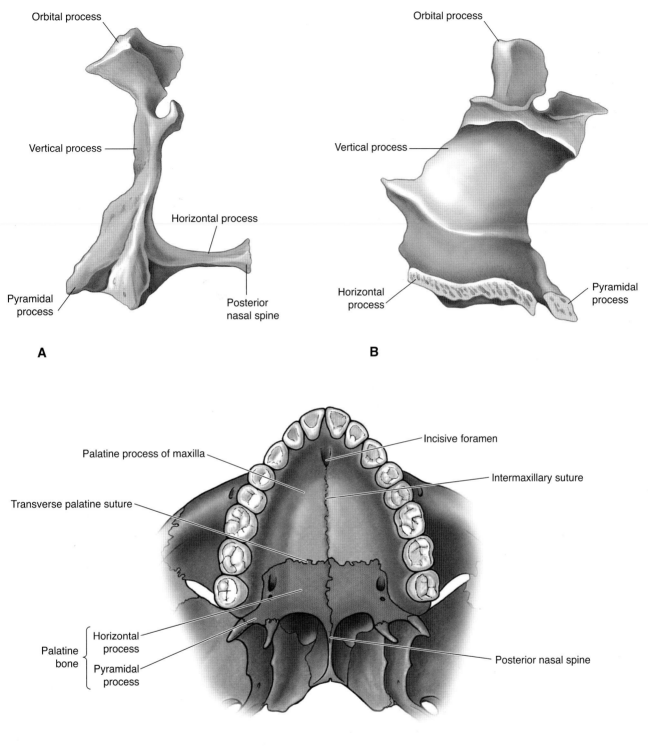

Figure 10-6   The palatine bones. **A**. Anterior view. **B**. Sagittal view. **C**. Inferior view. (**C**: Adapted with permission from Agur, A.M., Dalley, A.F. (2008). *Grant's atlas of anatomy* (12th ed.). Baltimore: Lippincott Williams & Wilkins.)

Although the outer surface of each parietal bone is somewhat smooth in appearance, the inner surface is marked by grooves resembling blood vessels. In fact, these grooves are called the middle meningeal vessel grooves where blood vessels that pass through the meningeal layers of the brain rest.

Occipital

The occipital bone makes up the posterior portion of the cranium (see Figure 10-13) and consists of two parts: the larger squamous portion and the smaller basilar portion. The squamous portion is relatively unremarkable except for the lambdoidal (or parietal)

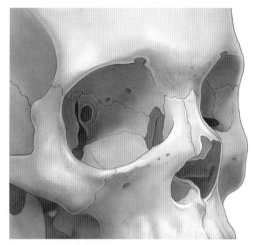

Anterolateral view

Figure 10-7   The lacrimal bone. (Adapted with permission from Agur, A.M., Dalley, A.F. (2008). *Grant's atlas of anatomy* (12th ed.). Baltimore: Lippincott Williams & Wilkins.)

the inion or external occipital protuberance. Running transversely along the occipital bone where the squamous portion ends and the basilar portion begins are two ridges called the superior and inferior nuchal lines.

The basilar portion of the occipital bone is more remarkable in terms of landmarks. Most obvious is the large hole in the basilar part called the foramen magnum. The spinal cord passes through the foramen magnum on its way down the spinal column. In the anterior region of the foramen magnum and lateral to it are two prominent **occipital condyles**. The occipital condyles are the points of articulation of the base of the skull to the first cervical vertebra (C1, or the atlas). Anterior to each condyle is a **hypoglossal canal**. Anterior and medial to the condyles is the **pharyngeal tubercle**, where the superiormost border of the pharynx attaches to the base of the skull. Finally, posterior to the condyles is a depression called the condylar fossa. Within this fossa is a small opening known as the condylar canal.

margin where the occipital bone articulates with the parietal bones and the mastoid margin where the occipital bone articulates with the temporal bones. The point where the squamous part of the occipital bone extends most posteriorly is called

Temporals

The temporal bones comprise the sides of the cranium (see Figure 10-14). These bones consist of two major parts and three subparts. The two major

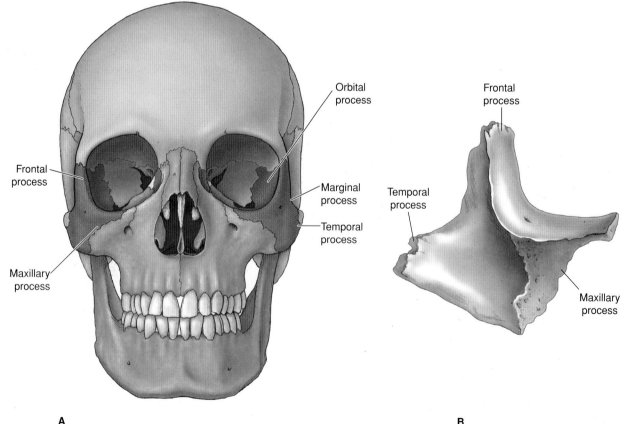

A

B

Figure 10-8   The zygomatic bones. **A.** Anterior view. **B.** Interior view. (**A**: Adapted with permission from Agur, A.M., Dalley, A.F. (2008). *Grant's atlas of anatomy* (12th ed.). Baltimore: Lippincott Williams & Wilkins.)

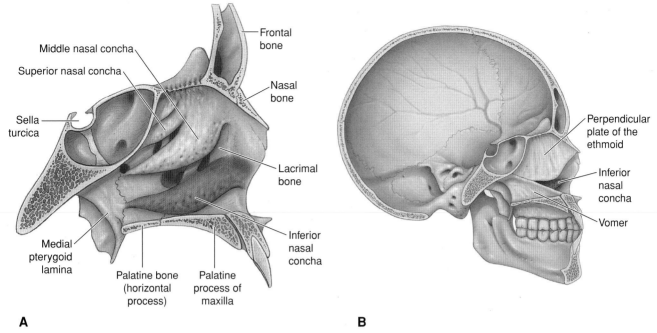

Figure 10-9   The inferior nasal conchae. **A**. Sagittal view. **B**. Midsagittal view. (Adapted with permission from Anatomical Chart Company.)

portions of the temporal bones are the squamous and petrous portions. The squamous portion is smooth in appearance and makes up the lateral, anterior, and superior portion of the temporal bone. Of particular note is the zygomatic process, a landmark of the squamous portion that articulates with the temporal process of the zygomatic bone to form the zygomatic arch, or cheekbone.

The petrous portion lies at the base of the skull between the sphenoid and occipital bones and can be further divided into tympanic and mastoid sections. The petrous portion gets its name from the fact that the bone is very hard. Within the tympanic section of the petrous portion reside the essential organs of hearing and balance—the cochlea and semicircular canals. Posterior to the tympanic section is the mastoid section,

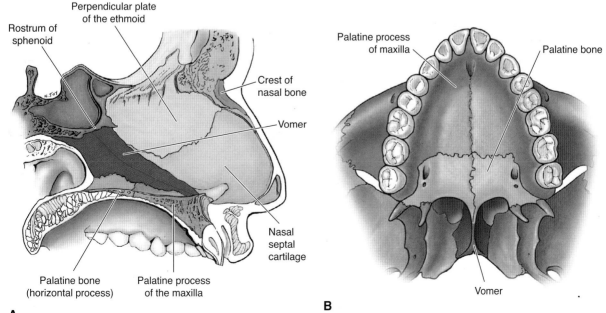

Figure 10-10   The vomer. **A**. Midsagittal view. **B**. Inferior view. (Adapted with permission from Agur, A.M., Dalley, A.F. (2008). *Grant's atlas of anatomy* (12th ed.). Baltimore: Lippincott Williams & Wilkins.)

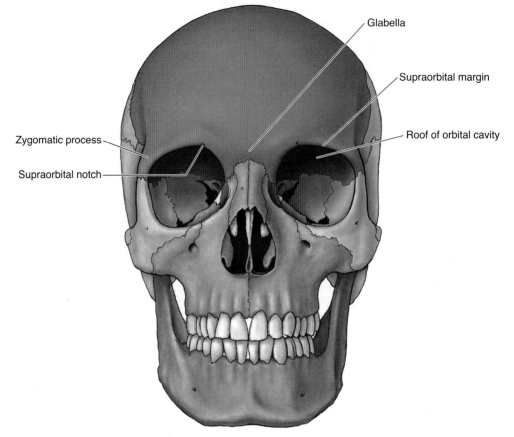

Anterior view

Figure 10-11 The frontal bone. (Adapted with permission from Agur, A.M., Dalley, A.F. (2008). *Grant's atlas of anatomy* (12th ed.). Baltimore: Lippincott Williams & Wilkins.)

which includes the mastoid process. The mastoid section is not solid bone but rather composed of numerous irregularly shaped cavities referred to as the **mastoid air cells**. In the inferior part of the mastoid section, these air cells are relatively small and diminish in size until all that remains is bone marrow. In the anterior and superior regions of the mastoid section, the air cells are progressively larger until they give way to the **tympanic antrum**. The upper limit of the tympanic antrum is the **tegmen tympanum**, which is the roof of the tympanic cavity. These structures will receive a more detailed discussion in Chapter 12.

Two final landmarks of note are the styloid process and the **mandibular fossa**. The styloid process roughly resembles a sharpened pencil tip. It is located in the petrous portion of the temporal bone, posterior and inferior to the zygomatic process. The styloid process is the point of attachment of three muscles (styloglossus, stylohyoid, and stylopharyngeus) and two ligaments (stylomandibular and stylohyoid). The mandibular fossa is a depression located on the inferior surface of the temporal bone between the styloid and zygomatic processes. The condylar pro-

cess of the mandible rests within this fossa forming the temporomandibular joint (TMJ).

Ethmoid

The ethmoid bone is interesting in that although it is classified as a bone of the cranium, it also contributes to the facial part of the skull. The ethmoid contributes to the orbits of the eyes and nasal cavity as well as makes up the medial portion of the anterior cranial base. Figure 10-15 provides an illustration of this bone, which consists of five parts: **cribriform plate, crista galli**, perpendicular plate, and two **ethmoidal labyrinths**. The cribriform plate is horizontally oriented, whereas the crista galli and perpendicular plates comprise one piece that is oriented vertically (the crista galli rises above, while the perpendicular plate extends below the cribriform plate). The ethmoidal labyrinths are also inferior to the cribriform plate but have a lateral orientation.

The cribriform plate serves as a partition between the nasal and cranial cavities (the nasal cavity is below and the cranial cavity is above). It is perforated by small openings. The olfactory nerve (cranial nerve I)

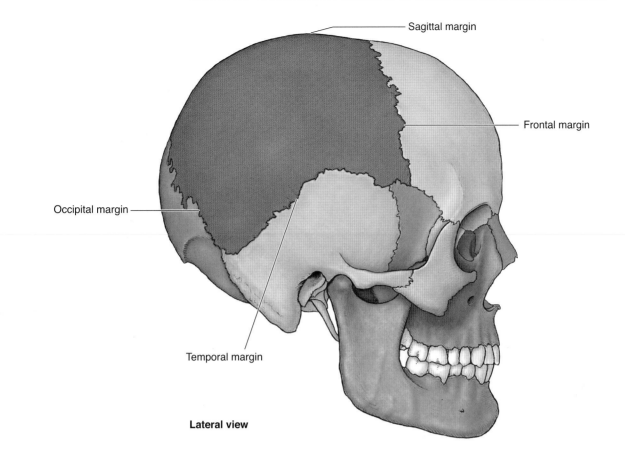

Sagittal margin

Frontal margin

Occipital margin

Temporal margin

Lateral view

Figure 10-12 The parietal bone. (Adapted with permission from Agur, A.M., Dalley, A.F. (2008). *Grant's atlas of anatomy* (12th ed.). Baltimore: Lippincott Williams & Wilkins.)

rests upon the cribriform plate, and nerve fibers from it pass through the perforations into the nasal cavity to course along the surfaces of the nasal conchae.

Rising above the cribriform plate in a vertical plane is the crista galli (translated literally as "cock's comb"). Therefore, the crista galli is housed within the cranial cavity. This somewhat triangular process serves as the anterior point of attachment for the **falx cerebri**, a fold of dura mater that separates the two cerebral hemispheres of the brain.

The perpendicular plate of the ethmoid extends inferiorly from the cribriform plate in a vertical plane. It articulates with the frontal and nasal bones anteriorly and the vomer and rostrum of the sphenoid posteriorly. The cartilaginous nasal septum is also attached to the anterior perpendicular plate.

The ethmoidal labyrinths contain highly irregular air cells that form the paired **ethmoid paranasal sinuses**. These sinuses are present at birth. The labyrinths are separated from the medial walls of the orbits of the eyes by a very thin layer of bone (the **lamina papyracea**). Thin scroll-like layers of bone also extend from the labyrinths. These are known as the superior and middle nasal con-

chae (recall that the inferior nasal conchae are independent bones of the facial part of the skull). In total then, there are three scrolls of bone along the lateral walls of each of the two chambers of the nasal cavity.

Sphenoid

The sphenoid bone is perhaps the most complex of all the bones of the skull. When removed from the skull, it somewhat resembles a butterfly (see Figure 10-16). Within the skull, it can be found immediately posterior to the ethmoid and immediately anterior to the foramen magnum and basilar portion of the occipital bone. The sphenoid has seven major parts: a singular corpus and paired greater wings, lesser wings, and pterygoid processes. The greater and lesser wings extend laterally from the corpus while the pterygoid processes extend inferiorly. The anterior surface of the corpus forms the posterior wall of the nasal cavity. The inferior surface of the corpus has a small ridge called the rostrum, which articulates with the vomer.

The two lesser wings extend laterally from the superior–anterior aspect of the corpus. The inferior surfaces of the lesser wings form the upper boundaries

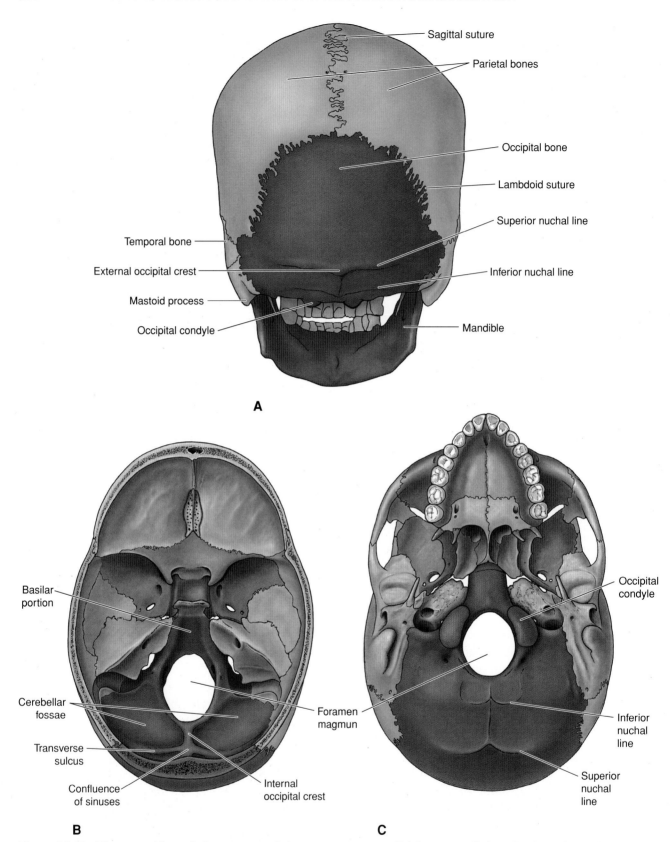

Figure 10-13 The occipital bone. **A**. Posterior view. **B**. Interior superior view. **C**. Inferior view. (Adapted with permission from Agur, A.M., Dalley, A.F. (2008). *Grant's atlas of anatomy* (12th ed.). Baltimore: Lippincott Williams & Wilkins.)

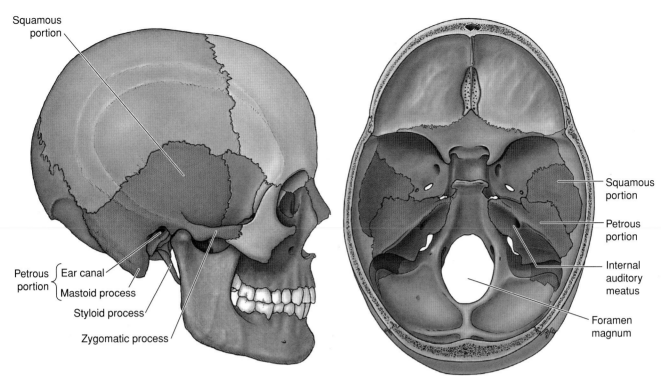

Figure 10-14 The temporal bone. **A**. Lateral view. **B**. Internal superior view. (Adapted with permission from Agur, A.M., Dalley, A.F. (2008). *Grant's atlas of anatomy* (12th ed.). Baltimore: Lippincott Williams & Wilkins.)

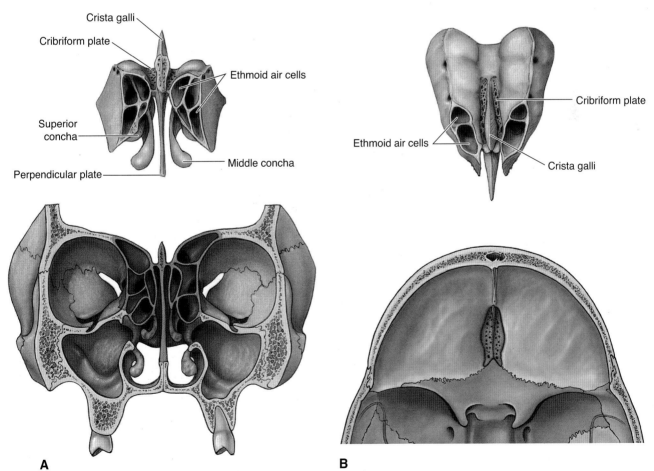

Figure 10-15 The ethmoid bone. **A**. Coronal view. **B**. Superior view. (**A** and **B1**: Adapted with permission from Anatomical Chart Company; **B2**: Adapted with permission from Agur, A.M., Dalley, A.F. (2008). *Grant's atlas of anatomy* (12th ed.). Baltimore: Lippincott Williams & Wilkins.)

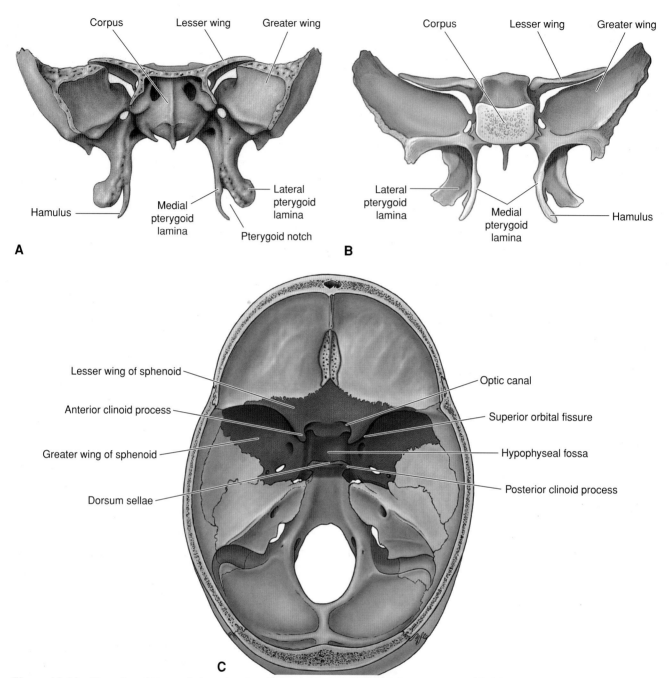

Figure 10-16 The sphenoid bone. **A**. Anterior view. **B**. Posterior view. **C**. Internal superior view. (**A**: Adapted with permission from Anatomical Chart Company; **B**: Adapted with permission from Oatis, C.A. (2008). *Kinesiology* (2nd ed.). Baltimore: Lippincott Williams & Wilkins; **C**: Adapted with permission from Agur, A.M., Dalley, A.F. (2008). *Grant's atlas of anatomy* (12th ed.). Baltimore: Lippincott Williams & Wilkins.)

of the **superior orbital fissures**. The anterior margins of the lesser wings articulate with orbital plates of the frontal bone. The lesser wings come together at the jugum. Posterior to the jugum is the chiasmatic sulcus which houses the optic chiasma where the two optic nerves (cranial nerve II) cross over after they have exited the retinal area of the eyeballs and passed through the **optic canals**. Immediately posterior to the chiasmatic sulcus is the **sella turcica** which houses the pituitary gland.

The greater wings also extend laterally from the corpus of the sphenoid. These wings contribute primarily to the orbits of the eyes as part of their superior, lateral, and inferior walls. The lateral margins of the greater wings articulate with the zygomatic bones. At the point where the greater wings meet the corpus of the sphenoid, the pterygoid processes extend vertically in a downward direction.

Each of the two pterygoid processes is composed of two laminae. These are the medial and lateral pterygoid lamina, which are separated from each other by the pterygoid notch. Along their anterior aspects, the pterygoid notches articulate with the palatine bones. The lateral pterygoid lamina is wider than the medial pterygoid lamina and serves as the point of articulation for the medial and lateral pterygoid muscles. The medial pterygoid lamina is more narrow and terminates in a small hook-like structure called the **hamulus**.

The corpus of the sphenoid is hollow. Two chambers can be found within; these chambers are separated by a thin midline septum creating a pair of **sphenoid paranasal sinuses**. These sinuses are not present at birth, but rather start to form around the third year of life. The sphenoid paranasal sinuses, along with the frontal, ethmoid, and maxillary paranasal sinuses (mentioned in earlier sections), are lined with a membrane created by a fusion of periosteum and mucous membrane (this membrane is referred to as the **mucoperiosteum**). The lining of these paranasal sinuses is continuous with the mucous membrane lining of the nasal cavity.

All of the paranasal sinuses drain into the nasal cavity proper. The sphenoid paranasal sinuses open into spaces above the superior nasal conchae. The frontal and maxillary sinuses open into the medial nasal meatus, and the ethmoid paranasal sinuses open into the superior and medial nasal meatuses.

> ### Why You Need to Know
>
> *Sinusitis is a condition where the mucous membranes of the paranasal sinuses and nasal cavity become inflamed. As the inflammation continues, the paranasal sinuses may not be able to drain into the nasal cavity. Mucous is then trapped within the paranasal sinuses, creating tenderness and pain. If the condition is chronic, a surgeon may have to drill larger holes (called windows) in the nasal cavity to allow the mucous to drain more freely.*

In all, the sphenoid bone articulates with all of the other cranial bones of the skull as well as several of the facial bones (maxillae, palatines, vomer, and zygomatics). This bone contributes to the orbits of the eyes as well as the nasal and pharyngeal cavities.

THE ORAL CAVITY

The oral cavity is the most active of the cavities involved in speech production. It consists of several anatomical structures including the lips, cheeks, teeth, alveolar ridge, hard palate, velum, tongue, and mandible. The **faucial pillars**, tonsils, **velopharyngeal (V-P) mecha-nism**, and muscles of facial expression will also be included here as part of the oral cavity. One will quickly realize that excluding the muscles of facial expression, these structures collectively make up the mouth. The mouth has both primary (i.e., biological) and secondary (i.e., nonbiological) functions. In terms of biological function, the mouth serves as the conduit by which the respiratory and digestive systems communicate with the external environment. As part of the digestive system, the mouth is used during the processes of **mastication** (chewing) and deglutition (swallowing). The digestion of food begins in the oral cavity.

> ### Why You Need to Know
>
> *Although mothers often tell their children to breathe through their nose, many tend to be "mouth breathers," that is, they take in oxygen primarily through the mouth. The problem with such breathing is that inhaled air is not moistened and heated quite as efficiently as it is when breathed in through the nose. To some degree, the nose also filters the air as it passes through on its way to the pharynx and beyond. The oral cavity performs this task less effectively.*

The nonbiological or secondary function of the oral cavity is to generate speech sounds and to modify the pitch characteristics of the vocal tone through the process of resonance. These secondary functions will be discussed in greater detail in the physiology section of this chapter. In the paragraphs that follow, a closer inspection will be made of the individual structures that comprise the oral cavity.

The Lips

The lips, or **rima oris**, are illustrated in Figure 10-17. The lips are composed of four layers of tissue; from

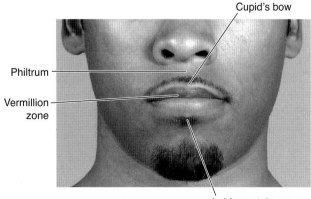

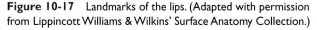

Figure 10-17 Landmarks of the lips. (Adapted with permission from Lippincott Williams & Wilkins' Surface Anatomy Collection.)

superficial to deep, these include the cutaneous, muscular, glandular, and mucous layers. Fat, in differing amounts depending upon the individual, may also be deposited within these layers. The cutaneous layer is simply skin. Deep to the cutaneous layer is a layer of muscle tissue. This muscle is the *orbicularis oris*, a sphincter muscle that completely encircles the lips. The orbicularis oris has a deep and a superficial layer. The deep layer consists of muscle fibers arranged in concentric rings, while the superficial layer receives muscle fibers from other facial muscles (these muscles will be discussed later). The glandular layer contains labial glands that are similar to saliva glands in structure. Finally, the mucous layer of the lips is continuous with the mucous membrane of the oral cavity and pharynx. On their inner (or lingual) surface, the lips are anchored at midline to the alveolar region (upper lip) and mandible (lower lip) by the superior and inferior labial frenula (singular: frenulum).

A view of the external surface of the lips reveals several landmarks. The lips are darker in hue than the rest of the face due to the transparency of the **vermilion zone** (this transparency is created by an abundance of **eleidin** in the epithelium). The transparency of the vermilion zone allows the vascular tissue below to be more prominently displayed. Running from the septum of the nose to the middle of the upper lip are two vertically oriented ridges with a deep furrow between them. This furrow is called the **philtrum**. The philtrum terminates on the upper lip, creating a midline depression that makes the upper lip appear like an archer's bow. Hence, the upper margin of the upper lip is referred to as **Cupid's bow**.

The Cheeks

The cheeks, or **buccae**, are similar in structure to, and are continuous with, the lips. The external layer is skin (i.e., cutaneous), the innermost layer is a mucous membrane, and muscular and glandular layers reside within. Several facial muscles (whose functions are to assist in mastication and to mediate facial expression) can be found in the muscular layer of the cheeks. Within the glandular layer reside five or six glands corresponding to the molar region of the teeth. Appropriately enough, they are referred to as the molar glands. Stenson's duct (a part of the parotid salivary gland) also opens into the buccal region. Finally, a buccal fat pad may exist to some degree. In infants, this pad is quite prominent, but it tends to dissipate somewhat as the individual develops. The cheeks and lips, along with the gums and posterior teeth, form a secondary cavity within the oral cavity called the buccal cavity.

The Teeth

The complete set of teeth for an adult numbers 32, but for a child, it is only 20. Obviously then, humans have two sets of teeth. The first set that develops during early childhood is called the deciduous set (but is also referred to by some people as the baby, milk, primary, or temporary teeth). These teeth eventually shed and are replaced by the permanent teeth. There are more teeth in the permanent set because the maxillae and mandible have grown large enough to accommodate the additional teeth.

Morphologically, there are four basic types of teeth: incisors, cuspids (also known as canines), premolars, and molars. Incisors are chisel shaped, allowing them to efficiently cut and shear food. Cuspids are more tusk-like in appearance. This arrangement allows these teeth to rip and tear. Finally, the premolars and molars are flat with broad surfaces; this makes them ideal for crushing and grinding.

A Typical Tooth

A typical tooth consists of several structures (see Figure 10-18). Gross anatomy of the external surface reveals a crown, neck, and root. The crown is the part of the tooth that can be seen (approximately one-third of the tooth). The root lies below the gum line

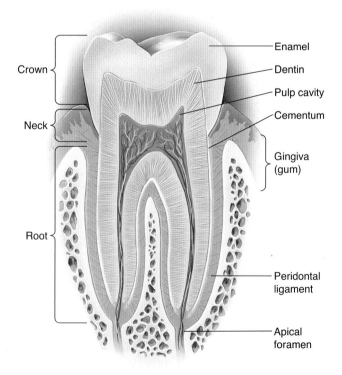

Figure 10-18 Anatomical structure of a typical tooth. (Adapted with permission from Anatomical Chart Company.)

and therefore cannot be seen (approximately two-thirds of the tooth). The neck is an ill-defined region between the crown and root, generally at the gum line. The crown is covered by a very hard substance called **enamel** (approximately 96% mineral by weight), while the root is covered by **cementum** (approximately 50% mineral by weight). The neck region corresponds to the **cementoenamel junction**, where the enamel ends and the cementum begins. The bulk of the solid portion of a tooth is referred to as **dentin**.

The tooth is anchored within its dental alveolus (tooth socket) by a **periodontal ligament** or membrane. The articulation of tooth and alveolus is a joint called a **gomphosis**. This type of joint holds the tooth in its socket while allowing the periodontal ligament to absorb the mechanical forces placed on the tooth through chewing or other activity where the teeth come into contact with each other.

An internal view of a typical tooth will also reveal several landmarks and structures. The interior of a tooth is hollow, forming a pulp canal. The larger portion of the pulp canal is referred to as the **pulp cavity**. The pulp cavity is filled with dental pulp, specialized tissue that is rich in nerve endings and blood vessels. The nerve fibers and blood vessels make their way into the pulp cavity through the **apical foramen**, which is actually at the bottom of the tooth root(s).

Depending on its type, a tooth can have any number of surfaces. The contact surface of an incisor is called the incisal edge, but for the other teeth, it is called the occlusal surface. The posterior surface (facing the oral cavity) is called the lingual surface, in reference to the tongue. The anterior surface of the incisors and cuspids is referred to as the labial surface in reference to the lips. For the premolars and molars, this surface is called the buccal surface in reference to the cheeks. Finally, adjacent teeth have approximal surfaces. If one divides the upper and lower sets of teeth into left and right halves (i.e., starting at midline between the two central incisors), the approximal surfaces will be classified as either mesial (facing toward the midline) or distal (facing away from the midline). This means that the surfaces of the two central incisors that face each other are both mesial surfaces.

The Development of Teeth

The life cycle of teeth involves four stages: growth, calcification, eruption, and attrition. During the growth stage, the tooth buds form along with the enamel and dentin. The enamel and dentin harden during the calcification stage. These two stages take place while the teeth are still embedded within the maxillae and mandible. The eruption stage takes place when the teeth begin to migrate into the oral cavity. This stage has two substages: intraosseous and clinical. During intraosseous eruption, the teeth make their way through the bony alveolar ridge. At this point, the teeth are still not completely calcified and the roots have not fully formed. Through a process known as resorption, specialized cells called **osteoclasts** break down the bone tissue within the alveolar ridge and the teeth migrate. Once the teeth have clinically erupted, **osteoblasts** reform the bone to create the alveoli. Clinical eruption is evidenced by the teeth cutting through the **gingivae**. The final stage, attrition, takes place throughout life. As mechanical forces of chewing act upon the teeth, they wear down. However, the teeth still maintain their spatial relationships because eruption also continues throughout life.

The deciduous or primary teeth are 20 in number but do not all erupt at once. Eruption of the complete deciduous set takes approximately 14 to 18 months to accomplish, although this can vary considerably from child to child. Typically, the first teeth that erupt are the lower central incisors. This takes place between approximately 6 to 9 months of age. The upper central and upper lateral incisors tend to be the next teeth to erupt, at approximately 8 to 10 months of age. Eruption then continues anteriorly to posteriorly until the second molars erupt at approximately 20 to 24 months of age. When all deciduous teeth have erupted, the child will have 20 teeth: two upper central incisors; two upper lateral incisors; two upper cuspids; two upper first molars; two upper second molars; two lower central incisors; two lower lateral incisors; two lower cuspids; two lower first molars; and two lower second molars (see Figure 10-19A).

Before the complete permanent set of teeth comes in, there is a period of time when the child may have some deciduous teeth and some permanent teeth. This is referred to as the mixed dentition stage. The same process that causes the deciduous teeth to erupt is responsible for eruption of the permanent teeth. A bony partition separates the deciduous teeth from the permanent teeth below them. At the appointed time, osteoclasts resorb bone allowing the permanent teeth to migrate. The deciduous teeth above are shed. Once the permanent teeth are in place, osteoblasts reform bone. The mixed dentition stage spans approximately 6 years. It begins typically when the deciduous lower central incisors are shed at 6 to 8 years of age, and ends when the deciduous second molars are shed at approximately 10 to 12 years of age.

The permanent set of teeth begins to erupt with the lower central incisors and upper and lower first

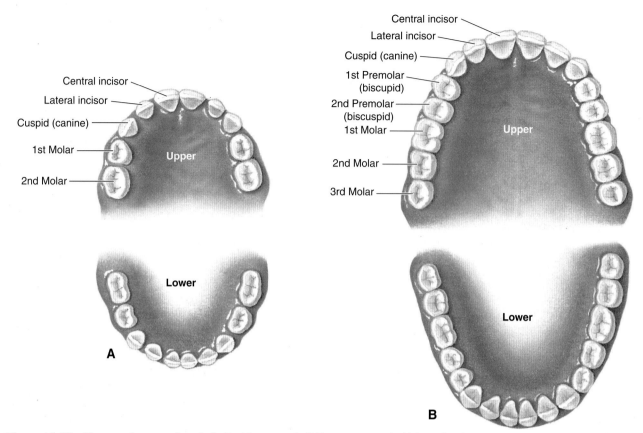

Figure 10-19 The complete set of teeth. **A.** Deciduous teeth. **B.** Permanent teeth. (Adapted with permission from Anatomical Chart Company.)

molars at approximately 6 to 7 years of age. Eruption then continues for the anterior teeth (incisors and cuspids) and eventually for the posterior teeth (bicuspids and molars). Eruption of the permanent teeth spans approximately 11 to 19 years. The upper and lower third molars (also known as "wisdom teeth") may not erupt until the individual is in his or her mid-20s.

When the complete permanent set has erupted, there will be 32 teeth, 12 more than were in the deciduous set (see Figure 10-19B). Some permanent teeth have a deciduous partner, while some permanent teeth do not. The permanent teeth that have a deciduous partner are referred to as successional teeth, whereas permanent teeth that do not have a deciduous partner are called superadded teeth. The superadded teeth include two upper first and two upper second bicuspids (also known as premolars), two lower first and two lower second bicuspids, and two upper and two lower third molars. Figure 10-19B illustrates a complete permanent dental set. Each dental arch (upper and lower) has 16 teeth with the left and right halves of each arch being mirror images of each other. Each half arch has a central incisor, lateral incisor, cuspid, first bicuspid, second bicuspid, first molar, second molar, and third molar. The incisors, cuspids,

and bicuspids tend to have a single root although the upper first bicuspids may have two roots. The lower molars typically have two roots, but the upper molars typically have three roots. The occlusal surfaces of bicuspids and molars tend to be flat by comparison with the incisors and cuspids. The flat surface of these teeth is divided into sections created by grooves along the surface. These sections are called cusps. As the term implies, bicuspids have two cusps. The first molars typically have four cusps; the second molars may have three or four cusps; and finally the third molars typically have three cusps.

Why You Need to Know

There is a relationship between the development of the teeth and development of speech. In general, the first consonant sounds to emerge (at about 6 to 9 months) are produced by either the lips (/p, m/) or the tongue and alveolar ridge (/t, d, n/). The first primary teeth (lower and upper central incisors and upper lateral incisors) emerge between 6 and 10 months. The 20 primary teeth are in place by approximately 30 months of age. The first consonant sound to emerge that involves the teeth (and lower lip) is usually the /f/

at around 30 to 36 months. This is followed by the /v/ at around 48 months, and finally the two "th" sounds (where the tongue tip is placed between the upper and lower teeth) at around 54 to 60 months. Incidentally, when the primary upper and lower central and lateral incisors are shed at approximately 6 to 8½ years, some children may exhibit a bit of a regression in the ability to produce the two "th" sounds correctly. These errors usually dissipate once the permanent central and lateral incisors are in place.

Of some importance to speech–language pathologists are the spatial relationships of the teeth. A certain amount of maxillary overbite and overjet is normal. Because the maxillary arch is larger than the mandibular arch, the anterior mandibular teeth (incisors and cuspids) will rest inside of their maxillary counterparts when the jaw is closed (this is maxillary overbite). The upper incisors are also angled a little more toward the lips than the lower incisors, resulting in a normal degree of overjet.

Over 100 years ago, Angle (1899) proposed a system for classifying the relationship of the upper jaw to the lower jaw that is still used today. The reference point for this relationship is centric occlusion where the mandible is central to the maxilla and there is complete occlusal contact of the upper and lower teeth (i.e., the jaw is "clenched"). Angle suggested three basic types of occlusion (Class I occlusion and Class I malocclusion are considered one type of occlusion, with Class II and Class III malocclusion viewed as the other two types). Class I occlusion, which is considered normal, is evidenced by the cusps of the mandibular (lower) first molars resting ahead and inside the cusps of the maxillary (upper) first molars. With this normal profile, one can then describe three types of malocclusion. With Class I malocclusion, the first molar relationship is intact, but some type of anomaly exists in the anterior region of the dental arch. With Class II malocclusion, the cusps of the mandibular first molars are behind and inside their counterparts in the maxillary dental arch. The chin will appear to be receding and the individual with this type of malocclusion will be said to have an "overbite." Interestingly, almost half the world's population has a Class II malocclusion! With Class III malocclusion, the cusps of the mandibular first molars rest ahead of the maxillary first molars, giving the chin the appearance that it is jutting out. A person with this type of malocclusion is said to have an "underbite." Finally, in addition to the overall occlusal relationship of the teeth, there may be any number of teeth that are not positioned properly. Any number of teeth may exhibit **distoversion, infraversion, labioversion, mesioversion, supraversion**, and/or **torsiversion**.

The Alveolar Ridge

The alveolar ridge is the bony part of the mandible and maxilla where the alveoli (tooth sockets) reside. This ridge continues behind the upper and lower teeth and is more prominent in the maxillary arch. A layer of mucous membrane covers the bony ridge. This mucous membrane is continuous with the membrane that lines the rest of the oral cavity. The maxillary alveolar ridge is more clinically important for speech–language pathologists because it is the site of production of several of the consonant sounds in the English language.

The Hard Palate

The hard palate makes up the bony part of the ceiling of the oral cavity as well as the floor of the nasal cavity. As mentioned previously, it is not a singular bone but instead is actually formed by the processes of four bones. More specifically, the anterior three-fourths of the hard palate is formed by the palatine processes of the maxillae, whereas the posterior one-fourth is formed by the horizontal processes of the palatine bones. The palatine and horizontal processes from the left fuse with their partners on the right along the intermaxillary suture. At midline where the two horizontal processes meet, the posterior nasal spine is formed. A palatal arch is created by the fact that the palatine processes are thicker anteriorly and laterally but thinner medially. This arch is highly variable from person to person and is somewhat dependent upon the status of the maxillary dental arch.

The maxillary alveolar ridge and hard palate are covered with a mucous membrane. Immediately behind the alveolar ridge is a series of transversely oriented wrinkles called rugae. Extending beyond the rugae along the length of the hard palate is a midline raphe. The prominence of the rugae and midline raphe is also highly variable from person to person. Finally, in approximately one-fifth of the population, there may be a visible bulge on the hard palate. This bulge is known as a torus palatinus, which is typically an outgrowth of bone along the intermaxillary suture. The tissue surrounding the torus palatinus is likely to have a bluish tint.

The Velum

The velum, or soft palate, is a three-layered structure. The deepest layer is a **palatal aponeurosis** that attaches onto the posterior free border of the horizontal processes of the palatine bones. This aponeurosis can be considered the "skeleton," and along with other connective tissues, it makes up approximately one-third of the bulk of the velum. The intermediate layer has muscle fibers from several muscles. Laterally, muscle fibers from the velum are continuous with the muscles that comprise the superior pharyngeal constrictor. Otherwise, the bulk of velar muscle tissue is confined to its mid-region. The superficial layer of the velum is a mucous membrane that is continuous with the rest of the oral cavity.

The muscles of the velum are summarized in Table 10-1. When these muscles contract, they will elevate, lower, or tense the velum. The *palatoglossus* and *palatopharyngeus* muscles serve to lower and relax the velum. The *tensor veli palatini (TVP)* muscle also lowers the velum but tenses it as well. Finally, the *levator veli palatini (LVP)* (which makes up the bulk of the muscular tissue of the velum) and the *musculus uvulae* raise the velum (see Figure 10-20 for views of these muscles). The actions of these muscles will be described more fully when the V-P mechanism is discussed in the section on physiology. At rest, the velum hangs down into the upper posterior region of the oral cavity. At midline, one will see a singular structure known as the **uvula**. If you start at the uvula and move laterally, you will see two folds of mucous membrane along the sides of the posterior oral cavity. These are the faucial pillars, which will be described in more detail below.

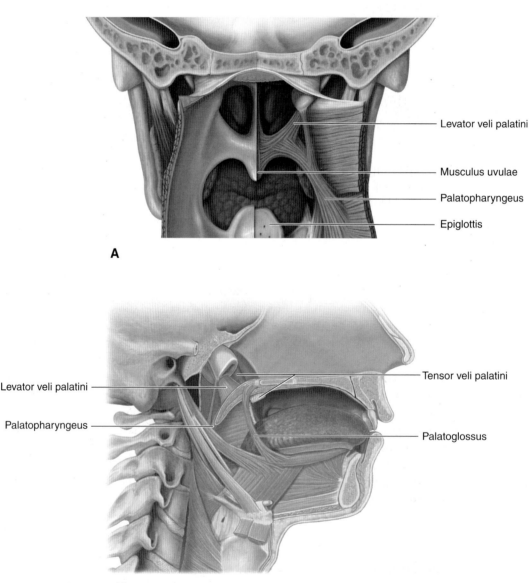

A

Levator veli palatini

Musculus uvulae

Palatopharyngeus

Epiglottis

Levator veli palatini

Palatopharyngeus

Tensor veli palatini

Palatoglossus

B

Figure 10-20 Muscles of the velum. **A**. Posterior view. **B**. Sagittal view. (Adapted with permission from Tank, P.W., Gest, T.R. (2008). *Lippincott Williams & Wilkins atlas of anatomy*. Baltimore: Lippincott Williams & Wilkins.)

TABLE 10-1

ORIGINS, INSERTIONS, AND ACTIONS OF THE VELAR MUSCLES

Muscle	Origin	Insertion	Action
Levator veli palatini	Apex of petrous portion of temporal bone and cartilaginous framework of the auditory tube	Fibers interdigitate at the velum	Primary velar elevator; raises the velum up and back to close off the nasal cavity from the oral cavity; may assist in triggering the pharyngeal swallow reflex
Musculus uvulae	Nasal spines of the palatine bones and adjacent palatine aponeurosis	Uvula of the velum	Shortens and elevates the velum for a stronger seal of the velopharyngeal port than what the levator veli palatini can accomplish alone
Palatoglossus (glossopalatine)	Anterior surface of velum	Lateral tongue	With tongue anchored, depresses velum, but with not as much force as the palatopharyngeus; may assist in triggering the pharyngeal swallow reflex
Palatopharyngeus (pharyngopalatine)	Velum, pterygoid hamulus, and cartilage of the auditory tube	Superior cornu of thyroid cartilage and lateral wall of the pharynx	Provides greater force than the palatoglossus in lowering the velum; also pulls the velum backward; aids in guiding the bolus to the lower pharynx
Superior pharyngeal constrictor	Medial pterygoid plate, pterygomandibular raphe, mylohyoid line, lateral tongue	Medial pharyngeal raphe	Assists the levator veli palatini in creating greater seal of the velopharyngeal port by pulling the posterior pharyngeal wall forward while pulling the lateral walls inward
Tensor veli palatini	Hamulus, spine, and angle of the sphenoid bone	Posterior border of the palatine bone and the connective tissue and musculature of the velum	Unilateral contraction will pull the velum to the side and slightly downward; bilateral contraction will flatten the velum and pull it down slightly and increase tension on the palatal aponeurosis; also opens the lumen of the Eustachian tube; may assist in triggering the pharyngeal swallow reflex

The Tongue

The tongue is an intricate structure whose importance cannot be understated. Its biological functions are to serve as the primary organ of taste as well as to participate in the processes of mastication and deglutition. Secondary to these functions is the formulation of speech sounds. The tongue is the major structure responsible for modifying the resonant characteristics of the vocal tract and is also the primary articulator in the production of many of the consonant sounds of English.

Gross Anatomy

Figure 10-21 provides an illustration of the gross anatomy of the tongue. The two primary parts of the tongue are the blade and root. The blade is that part of the tongue that is readily visible, while the root is below the blade and cannot be seen easily. The blade is further divided into a tip, blade, front, and back. If the tongue is pressed flat against the ceiling of the oral cavity, the tip will rest against the anterior teeth, the blade will rest against the alveolar ridge, the front will rest against the hard palate, and the back will rest against the velum. Running lengthwise down the center of the tongue is a furrow called the **longitudinal median sulcus**. Approximately two-thirds of the way down the length of the dorsum of the tongue from its tip, the longitudinal median sulcus intersects with a chevron-shaped landmark called the **sulcus terminalis**, which courses transversely and is perpendicular to the longitudinal median fissure. At the point where the longitudinal median sulcus intersects the sulcus terminalis, a small pit known as the **foramen cecum** resides. At the posterior limit of the root of the tongue,

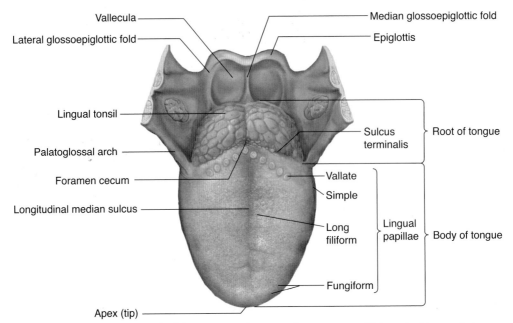

Figure 10-21 Gross anatomy of the tongue and surrounding structures. (Adapted with permission from Tank, P.W., Gest, T.R. (2008). *Lippincott Williams & Wilkins atlas of anatomy.* Baltimore: Lippincott Williams & Wilkins.)

three slips of tissue arise and anchor the base of the tongue to the anterior (lingual) surface of the epiglottis. These are the **median** and **lateral glossoepiglottic folds**. Between the median glossoepiglottic fold and each of the lateral glossoepiglottic folds are small depressions called **valleculae**. The surface of the tongue has somewhat of a rough appearance. This is due to the presence of papillae all over the surface of the tongue anterior to the sulcus terminalis. There are four types of papillae: **filiform, fungiform, simple,** and **vallate**. The papillae house the taste buds which are the essential organs for the sense of taste.

The posterior one-third of the tongue is smoother in appearance than the anterior portion. Several mucous glands are found here along with lymphoid tissue known as the lingual tonsil. Anteriorly on the undersurface of the tongue, you will note a vertically oriented slip of mucous membrane that courses from the inferior surface of the tongue to the floor of the oral cavity. This is the **lingual frenulum**.

Why You Need to Know

At one time or another, you may have heard another person say something to the effect that "that person is tongue tied." Obviously we do not possess the ability to tie our tongues into knots! The term "tongue tied" generally means that the person is having difficulty speaking. In fact, the individual may have a lingual frenulum that is too short so that it may not provide the tongue the mobility to approximate the alveolar

ridge, hard palate, and/or velum. This indeed could very likely cause imprecise or incorrect articulation of speech sounds that require the tongue to move toward the ceiling of the oral cavity.

The outer surface of the tongue is a mucous membrane that is continuous with the covering of all other structures in the oral cavity. On the inferior surface of the tongue, the mucous membrane is relatively thin. It is thick, loose, and freely movable in the region posterior to the sulcus terminalis. Anterior to the sulcus terminalis, the mucous membrane is thin and closely adheres to the underlying muscle tissue. The mucous membrane consists of a basement layer of connective tissue called the **corium**. The corium is dense and somewhat felt-like in consistency. It can be thought of as the "skeleton" of the tongue.

The Tongue as a Muscular Hydrostat

The bulk of the tongue is composed of muscle tissue. Some of the muscles are housed completely within the tongue itself and are referred to as intrinsic muscles. Other muscles originate on anatomical structures outside the tongue but attach to some part of the tongue (and hence are known as extrinsic muscles). Other than the hyoid bone and the corium, there is relatively little skeletal support for the tongue. Instead, the tongue has the ability to change its shape and position without diminishing its volume in the process. As such, the tongue acts like a fluid-filled structure that is

TABLE 10-2

ORIGINS, INSERTIONS, AND ACTIONS OF THE INTRINSIC TONGUE MUSCLES

Muscle	Origin	Insertion	Action
Inferior longitudinal	Hyoid bone and root of the tongue	Apex of the tongue and styloglossus	Primarily works to depress the tongue tip, but also assists in shortening, protruding, and retracting the tongue, and moving the tip from side to side
Superior longitudinal	Submucous fibrous tissue of the tongue root and the median fibrous septum	Edges of the tongue and the fibrous membrane	Primarily works to elevate the tongue tip, but also assists in protruding and retracting the tongue, relaxing the lateral margins of the tongue, and moving the tip from side to side
Transverse	Median fibrous septum	Submucous fibrous tissue at the lateral margins of the tongue	Primarily works to narrow and elongate the tongue, but also assists in relaxing the lateral margins of the tongue and elevating the posterior part of the tongue
Vertical	Mucous membrane of the dorsum of the tongue	Lateral and inferior surfaces of the tongue	Primarily works to flatten the tongue, but also assists in protruding the tongue and creating a longitudinal groove along the middle of the tongue

incompressible. Of course, the tongue is not filled with fluid but instead is composed of muscle tissue. This architecture is referred to as a muscular **hydrostat** (Kier & Smith, 1985; Smith & Kier, 1989).

The corium of the tongue provides the leverage for eight muscles (four intrinsic and four extrinsic) to play off each other to effect the movements the tongue is capable of making (Miller, Watkin, & Chen, 2002). As it changes its shape and position, inward displacement in one area of the tongue results in outward displacement of another area, thereby preserving the tongue's volume. The hydrostatic property of the tongue allows it to perform a myriad array of movements including bulging, centralizing, curling, flattening, grooving, lateralizing, pointing, protruding, retracting, and moving from side to side, among others.

The intrinsic tongue muscles include the following: *inferior longitudinal, superior longitudinal, transverse,* and *vertical.* Table 10-2 summarizes the origins, insertions, and actions of these muscles, while Figure 10-22 provides illustrations of them. It should be noted that the intrinsic muscles are all considered paired because of the presence of a vertically oriented cavity within the tongue called the **fibrous midline septum.** Fibers of the superior longitudinal muscles are confined primarily to the mid-region of the tongue, while the inferior longitudinals can be found more laterally. The fibers of both of these muscles course along the length of the tongue. As the terms transverse and vertical imply, these two muscles have fibers that are arranged in the transverse and vertical planes. Upon inspection of Table 10-2, you

will observe that the intrinsic muscles are responsible primarily for refined tongue movements and postures (e.g., elongating, flattening, narrowing, shortening).

> *Why You Need to Know*
>
> *The two halves of the interior of the tongue also receive independent neural innervation and blood supply. In neurological disorders where half of the tongue is affected (i.e., unilateral paralysis), the unaffected half will still function properly. A clinical sign of unilateral paralysis of the tongue is deviation of the tongue to the paralyzed side when the patient is asked to stick out the tongue. This is because the unaffected muscles will overbalance and mechanically turn the tongue to the side of least resistance—the paralyzed side.*

The extrinsic muscles are responsible for gross posturing of the tongue. These muscles include the *genioglossus, styloglossus, palatoglossus,* and *hyoglossus.* The origins, insertions, and actions of these muscles are summarized in Table 10-3. The palatoglossus was mentioned as a muscle of the velum (refer back to Figure 10-20). The remaining extrinsic muscles are illustrated in Figure 10-23. Being an astute student, you will note that all of these muscles have the term "-glossus" (referring to the tongue) as the second half of their name. The first half of the name refers to the other structure to which the muscle is attached (e.g., "genio-" = chin or inside of the mandible; "stylo-" = styloid process; "palato-" = velum; "hyo-" = hyoid bone).

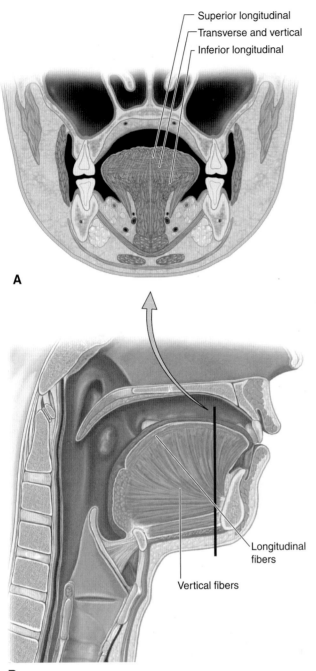

Figure 10-22   The intrinsic tongue muscles. **A**. Coronal view. **B**. Sagittal view. (Adapted with permission from Tank, P.W., Gest, T.R. (2008). *Lippincott Williams & Wilkins atlas of anatomy*. Baltimore: Lippincott Williams & Wilkins.)

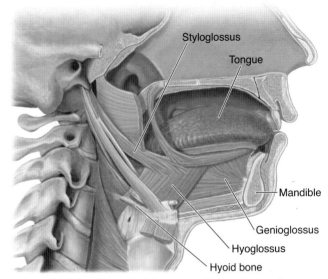

Figure 10-23   The genioglossus, styloglossus, and hyoglossus muscles. (Adapted with permission from Tank, P.W., Gest, T.R. (2008). *Lippincott Williams & Wilkins atlas of anatomy*. Baltimore: Lippincott Williams & Wilkins.)

or velum) is anchored, or upon both structures being free to move.

The hydrostatic interplay between and among the intrinsic and extrinsic muscles allows for intricate posturing and maneuvering of the tongue. The superior longitudinal is responsible for elevating the tongue tip while the inferior longitudinal performs the opposite function. The transverse muscle narrows the tongue. Tongue protrusion is accomplished primarily by contraction of the posterior fibers of the genioglossus; however, this muscle contracting alone will simply cause the tongue to hang downward as it protrudes. The superior longitudinal, inferior longitudinal, and vertical muscles assist in protrusion by pointing the tongue tip and narrowing the tongue body. Retraction of the tongue is effectuated primarily by the anterior fibers of the genioglossus. The superior and inferior longitudinals shorten the tongue as it retracts and the hyoglossus depresses the sides of the tongue during retraction. If you wanted to retract the tongue all the way back into the pharynx (as in swallowing), you would contract the styloglossus muscle.

Movement of the tongue from side to side is accomplished by contraction of the superior and inferior longitudinals. The two muscles on the right acting together will turn the tongue tip to the right. Similarly, simultaneous contraction of the superior and inferior longitudinals on the left will turn the tongue tip to the left. Depression of the body of the tongue is accomplished by contraction of the genioglossus (medial portion of the tongue) and hyoglossus (lateral edges of the tongue). To elevate the posterior tongue, contraction of the palatoglossus muscle is necessary. The

The genioglossus has anterior and posterior muscle fibers. This muscle makes up the bulk of the tongue tissue. It is the largest and strongest of all tongue muscles. The styloglossus is an antagonist of the genioglossus (i.e., its action is the opposite of the genioglossus). The palatoglossus (also referred to sometimes as the glossopalatine) has three functions: (a) it pulls the velum down; (b) it elevates the posterior portion of the tongue; or (c) it does both. Which action is performed is dependent upon which structure (tongue

TABLE 10-3

ORIGINS, INSERTIONS, AND ACTIONS OF THE EXTRINSIC TONGUE MUSCLES

Muscle	Origin	Insertion	Action
Genioglossus	Superior mental spine of the posterior mandibular symphysis	Upper corpus of the hyoid, some to the dorsum of the tongue, and some to the upper pharynx	Posterior fibers assist in protruding the tongue tip and relaxing the lateral margins of the tongue; anterior fibers retract the tongue; contraction of the entire muscle depresses the medial portion of the tongue and assists in creating a longitudinal groove along the middle of the tongue
Hyoglossus	Greater cornu and corpus of hyoid	Lateral submucous tissue of posterior tongue	Depresses the sides of the tongue; assists in retracting the tongue
Palatoglossus	Anterior surface of velum	Lateral tongue	Assists in elevating the posterior part of the tongue
Styloglossus	Styloid process of temporal bone	Lateral area of dorsum of tongue	Assists in retracting the tongue by pulling it toward the pharynx for swallowing

transverse muscle assists the palatoglossus by bunching up the back of the tongue.

If you wanted to create a longitudinal groove along the middle of the tongue, you'd have to contract the geniohyoid and vertical muscles. To create a shallow groove, you'd contract only a part of the geniohyoid. Contraction of the entire geniohyoid would create a deep groove. Finally, relaxation of the lateral edges of the tongue is accomplished by contracting the posterior fibers of the genioglossus as well as the superior longitudinal and transverse muscles. You no doubt are getting the impression that the tongue is capable of refined movement and posturing, and this requires a sophisticated dance between and among the intrinsic and extrinsic tongue muscles!

The Mandible

The mandible (illustrated in Figure 10-4) was described in detail along with the other bones of the skull. In this section, instead of describing the mandible, we will examine more closely the joint that is created by the articulation between the mandible and temporal bone of the skull. As was mentioned earlier in this chapter, this is referred to as the temporomandibular joint (TMJ).

The Temporomandibular Joint

The TMJ is formed specifically by the articulation of the condylar process of the mandible with the mandibular fossa of the temporal bone. The mandibular condyle only indirectly articulates with the mandibular fossa because it is separated from it by the articular meniscus. The parts of the condyle and mandibular fossa that

actually articulate with each other are covered by a fibrocartilage. This deviates from typical joint architecture because most bones that articulate with each other are padded with hyaline cartilage. The primary difference between hyaline cartilage and fibrocartilage is that the latter is devoid of vascular tissue. This is important for the TMJ because blood vessels would be crushed by the action of the TMJ during chewing and vocal activity if the articular surfaces were lined with hyaline cartilage. Finally, the entire TMJ is encapsulated by a membrane called the articular capsule. The condyle is held in place by a series of ligaments. These include the temporomandibular (or lateral), sphenomandibular, and stylomandibular ligaments.

The TMJ is classified as a ginglymoarthrodial joint. This type of joint allows for a hinge-like movement with some limited gliding. In actuality, there are two TMJs but if functioning properly the two act as a single bilateral unit. The joint is set in such a way that the mandible is able to move vertically (i.e., opening and closing), anteroposteriorly (i.e., protruding and retracting), and transversely (i.e., from side to side). All these three dimensions of movement take place to some degree during chewing and speaking.

Why You Need to Know

TMJ dysfunction syndrome can severely restrict one's ability to utilize the mandible for chewing or speech purposes. Symptoms may include facial pain and spasm, reduced mandibular movement, and noises in the joint. Treatment may include surgery or the use of an orthodontic prosthesis to reduce grinding of the teeth.

TABLE 10-4

ORIGINS, INSERTIONS, AND ACTIONS OF THE MANDIBULAR ELEVATOR MUSCLES

Muscle	Origin	Insertion	Action
Masseter (external body)	Anterior portion of zygomatic arch	Angle and lateral surface of the mandibular ramus	Along with the medial (internal) pterygoid straps the mandible to the skull; primarily closes and retracts the jaw; may assist in lateral jaw movement
Masseter (internal body)	Posterior and medial portion of zygomatic arch	Upper half of ramus and lateral surface of coronoid process of the mandible	
Medial (internal) pterygoid	Pterygoid fossa and medial surface of lateral pterygoid plate	Inner surface of the ramus and angle of the mandible	Along with the masseter, straps the mandible to the skull; primarily elevates the mandible; assists in protruding the mandible
Temporalis	Entire temporal fossa	Anterior border of the ramus and coronoid process of the mandible	Primarily elevates the mandible; assists in retracting the mandible and moving the mandible laterally

Mandibular Movements

The primary movement of the mandible is elevation and depression. When the mandible is elevated, the mouth is closed. By the same token, when the mandible is depressed, the mouth is open. Two sets of muscles are responsible for these movements, and they are referred to as the mandibular elevator and mandibular depressor muscles. Tables 10-4 and 10-5 provide summary information about the elevator and depressor muscles, respectively.

The mandibular elevator muscles include the *masseter, medial* (or *internal*) *pterygoid,* and *temporalis.* The masseter and temporalis muscles are illustrated in Figure 10-24, and the medial pterygoid is illus-

trated in Figure 10-25. The masseter has both internal and external fibers. Although it is a relatively slow muscle, it is the most powerful of all muscles of mastication. The temporalis is a quicker muscle whose action is snapping. The medial pterygoid along with the masseter are referred to as the mandibular sling muscles because they suspend the mandible in place along with the mandibular ligaments mentioned in the previous section.

The mandibular depressor muscles include the *digastricus, mylohyoid, geniohyoid,* and *lateral* (or *external*) *pterygoid.* The first three of these muscles were described in Chapter 8 as suprahyoid laryngeal muscles, but they also have the ability to pull the man-

TABLE 10-5

ORIGINS, INSERTIONS, AND ACTIONS OF THE MANDIBULAR DEPRESSOR MUSCLES

Muscle	Origin	Insertion	Action
Digastricus (anterior belly)	Inside lower border of mandible	Lesser cornua of hyoid bone	With the hyoid anchored, primarily depresses mandible; anterior digastricus assists in retracting the mandible
Digastricus (posterior belly)	Mastoid process of temporal bone	Lesser cornua of hyoid bone	
Geniohyoid	Lower part of mental symphysis of mandible	Anterior corpus of hyoid	With the hyoid anchored, primarily depresses mandible; assists in retracting the mandible
Lateral (external) pterygoid	Lateral greater wing of sphenoid and lateral pterygoid plate	Pterygoid fossa on the anterior neck of mandibular condyle	Primarily depresses the mandible; bilateral contraction assists in protruding mandible; unilateral contraction will assist in lateral mandibular movement (i.e., a grinding action)
Mylohyoid	Inner surface of corpus of mandible	Midline raphe; posterior fibers to corpus of hyoid	With the hyoid anchored, primarily depresses mandible; assists in retracting the mandible

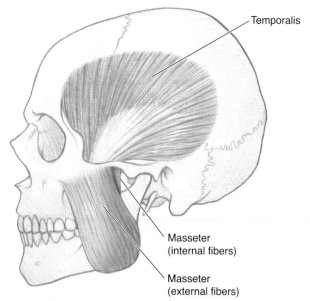

Figure 10-24 The masseter and temporalis muscles. (Adapted with permission from Scheumann, D.W. (2002). *The balanced body: A guide to deep tissue and neuromuscular therapy* (2nd ed). Baltimore: Lippincott Williams & Wilkins.)

dible down. The lateral pterygoid muscle is illustrated in Figure 10-25 along with the medial pterygoid so that you can see the relationship between them. The digastricus, geniohyoid, and mylohyoid muscles are illustrated in Figure 10-26.

As was mentioned in the section above, the mandible not only has the ability to raise and lower but can also protrude, retract, and move from side to side. The same muscles that elevate and depress the mandible

are responsible for these movements. Anteroposterior and transverse movement of the mandible is dependent upon which of these muscles is contracting at a given time. Mandibular protrusion is dependent upon simultaneous contraction of the medial and lateral pterygoid muscles. Retraction is mediated by simultaneous contraction of the posterior fibers of the temporalis and the anterior belly of the digastricus as well as the mylohyoid and geniohyoid muscles. Finally, transverse (i.e., lateral) movement is dependent upon simultaneous contraction of the lateral pterygoid and the posterior portion of the temporalis. Imagine how intricate the interplay of muscular contraction must be to effect the rotary movements of the mandible that are seen during chewing and to a lesser extent, speaking!

Other Structures of the Oral Cavity

Faucial Pillars

The faucial pillars can be seen quite clearly when you open your mouth and examine the back of your oral cavity in a mirror. As a reference point, at midline of the ceiling along the posterior limit of the oral cavity is the uvula, the singular bulb-like structure at the terminus of the velum. If you start at the uvula and follow either side along the back of the oral cavity, two folds of skin will become apparent on each side. These folds are the anterior and posterior faucial pillars. Although you will see only the mucous membrane of these folds, within them are muscle fibers. The anterior faucial

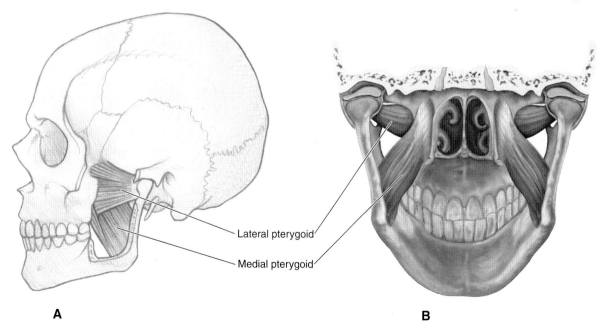

Figure 10-25 The medial and lateral pterygoid muscles. **A**. Lateral view. **B**. Posterior view. (**A**: Adapted with permission from Scheumann, D.W. (2002). *The balanced body: A guide to deep tissue and neuromuscular therapy* (2nd ed). Baltimore: Lippincott Williams & Wilkins; **B**: Adapted with permission from Anatomical Chart Company.)

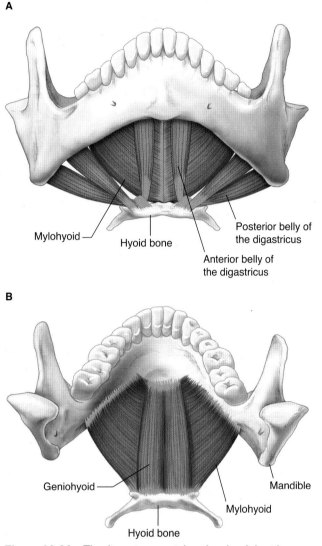

A

Mylohyoid

Hyoid bone

Posterior belly of the digastricus

Anterior belly of the digastricus

B

Geniohyoid

Mylohyoid

Mandible

Hyoid bone

Figure 10-26 The digastricus, geniohyoid, and mylohyoid muscles. **A**. Anterior-inferior view. **B**. Posterior-superior view.

pillars house fibers of the palatoglossus muscles. The posterior pillars contain fibers from the palatopharyngeus muscles. As such, the anterior pillars are sometimes referred to as the palatoglossal folds, while the posterior pillars are known as the palatopharyngeal folds. A space—the **tonsillar fossa**—exists between these two folds.

Tonsils

At the posterior limits of the oral cavity are a series of lymphoid masses called tonsils. These masses are arranged somewhat in a circle and are therefore referred to as **Waldeyer's ring**. One of these masses was mentioned in the section on the tongue: the lingual tonsil. This tonsil, found at the base of the posterior tongue, is the floor of Waldeyer's ring. The lateral walls of the ring are created by the palatine tonsils. These are housed within the tonsillar fossae between the ante-

rior and posterior faucial pillars. Some of the tonsillar fossae still remains immediately superior to the palatine tonsils. This space is called the **supratonsillar fossa**. Finally, the ceiling of Waldeyer's ring is formed by the pharyngeal tonsil, or adenoids. The adenoids are found along the posterior pharyngeal wall in the region of the velum.

Being lymphoid tissue, the tonsils are responsible for fighting infection. As bacteria are introduced into the oral and pharyngeal cavities, the tonsils trap as much of the invaders as possible so that the upper respiratory tract will remain healthy. However, sometimes, the tonsils become inflamed and infected. This is usually evident by pus accumulating in the supratonsillar fossae. Because the pharyngeal ostium (opening) of the Eustachian tube is proximal to the adenoids, any infection of the adenoids may reflux into the Eustachian tube and through it enter the middle ear cavity.

> ### Why You Need to Know
>
> *Chronic hypertrophy (swelling) of the adenoids may result in obstruction of the nasopharynx, which in turn may result in mouth breathing and denasality of the voice. The individual's speech will sound dull, especially for the nasal consonants /m/, /n/, and /ŋ/. Words like "mom," "nice," and "song" will sound like "bob," "dice," and "sog." At some point, the doctor may decide to perform a "T & A" procedure— removal of the tonsils and adenoids.*

Velopharyngeal Mechanism

Most of the structures of the velopharyngeal (V-P) mechanism, or port, were described in the section on the velum. The V-P mechanism is responsible for regulating the communication between the oral and nasal cavities. This is important for both digestive and speech functions, as will become evident when the V-P mechanism is revisited later in this chapter in the section on physiology. The V-P mechanism consists of the velum and posterior pharyngeal wall. When the velum is raised to approximate the posterior pharyngeal wall, the V-P port is closed. Separation between the velum and posterior pharyngeal wall means that the V-P port is open. The muscles that mediate movement of the velum (refer back to Table 10-1) are involved in V-P mechanics.

In some individuals, a bulging of the posterior pharyngeal wall, called **Passavant's pad**, may exist to assist the velum in approximating the posterior wall of the pharynx. Whether Passavant's pad actually exists is a topic of debate among anatomists. Some believe it does not, while others believe it does. Still others hold the position that Passavant's pad may exist for some individuals, especially for persons whose velum is shorter than normal so that it cannot adequately approximate the posterior pharyngeal wall without some assistance from the pharynx.

V-P Closure

The primary muscle of velar elevation is the levator veli palatini (LVP). Fibers of this muscle comprise approximately 40% or more of the velum (Boorman & Sommerlad, 1985; Kuehn & Kahane, 1990). The fibers extend from just behind the hard palate to the front of the uvula and then proceed laterally at an angle of about 45 degrees to their cranial attachments, in essence forming a superiorly oriented sling with the velum serving as the cradle. Bilateral contraction of the LVP will lift the velum toward the posterior pharyngeal wall in an angular fashion. Contraction affects a large area of the velum, thereby allowing for a broad seal between the velum and posterior pharyngeal wall.

The musculus uvulae assists in elevating the velum when a tighter seal is required. This muscle accounts for the lengthwise convexity of the upper surface of the velum. When it contracts, it serves three purposes: (1) it shortens the velum; (2) it elevates the velum; and (3) it increases the thickness of the velum throughout a portion of its length. The musculus uvulae assists in shortening the distance between the velum and posterior pharyngeal wall while creating greater contact force between the two.

Finally, the superior constrictor muscle (a pharyngeal wall muscle in the region of the nasopharynx) may also assist in closure of the V-P port. When this muscle contracts, it pulls the posterior pharyngeal wall forward as it pulls the lateral walls inward. This action, in concert with action of the LVP and in some cases the musculus uvulae, creates a seal between the velum and posterior pharyngeal wall.

It should be noted that as the velum slides up and down the posterior pharyngeal wall, friction is generated. The frictional forces generated by this activity causes velar glands to secrete a lubricating substance to reduce the friction (Kuehn & Moon, 2005).

V-P Opening

To open the V-P port, the velum must be lowered. This is accomplished through the contraction of the palatopharyngeus, palatoglossus, and, to some extent, the tensor veli palatini (recall that the first two muscles comprise the faucial pillars). Of these three muscles, the palatopharyngeus muscles provide the greatest force of depression. The prevailing thought is that the palatopharyngeus acts like a sling that is oriented in the opposite direction of the LVP (Hixon, Weismer, & Hoit, 2008). With the pharyngeal attachment of the muscle stabilized, the vertical fibers of the palatopharyngeus pull downward and backward on the velum when they contract. With the tongue stabilized, contraction of the palatoglossus muscles will also depress the velum but with less force than what the palatopharyngeus muscles provide (Moon & Kuehn, 2004).

Finally, the TVP muscle plays a minor role in velar depression. Fibers of the TVP originate at the sphenoid bone and the cartilaginous part of the Eustachian tube and then course downward in a vertical direction to terminate in a tendon. The tendon then wraps around the hamulus of the medial pterygoid lamina where the muscle changes to a more horizontal direction, terminating at the hard palate and velum (Barsoumian, Kuehn, Moon, & Canady, 1998). This arrangement allows the TVP to act similarly to a rope being pulled around a pulley (the hamulus being the pulley). TVP contraction causes three things to happen: (1) it lowers the velum slightly; (2) it flattens the velum; and (3) it applies tension to the palatal aponeurosis in much the same way as a drumhead tightens on a drum.

Other Functions of the V-P Mechanism

Not only do the muscles of the V-P mechanism work to mediate the degree of coupling between the oral and nasal cavities, but they perform other important tasks. First, the V-P mechanism is thought to assist in swallowing. Not only is the V-P port activated during a swallow, but Kuehn, Templeton, and Maynard (1990) and Liss (1990) found that the TVP, LVP, and palatoglossus muscles contain muscle spindles. They believed that these spindles house special receptors that aid in initiating the pharyngeal swallow reflex.

The other task that the V-P mechanism performs is related to phonation. Recall from Chapter 8 that the vocal folds are set into vibration when subglottic pressure overcomes their resistance. Prior to phonation, subglottic pressure is greater than supraglottic pressure so that when phonation commences, the air passes upward and outward through the vocal folds. However, as soon as the vocal folds begin to vibrate, subglottic pressure diminishes. To maintain vocal fold vibration once it has been initiated, subglottic pressure must remain greater than supraglottic pressure. As the vocal folds vibrate, the velum increases its height. The increase in velar height results in greater supraglottic volume. The increased supraglottic volume causes a drop in supraglottic pressure so that it remains less than subglottic pressure.

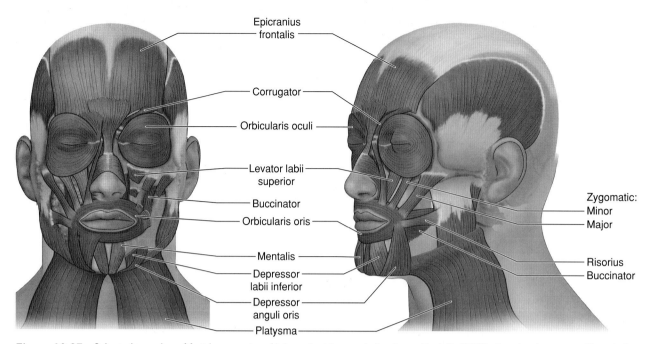

Figure 10-27 Selected muscles of facial expression. (Adapted with permission from Cael, C. (2009). *Functional anatomy: Musculoskeletal anatomy, kinesiology, and palpation for manual therapists.* Baltimore: Lippincott Williams & Wilkins.)

Muscles of Facial Expression

A thorough discussion of the oral cavity would not be complete without at least mentioning the muscles of the face. Not only do humans communicate primarily through an acoustic signal (i.e., speech), they also communicate through facial expression. Furthermore, the production of some speech sounds requires contraction of at least some of the facial muscles. Therefore, this final section of our journey through the oral cavity will provide you with an overview of the muscles that mediate facial expression.

The *orbicularis oris,* which was described in the section concerning the lips, is the reference point for most of the muscles of facial expression. Many of the muscles listed in Table 10-6 make their insertion into its superficial layer from various angles. Five muscles (*depressor labii inferior, levator labii superior, levator labii superior alaeque nasi, zygomatic major,* and *zygomatic minor*) approach the orbicularis oris from an oblique direction above or below. Two muscles, the *buccinator* and *risorius,* insert into the orbicularis oris from a horizontal direction. Three muscles (*depressor anguli oris, levator angli oris,* and *mentalis*) course in a perpendicular fashion toward the orbicularis oris before inserting into it. The *incisivus labii inferior* and *incisivus labii superior* are not true lip muscles, but they course in a direction parallel to the length of the orbicularis oris. The remaining muscles (*corrugator, epicranius frontalis, orbicularis oculi,* and *platysma*) are supplementary muscles of facial expression. Many of these muscles are illustrated in Figure 10-27.

All of these muscles act as a unit to mediate facial expression. The full gamut of facial expressions can be represented by contraction of any number of these muscles. This includes blinking and winking the eyes; raising and lowering the eyelids; pursing the lips; frowning; and smiling. Indeed, these expressions can be accomplished with varying intensity (e.g., a "gentle" frown versus a "heavy" frown). A closer inspection of Table 10-6 will reveal the complexity of muscle activity that is involved in facial expression.

THE NASAL CAVITY

When one thinks of the nose, the first thing that comes to mind is breathing or smelling. If you believe that these are the only functions of the nose, you'd be in error. The nose—or more specifically the nasal cavity—plays an important role in speech production. This function will be described in more detail in the section on physiology; for now, we will turn our attention to the anatomical structures of the nose and nasal cavity. The nasal cavity begins at the nose and terminates in the region of the **nasopharynx,** immediately above the velum and anterior to the posterior pharyngeal wall. The structures that will be discussed in this section include the nose, nasal septum, nasal conchae and meatuses, and mucous membrane.

TABLE 10-6

ORIGINS, INSERTIONS, AND ACTIONS OF THE MUSCLES THAT MEDIATE FACIAL EXPRESSION

Muscle	Origin	Insertion	Action
Buccinator	Pterygomandibular raphe, lateral surface of the alveolar process of the maxilla, and the mandible in the region of the third molars	Muscle fibers of both the upper and lower lips	Compresses the lips and cheeks against the teeth and draws the corners of the mouth outward
Corrugator	Superciliary arch of the frontal bone	Skin above the medial arch of the eyebrows	Pulls the eyebrows downward and inward, thereby wrinkling the skin of the forehead between the eyes
Depressor anguli oris	Oblique line of the mandible	Orbicularis oris at the angle of the mouth and the upper lip	Depresses the angle of the lip and assists in compressing the upper lip against the lower lip
Depressor labii inferior	Oblique line of the mandible near the mental foramen	Orbicularis oris of the lower lip	Pulls the lower lip downward and outward
Epicranius frontalis	Epicranial aponeuroses	Skin of the forehead near the eyebrows	Raises the eyebrows and causes the skin on the forehead to wrinkle horizontally
Incisivus labii inferior	Mandible in the region of the lateral incisor teeth	Orbicularis oris at the angle of the mouth	Pulls the corner of the mouth inward and downward
Incisivus labii superior	Maxilla immediately above the canine teeth	Orbicularis oris at the angle of the mouth	Pulls the corner of the mouth inward and upward
Levator anguli oris	Canine fossa of the maxilla	Upper lip and angle of the lower lip	Pulls the corner of the mouth upward and assists in closing the mouth by pulling the lower lip upward
Levator labii superior	Lower margin of the orbit of the eye, maxilla, and zygomatic bone	Upper lip between the levator anguli oris and levator labii superior alaeque nasi	Elevates and everts the upper lip
Levator labii superior alaeque nasi	Frontal process and infraorbital margin of the maxillae	Lateral cartilages of the nose and the orbicularis oris	Elevates the upper lip
Mentalis	Incisive fossa of the mandible	Skin of the chin	Elevates, protrudes, and everts the lower lip, and wrinkles the skin of the chin
Orbicularis oculi	Nasal process of the frontal bone, frontal process of the maxilla, and palpebral ligament	Lateral palpebral raphe	Closes the eyelids, draws tears from the lacrimal glands into the eyes
Orbicularis oris	Near midline on the anterior surfaces of the maxilla and mandible	Mucous membrane of the margin of the lips and raphe with the buccinator	Closes the mouth and puckers the lips
Platysma	Skin over the lower neck and upper lateral chest	Inferior border of the mandible and skin over the lower face and angle of the mouth	Depresses and wrinkles the skin of the lower face and mouth; aids in the forced depression of the mandible
Risorius	Fascia of the masseter muscle	Skin of the corner of the mouth and muscle fibers of the lower lip	Pulls the mouth angle outward
Zygomatic major	Anterior surface of the zygomatic bone, immediately lateral to the zygomatic minor muscle	Orbicularis oris of the upper lip and skin of the corner of the mouth	Pulls the angle of the mouth upward and outward
Zygomatic minor	Anterior surface of the zygomatic bone, immediately medial to the zygomatic major muscle	Orbicularis oris of the upper lip	Elevates the upper lip

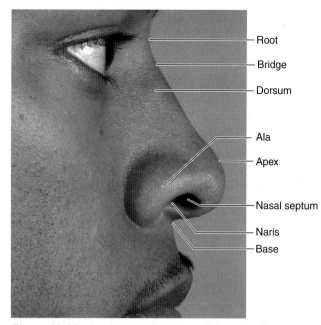

Figure 10-28 Landmarks of the nose. (Adapted with permission from Lippincott Williams & Wilkins' Surface Anatomy Collection.)

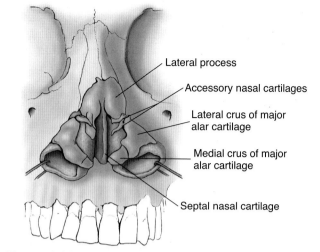

Figure 10-29 Nasal cartilages. (Adapted with permission from Agur, A.M., Dalley, A.F. (2008). *Grant's atlas of anatomy* (12th ed.). Baltimore: Lippincott Williams & Wilkins.)

As illustrated in Figure 10-28, the nose can be divided into several parts. These include the root, bridge, dorsum, apex, base, nares, and columella nasi. The root of the nose corresponds to the point where the nasal bones articulate with the frontal bone. The bridge is that part of the nose that corresponds to the nasal bones. Extending from the nasal bones is cartilage; the dorsum is this part of the nose. The apex (or tip) is the part of the nose that protrudes furthest from the face. The base is the bottom of the nose where it joins the face above the upper lip. Along the base are two openings called the anterior nares, which are more commonly referred to as nostrils. The anterior nares are separated by a partition called the columella nasi. The columella nasi is simply a continuation of the dorsum to the base of the nose.

The outer lining of the nose is epithelial tissue (i.e., skin). Underlying the mucous membrane are several cartilages that give the nose its shape (see Figure 10-29). The **septal cartilage** is a vertically oriented partition that extends outward from the nasal orifice at midline. It not only serves as the dorsum of the nose but also completes the nasal septum that separates the nasal cavity into two chambers. Its posterior attachment is the bony nasal septum. Recall that the bony nasal septum is formed by the perpendicular plate of the ethmoid (the superior part) and the vomer (the inferior part). The lateral nasal cartilages make up the sides of the nose, while the alar cartilages (major and minor) complete the framework by assisting in the formation of the nares. The lateral

nasal cartilages articulate with the septal cartilage and the nasal bones. The alar cartilages articulate with the lateral nasal cartilages.

Superimposed upon the nasal cartilages are several muscles that assist in the process of breathing and to a lesser extent play a role in facial expression. Table 10-7 summarizes the muscles of the nose in terms of their origins, insertions, and actions. Figure 10-30 illustrates these muscles, which include the *anterior nasal dilator, depressor alae nasi, levator labii superior alaeque nasi, nasalis, posterior nasal dilator,* and

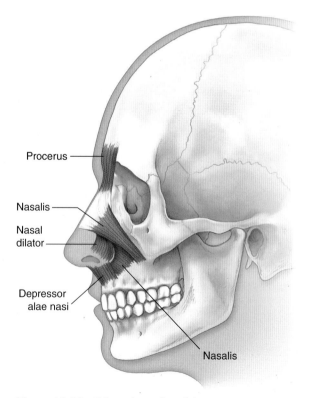

Figure 10-30 Selected muscles of the nose.

TABLE 10-7

ORIGINS, INSERTIONS, AND ACTIONS OF THE MUSCLES OF THE NOSE

Muscle	Origin	Insertion	Action
Anterior nasal dilator	Lower edge of the lateral nasal cartilage	Deep tissue of the skin that covers the nasal alae	Dilates the nostrils
Depressor alae nasi	Incisive fossa of the maxillae	Lower region of the cartilaginous nasal septum and adjacent alae of the nose	Depresses the alae of the nose which constricts the nostrils
Levator labii superior alaeque nasi	Frontal process and infraorbital margin of the maxillae	Lateral cartilages of the nose and the orbicularis oris	Dilates the nostrils
Nasalis	Superior and lateral to the incisive fossa of the maxillae	An aponeurosis of the procerus muscle as well as an aponeurosis of the nasalis from the opposite side	Depresses the cartilages of the nose, which narrows the nostrils
Posterior nasal dilator	Nasal aperture of the maxillae and adjacent sesamoid cartilages	The skin of the inferior and posterior alar cartilages	Dilates the nostrils
Procerus	Lower nasal bones and upper lateral nasal cartilages	Skin of the lower forehead between the eyebrows	Depresses the medial angle of the eyebrow and wrinkles the skin over the bridge of the nose

procerus. With the exception of the procerus, these muscles serve to either dilate or constrict the nostrils.

The interior of the nasal cavity consists of two chambers separated by the nasal septum. The open space immediately inside the anterior nares is the vestibule (children stick their finger here when "picking their nose"). Along the lateral walls of each chamber are three scrolls of bone that extend into the cavity space and form longitudinal channels along the length of the nasal cavity. The scrolls of bone are the superior, medial, and inferior nasal conchae or turbinates. You may recall from a previous discussion in this chapter that the superior and medial nasal conchae come from the ethmoid, while the inferior nasal conchae is an independent bone.

Why You Need to Know

Many people have a "deviated" septum from trauma to the nose (e.g., being hit in the nose while boxing) or disease. This means that the cartilaginous portion of the nasal septum is bent so that it deviates to one side instead of remaining midline. The deviation is usually to the left. A deviated septum can pose problems for a person in terms of breathing through one nostril or drainage of mucous on one side of the nose.

The longitudinal channels formed by the conchae are the nasal meatuses. As there are three conchae, there are three meatuses in each chamber. Referred to as the superior, medial, and inferior meatuses, they correspond to their like-named conchae. Each meatus lies below its corresponding concha. The lateral walls of the nasal cavity also contain the openings through which the paranasal sinuses drain into the nasal cavity.

The ceiling of the nasal cavity is composed primarily of the cribriform plate of the ethmoid. The cribriform plate is perforated so that fibers from the olfactory nerve (cranial nerve I) can pass into the nasal cavity. The posterior limit of the nasal cavity opens into the uppermost region of the pharynx—the appropriately named nasopharynx. The nasal cavity communicates with the nasopharynx via the posterior nares, or **choanae**.

The interior of the nasal cavity is covered by a mucous membrane. As with the rest of the respiratory passageway, the mucous membrane is ciliated. That is, tiny hairs project from the surface of the mucous membrane. A thin layer of mucous blankets the interior of the nasal cavity. This protective blanket traps organisms and contaminants. The cilia continually sweep the mucous and trapped invaders toward the nasopharynx. Eventually, the polluted mucous makes its way down the throat and into the stomach.

THE PHARYNGEAL CAVITY

The pharyngeal cavity is more commonly referred to as the throat, although it actually extends all the way to the base of the skull superiorly and to the esophagus inferiorly (refer back to Figure 10-1). Its composition is similar to that of the velum; it has a basement "skeleton" known as the **pharyngeal aponeurosis**, an intermediate layer of muscle tissue, and finally a superficial layer of mucous membrane.

Pharyngeal Aponeurosis

The pharyngeal aponeurosis is a funnel-shaped sheet of connective tissue that originates at the base of the skull, and more specifically, the pharyngeal tubercle of the occipital bone (immediately anterior to the foramen magnum), petrous portion of the temporal bone, cartilage of the Eustachian tube, and medial pterygoid lamina of the sphenoid. In an adult male, this tube is approximately 12 cm in length. The greatest width of the pharynx is approximately 4 cm and the greatest depth is approximately 2 cm. This is at the superior end of the tube, at the base of the skull. The pharynx then narrows considerably until by the time it terminates at esophagus, it has a width of only approximately 2½ cm and virtually zero depth (i.e., the anterior and posterior pharyngeal walls touch each other and do not separate until food or drink passes through on the way to the esophagus).

Pharyngeal Muscles

The pharyngeal aponeurosis is superimposed by muscle tissue. The muscular pharynx is highly complex. Muscles interdigitate to such an extent that it is difficult to parse out the individual muscles. Therefore, the muscular layer of the pharynx is typically divided into three overlapping regions referred to as the superior, medial, and inferior constrictor muscles. Each of the constrictor muscles consists of between two and four individual muscles. In addition to the constrictor muscles, secondary muscles also play a role in pharyngeal mechanics. Table 10-8 provides summary information for the pharyngeal muscles. The constrictor muscles are illustrated in Figure 10-31. The superior pharyngeal constrictor consists of four muscles: *buccopharyngeus, glossopharyngeus, mylopharyngeus,* and *pterygopharyngeus*. The medial pharyngeal constrictor consists of two muscles: *ceratopharyngeus* and *chondropharyngeus*. The inferior pharyngeal constrictor consists of two muscles: *cricopharyngeus* and *thyropharyngeus*. Although the superior pharyngeal constrictor is the most complex of the constrictor muscles, it also is the weakest. All three of the constrictor muscles influence the volume of the pharyngeal

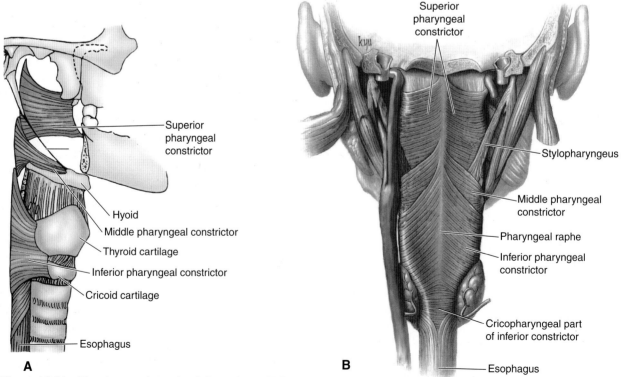

Figure 10-31 The pharyngeal muscles. **A**. Lateral view. **B**. Posterior view. (Adapted with permission from Moore, K.L., Agur. A.M., Dalley, A.F. (2009). *Clinically oriented anatomy* (6th ed.). Baltimore: Lippincott Williams & Wilkins.)

TABLE 10-8

ORIGINS, INSERTIONS, AND ACTIONS OF THE PHARYNGEAL MUSCLES

Muscle	Origin	Insertion	Action
Inferior constrictor: Cricopharyngeus Thyropharyngeus	Thyroid cartilage, cricoid cartilage, inferior cornu of hyoid bone	Medial pharyngeal raphe and the esophagus	Assists in swallowing and vocal resonance by reducing the cross-sectional area of the pharyngeal lumen in the laryngopharyngeal region (by forward movement of the posterior pharyngeal wall and medial movement of the lateral pharyngeal walls in a sphincter-like fashion)
Middle constrictor: Ceratopharyngeus Chondro-pharyngeus	Greater and lesser cornua of hyoid bone	Medial pharyngeal raphe; fibers overlap with inferior fibers from the superior constrictor and superior fibers of the inferior constrictor	Performs a similar function as the inferior constrictor except the action is confined to the oropharyngeal region
Palatopharyngeus (pharyngopalatine)	Soft palate, pterygoid hamulus, and the cartilage of the auditory tube	Superior cornu of the thyroid cartilage and lateral wall of the pharynx	With the velum stabilized, the upper fibers assist the superior constrictor in drawing the lateral pharyngeal walls medially; lower fibers elevate the pharynx and larynx
Salpingopharyngeus	Inferior border of the medial aspect of the cartilage at the orifice of the auditory tube	Blends with fibers of the palatopharyngeus muscle	Pulls the lateral walls of the pharynx upward and inward, thereby decreasing the width of the pharynx
Stylopharyngeus	Medial side of the base of the styloid process	Between the superior and middle constrictors	Pulls upward on the pharynx and draws the lateral walls even more laterally, thereby increasing the width of the pharynx; pulls upward on the pharynx and larynx
Superior constrictor: Buccopharyngeus Glossopharyngeus Mylopharyngeus Pterygopharyngeus	Medial pterygoid plate, pterygomandibular raphe, mylohyoid line, lateral tongue	Medial pharyngeal raphe	Performs a similar function as the inferior and middle constrictors except the action is confined to the nasopharyngeal region

tube. When bilateral contraction of these muscles occurs, they act as a sphincter that serves to narrow the pharyngeal lumen. This action has implications for swallowing and vocal resonance.

Why You Need to Know

Of particular importance is the cricopharyngeus muscle which is part of the inferior constrictor. In many cases of laryngectomy (removal of the larynx, usually due to cancer), a portion of the cricopharyngeus is preserved, if possible. The cricopharyngeus will serve as the laryngectomee's sound source for "voicing" by vibrating as air is forced across it.

Although not part of the pharyngeal constrictor complex, the *palatopharyngeus* (also known as the pharyngopalatine), *salpingopharyngeus*, and *stylopharyngeus* muscles also play a part in pharyngeal mechanics. The palatopharyngeus muscle was described earlier as a velar depressor, but some of its fibers blend with fibers of the pharynx. This muscle shortens the distance between the velum and pharynx, thereby narrowing the posterior faucial pillars. With the velum stabilized, the palatopharyngeus assists the superior constrictor in drawing the lateral pharyngeal walls medially, thereby narrowing the pharyngeal lumen. The salpingopharyngeus muscle also assists in narrowing the pharyngeal lumen. When it contracts, it pulls the lateral walls of the pharynx upward and inward, thereby decreasing the width of the pharynx.

The stylopharyngeus has the opposite effect on the pharynx as the constrictors, palatopharyngeus and salpingopharyngeus. This muscle elevates the pharynx and pulls the lateral walls even more laterally, thereby widening the pharyngeal lumen. This muscle, along with the palatopharyngeus, also elevates the pharynx and larynx, which is an action necessary in swallowing.

Mucous Membrane

The superficial layer of the pharynx is a mucous membrane that is continuous with the mucous membrane of the oral cavity, larynx, and esophagus. In the uppermost region of the pharynx, the membrane consists of columnar ciliated epithelium. In the lower (i.e., oral and laryngeal) regions, the membrane consists of stratified squamous cells. Clusters of mucous glands lie immediately beneath the mucous membrane. These clusters are more numerous around the orifice of the Eustachian tube than elsewhere in the pharynx.

Pharyngeal Regions

As illustrated in Figure 10-1, the pharynx is divided into three regions: the nasopharynx, **oropharynx**, and **laryngopharynx**. The nasopharynx is superior to the velum and extends from the choanae to the posterior pharyngeal wall. This part of the pharynx contains several landmarks. These include the **torus tubarius**, pharyngeal ostium of the Eustachian (auditory) tube, adenoids, and pharyngeal bursa. The torus tubarius is a comma-shaped ridge in the lateral walls of the nasopharynx. It is composed of two muscles lying beneath the mucous membrane: the salpingopalatine (anterior portion) and salpingopharyngeus (posterior portion). The ostium of the Eustachian tube resides under the curved part of the torus tubarius. The adenoids are found along the posterior pharyngeal wall, superior to the velum. Finally, the pharyngeal bursa is a groove in the mucous membrane that runs vertically at midline from the adenoids to the base of the skull.

By comparison with the nasopharynx, the oro- and laryngopharynges are relatively void of landmarks. The oropharynx extends from the velum superiorly to the hyoid bone inferiorly. The laryngopharynx then extends from the hyoid bone superiorly to the aditus laryngis inferiorly.

NEURAL INNERVATION

Because all structures of the vocal tract are in the head and neck, you might surmise correctly that cranial nerves will be responsible for innervating the muscles of the velum, tongue, mandible, face, nose, and pharynx. Table 10-9 summarizes the neural innervation of most of the muscles that were discussed in this chapter. In total, half of the 12 cranial nerves serve the structures of the face and the oral, nasal, and pharyngeal cavities. These include the trigeminal (cranial nerve V), facial (VII), glossopharyngeal (IX), vagus (X), spinal accessory (XI), and hypoglossal (XII) nerves.

All of the muscles of the velum are innervated by the vagus nerve except the tensor veli palatini (TVP), which is innervated by the trigeminal. The musculus uvulae, palatoglossus, and palatopharyngeus may also be innervated by the spinal accessory nerve.

All of the intrinsic muscles of the tongue are innervated by the hypoglossal nerve. The same is true for all of the extrinsic tongue muscles except the palatoglossus, which is innervated by the vagus and possibly the spinal accessory nerve.

The mandibular elevator muscles are all innervated by the anterior trunk of the mandibular branch of the trigeminal nerve. Three cranial nerves innervate the mandibular depressor muscles. The anterior belly of the digastricus, the lateral pterygoid, and the mylohyoid muscles are innervated by the trigeminal nerve. The posterior body of the digastricus is innervated by the facial nerve. Finally, the geniohyoid muscle is innervated by the hypoglossal nerve.

All three pharyngeal constrictor muscles receive their innervation from the vagus nerve. The spinal accessory nerve may also be involved, but its role in the innervation of these muscles is not as clear as the vagus. This is also true of the palatopharyngeus and salpingopharyngeus muscles. The only exception to pharyngeal innervation is the stylopharyngeus muscle, which is innervated by the glossopharyngeal nerve.

The muscles of the nose and face are not included in Table 10-9. However, as a general rule, the muscles of the nose and face receive motor innervation from the facial nerve. The skin, glands, and other soft tissues receive primarily sensory innervation from the trigeminal nerve. Although virtually all muscles of the nose and face are innervated by the facial nerve, they receive their innervation from various branches of the nerve. For example, the stylohyoid muscle receives innervation from the stylohyoid branch of the facial nerve. The corrugator, frontalis, and orbicularis oculi muscles are innervated by the temporal branch, and the last of these three muscles also is innervated by the zygomatic branch. The buccinator, procerus, and orbicularis oris muscles are innervated by the buccal branch of the facial nerve. Finally, the platysma muscle receives innervation from the mandibular and cervical branches of the facial nerve.

TABLE 10-9

INNERVATION OF SELECT MUSCLES OF THE ARTICULATORY/RESONANCE SYSTEM

Muscle	Innervation
Mandibular Muscles	
Elevator Muscles	
Masseter (internal and external branches)	Trigeminal (cranial nerve V), anterior trunk of mandibular branch
Medial (internal) pterygoid	Trigeminal (cranial nerve V), anterior trunk of mandibular branch
Temporalis	Trigeminal (cranial nerve V), anterior trunk of mandibular branch
Depressor Muscles	
Digastricus	Anterior belly—trigeminal (cranial nerve V); posterior belly—facial (cranial nerve VII)
Geniohyoid	Hypoglossal (cranial nerve XII)
Lateral (external) pterygoid	Trigeminal (cranial nerve V), mandibular branch
Mylohyoid	Trigeminal (cranial nerve V), mylohyoid branch
Tongue Muscles	
Extrinsic Muscles	
Genioglossus	Hypoglossal (cranial nerve XII)
Hyoglossus	Hypoglossal (cranial nerve XII)
Palatoglossus	Vagus (cranial nerve X); possibly spinal accessory (cranial nerve XI)
Styloglossus	Hypoglossal (cranial nerve XII)
Intrinsic Muscles	
Inferior longitudinal	Hypoglossal (cranial nerve XII)
Superior longitudinal	Hypoglossal (cranial nerve XII)
Transverse	Hypoglossal (cranial nerve XII)
Vertical	Hypoglossal (cranial nerve XII)
Velar Muscles	
Levator veli palatini	Vagus (cranial nerve X)
Musculus uvulae	Vagus (cranial nerve X); possibly spinal accessory (cranial nerve XI)
Palatoglossus	Vagus (cranial nerve X); possibly spinal accessory (cranial nerve XI)
Palatopharyngeus	Vagus (cranial nerve X); possibly spinal accessory (cranial nerve XI)
Tensor veli palatini	Trigeminal (cranial nerve V)
Pharyngeal Muscles	
All pharyngeal constrictor muscles	Vagus (cranial nerve X); possibly spinal accessory (cranial nerve XI)
Palatopharyngeus	Vagus (cranial nerve X); possibly spinal accessory (cranial nerve XI)
Salpingopharyngeus	Vagus (cranial nerve X); possibly spinal accessory (cranial nerve XI)
Stylopharyngeus	Glossopharyngeal (cranial nerve IX)

Physiology of the Articulatory/Resonance System

In this section, we turn our attention to the physiology of the articulatory/resonance system. First, you will learn the mechanics that are involved in speech production. Related to this is a discussion of how the vocal tone produced by the vocal folds is shaped and formed into the acoustic signal we recognize as human speech. Finally, because **dysphagia** is an important area of clinical practice in speech–language pathology, you will be provided the basic mechanics of mastication and deglutition.

THE MECHANICS OF SPEECH PRODUCTION

When one comes to an understanding of the mechanics of speech production, one begins to appreciate the complexity of the event. A typical human produces conversational speech at a rate of approximately 175 words per minute. This equates to approximately 20 speech sounds per second. To be able to produce speech at such a rapid rate, the structures that make up the vocal tract must work cooperatively and in synchrony. This involves the coordinated effort of literally hundreds of neural impulses and muscle contractions. Although it is not the purpose of this text to provide you a thorough descrip-

TABLE 10-10

VOWELS AND CONSONANTS OF ENGLISH AND THE IPA CHARACTERS THAT REPRESENT THEM

Vowels		Consonants			
Character	*Example*	*Character*	*Example*	*Character*	*Example*
i	b<u>ee</u>t	p	<u>p</u>ig	tʃ	<u>ch</u>eap
ɪ	b<u>i</u>t	b	<u>b</u>ig	dʒ	<u>j</u>eep
eɪ, e	b<u>ai</u>t	t	<u>t</u>oo	m	<u>m</u>ice
ɛ	b<u>e</u>t	d	<u>d</u>ue	n	<u>n</u>ice
æ	b<u>a</u>t	k	<u>K</u>ate	ŋ	si<u>ng</u>
u	b<u>oo</u>t	g	<u>g</u>ate	j	<u>y</u>ell
ʊ	b<u>oo</u>k	f	<u>f</u>ace	w	<u>w</u>ell
oʊ, o	b<u>oa</u>t	v	<u>v</u>ase	r	<u>r</u>ake
ɔ	b<u>ou</u>ght	s	<u>S</u>ue	l	<u>l</u>ake
a	y<u>a</u>cht	z	<u>z</u>oo		
ɝ	b<u>ir</u>d	θ	<u>th</u>in		
ɚ	moth<u>er</u>	ð	<u>th</u>en		
ʌ	b<u>u</u>t	ʃ	<u>sh</u>ock		
ə	<u>a</u>bout	ʒ	mea<u>s</u>ure		
aɪ	n<u>i</u>ce	h	<u>h</u>ow		
aʊ	c<u>ow</u>				
ɔɪ	<u>oi</u>l				

tion of speech production, a basic discussion of the physiology of the articulatory/resonance system should drive home the complexity of human vocal communication.

In the foregoing section on the anatomy of the vocal tract, you may have realized that some structures are relatively benign in terms of their contribution to articulation and resonance, while other structures play a more active role. Some structures are immovable, whereas others are moveable due to muscle contraction. In the sections that follow, a brief description will be provided for each of the structures that comprise the vocal tract: lips, teeth, alveolar ridge, hard palate, velum, tongue, mandible, and pharynx.

In the sections that follow, you will be presented the vowels and consonants that make up the sound system of the English language. There are 26 letters of the alphabet, but approximately 43 speech sounds in English. Because there are more speech sounds than alphabet letters in English, speech–language pathologists use a special character set to represent each of the speech sounds. This character set comes from the International Phonetic Alphabet (IPA). The IPA uses alphabet letters to represent some of the speech sounds but relies on special characters to represent others. Table 10-10 provides a list of the English vowels and consonants and the IPA characters that are used to represent them. As you read the sections below, if you encounter an IPA character you are not familiar with, simply consult Table 10-10 to see how that particular sound is pronounced.

The Lips

The lips are composed of the orbicularis oris muscles. The orbicularis oris muscles, in turn, serve as the insertion for several facial muscles. The buccinator, depressor anguli oris, depressor labii inferior, incisivus labii inferior, incisivus labii superior, levator anguli oris, levator labii superior, levator labii superior alaeque nasi, mentalis, risorius, zygomatic major, and zygomatic minor muscles all act upon the lips in one fashion or another. These muscles work together in various combinations to mediate a wide range of lip movements during vocal activity. One particular movement seen in speech production is lip rounding. This is accomplished primarily through action of the orbicularis oris muscles, which act in a sphincter-like manner when they contract. Lip rounding is necessary for the production of certain vowel sounds (e.g., /u/ and /oʊ/) as well as the consonant sound /w/. Lip rounding and protrusion results in elongation of the oral cavity, which in turn changes the resonant properties of the vocal tract. Lip protrusion is accomplished by simultaneous contraction of the depressor labii inferior, levator labii superior, mentalis, and zygomatic minor muscles.

The lips are also involved in the production of other consonant sounds referred to as bilabials. As the term implies, the two lips come into contact with each other during the production of these sounds, which include the /p/, /b/, and /m/. You can see right away that the lips are actively involved in speech production.

The Teeth

The teeth are involved in speech production to a certain extent, although their contribution to the process is more benign than the lips or other structures of the oral cavity. With the exception of the lower set of teeth during mandibular movement, the teeth are immovable. However, the teeth are involved in the production of some speech sounds such as the linguadental consonants /θ/ and /ð/ (referred to as the soft and hard "th" sounds, respectively) and the labiodental consonants /f/ and /v/. As the name implies, linguadental consonants are produced by placing the tongue tip between the upper and lower teeth. By the same token, labiodental sounds are produced by compressing the upper teeth onto the lower lip. In either case, the teeth do not initiate the production of the consonant but rather serve as the secondary articulators (the tongue and lips are the primary articulators).

The Alveolar Ridge

One may recall from the discussion in the anatomy section of this chapter that the alveolar ridge is the bony part of the upper and lower gums where the tooth sockets reside. They are covered by a layer of mucous membrane. In terms of speech production, the maxillary alveolar ridge deserves mention. Being benign in terms of its contribution to speech production, it serves as the secondary articulator of consonant sounds referred to as alveolar sounds. The tongue is the primary articulator in the production of these sounds, which includes the /t/, /d/, /s/, /z/, /l/, and /n/. For some people, the /r/ sound may also be produced in the region of the alveolar ridge.

The Hard Palate

The hard palate is also a benign structure and therefore serves as a secondary articulator in the production of some speech sounds. In some cases, the tip of the tongue approximates the anteriormost part of the hard palate (at its juncture with the alveolar ridge). This includes the consonants /ʃ/, /ʒ/, /tʃ/, and /dʒ/. The /r/ may also be produced in this region by some people. One consonant sound in English is a true palatal sound—the /j/. In this case, the blade of the tongue articulates with the bulk of the hard palate.

The Velum

Being composed partly of muscular tissue, you can surmise that the velum is an active structure in speech production. It is the secondary articulator for the production of the velar consonant sounds /k/, /g/, and /ŋ/. In these cases, the back of the tongue elevates to approximate the velum. However, in speech production, the primary purpose of the velum is to assist in regulating oral/nasal resonance. Along with the posterior pharyngeal wall, the velum does this as part of the V-P mechanism or port.

When the V-P port is open, some of the vocal tone is diverted into the nasal cavity to resonate there while the remainder of the vocal tone resonates in the oral cavity. When the V-P port is closed, the nasal cavity is sealed off from the oral cavity so that all of the vocal tone passes into the oral cavity to resonate. This mechanism is very important because in English, all speech sounds are produced through oral resonance except for three consonants. These three are referred to as the nasal consonants and include the /m/, /n/, and /ŋ/. You will note that these three sounds were presented above. That is, the /m/ is a bilabial consonant, the /n/ is an alveolar consonant, and the /ŋ/ is a velar consonant. What distinguishes these three sounds from all the others is that not only is there resonance taking place in the oral cavity but in the nasal cavity as well. The resonance of part of the vocal tone within the nasal cavity gives these three sounds a distinctive nasal quality or "twang." This is referred to as **nasal murmur**.

For the V-P port to be open so that nasal resonance can occur for the /m/, /n/, and /ŋ/, the soft palate must be depressed. You will recall that the V-P mechanism acts in a sphincter-like fashion so that the velum does not lower like a door on a hinge but rather separates from the posterior pharyngeal wall. The muscles that are responsible for depressing the velum are the palatoglossus and palatopharyngeus muscles, and to a lesser extent possibly the tensor veli palatini (TVP) muscles. Any time one of the nasal consonants is encountered in conversational speech, these muscles must contract to depress the velum and open the V-P port. All the other speech sounds in English require some degree of V-P closure.

The degree of V-P closure during speech varies according to the phonetic context. Obviously, the V-P port is open considerably for the nasal consonants. However, V-P closure is not necessarily complete for the production of nonnasal speech sounds. There is a degree of V-P opening for the low vowels (/ɛ/, /æ/, /ɔ/, /a/) although not as much as for the nasal consonants. Similarly, there is a smaller degree of V-P opening for the high vowels (/i/, /ɪ/, /u/, /ʊ/) than the low vowels, and even greater closure of the V-P port for the oral consonants than either the low or high vowels. The degree of V-P closure is greatest for the plosives (/p/, /b/, /t/, /d/, /k/, /g/) than other speech sounds because these require the greatest **intra-oral air pressure** for production. The V-P port must be closed to allow you to generate the intra-oral pressure that is necessary for production of the plosives. V-P port closure is accomplished by contraction of the levator veli palatini (LVP) and musculus uvulae muscles.

From the foregoing discussion, you can see that V-P closure does not have to be absolute to effectuate the proper balance between oral and nasal resonance. Moll (1962) estimated that normal speakers exhibit 14% opening of the V-P port during production of the isolated /i/ vowel, 37% opening for the /a/ vowel, and as much as 38% V-P opening for the /æ/ vowel. According to Raphael, Borden, and Harris (2007), no apparent nasality is perceived during speech if the velum comes within 2 mm (approximately 20 mm² of open area) of the posterior pharyngeal wall. On the other hand, there is a definite perception of nasality once the velum exceeds 5 mm (approximately 50 mm² of open area) of distance from the posterior pharyngeal wall.

When you consider the rapidity of human speech and the relatively random nature in which the nasal consonants are dispersed throughout a person's speech, you will quickly realize that more critically important is the *timing* of V-P opening and closure. Poor timing of the V-P mechanism may result in an imbalance between oral and nasal resonance. To drive home the point, recall that the average rate of speech is approximately 175 words per minute (roughly 20 speech sounds per second). The duration of an English nasal sound is approximately 70 msec and the duration of other speech sounds may be somewhat longer (e.g., vowels) or shorter (e.g., plosives) than that. You should have no problem appreciating how quickly the velum must move to provide the proper balance between oral and nasal resonance at such high rate of speech.

> **Why You Need to Know**
>
> *When the degree and/or timing of V-P closure are adversely affected, the result may be a condition of hypernasality or denasality. With hypernasality, there is too much nasal resonance during the production of nonnasal speech sounds. With denasality, there is not enough nasal resonance during the production of /m/, /n/, and /ŋ/. Some structural anomalies that may result in poor oral/nasal resonance will be discussed in Chapter 11.*

The Tongue

The tongue is the primary articulator during the production of most consonant sounds and is also the primary structure responsible for the production of vowel sounds. The tongue is involved in the production of 18 of the 24 consonant sounds in the English language (the consonants that are produced without tongue involvement are the /p/, /b/, /m/, /f/, /v/, and /h/). In the case of the linguadental consonants (/θ/ and /ð/), the tip of the tongue is placed between the upper and lower teeth. For the alveolar consonants (/t/, /d/, /s/, /z/, /n/, /l/, and for some people /r/), the tip of the tongue comes into proximity with the maxillary alveolar ridge. In the case of the palatal consonants (/j/, /ʃ/, /ʒ/, /tʃ/, /dʒ/, and for some people /r/), the blade and/or front of the tongue articulates with the hard palate. Finally, for the velar consonants (/k/, /g/, and /ŋ/), the back of the tongue raises to approximate the velum. Although the /w/ sound is considered by many to be a bilabial sound, the back of the tongue may also come into proximity with the velum during its production.

The tongue is also involved in the production of all of the vowel sounds. In English, there are 14 **monophthongs** (also known as pure vowels) and five **diphthongs**. A more thorough discussion of the acoustic qualities of the vowels will be presented in the section below. For now, you are referred to Figure 10-32. This figure illustrates what is commonly known as the vowel quadrilateral. The left side of the quadrilateral represents the anterior region of the oral cavity (i.e., the lips and alveolar ridge). The right side represents the posterior region (i.e., the velum and pharynx). You will note two dimensions: horizontal and vertical.

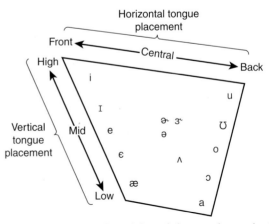

Figure 10-32 The vowel quadrilateral showing the result of vertical and horizontal tongue placement within the oral cavity. (Adapted with permission from Raphael, L.J., Borden, G.J., Harris, K.S. (2006). *Speech science primer* (5th ed.). Baltimore: Lippincott Williams & Wilkins.)

The horizontal dimension represents protraction and retraction of the tongue within the oral cavity. That is, the tongue is able to move toward the lips, toward the pharynx, or any point between the two. The terms front, central, and back are used to indicate the relative position of the tongue horizontally. The vertical dimension represents movement of the tongue toward the floor of the oral cavity, toward the ceiling (i.e., hard palate), or any point between the two. The terms high, mid, and low are used to indicate the relative position of the tongue vertically. The vowel sounds are classified then, according to these two dimensions. For example, the /i/ vowel is classified as a high front vowel. This means that the tongue tip and blade move forward and up toward the alveolar ridge. In the case of the /a/ vowel, the tongue moves backward and down toward the lower oropharynx. All monophthongs are classified in this manner.

The diphthongs are single vowel sounds consisting of a blending of two monophthongs produced in a rapid fashion. In other words, the tongue rapidly transitions from its placement for one vowel (the onglide) to the placement for a second vowel (the offglide). For example, the diphthong /ɔɪ/ is produced when the tongue initiates its placement for the vowel /ɔ/ (low and toward the back of the oral cavity) and then moves rapidly to the articulatory position for the /ɪ/ vowel (high and toward the front of the oral cavity). This process occurs so rapidly that acoustically we perceive a singular vowel sound.

Naturally, muscle activity is necessary for allowing the tongue to move to the various regions of the oral cavity to produce most of the consonants and all of the vowel sounds. Recall in the previous section that tongue muscles are classified as either extrinsic or intrinsic. The extrinsic muscles are responsible for gross positioning of the tongue within the oral cavity. For example, the hyoglossus muscles and anterior fibers of the genioglossus muscles retract the tongue while posterior fibers of the genioglossus muscles protrude the tongue. The palatoglossus and styloglossus muscles elevate and retract the back of the tongue. Finally, the hyoglossus muscles along with the entire genioglossus muscles depress the tongue within the oral cavity.

The intrinsic tongue muscles are responsible for making fine adjustments to the tongue but also assist in positioning the tongue within the oral cavity. The inferior longitudinal and superior longitudinal muscles shorten the tongue. However, the inferior longitudinal muscles can also pull the tongue tip downward and the superior longitudinal muscles can also raise the tongue tip upward. The transverse muscles narrow and elongate the tongue, while the vertical muscles flatten it. These muscles allow the tongue to move rapidly within the oral cavity, which is essential for speech production. The tongue tip is able to produce more than eight repetitive movements per second (e.g., "tah-tah-tah-tah . . . ")! This makes the tongue a very efficient articulator.

The Mandible

The mandible or lower jaw is also actively involved in speech production. Its movements are accomplished by way of the temporomandibular joints (TMJs). As was mentioned in an earlier section of this chapter, although there are two TMJs, they act as a unit when elevating and depressing the mandible. Mandibular elevator (i.e., masseter, medial pterygoid, and temporalis) muscles close the mouth by raising the mandible, and mandibular depressor (i.e., digastricus, geniohyoid, lateral pterygoid, and mylohyoid) muscles open the mouth by depressing the mandible. Not only does the mandible move in a vertical dimension (i.e., opening and closing), but it can also move in an anteroposterior, lateral, and rotary fashion. These actions are accomplished through differential contractions of the elevator and depressor muscles. Seldom does the mandible completely close during speech production. Movement of the mandible during vocal activity is approximately 7 to 18 mm vertically and 2 to 3 mm anteroposteriorly. You will note that as one produces the front (/i/, /ɪ/, /e/, /ɛ/, /æ/) and back (/u/, /ʊ/, /o/, /ɔ/, /a/) vowels from high to low position, mandibular depression becomes greater and greater. Like the tongue, the mandible is also capable of rapid repetitive movements. On average, the mandible can produce approximately 7.5 repetitive movements (e.g., "pah-pah-pah-pah . . .") per second. This makes the mandible capable of handling the demands placed upon it by speech production.

The Pharynx

The pharynx is a funnel-shaped tube that courses from the base of the skull to the esophagus. It is typically divided into three regions: the nasopharynx, oropharynx, and laryngopharynx. The pharynx houses a complex array of muscles collectively referred to as the superior, middle, and inferior constrictor muscles. In terms of speech production, the pharynx is somewhat static, that is, it does not appear to contribute significantly to the production of speech sounds. However, being a cavity, it does have resonant properties (and the same can be said of the oral and nasal cavities as well, although the contribution of the nasal cavity is also static while the oral cavity is highly dynamic). The action of the constrictor muscles appears to be more important in swallowing than in the production of speech.

The Integration of Oral Structures

It should be emphasized that the lips, mandible, tongue, velum, and pharynx do not perform isolated movements. That is, movements of these structures are interrelated and integrated to an extent. For example, the mandible is coupled to the tongue and lower lips and teeth. It assists these structures in meeting their articulatory contacts with other anatomical structures. The velum, tongue, and faucial pillars also seem to act as an integrated unit. Stimulation of the larynx, palate, or pharynx will cause the tongue to protrude, and stimulation of the anterior oral region will result in tongue retraction.

Finally, the width of the pharyngeal lumen can also be influenced by the epiglottis, tongue, and velum. The oral and pharyngeal cavities are coupled by these structures. For example, upward movement of the tongue, downward movement of the velum, and medial movement of the palatoglossal arches will cause a reduction in the coupling between the oral and pharyngeal cavities. Therefore, you should be cognizant of the fact that the articulators do not perform their tasks in a serial order; rather, their movements are often dependent upon the movements of other structures.

ACOUSTICS, ARTICULATION, AND RESONANCE

With the anatomy and physiology of the vocal tract described, it is now time to turn your attention to how the anatomy and physiology act to shape the vocal tone into an acoustic signal we perceive as human speech. Recall from Chapter 8 that the human larynx is capable of producing a complex tone that is rich in harmonic structure. Humans possess the ability to vary the vocal tone in its frequency and intensity. Variations in vocal frequency are evident in the intonational patterns that are used during conversational speech.

The vocal tone is simply a buzzing sound. The structures that are superior to the larynx (i.e., the structures that make up the vocal tract) are responsible for transforming the vocal tone into speech. It is the purpose of this section of the chapter to describe the transformation process. It is beyond the scope of this chapter to offer a detailed and thorough account of articulation and resonance (that can be accomplished through a basic course in speech science). The purpose of the foregoing discussion then is to provide you with a very basic understanding of these processes.

Basic Principles of Acoustics

Before the transformation process can be described, you must have an understanding of some basic concepts related to acoustics. First, you must understand the concept of resonance. In general, resonance is simply a response to an outside force. The response is typically vibration. When something resonates, it vibrates. The object that vibrates is called a **resonator**. When a resonator is acted upon by an outside force, it responds to that outside force by vibrating. Practically everything on this planet vibrates and has its own **natural resonant frequency**. When an outside force matches a resonator's natural resonant frequency, it vibrates at its greatest amplitude and is said to be "in resonance." Anyone who has ever placed their lips over the mouth of an empty bottle and blown into it has witnessed resonance. When the force of exhaled air reaches the natural resonant frequency of the bottle, the bottle responds by vibrating at its greatest amplitude. The result is a loud sound.

The vocal tract is similar in structure to a bottle or tube that is closed at one end (i.e., the vocal folds) and open at the other (i.e., the lips). If an outside force acts upon the vocal tract, it will resonate. However, because of the placement of the tongue and other anatomical structures, the vocal tract can be partitioned into a series of chambers, each one having its own natural resonant frequency that responds to the outside force acting upon it. In the case of the vocal tract, what is the outside force? Quite simply, the outside force is the vocal tone being generated by the larynx. As the vocal tone passes through the vocal tract, it sets the air within the vocal tract into vibration, resulting in resonance within the partitioned chambers. Which frequencies resonate depends upon the volumes of these chambers.

There is a predictable relationship between chamber volume and resonance. This relationship can be easily demonstrated by using the same bottle mentioned above. If you blow with enough force into the empty bottle, the result will be a loud sound of relatively low frequency. However, if you fill the bottle halfway with water and then blow into it, the loud sound is now relatively higher in frequency. By filling it halfway with water, you have lessened the effective

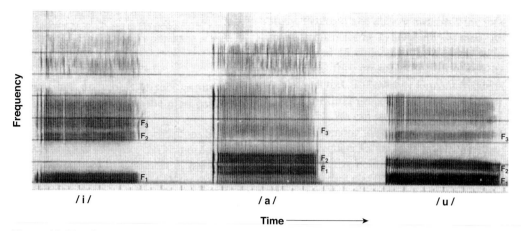

Figure 10-33 A spectrogram showing the formants for the vowels /i/, /a/, and /u/. (Adapted with permission from Raphael, L.J., Borden, G.J., Harris, K.S. (2006). *Speech science primer* (5th ed.). Baltimore: Lippincott Williams & Wilkins; Courtesy of Kay Elemetrics.)

vibrating volume of the bottle. In other words, the volume of the bottle is smaller. Therefore, the relationship between volume and frequency is an inverse one. As volume decreases, frequency increases and vice versa.

Returning to the vocal tract you may quickly surmise that its partitioned chambers can be adjusted in terms of their volumes; the result then would be changes in the natural resonant frequencies of those chambers. In other words, humans have the ability to manipulate and change which frequencies of the vocal tone will resonate. As such, the vocal tract can be thought of as an acoustic **filter**. Depending on vocal tract configuration, certain frequencies of the vocal tone will resonate while other frequencies will lose energy or dampen.

In fact, large *bands* of frequencies will resonate at any given time. These bands are called **formants**. When the partitioned cavities of the vocal tract resonate, several formants are produced. The first formant (F_1) is the band of lowest frequency; the second formant (F_2) is the next higher frequency band; the third formant (F_3) is composed of even higher frequencies, and so on. Formants can be seen clearly on a spectrogram—the output of a spectrograph, an electronic instrument that analyzes sound according to frequency and intensity. Figure 10-33 provides a spectrogram showing the vowels /i/, /a/, and /u/. The formants are the dark horizontal bars. The darkness of the bars indicates that they are of relatively great amplitude (in other words, they are in resonance). The "thickness" of the bars shows that the formants are not just individual frequencies but bands of frequencies.

A distinction should be made between **periodic sounds** and **aperiodic sounds**. When a sound is generated, it creates waves of acoustic energy. If the waves repeat themselves consistently and predictably over time, the result is a periodic sound. If, however, the waves emanate in a random fashion so that there is no discernible pattern to their behavior, the result is an aperiodic sound. The vocal tone is a periodic, complex tone. An example of an aperiodic sound is noise (e.g., a hissing sound). When the vocal tract is relatively open (i.e., very little constriction exists along its length), the acoustic signal that is produced is periodic. However, when an obstruction or constriction exists anywhere along the vocal tract, the result will be a sound that is aperiodic. Periodicity of sound will be described in more detail below.

Finally, one should understand the difference between **voiced** and **unvoiced** speech sounds. When a sound is voiced, it means that the vocal folds are vibrating and generating a vocal tone during its production. In contrast, the vocal folds do not vibrate during the production of unvoiced sounds; this means that there is no vocal tone being generated during the production of unvoiced sounds. In English, all vowel sounds are voiced. Fifteen of the 24 English consonant sounds are voiced. This means that the voiced consonants will have some degree of periodicity because of the vocal tone being generated as they are being articulated.

Articulation and Resonance

The purpose of this section is to provide you with a basic understanding of how articulation and resonance results in the transformation of the vocal tone into an acoustic signal recognized as speech. In 1960, Gunnar Fant developed the Acoustic Theory of Speech Production to describe how vowels are produced. Over the years, his theory has become more widely known as the Source-Filter Theory (see Figure 10-34).

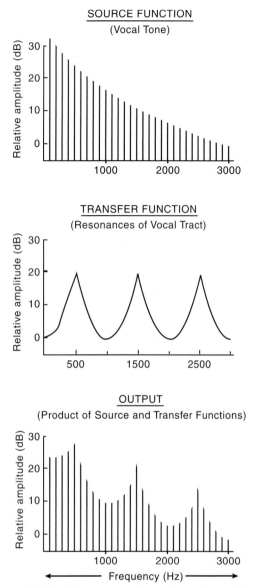

Figure 10-34   The source and transfer functions of Source-Filter Theory, with resulting output (a vowel sound). (Adapted with permission from Raphael, L.J., Borden, G.J., Harris, K.S. (2006). *Speech science primer* (5th ed.). Baltimore: Lippincott Williams & Wilkins.)

As its more common name implies, speech production is a result of two components—a source and a filter. Anatomically, the source is the vibrating vocal folds while the filter is the vocal tract. As illustrated in Figure 10-34, when the vocal folds vibrate, they create a complex tone that is rich in harmonics (as illustrated by the vertical lines in the top-most graph). These harmonics diminish in intensity for the higher frequencies. The vocal tone produced by the vibrating vocal folds is referred to as the source function. The vocal tract, as a filter, causes certain bands of frequencies to resonate. As shown in the middle graph of Figure 10-34, this is referred to as the transfer function. The peaks you see are formants. In the graph,

there is a peak at 500 Hz, another at 1500 Hz, and another at 2500 Hz. The peak at 500 Hz represents the natural resonant frequency for the first formant, the peak at 1500 Hz represents the natural resonant frequency for F_2, and the peak at 2500 Hz represents the natural resonant frequency for F_3. It should be noted that although Figure 10-34 shows only one example of a transfer function, there are actually many transfer functions—each one associated with a different configuration of the vocal tract. If the configuration of the vocal tract is changed even minimally (e.g., by tongue movement), a different transfer function will result, that is, the resonant characteristics of the vocal tract will change and a different sound will emerge.

As the vocal tone makes its way through the vocal tract, it is passed through the filter and the transfer function modifies the vocal tone so that the resulting **spectrum** resembles both the source and the filter. The harmonic structure of the vocal tone remains intact, but instead of a steady and gradual decrease in amplitude from the lower to higher frequencies, there are amplitude peaks superimposed upon the vocal tone by the transfer function. These peaks correspond to the format frequencies of the transfer function. The various speech sounds in a language are created by changing the filter (i.e., vocal tract configuration), thereby changing the transfer function. The source function remains relatively the same; it is the transfer function that causes a change in speech sound. In other words, each speech sound has its own transfer function created by a different configuration of the vocal tract.

Vowels

According to the Source-Filter Theory, vowels are produced simply by changing the configuration of the vocal tract, which is accomplished primarily by placement of the tongue. As you may recall from an earlier section of this chapter, vowels are classified as front to back and high to low. These terms describe what the tongue is doing during vowel production. Shifting the position of the tongue changes the configuration of the vocal tract, which in turn sets up changes in resonance. In other words, formant frequencies can be adjusted by the position of the tongue. Although each vowel in English has several formants, only the first two (F_1 and F_2) are of critical importance for discriminating most of the vowel sounds.

The first format (F_1) is affected primarily by tongue height. Movement of the tongue toward the ceiling of the oral cavity (as for the high vowels) will result in a lowering of frequencies associated with F_1, and movement of the tongue toward the floor of the oral cavity will result in a rise in frequencies associated with F_1. The second formant (F_2) is affected primarily by the anterior-to-posterior placement of the tongue. As the tongue moves in an anterior direction (as for the front vowels), the frequencies associated with F_2 rise, and as the tongue moves in a posterior direction, the frequencies associated with F_2 lower.

To understand this, you should consider that the tongue essentially divides the oral cavity into two chambers, one anterior to the position of the tongue and the other posterior to it. The first formant is associated with resonance within the chamber that is posterior to the tongue and the second format is associated with resonance within the chamber that is anterior to the tongue. If the tongue is moved toward the ceiling of the oral cavity, the chamber posterior to the tongue will enlarge, thereby causing the frequencies associated with F_1 to lower. If one moves the tongue forward (i.e., towards the lips), it causes the anterior chamber to become smaller, thereby resulting in a rise in frequencies associated with F_2 (remember the relationship between chamber volume and frequency).

To illustrate, consider the vowels /i/ and /a/, which are high-front and low-back vowels, respectively. For the vowel /i/, the tongue moves forward and toward the ceiling of the oral cavity. For the vowel /a/, the tongue moves backward and toward the floor of the oral cavity. One would expect then that F_1 for the vowel /i/ would be lower than F_1 for the vowel /a/ because the tongue is in a higher position for /i/. Similarly, one would expect that F_2 would be higher for /i/ than for /a/ because the tongue has a more anterior placement for /i/ than for /a/. Indeed, the average F_1 frequency for an adult male is 270 Hz for /i/ and 730 Hz for /a/; the average F_2 frequency is 2290 Hz for /i/ and 1090 Hz for /a/ (see the formant comparisons for these vowels in Figure 10-35). All the other vowel sounds are a result of changes in formant frequencies brought on by changes in tongue height and advancement. With each change in tongue height and/or advancement, a different filter is created and hence, a different transfer function is created as well. Each vowel has its own acoustic spectrum.

Consonants

The production of consonant sounds differs from that of vowels. Although some consonants resemble vowels in terms of their spectral properties, most of them do not look much like vowels. In general, vowel sounds are produced by relatively little constriction anywhere along the vocal tract. In other words, the vocal tract tends to be open. Most of the consonants, on the other hand, are produced by creating either a complete obstruction or a narrow constriction somewhere in the vocal tract.

In the physiology section of this chapter, you learned that consonants are classified according to the place where they are created. Bilabial consonants are produced by the lips; labiodental consonants by the lips and teeth; linguadental consonants by the tongue and teeth; alveolar consonants by the tongue and alveolar ridge; palatal consonants by the tongue and hard palate; velar consonants by the tongue and soft palate; and finally the one glottal consonant by the open vocal folds. Consonant sounds are also classified according to the manner in which they are created.

Plosives (also known as stops) are produced by creating a complete obstruction of the expired breath stream so that intra-oral air pressure builds up behind the obstruction. The air pressure is then released abruptly, creating an explosive sound. The plosives include the /p/, /b/, /t/, /d/, /k/, and /g/ sounds. For the /p/ and /b/, the obstruction is at the lips (recall that they are classified as bilabial sounds). For /t/ and /d/, the obstruction is at the alveolar ridge. Finally, for /k/ and /g/, the obstruction is at the velum. The abrupt release of air pressure results in a spike of acoustic energy that is aperiodic. The /b/, /d/, and /g/ sounds are voiced, so there is at least a small degree of periodicity associated with the vocal tone during the production of these consonants.

Fricative consonants are produced by creating a narrow constriction somewhere in the vocal tract. Instead of completely obstructing the breath stream, the breath stream is forced through the narrow constriction, thereby creating turbulence or friction. The fricatives are the largest class of consonants according to manner of production in English. They include the /s/, /z/, /f/, /v/, /θ/, /ð/, /ʃ/, /ʒ/, and /h/ sounds. The turbulence created by these sounds results in a

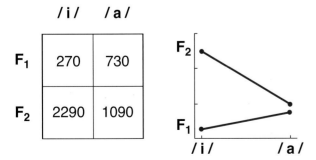

	/i/	/a/
F_1	270	730
F_2	2290	1090

Figure 10-35 Comparison of formants for the vowels /i/ and /a/ for an adult male. (Adapted with permission from Raphael, L.J., Borden, G.J., Harris, K.S. (2006). *Speech science primer* (5th ed.). Baltimore: Lippincott Williams & Wilkins.)

very noticeable aperiodic component. The voiced fricatives (/z/, /v/, /ð/, and /ʒ/) also have a periodic component due to generation of the vocal tone during their articulation. You are referred back to the section on physiology to determine where in the vocal tract the constriction occurs for the various fricative sounds.

Two consonant sounds are classified as affricates (/tʃ/ and /dʒ/). An affricate is a combination of a plosive and fricative sound. During their production, a total obstruction is first created, but then instead of an abrupt release of intra-oral air pressure, there is a transition to a narrow constriction through which the air pressure is forced. These sounds also have a fricative component that is aperiodic. The /dʒ/ is voiced, and therefore has at least some degree of periodicity.

In terms of place, the nasal consonants (/m/, /n/, and /ŋ/) are similar to the plosives /b/, /d/, and /g/. In terms of manner, however, there is an added characteristic of the nasals that does not exist for the plosives (or any other speech sounds for that matter). During the production of the nasals, the V-P port is opened (for all other speech sounds, including the vowels, the V-P port is closed). This allows some of the breath stream to be diverted into the nasal cavity to resonate there, while some of the breath stream resonates within the oral cavity. Nasal cavity resonance gives these three sounds a distinctive nasal "twang." All three nasal sounds have a vowel-like resonant quality. All three are also voiced so that the vocal tone provides an even greater degree of periodicity.

The remaining consonant sounds are the semivowels because their spectral characteristics are very similar to the vowel sounds. The semivowels are further classified as either liquids or glides. The liquids include the /r/ and /l/, and the glides include the /w/ and /j/. The /r/ and /l/ are referred to as liquids because their acoustic properties change depending on what other speech sounds are adjacent to them. For example, an /r/ sound before a vowel is a slightly different sound than an /r/ after a vowel (e.g., compare the /r/ in "ring" to the /r/ in "car"). The /w/ and /j/ are called glides because there are actually two articulatory positions when they are produced. The articulators move into a particular position but then glide to a second position during production. The semivowels are periodic not only because of their vowel-like resonant qualities but also because they are all voiced.

THE PROCESS OF SWALLOWING

Swallowing, or deglutition, is a highly complex process that requires the integrated activity of many anatomical structures, muscles, and nerves. Practically, the entire vocal tract is involved in the process—the lips, tongue, mandible, hard palate, velum, pharynx, and larynx are all part of the event. Muscles of the lips, tongue, mandible, velum, pharynx, and larynx are also involved. Finally, cortical and brainstem centers, as well as 6 of the 12 cranial nerves, play a part in swallowing.

The process of swallowing has three distinct phases: oral, pharyngeal, and esophageal. Some would add a fourth phase—the **oral preparatory phase**—to the list, but technically, this phase is an antecedent to the actual process of swallowing. It will be included here to give you a better understanding of the complete process, from activity leading up to the swallow to the swallow proper.

The oral preparatory and oral phases are under voluntary control, that is, an individual has the ability to start or stop the process at any time. The muscles that are involved in these phases are striated, or voluntary, muscles. The motor and premotor areas of the frontal lobe cortex are responsible for controlling these muscles. Once a swallow enters the pharyngeal phase, the process is switched over to autonomic control primarily. Striated and smooth muscles receive innervation during these phases of swallowing. Food is transported through the pharynx by contraction of striated muscles and then through the esophagus through **peristalsis** (which takes place via contractions of smooth muscles). The involuntary phases of swallowing are regulated by subcortical areas, more specifically the medulla oblongata and pons. During the brief time a swallow takes place, the swallowing center of the medulla oblongata and pons inhibits the respiratory center of the medulla. In other words, the person does not breathe during a swallow.

The Phases of Swallowing

Oral Preparatory Phase

The oral preparatory phase involves the preparation of food so that it can be swallowed. The tongue, teeth, mandible, and salivary glands are primarily involved in the process, and the lips and cheeks play a secondary role. The lips seal the oral cavity so that food is not ejected back out of the mouth and the cheeks compress themselves upon the teeth to prevent food from being pushed into the buccal cavity.

As the food is chewed (i.e., masticated), the salivary glands release saliva to begin the process of breaking down the food. The anterior tongue manipulates the food by pushing it into the teeth, pulling it back to be mixed with saliva, and then pushing it back into the teeth again (this occurs between 20 and 30 times before the swallow is initiated). The posterior tongue is raised by the palatoglossus muscles to prevent food from being forced into the pharynx. With assistance from the hard palate, the tongue forms a **bolus** of appropriate size so that it can be passed into the pharynx and eventually the esophagus. Mastication involves the elevator and depressor muscles of the mandible, the intrinsic and extrinsic muscles of the tongue, and the muscles of the lips and cheeks.

While the food is being chewed, the individual must breathe through the nose. To be able to do so, the palatoglossus muscles must contract to lower the velum and establish communication between the nasal and pharyngeal cavities. You will note that during the oral preparatory phase, the palatoglossus performs a dual function—lowering the velum while raising the back of the tongue.

Oral Phase

The oral, or buccal, phase is the first true stage of swallowing. In this phase, chewing stops. With the bolus prepared, activity shifts to the transport of the bolus to the pharynx. The posterior tongue lowers while the anterior tongue elevates toward the hard palate. The tongue then retracts in a posterior direction to squeeze the bolus back toward the pharynx. The muscles of the lips and cheeks remain contracted to narrow the oral cavity to facilitate bolus transit. As the bolus approaches the oropharynx, the back of the tongue and uvula elevate primarily through contraction of the palatoglossus and styloglossus muscles. This action seals the nasopharynx to prevent the bolus from being injected into it. Muscles of the lips, face, tongue, and uvula are involved in the oral phase of swallowing, requiring neural innervation from the trigeminal (V), facial (VII), and hypoglossal (XII) cranial nerves. The glossopharyngeal (IX) cranial nerve provides sensory fibers to the tongue. Once the bolus makes contact with the faucial pillars, the oral phase terminates and the pharyngeal phase begins. At this point, swallowing becomes involuntary, as the autonomic nervous system takes primary control of the process.

Pharyngeal Phase

As the bolus enters the oropharynx, the velum elevates toward the posterior pharyngeal wall, primarily by contraction of the levator veli palatini (LVP) muscles. The muscles making up the superior constrictor contract, thereby narrowing the faucial pillars to prevent the bolus from being ejected into the oral cavity. As this is taking place, the hyoid bone and larynx elevate and move anteriorly through action of the suprahyoid muscles. The anterior and superior positioning of the

larynx relaxes the cricopharyngeus muscles, which relaxes the upper esophageal sphincter (UES) at the upper end of the esophagus. The epiglottis passively seals the aditus laryngis while the vocal folds adduct to seal the lower respiratory passageway. The bolus is forced down the pharynx by contraction of the constrictor muscles. As it approaches the epiglottis, the bolus divides into two masses that are then forced around the larynx and through the pyriform sinuses in preparation of entry into the esophagus. The masses meet again at the UES and are forced by the inferior constrictor into the esophagus. Breathing ceases during the second it takes for the bolus to be transported through the pharynx to the esophagus. The pharyngeal phase involves neural innervation from four cranial nerves: trigeminal (V); vagus (X); spinal accessory (XI); and hypoglossal (XII).

Esophageal Phase

Esophageal transit time is approximately 10 to 20 seconds. Once the bolus enters the esophagus, the cricopharyngeus muscles contract to seal the UES. In the upper third of the esophagus, the constrictor muscles force the bolus down until the striated muscles give way to involuntary muscles. Peristalsis and gravity continue to push the bolus of food toward the stomach. As the lower esophageal sphincter is approached, it relaxes and the bolus is emptied into the stomach. At the same time the bolus enters the esophagus, the larynx and velum lower to allow respiration to resume.

The vagus (X) cranial nerve appears to be most actively involved in the esophageal phase of swallowing. For the upper one-third of the esophagus, the vagus nerve has more of a direct role by innervating the voluntary muscles fibers found there. For the remainder of the esophagus, the vagus plays more of a modulatory role as the autonomous nervous system innervates the smooth muscle fibers in this region.

Why You Need to Know

Treatment for swallowing disorders includes compensatory swallowing strategies, dietary modifications, exercises to improve muscle function, medications and/or surgery, and neuromuscular electrical stimulation. The last treatment option involves stimulation of paralyzed muscles with electric current to trigger a swallowing response. The speech–language pathologist is an integral member of the dysphagia team. If you are interested in the topic of neuromuscular electrical stimulation, an example of research in this area can be found in Baijens, Speyer, Roodenburg, and Manni (2008).

Summary

This chapter described the anatomy and physiology of the articulatory/resonance system. Chapters 6 and 8 described the anatomy and physiology of the respiratory and phonatory systems, respectively. In those chapters, you learned how respiration is used to set the vocal folds into vibration. Vibration of the vocal folds, in turn, generates a complex tone that is rich in harmonic structure. However, the vocal tone is nothing more than a buzzing sound. This chapter provided you with the final piece of the puzzle—how articulation and resonance act to transform the vocal tone into the acoustic signal humans recognize as speech. This chapter also provided you with a basic understanding of the swallowing process. A typical speech–language pathologist may have a number of individuals on her caseload who have a diagnosis of dysphagia. A good understanding of the normal process of deglutition is necessary to understand how dysphagia may adversely affect a person's ability to swallow.

CHAPTER 11

Pathologies Associated with the Articulatory/Resonance System

Knowledge Outcomes for ASHA Certification for Chapter 11
- Demonstrate knowledge of the etiologies of articulation disorders (III-C)
- Demonstrate knowledge of the characteristics of articulation disorders (III-C)
- Demonstrate knowledge of the etiologies of swallowing disorders (III-C)
- Demonstrate knowledge of the characteristics of swallowing disorders (III-C)

Learning Objectives
- You will be able to describe how a knowledge of articulatory phonetics can assist you in understanding the various pathologies that may affect the articulatory/resonance system.
- You will be able to discuss the etiology and characteristics of cleft lip and palate and other craniofacial anomalies, and how these anomalies may adversely affect articulation and resonance.
- You will be able to define velopharyngeal incompetence and provide examples of pathological conditions that may result in this disorder.
- You will be able to evaluate how articulation and resonance may be adversely affected by cranial nerve damage.
- You will be able to recite some of the differences between apraxia of speech and dysarthria.
- You will be able to discuss how apraxia of speech and dysarthria affect the articulatory/resonance system.
- You will be able to describe several progressive and nonprogressive neurological pathologies and how their characteristics may adversely affect articulation and resonance.
- You will be able to differentiate the different types of hearing impairment and describe how hearing impairment may adversely affect speech production.

AFFIX AND PART-WORD BOX

TERM	MEANING	EXAMPLE
acro-	peak	**acro**cephalosyndactyly
arthro-	pertaining to the joints	**arthro**-ophthalmopathy
cardio-	pertaining to the heart	velo**cardio**facial syndrome
cephalo-	referring to the head	acro**cephalo**syndactyly
cranio-	referring to the head or skull	**cranio**facial anomaly
dactyl-	pertaining to the fingers	acrocephalosyn**dactyl**y
dermal	pertaining to the skin	ecto**dermal**
dys-	abnormal	**dys**ostosis

TERM	MEANING	EXAMPLE
ecto-	outer	**ecto**derm
ectro-	congenital absence of	**ectro**dactyly
-gnathia	a condition of the jaw	micro**gnathia**
hemi-	partial	**hemi**paresis
hyper-	an excessive amount of	**hyper**nasality
micro-	abnormally small	**micro**gnathia
ophthalmo-	pertaining to the eyes	**ophthalmo**pathy
-osis	a condition	dysost**osis**
ost-	pertaining to bone(s)	dys**ost**osis
-pathy	a pathological or diseased condition	ophthalmo**pathy**
syn-	together (i.e., fused)	**syn**dactyly
velo-	pertaining to the velum, or soft palate	**velo**pharyngeal

A Brief Review of Articulation and Resonance

ARTICULATORY PHONETICS

As you learned in Chapter 10, the vocal tract comprises the articulatory/resonance system. The vocal tract consists of three cavities (i.e., nasal, oral, and pharyngeal) and several anatomical structures. These include the lips, teeth, alveolar ridge, hard palate, velum, tongue, and pharynx. As the vocal tone passes through the vocal tract, it is molded and shaped into the various speech sounds of a language by action of these structures.

To understand how the articulatory/resonance system can be affected by pathologies, you must first have a basic understanding of articulatory or physiological phonetics—the study of the sounds of a language in regard to the physiological movements that are necessary to produce them. You were introduced to articulatory phonetics in Chapter 10. Although we provided a brief description of articulatory phonetics in that chapter (especially as it related to the movements that are required of the various articulators), it is probably not a bad idea to reintroduce the topic (in condensed form) at the beginning of this chapter so that you will have a point of reference in terms of "normal" articulation and resonance when the disorders are presented later in this chapter.

It should be mentioned that it is not within the scope of this textbook to provide you a comprehensive discussion of articulatory phonetics. Our purpose in including this discussion is simply to provide you the basic framework behind articulation and resonance. As such, the discussion will focus on the production of individual speech sounds and not on connected (or conversational) speech. For example, the effects of **coarticulation** on connected speech will be reserved for a course in speech science and therefore will not be presented in this chapter. Only a brief overview of basic articulatory phonetics will be provided here.

You should make the distinction between **articulation** and **resonance**. Articulation involves the accuracy, direction, and timing of the movements of the vocal tract structures to produce speech sounds. Resonance involves modification of the vocal tone as a result of forced vibration as the tone passes through the cavities of the vocal tract. Both processes (i.e., articulation and resonance) occur simultaneously, resulting in the production of speech sounds.

Refer to Table 11-1. This table provides a classification of the consonant sounds in the English language. Consonant sound production can be classified according to the place and manner of articulation, as well as whether or not the vocal folds vibrate during their production. Place refers to where the articulators go during consonant production, while manner refers to how the consonant sound is actually produced. As the term implies, bilabial means two lips. Consonants classified as bilabial are produced at the lips. Labiodental refers to the lips and teeth. Interdental means "between the teeth." Alveolar refers to the alveolar ridge; palatal refers to the hard palate; velar refers to the soft palate; and glottal refers to the glottis.

In terms of manner, plosive sounds are created by completely occluding the expired breath stream and

TABLE 11-1

TRADITIONAL (PLACE/MANNER) CLASSIFICATION OF ENGLISH CONSONANT SOUNDS

		Place of Production						
		Bilabial	Labiodental	Interdental	Alveolar	Palatal	Velar	Glottal
Manner of Production	Plosive	p, b			t, d		k, g	
	Fricative		f, v	θ, ð	s, z	ʃ, ʒ		h
	Affricate					ʧ, ʤ		
	Nasal	m			n		ŋ	
	Glide	(w)				j	w	
	Liquid				l	r		

Note: All of the characters above represent their corresponding sounds, except the following:

θ = soft "th" as in breath   ð = hard "th" as in breathe
ʃ = "sh" as in shoe   ʒ = "zh" as in measure
ʧ = "ch" as in chew   ʤ = "j" as in jury
ŋ = "ng" as in sing   j = "y" as in yellow

then releasing it abruptly, resulting in an explosive type of sound. Fricative sounds are produced by creating a narrow constriction that the expired breath stream is forced through or around, creating turbulence or a friction type of sound. Affricates are a combination of plosives and fricatives. First, a complete obstruction is created in the vocal tract, but the obstruction gives way rapidly to a constriction that the breath stream is forced through. The nasal consonants are produced in much the same way as voiced plosives, but there is the added feature of resonance within the nasal cavity due to the opening of the velopharyngeal (V-P) port during their production. Opening of the V-P port allows some of the breath stream to be diverted to the nasal cavity while the balance of the breath stream continues through the oral cavity. Glides are consonant sounds that are somewhat similar to diphthongs. There is a rapid transition from one articulatory position to another that creates these sounds (i.e., the /w/ and /j/). Finally, the /r/ and /l/ sounds are given the name "liquid" because like liquid (e.g., water), they change depending on the context in which they are produced (i.e., as water changes its shape and form depending on the container in which it is poured, the liquid consonants also change their shape and form depending on what other speech sounds are produced adjacent to them).

Finally, 9 of the 24 consonant sounds are produced without vocal fold vibration. In Table 11-1, you will note that in several of the cells there are two consonants separated by a comma. In each of these cases, the consonant on the left is an unvoiced consonant; in other words, the vocal folds do not vibrate during their production. The consonant on the right of the comma is voiced. All of the single consonants in Table 11-1 are voiced with the exception of the /h/

sound, which is the only unvoiced consonant that does not have a voiced partner. As a final word, it should be noted that resonance is involved in consonant production (especially for the nasals, glides, and liquids), but consonant production is more a result of breath stream obstruction or constriction than resonance.

The tongue is involved in the production of three-fourths of the consonant sounds. The consonant sounds that do not require involvement of the tongue are the bilabials (/p/, /b/, and /m/), labiodentals (/f/ and /v/), and the fricative /h/. The bilabials are produced by compressing the upper and lower lips. The labiodentals are produced by compressing the upper teeth onto the lower lip. The /h/ sound is produced by forcing air through the open glottis, creating turbulence at the level of the vocal folds. As far as all of the other consonants (i.e., alveolars, interdentals, palatals, and velars) go, the tongue works with the alveolar ridge, teeth, hard palate, or velum to produce the consonant. In the case of the interdentals (the "th" sounds /θ/ and /ð/) for example, the tongue tip is placed behind or between the upper and lower teeth. From this example, you should be able to determine how the other consonants are produced. The /w/ sound is interesting because it has two simultaneous places of articulation. Note as you produce the /w/ sound (as in "wood") that your lips round as the body of the tongue moves up toward the soft palate.

There are eight **cognate pairs** of consonants in English. For these cognate pairs, both the place and manner of articulation are identical. The only difference between the two sounds in each pair is that one is produced without vocal fold vibration, whereas the other is produced simultaneously with vocal fold vibration.

TABLE 11-2

CLASSIFICATION OF ENGLISH VOWEL SOUNDS ACCORDING TO TONGUE HEIGHT AND ADVANCEMENT

		Front	Central	Back–Central	Back
		Tongue Advancement			
Tongue Height	High	i ɪ			u ʊ
	High–mid	e			o
	Mid		ɝ ɚ ə		
	Low–mid	ɛ		ʌ	ɔ
	Low	æ			a

Key:
i = see   ɝ = bird   u = moon
ɪ = hit   ɚ = teacher   ʊ = would
e = cake   ʌ = mud   o = boat
ɛ = red   ə = about   ɔ = bought
æ = sad   a = mop

Vowel sounds are typically classified according to where the tongue is placed within the oral cavity. Tongue placement can be accomplished within the vertical and horizontal dimensions. Vertical placement is referred to as tongue height. Horizontal placement is referred to as tongue advancement. Both height and advancement of the tongue determine vowel sound production. Vowel sounds are not differentiated according to the unvoiced/voiced scheme because all vowels are produced with vocal fold vibration (hence, they are all voiced).

Referring to Table 11-2, you can see that tongue height is described using such terms as high, mid, and low. A high vowel is produced by elevation of the tongue toward the ceiling of the oral cavity. By the same token, a low vowel is produced by lowering the tongue toward the floor of the oral cavity. In terms of tongue advancement, the terms front, central, and back are used. Front vowels are produced by placing the tongue in the vicinity of the teeth. Back vowels then are produced by placing the tongue in the vicinity of the soft palate and pharynx. When you combine both tongue height and advancement, you get a wide range of possible tongue positions. For example, the /i/ vowel (as in the word "heat") is classified as a high front vowel because the tongue is placed in a position that approximates the alveolar ridge. The /æ/ vowel (as in the word "cat") is also produced by placing the tongue in an anterior position, but the tongue is also placed at the floor of the oral cavity. As one produces the front and back vowels from high to low, the mandible also lowers a bit more and more. You can test this out yourself. Say the words "beat," "bit," "bait," "bet," and "bat" in succession. Make a mental note of what the

tongue and mandible are doing when you say these words (you are producing the front vowels in succession from high to low). It should be noted that tongue height and advancement function to create the various vowel sounds by modifying the resonant characteristics of the oral cavity. With each change in placement of the tongue, the oral cavity becomes a different resonator and thus, a different vowel sound is produced (recall the Source-Filter Theory described in Chapter 10).

The tongue is also the primary structure involved in the production of diphthongs (/aɪ/ as in "nice"; /aʊ/ as in "how"; /ɔɪ/ as in "boy"). However, in the case of the diphthongs, the tongue rapidly shifts from the articulatory position for one vowel to the articulatory position for a second vowel. Note the characters that are used to represent the diphthongs. Go back to Table 11-2 and you can see which two vowels are involved in the production of each diphthong. Take the /aʊ/ diphthong. This sound is produced by having the tongue first assume the position for the /a/ vowel and then rapidly transitioning the tongue to the position for the /ʊ/ vowel. Note that in this case, the shift is from a low back vowel to a high back vowel, and indeed, /aʊ/ is produced by shifting from a low tongue position to a high tongue position. The advancement of the tongue remains back throughout the production of /aʊ/. In the case of /aɪ/ and /ɔɪ/, both tongue height and advancement change. Both of these sounds start with a low back tongue position but then move quickly to a high front tongue position. Shifts from one articulatory position to another create a gliding acoustic quality that is distinctive of the diphthongs.

RELATING ARTICULATORY PHONETICS TO DISORDERS OF ARTICULATION AND RESONANCE

Why should you be concerned with this crash course in articulatory phonetics? The answer is simple. If you understand how speech sounds are produced, that is, which anatomical structures are involved and the physiological processes that play a part in articulation and resonance, you can easily determine how aberrations in structure and/or function will affect the production of speech sounds. Many articulation and resonance disorders have an anatomical, neurological, or physiological etiology. It is the relationship between these etiologies and the resulting articulation and/or resonance disorder to which we now turn our attention.

Pathologies Affecting Articulation and Resonance

DEFINITIONS AND ORGANIZATION OF DISORDERS

Before we begin an extended discussion of the relationship between anatomical and physiological impairments and articulation/resonance disorders, we must begin with some basic definitions. First and foremost, you should understand the distinction between an **articulation disorder** and a **phonological disorder**. An articulation disorder results from "[i]ncorrect production of speech sounds due to faulty placement, timing, direction, pressure, speed, or integration of the movement of the lips, tongue, velum, or pharynx." (Nicolosi, Harryman, & Kresheck, 2004, p. 21) In other words, an articulation disorder is a physical impairment of the ability to correctly move and position the articulators for the correct production of speech sounds. A phonological disorder, on the other hand, not only involves incorrect production of speech sounds but also involves violations of the rules that govern the speech sound system. In fact, it is typically the violations of underlying rules that results in speech sound errors. To put it another way, phonology is one component of language; articulation is one component of phonology. Therefore, a phonological disorder is a broader disorder than an articulation disorder. It is not within the scope of this textbook to discuss phonological disorders but rather to help you see the relationship between abnormal anatomy and/or physiology and articulation/resonance disorders.

A distinction also needs to be made between an **organic disorder** and a **functional disorder**. An organic disorder (whether articulation, language, voice, or any other communication disorder) can be traced back to an observable etiology such as a biochemical aberration, genetic variation, illness, injury, or neurological impairment. By contrast, a functional disorder exists in the absence of any known or observable organic pathology. In the case of articulation, a disorder may exist simply due to the habituation of faulty motoric patterns (i.e., the child habitually makes incorrect placements of the articulators). A functional articulation disorder may also be referred to as a **developmental articulation disorder** because the errors tend to occur during childhood during the developmental period. It is not within the scope of this chapter to discuss functional disorders because of the fact that no known anatomical or physiological etiology is apparent. We will instead turn our attention to articulation disorders of an organic nature.

For the remainder of this chapter, you will be acquainted with a variety of organic disorders that may result in impaired articulation and/or resonance. These organic disorders will be discussed in relation to their underlying etiology—structural, neurological, and sensory. **Structural disorders** involve aberrations of anatomy such as cleft lip and/or palate. The etiology of **neurological disorders** is within the nervous system. Neurological disorders include nerve damage (especially to the cranial nerves), **motor speech disorders**, and other neurological disorders affecting the central and/or peripheral nervous systems. Motor speech disorders affect the proper execution of movements that are necessary for correct speech production and include apraxia of speech (AOS) and dysarthria. Other neurological disorders may include **progressive neurological disorders** (e.g., amyotrophic lateral sclerosis [ALS], multiple sclerosis [MS]) or nonprogressive neurological disorders (e.g., cerebral palsy [CP]). Finally, **sensory disorders** involve impairments of sensory systems that are essential for proper articulation and resonance. These include the auditory, **tactile**, and **kinesthetic** systems. The discussion of sensory disorders that takes place later in this chapter will only focus on the auditory system.

It must be emphasized that you should not be too overly concerned with the classification scheme mentioned above. There are other ways of classifying impairments that affect the articulatory and resonance systems. It should also be noted that within the classification system mentioned earlier, there is considerable overlap. For example, AOS will be discussed as a motor speech disorder although it could just as easily be discussed as a neurological disorder. Similarly, nerve damage (e.g., trauma) could be viewed as a structural disorder although it will be discussed here as a neurological disorder. Your focus then should not be on how impairments are classified but rather on the relationship between these impairments and the potential articulation and/or resonance disorders that may result. That said, let us turn our attention to these impairments.

STRUCTURAL DISORDERS THAT MAY AFFECT ARTICULATION AND RESONANCE

Perhaps, the most obvious structural disorder that will likely have a detrimental effect on articulation and resonance is cleft lip and palate. Similarly, there are several other craniofacial anomalies that may also manifest themselves as deviations of articulation and/or resonance. In the case of structural disorders, the probability that articulation and resonance will both be adversely affected is high.

Cleft Lip and/or Palate

Cleft lip and palate are among the most common congenital anomalies (American Cleft Palate-Craniofacial Association and Cleft Palate Foundation, 1997). The incidence of clefting differs according to race. Cleft lip with or without cleft palate occurs in approximately one in 1000 live births among Caucasians; approximately 1.7 in 1000 live births among Asians; approximately 3.6 in 1000 live births among Native Americans; and 1 in 2500 live births among African Americans (Harold, 2009). In Chapter 10, you learned that the two maxillary bones fuse together medially at the intermaxillary suture. A cleft occurs when the maxillary bones do not fuse between the eighth and twelfth weeks of embryonic development. There are several classification schemes for cleft lip and palate, but these are not important for the purpose of this discussion. As you can see in Figure 11-1, clefts may involve the upper lip only (referred to as cleft lip); the hard palate only

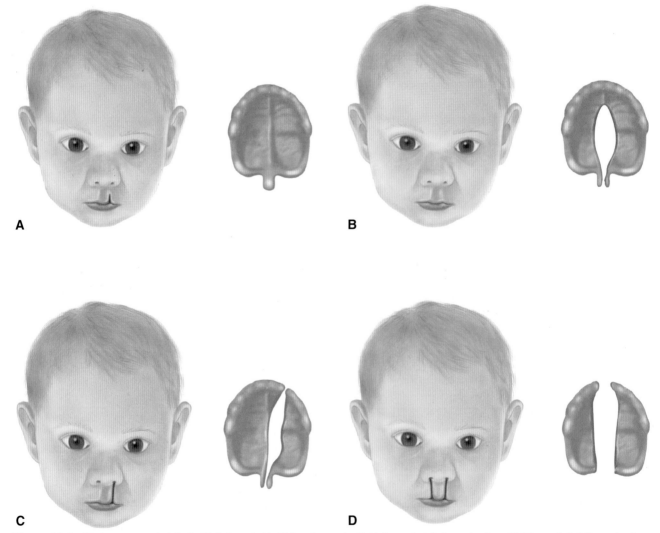

Figure 11-1 Various types of cleft. **A.** Cleft lip only. **B.** Cleft palate only. **C.** Unilateral cleft lip and palate. **D.** Bilateral cleft lip and palate. (Modified with permission from Anatomical Chart Company.)

(referred to as cleft palate); the upper lip and hard palate (referred to as cleft lip and palate); or the upper lip, hard palate, and velum (referred to as complete cleft lip and palate). Clefts of the prepalatal region (i.e., the lip and alveolar ridge) can be unilateral or bilateral.

Possessing an understanding of the anatomy of the lips, teeth, hard palate, and velum, you should be able to surmise that a cleft will likely have an adverse effect on articulation and/or resonance. Clefts of the lip and/or alveolar ridge without involvement of the hard or soft palate may result in some articulation errors due to the likelihood that the individual's dentition is adversely affected. Similarly, a cleft of the lip may affect the individual's ability to round the lips for the /w/ consonant or the vowels that require lip rounding (mainly several of the back vowels). However, there will probably not be a problem with resonance as the hard and soft palates are essentially intact.

When the hard palate and/or velum are involved, both articulation and resonance may be detrimentally affected. From the standpoint of articulation, a cleft of the hard or soft palate may prevent the individual from being able to generate sufficient intraoral air pressure to produce the **pressure consonants**—primarily the plosives and affricates, but also the fricatives to a lesser extent. The individual's productions of the plosives, fricatives, and affricates may be distorted, weak, or absent. From the standpoint of resonance, a cleft of the hard and/or soft palate will compromise the integrity of the oral and nasal cavities. There will not be a separation between the oral and nasal cavity, so a portion of the breath stream may pass unimpeded into the nasal cavity and resonate there. The result is a condition known as **hypernasality**, a resonance disorder in which nonnasal speech sounds (all of the vowels and diphthongs and all but three of the consonants in English) may become heavily nasalized. The air that passes into the nasal cavity, if under sufficient pressure, may also create turbulence as it exits the nostrils, creating nasal air emission. In the more extreme cases of cleft lip and palate, the individual typically develops compensatory strategies in an attempt to produce the pressure consonants and to reduce hypernasality. Of these, the **glottal stop** and **pharyngeal fricative** are commonly used to substitute for the plosives and fricatives, respectively. The pharyngeal fricative (which is produced by creating turbulence of the breath stream in the pharynx) does not occur in English, not even for persons who have an intact speech sound system. The glottal stop also is not recognized as an English speech sound, but it is used in certain linguistic contexts by persons who have an intact speech sound system (e.g., in saying the word "curtain," we seldom enunciate the /t/ sound; instead, we substitute a glottal stop and pronounce the word as "ker-n" with a very slight pause between the two syllables). The difference between a person with an intact speech sound system and an individual who has a cleft palate is that the glottal stop tends to be pervasive in the speech of the individual with cleft palate.

It should be noted that many children with cleft palate also have chronic bouts of **conductive hearing loss**. As you may recall from Chapter 10, the Eustachian (or auditory) tube runs from the middle ear cavity to the nasopharynx. In the case of cleft palate, food or drink that is swallowed may be injected into the nasopharynx because of the opening created by the cleft. If the food or drink gets injected into the Eustachian tube, it can lead to middle ear infections, known as **otitis media**. The result could be a conductive hearing loss. The hearing loss could also adversely affect speech production (this will be discussed more fully below).

Other Craniofacial Anomalies

Cleft lip and palate is classified as a **craniofacial anomaly** because the structures of the skull and face deviate from what would be considered normal anatomy. Although trauma to the face and/or skull could certainly result in an anomaly, we typically think of craniofacial anomalies as having a genetic etiology. There are literally hundreds of genetically based craniofacial anomalies or syndromes. Many of these syndromes have little effect on speech production, but there are many that may have an adverse effect on speech. Cohen and Bankier (1991) estimated that there are nearly 350 syndromes in which orofacial clefting is a characteristic. It is outside the scope of this textbook to provide an exhaustive discussion of these syndromes; instead, you will be exposed to a small sample of craniofacial syndromes that may affect speech sound production.

> ### Why You Need to Know
> Many craniofacial syndromes have a genetic etiology. The etiology is typically autosomal, meaning that chromosomes other than those that determine gender and sexual characteristics are affected. In some cases, the syndrome can be traced back through the family history. These are known as familial cases. When new mutations of the syndrome occur, they are referred to as sporadic. The proportion of cases that are familial versus sporadic differs from syndrome to syndrome.

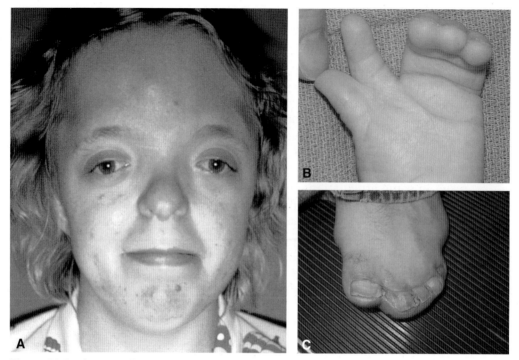

Figure 11-2 Apert syndrome. **A**. Typical facial features seen in the syndrome. **B**. Syndactyly of the fingers. **C**. Syndactyly of the toes. (**A**: Modified with permission from Gold, D.H., Weingeist, T.A. (2001). *Color atlas of the eye in systemic disease*. Baltimore, MD: Lippincott Williams & Wilkins; **B**: Modified with permission from Strickland, J.W., Graham, T.J. (2005). *Master techniques in orthopedic surgery: The hand* (2nd ed.). Philadelphia, PA: Lippincott Williams & Wilkins; **C**: Image provided by Stedman's [Dr. Barankin's Collection].)

Apert Syndrome

Apert syndrome, or **acrocephalosyndactyly**, is a craniofacial anomaly that occurs in approximately one of every 100,000 live births (Gorlin, Cohen, & Levin, 1990). As the more technical name implies, persons with this disorder exhibit two prominent features— an unusually peaked head and webbed fingers and/or toes (see Figure 11-2). This disorder primarily affects the mandible and maxilla, and the face may be flat or concave. There may be unusual deformities of the palate, including clefts. The pharynx tends to be shallow, which may result in a compromised airway. Hearing loss is common. In terms of speech production, there could be numerous speech sound errors due to several factors: compromised integrity of the **velopharyngeal mechanism**; malformed oral structures; and hearing impairment.

Crouzon Syndrome

Crouzon syndrome (technically referred to as **craniofacial dysostosis**) is similar to Apert syndrome but is less severe. It occurs more often than Apert syndrome, in approximately 1 of every 25,000 live births (Gorlin et al., 1990). The webbing of the fingers and toes that is seen in Apert syndrome is not seen in craniofacial dysostosis. However, the premature fusion of cra-nial bones seen in Apert syndrome is also seen here. Additional facial features typically seen in Crouzon syndrome are widely spaced eyes, shallow orbits, a beak-like nose, and a flattened nasal bridge. The shallow orbits make the eyes appear as if they are protruding (see Figure 11-3). In terms of oral structures, the person with Crouzon syndrome will have a small maxilla and a shorter nasopharyngeal space. Kreiborg (1981) found that cleft lip and/or palate are rare but not impossible in this syndrome. If clefting does occur, you can expect deviations in oral–nasal resonance. Similarly, malformation of oral structures may be manifested by a variety of articulation errors.

Ectrodactyly-Ectodermal Dysplasia-Clefting Syndrome

Ectrodactyly-ectodermal dysplasia-clefting syndrome—or simply EEC syndrome—is primarily manifested by "lobster-claw" deformities of the hands and feet, a paucity of body hair, dry skin, and missing or malformed nails and teeth. In the case of the hands and feet, one or more central digits may be missing (i.e., ectrodactyly), giving the appearance of claws. The malformation of teeth and nails, sparse hair, and dry skin (due to the absence of sweat glands) is known as ectodermal dysplasia. As you can see from the name

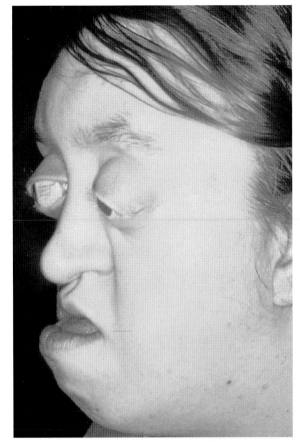

Figure II-3 Typical facial features seen in Crouzon syndrome. Note the protruding eyes, beak-like nose, and a flattened nasal bridge. (Modified with permission from Gold, D.H., Weingeist, T.A. (2001). *Color atlas of the eye in systemic disease.* Baltimore, MD: Lippincott Williams & Wilkins.)

of the syndrome, clefting is also a prominent characteristic. Cleft lip and palate occur in approximately three-fourths of cases of EEC syndrome. A conductive hearing loss (due to anomalies of the middle ear bones—malleus, incus, and stapes) occurs in just under one-third of cases of this disorder. If a cleft does exist, the individual will likely have difficulty in gener-

ating sufficient intraoral air pressure to produce the pressure consonants. There may also be hypernasality with concomitant nasalization of nonnasal speech sounds. Dental anomalies and other oral variations may result in numerous speech sound errors. The individual with EEC syndrome may engage in compensatory articulatory strategies.

Pierre Robin Sequence

Pierre Robin sequence is technically not a syndrome because a genetic defect does not appear to be the etiology of the disorder. During fetal development, the mandible fails to grow properly so that the tongue is prevented from descending into the oral cavity. The tongue remains high in the oral cavity, preventing the palatal shelves from elevating and fusing. The result is a cleft palate, usually U or V shaped. In addition to a cleft palate, the individual with Pierre Robin sequence will exhibit habitual posterior displacement of the tongue into the pharynx, which in turn may cause upper airway obstruction and swallowing problems. Further deficits may be exhibited in the digits, ears, eyes, and heart. Pierre Robin sequence may occur in isolation but is just as likely to be one component of a broader craniofacial anomaly (see Figure 11-4).

Stickler Syndrome

An example of a syndrome that includes characteristics of Pierre Robin sequence is Stickler syndrome, or congenital progressive **arthro-ophthalmopathy**. Many of the signs of Pierre Robin sequence are manifested in this syndrome, with added pathology of the joints (e.g., arthritis, skeletal abnormalities) and visual system (e.g., **astigmatism**, **cataracts**, detached retinas, and severe **myopia**). Once again—as with other craniofacial anomalies involving clefting—the cleft will likely create problems in oral–nasal resonance. In severe cases, unusual articulatory strategies may be

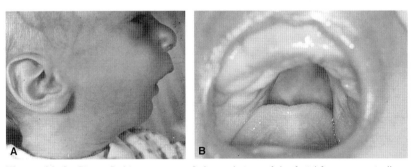

Figure II-4 Pierre Robin sequence. **A**. Lateral view of the facial features typically seen in the sequence. Note the micrognathia. **B**. Cleft palate in an individual with the sequence. (**A**: Reprinted with permission from Sadler, T.W. (2006). *Langman's medical embryology* (10th ed.). Philadelphia, PA: Lippincott Williams & Wilkins. Courtesy of Dr. R.J. Gorlin, Department of Oral Pathology and Genetics, University of Minnesota. **B**: Reprinted with permission from Chung, E.K. et al. (2006). *Visual diagnosis in pediatrics* (1st ed.). Philadelphia, PA: Lippincott Williams & Wilkins. Courtesy of Ellen Deutsch, MD.)

used to compensate for the inability to generate sufficient intraoral air pressure and/or to reduce hypernasality and nasal air emission.

Velocardiofacial Syndrome

Perhaps, the most frequently occurring craniofacial syndrome of which clefting is a characteristic is **velocardiofacial syndrome** (Peterson-Falzone, Hardin-Jones, & Karnell, 2001). As the name of this syndrome implies, the soft palate, heart, and structures of the face are typically involved. Individuals with this disorder tend to have cardiac problems and atypical facial features such as a prominent nose, long face, retruded chin, and unusually small head (known as microcephaly). Of primary concern to the speech–language pathologist is the involvement of the velum. It may have a cleft or there may be congenital **velopharyngeal incompetence** due to a soft palate that is so short that it cannot approximate the posterior pharyngeal wall to provide proper balance between oral and nasal resonance. In either case, the likely outcome will be hypernasality. The nonnasal speech sounds (i.e., all English speech sounds except the /m/, /n/, and /ŋ/) may be highly nasalized. The individual may also exhibit compensatory articulatory substitutions such as the glottal stop and pharyngeal fricative.

> ### Why You Need to Know
>
> *Not included in this formal discussion of craniofacial anomalies, but worth mentioning, is Down syndrome. This syndrome is neither a craniofacial disorder nor a structural disorder as defined here. However, it is an autosomal genetic disorder resulting from a condition known as **trisomy-21**, the presence of an extra 21st chromosome. The primary characteristic of Down syndrome is intellectual impairment, but other characteristics tend to be present such as almond-shaped eyes, short limbs, poor muscle tone, and protruding tongue. This syndrome is mentioned here because speech production errors tend to occur in persons having this syndrome. Speech may be characterized as imprecise, sluggish, or slurred (Gordon-Brannan & Weiss, 2006). Omissions of final consonants in words are also common (Kumin, 1998; Stoel-Gammon, 1998). By comparison with the craniofacial anomalies described here, in the case of Down syndrome, speech sound errors do not appear to be a result of structural deformity. Finally, chronic ear infections and a conductive hearing loss may create further disturbances in speech production.*

Other Structural Anomalies

Velopharyngeal Incompetence Not Related to Craniofacial Anomalies

Velopharyngeal incompetence may occur congenitally in the absence of craniofacial anomalies. This condition results from a soft palate that is too short so that it cannot approximate the posterior pharyngeal wall in the region of the nasopharynx or from a nasopharyngeal space that is too deep or wide to allow the soft palate to gain an adequate seal. In terms of speech production, the result of velopharyngeal incompetence is similar to what you would expect for cleft palate—hypernasality. However, not all cases of velopharyngeal incompetence are a result of an underlying craniofacial anomaly. Some structural variations not associated with a particular syndrome may result in velopharyngeal incompetence. For example, the individual may simply have a hard palate that is too short. This may cause an otherwise normal velum to have an anterior displacement that does not allow it to approximate the posterior pharyngeal wall. On the other hand, the hard palate may be normal, but the velum may be too short. In many of these cases, the muscles that mediate movement of the soft palate may insert into the hard palate instead of the anterior portion of the soft palate. Finally, in some cases, there may be neurological damage to either the nerves or muscles that control movement of the velum so that it cannot elevate to meet the posterior pharyngeal wall (this condition will be discussed in more detail below). No matter the underlying cause, the result will be velopharyngeal incompetence and with that a likelihood of improper balance between oral and nasal resonance.

Glossectomy

According to the American Cancer Society (2004), there are approximately 30,000 new cases of oral cancer in the United States each year. Of these cases, nearly 7500 involve cancer of the tongue. The incidence then is approximately 2.5 per 100,000 population annually. The primary causes of oral cancer (and cancer of the tongue) are long-term alcohol and tobacco use. Although cancer of the tongue is fairly uncommon by comparison to other cancers, its effects can be devastating. In the most severe cases, the individual with tongue cancer will require a total **glossectomy**. Removal of all of the tongue will have a negative effect on speech production and swallowing.

As you have learned, the tongue is involved in the production of all of the vowels and diphthongs and 75% of the consonant sounds in English. It is also an integral structure in the process of swallowing as the tongue helps to shape and form the bolus during chewing and then forces the bolus to the pharynx for swallowing. Although a prosthetic tongue may be provided after total glossectomy, to this time medical technology has not been able to make a prosthesis flexible and mobile enough to do the work of the natural tongue.

In terms of articulation and resonance, with partial removal of the tongue you may be able to assist the patient in developing compensatory strategies to improve articulation of error speech sounds and improving oral resonance for the diphthongs and vowels. In some cases where only minor surgery is involved, you may even be able to restore the patient's speech production to its premorbid level. With total glossectomy, however, you can expect pervasive articulation errors involving practically the entire speech sound system as well as poor resonance of the diphthongs and vowels. The speech sound system may be so adversely affected that the patient's speech is highly unintelligible. In these cases, the only option may be to provide an **augmentative and alternative communication** (AAC) system for the individual. AAC systems may include gestural communication such as Amer-Ind or manual signs; basic communication displays with alphabetic letters, words, or symbols on them; or electronic devices that produce synthetic speech output.

NEUROLOGICAL DISORDERS THAT MAY AFFECT ARTICULATION AND RESONANCE

As mentioned previously in this chapter, the term "neurological disorder" encompasses a wide range of pathological conditions affecting the nervous system. Some of these conditions may affect only the central nervous system (i.e., the brain and spinal cord), whereas others may affect only the peripheral nervous system (i.e., the cranial nerves, spinal nerves, and other peripheral nerves). Still other conditions may affect both the central and peripheral nervous systems. For the purpose of further discussion, neurological disorders have been divided into three broad categories: cranial nerve damage; motor speech disorders; and other neurological disorders, including progressive and nonprogressive neurological disorders. Our discussion of neurological disorders will proceed in that order.

Cranial Nerve Damage

In Chapter 10, you learned that half of the 12 pairs of cranial nerves play some role in articulation and/or resonance. These include the trigeminal (cranial nerve V), facial (VII), glossopharyngeal (IX), vagus (X),

spinal accessory (XI), and hypoglossal (XII) nerves. As you can see by perusing Table 11-3, some of these cranial nerves have a major impact on articulation and resonance (as well as swallowing) while others play a relatively minor role.

The cranial nerves that are involved in speech production and swallowing can be affected by **neuropathy** or trauma. For example, if pressure is exerted upon the cranial nerves (e.g., due to inflammation), the result may be **neuralgia** and in some cases even **palsy**. Disease processes such as Lyme disease, **neoplasm**, or **sarcoidosis** may also result in nerve pathology. Two of the cranial nerves in particular—the trigeminal and facial nerves—may be affected by disorders that are specific to them (i.e., trigeminal neuralgia and Bell's palsy, respectively). Cerebrovascular accidents, or strokes, may also affect any of the cranial nerves.

Trauma can come in the form of gunshot or stab wounds to the head and/or neck or from surgical procedures that go awry. For example, the spinal accessory nerve is susceptible to damage from facelift surgery that is not performed properly. Similarly, the hypoglossal nerve may be damaged during surgery to remove a blockage in an artery in the neck.

Naturally, which body parts are affected depends on which cranial nerves are experiencing the neuropathy or trauma. As you can see from Table 11-3, the muscles that mediate lip movement are all innervated by the facial nerve (cranial nerve VII). The muscles that mediate elevation of the mandible (i.e., closing the jaw) are all innervated by the trigeminal (V) nerve, whereas the muscles that mediate depression of the mandible (i.e., opening the jaw) are innervated by the trigeminal, facial (VII), or hypoglossal (XII) nerve. The intrinsic tongue muscles (which primarily mediate its shape and form) are all innervated by the hypoglossal (XII) nerve, as are all of the extrinsic muscles (which depress, elevate, protrude, and retract the tongue) except the palatoglossus, which is innervated by the vagus (X) and possibly the spinal accessory (XI) nerve. The muscles that elevate and depress the soft palate are innervated primarily by the vagus nerve (and the spinal accessory nerve as well), with the exception of the tensor veli palatini which is innervated by the trigeminal nerve. As you can deduce, there is some degree of redundancy in terms of neural innervation. This redundancy is a protective mechanism of sorts. For many of the structures of the oral cavity, more than one cranial nerve would have to be affected to cause complete loss of function.

The signs and symptoms you would observe in a patient who has experienced head or neck trauma

TABLE 11-3

THE INFLUENCE OF CRANIAL NERVES ON SPEECH PRODUCTION AND SWALLOWING

Cranial Nerve		Innervates	Whose Action Is To
Number	*Name*		
V	Trigeminal	Digastricus (anterior belly)	Lower the jaw
		Lateral pterygoid	Lower and protrude the jaw
		Masseter	Raise and retract the jaw
		Medial pterygoid	Raise the jaw
		Mylohyoid	Lower the jaw
		Temporalis	Raise and retract the jaw
		Tensor veli palatini	Lower and tense the soft palate
VII	Facial	Buccinator	Compress the lips against the teeth
		Depressor anguli oris	Compress the upper lip onto the lower lip
		Depressor labii inferior	Pull the lower lip downward and outward
		Digastricus (posterior belly)	Lower the jaw
		Incisivus labii inferior	Pull corner of the mouth inward and downward
		Incisivus labii superior	Pull corner of the mouth inward and upward
		Levator anguli oris	Pull the corner of the mouth and lower lip upward
		Levator labii superior	Raise the upper lip
		Levator labii superior alaeque nasi	Raise the upper lip
		Mentalis	Protrude and turn the lower lip outward
		Orbicularis oris	Close the mouth and pucker the lips
		Risorius	Pull the mouth angle outward
		Zygomatic major	Pull the mouth angle upward and outward
		Zygomatic minor	Raise the upper lip
IX	Glossopharyngeal	Stylopharyngeus	Assist in swallowing and vocal resonance
X	Vagus	Levator veli palatini	Raise the soft palate
		Musculus uvulae	Raise the soft palate
		Palatoglossus	Lower the soft palate and raise the back of the tongue
		Palatopharyngeus	Lower the soft palate and assist in swallowing and vocal resonance
		Pharyngeal constrictors	Assist in swallowing and vocal resonance
		Salpingopharyngeus	Assist in swallowing and vocal resonance
XI	Spinal accessory	Musculus uvulae	Raise the soft palate
		Palatoglossus	Lower the soft palate and raise the back of the tongue
		Palatopharyngeus	Lower the soft palate and assist in swallowing and vocal resonance
		Salpingopharyngeus	Assist in swallowing and vocal resonance
XII	Hypoglossal	Geniohyoid	Lower the jaw
		Genioglossus	Protrude the tongue tip and retract and lower the tongue
		Hyoglossus	Retract and lower the tongue
		Inferior longitudinal	Shape the tongue
		Styloglossus	Raise the tongue in a posterior direction
		Superior longitudinal	Shape the tongue
		Transverse	Shape the tongue
		Vertical	Shape the tongue

or neuropathy are dependent upon which nerves are affected and the location where the damage is focused. In general, the higher up one goes toward the brain and brainstem, the more diffuse (i.e., widespread) the damage will be. By the same token, the lower one goes toward the periphery, the more focal (i.e., limited) the damage will be. In the paragraphs that follow, you should keep in mind that the discussion pertains to damage to the **lower motor neuron** (LMN) as opposed to the **upper motor neuron** (UMN). Signs and symptoms of cranial nerve damage differ considerably depending on whether the damage is in the central nervous system or peripheral nervous system. The effects of UMN damage on articulation and resonance will be discussed in more depth in the later section on progressive neurological disorders. Regardless of which cranial nerve is affected, the primary signs of LMN damage may include **fasciculations, flaccid paralysis**, loss of reflexes, muscle **atrophy**, and weakness.

Damage to the Trigeminal Nerve

Although there are many possible etiologies of trigeminal nerve damage, one neuropathy specific to this nerve that is worth mentioning is trigeminal neuralgia, which is also known as tic douloureux. It is the most frequently occurring of all neuralgias. The cause of this disorder is not fully understood, but it is thought that it may be due to degeneration of the trigeminal nerve or by pressure placed upon it by inflammation or some other source. The primary symptom of trigeminal neuralgia is a sharp, cutting sensation on one side of the face, usually in the area of the jaw. In some cases, the disorder may mimic the symptoms of dental disease. In younger people, there may be concern that the symptoms could be an early sign of multiple sclerosis (MS). The pain can last from several minutes to several hours at a time, and it can be triggered by such activities as smiling, chewing, blowing the nose, or brushing the teeth. The disorder may come and go in some individuals but may be more chronic in others. During periods of severe pain, the individual may experience difficulty in chewing or speaking.

According to Table 11-3, the trigeminal nerve is primarily responsible for innervating the muscles that raise and lower the jaw. This action is necessary for **mastication** as well as speaking. Only one other cranial nerve is involved in jaw movement—the facial nerve, which innervates the posterior body of the digastricus to assist in lowering (i.e., opening) the jaw. The trigeminal nerve also innervates the tensor veli palatini muscle, which assists in lowering the soft palate, but the majority of muscles that mediate movements of the soft palate are not innervated by the trigemi-

nal nerve. Therefore, damage to the trigeminal nerve will have a detrimental effect on an individual's ability to open and close the jaw, and a lesser effect on the ability of an individual to lower the soft palate. How much ability is diminished depends on whether the damage is unilateral or bilateral. If the damage is unilateral, the jaw will deviate to the side of the damage when the individual is instructed to open or close the jaw. If the damage is bilateral, there may be complete inability to open and close the jaw, thereby impeding the individual from chewing and also affecting speech production. The effect on speech production will involve primarily oral resonance (see what happens to the resonance of your voice when you speak with your jaw being closed or opened very wide). From an articulatory standpoint, the inability of the individual to close the jaw may affect production of the bilabials (i.e., /p/, /b/, /m/), interdentals (i.e., /θ/ and /ð/), and labiodentals (i.e., /f/ and /v/). Because of the functional relationship between the tongue and mandible, high anterior speech sounds (e.g., the alveolars and high front vowels) may be affected to a lesser extent.

Damage to the Facial Nerve

Bell's palsy is a neuropathology that is associated with the facial nerve (see Figure 11-5). It is the most common cause of facial paralysis and is always unilateral.

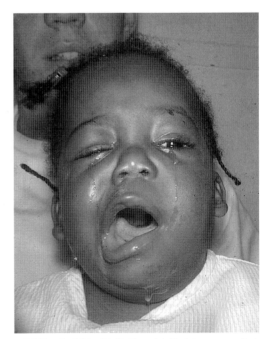

Figure 11-5 A child with Bell's palsy (facial nerve pathology) on the right side of her face. Note the drooping of the eye and corner of her mouth on the right. (Modified with permission from Bickley, L.S., Szilagyi, P. (2003). *Bates' guide to physical examination and history taking* (8th ed.). Philadelphia, PA: Lippincott Williams & Wilkins.)

The etiology is unknown although it is thought that a virus (e.g., herpes simplex) may be behind the disorder. For most sufferers, the condition is only temporary, typically lasting 3 to 8 weeks on average. However, for approximately 16% of persons who develop Bell's palsy, the condition may become chronic. The primary symptoms of this disorder include altered sense of taste; difficulty speaking; drooling from the mouth on the affected side; drooping of the ipsilateral eyelid and corner of the mouth; dryness or excessive tearing of the affected eye; and a heightened sense of hearing on the affected side.

As shown in Table 11-3, the facial nerve primarily innervates the muscles that mediate facial expression, although it also innervates the posterior belly of the digastricus, which assists in lowering the jaw. However, as you know from the forgoing discussion of the trigeminal nerve, jaw movement will more likely be affected adversely by cranial nerve V damage. The bad news is that the facial nerve is the only cranial nerve that innervates the facial muscles, so there is no neural redundancy to serve as a protective mechanism. As is true for the trigeminal nerve, unilateral damage will not affect speech production or swallowing as adversely as bilateral damage will. In the case of Bell's palsy, damage is always unilateral, so speech production and swallowing may be only mildly affected. Other forms of facial nerve damage can be bilateral.

Not all facial muscles are involved in speech production. For this discussion, we are only interested in the muscles that mediate movement of the lips. These include the buccinator, depressor anguli oris, depressor labii inferior, incisivus labii inferior and superior, levator anguli oris, levator labii superior, levator labii superior alaeque nasi, mentalis, orbicularis oris, risorius, and zygomatic major and minor. The net action of these muscles is to compress, evert, round, and pucker the lips as well as pull the corners of the mouth laterally, upward, and downward. Some of these actions are necessary for speech production and swallowing. In the case of speech production, inability to compress or round the lips may adversely affect production of the bilabials (i.e., /p/, /b/, /m/) and labiodentals (i.e., /f/ and /v/) as well as the rounded speech sounds (i.e., /w/, /u/, /ʊ/, /o/, /ɔ/, /ɝ/ and /ɚ/).

In terms of swallowing, you know from Chapter 10 that the lips compress to prevent the bolus from exiting the mouth as the tongue forces the bolus toward the pharynx. Therefore, damage to the facial nerve may disrupt the swallowing process. Depending on the severity of the problem, food and drink may eject from the mouth as the individual attempts to swallow. The individual may also exhibit drooling from one or both sides of the mouth.

Damage to the Glossopharyngeal Nerve

From Table 11-3, you can see that the glossopharyngeal nerve is involved minimally in the processes of resonance and swallowing. This nerve innervates only one muscle involved in these processes—the stylopharyngeus. This muscle plays a part along with several other muscles to dilate, elevate, relax, and tense the pharynx. Since several other muscles are also involved in these actions, damage to the glossopharyngeal nerve alone will likely have a minimal effect on resonance or swallowing. The vagus nerve, and possibly the spinal accessory nerve as well, would have to be damaged along with the glossopharyngeal nerve for there to be any measurable effect on resonance or swallowing.

Damage to the Vagus and Spinal Accessory Nerves

When it comes to the head and neck region, there is an almost inexorable link between the vagus and spinal accessory nerve. A controversy exists as to whether the spinal accessory nerve really innervates any of the head and neck muscles independently of the vagus nerve. Therefore, you will note in Table 11-3 that all of the muscles listed under the spinal accessory nerve are also listed under the vagus nerve. The vagus nerve does innervate some muscles that the spinal accessory nerve clearly does not—the levator veli palatini and all of the pharyngeal constrictor muscles. The discussion that immediately follows will focus on the vagus nerve, but keep in mind that for some of the structures mentioned later, the spinal accessory nerve may also be involved.

From Chapter 8, you learned that the vagus nerve plays a major role in phonation via the recurrent and superior laryngeal nerves. However, the vagus nerve also innervates several muscles that are integral in mediating movements of the pharynx, soft palate, and tongue. This nerve innervates the muscles that raise the soft palate as well as two of the three muscles that lower it (the third muscle—the tensor veli palatini—is innervated by the trigeminal nerve). The vagus nerve also innervates one muscle that assists in raising the back of the tongue. Finally, the vagus nerve innervates several muscles that mediate pharyngeal movements (the only exception is the stylopharyngeus muscle, which is innervated by the glossopharyngeal nerve). Clearly, the vagus nerve is the primary source of innervation for the muscles of the soft palate and pharynx. It plays a lesser role in the innervation of the muscles that mediate tongue movement. Therefore, damage to the vagus nerve is more likely to affect the soft palate and pharynx.

The site of nerve damage is very important in understanding which structures will be affected. Almost immediately upon exiting the base of the cranium, the inferior ganglion of the vagus nerve gives off three important branches along its journey through the neck. Most superior of these is the pharyngeal branch. Below the pharyngeal branch, the vagus gives off the superior laryngeal nerve, and finally below that the recurrent laryngeal nerve. If damage occurs at the level of the inferior ganglion, then all structures below that point will be affected, including the soft palate, pharynx, and larynx. If the damage is below the level where the pharyngeal branch comes off the vagus nerve, then the damage will be confined to the larynx since the nerve is still intact at the level of the pharyngeal branch (remember this mantra: "the higher up the lesion, the more widespread the damage"). If damage is confined to the pharyngeal branch alone, then the larynx will not be affected but the soft palate and pharynx will.

That said, if the pharyngeal branch of the vagus nerve is damaged, the result will likely be diminished movement of the soft palate and pharynx (see Figure 11-6). As you recall, the soft palate is part of the velopharyngeal mechanism. If the soft palate cannot raise and lower properly, the result will be improper oral–nasal resonance. An individual with paralysis of the soft palate will likely have some degree of hypernasality. The hypernasality will be more pronounced if there is bilateral damage because both sides will be paralyzed and the soft palate will not be able to

elevate at all. In the case of unilateral damage, the uvula will still be able to elevate on one side, so at least some degree of velopharyngeal closure can be accomplished.

> ### Why You Need to Know
>
> *Having the patient produce a staccato "ah" is a diagnostic test to determine where damage to the vagus nerve is occurring. If upon producing a staccato "ah" there is no movement of the soft palate at all, you can expect that there is bilateral damage to the vagus nerve. If upon producing a staccato "ah" the soft palate deviates to one side, then the damage is likely unilateral. In the case of unilateral damage, you can determine which side is affected by observing the uvula. The uvula will move to the unaffected side. This is because the muscles on the unaffected side are still able to contract, and thereby will "pull" the soft palate to that side. Figure 11-6 depicts vagus nerve damage on the patient's right side.*

In terms of swallowing, an inability to raise the soft palate may cause the bolus to be injected into the nasopharynx when it is forced into the pharynx by the tongue. Collection of food or drink within the nasopharynx may set the stage for bacteria to travel up the Eustachian tube and into the middle ear, potentially resulting in otitis media.

Similarly to the soft palate, the pharynx plays a role in resonance and swallowing. Therefore, paralysis of the pharyngeal muscles may adversely affect these processes. In the case of resonance, the voice may sound "muffled" or not as crisp as you would expect. In the case of swallowing, the lack of motility within the pharynx may prevent the bolus from being passed into the esophagus. Instead, the bolus may pocket in the inferior pharynx, most notably within the pyriform sinuses. In severe cases, aspiration of the bolus into the larynx can occur.

Damage to the vagus nerve (and to a lesser degree the spinal accessory nerve) will probably not have as negative an effect on articulation as it may on resonance and swallowing. The soft palate and pharynx are not actively involved in the articulation of speech sounds. The vagus nerve does innervate one extrinsic tongue muscle (the palatoglossus), but the action that this muscle performs on the tongue can also be accomplished by the styloglossus muscle, which is innervated by the hypoglossal nerve. Production of back consonants and vowels (i.e., /k/, /g/, /ŋ/, /u/, /ʊ/, /o/, /ɔ/, and /a/) may be affected somewhat, but

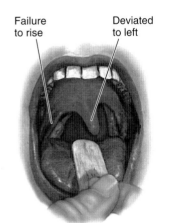

Failure to rise
Deviated to left

Figure 11-6 Hemiparesis of the soft palate due to right vagus nerve damage. The soft palate will deviate to the opposite side during the production of staccato "ah." (Modified with permission from Bickley, L.S., Szilagyi, P. (2003). *Bates' guide to physical examination and history taking* (8th ed.). Philadelphia, PA: Lippincott Williams & Wilkins.)

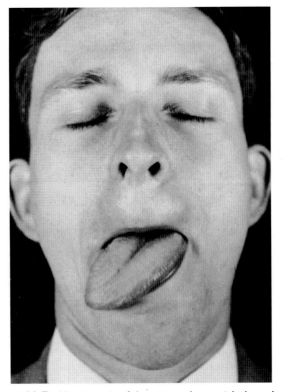

Figure 11-7 Hemiparesis of the tongue due to right hypoglossal nerve damage. The tongue will deviate to the affected side during protrusion. (Modified with permission from Campbell, W.W. (2005). *DeJong's the neurologic examination* (6th ed.). Philadelphia, PA: Lippincott Williams & Wilkins.)

ever, she can stick out her tongue but it deviates to one side of the mouth, the damage is unilateral. Which side the tongue deviates tells you which hypoglossal nerve is damaged. The tongue will deviate to the side of the damage. This is because unilateral damage to the genioglossus muscle means that only half of it is contracting—the half that causes the tongue to move toward the opposite side. The tongue will move away from the intact genioglossus, that is, toward the "bad" side. Figure 11-7 depicts damage to the right hypoglossal nerve.

in most cases the individual will still be able to produce these sounds.

Damage to the Hypoglossal Nerve

With the exception of the innervation of the geniohyoid muscle, the hypoglossal nerve's role is almost exclusively associated with movements of the tongue (see Figure 11-7). This nerve innervates all of the intrinsic muscles of the tongue as well as all of the extrinsic tongue muscles except the palatoglossus (which, as you have just learned, is innervated by the vagus and possibly even the spinal accessory nerve). Clearly, damage to this cranial nerve is going to have serious consequences for the primary structure of articulation and oral resonance.

> ### Why You Need to Know
>
> *Similarly to the vagus nerve and the soft palate, you can determine whether hypoglossal nerve damage is unilateral or bilateral, and if unilateral, which hypoglossal nerve is affected. In this case, ask the patient to stick her tongue out. If she cannot do this task at all, the damage is likely bilateral. If, how-*

Articulation, chewing, resonance, and swallowing will all be affected adversely by damage to the hypoglossal nerve, especially if the damage is bilateral. As has been mentioned several times, the tongue is the primary articulator, playing a role in the production of three-fourths of the consonant sounds in English (the *non*-tongue–influenced consonants are /p/, /b/, /m/, /f/, /v/, and /h/). In addition, the tongue is the primary structure involved in oral resonance for all of the vowels and diphthongs. For the processes of chewing and swallowing, the tongue also plays an important role. During deglutition, the tongue helps shape and form the bolus as it is being chewed. During swallowing, the tongue is responsible for "squeezing" the bolus back along the ceiling of the oral cavity, eventually forcing it through the oropharyngeal isthmus and into the pharynx. Just think of how adversely affected an individual's ability to chew, speak, and swallow would be if he had bilateral damage to the hypoglossal nerve!

Motor Speech Disorders

As you learned in Chapter 5, a motor speech disorder is the result of a neurological impairment in which motor planning, programming, neuromuscular control, or the execution of speech is adversely affected (Duffy, 2005). The more common etiologies of this condition are cerebrovascular accident (i.e., stroke), degenerative disease, traumatic brain injury, and neoplasm. Two neuropathologies are classified as motor speech disorders: **apraxia of speech** (**AOS**) and **dysarthria**. As you will learn in reading the paragraphs that follow, one of these disorders—dysarthria—in many cases is the result of cranial nerve damage and therefore the discussion of dysarthria is highly related to the foregoing discussion on cranial nerve damage. However, keep in mind that the discussion above centered on the likely outcome of *isolated* cranial nerve damage, and specifically damage that is more peripherally

TABLE 11-4

DIFFERENTIATING BETWEEN APRAXIA OF SPEECH AND DYSARTHRIA

Feature	Apraxia of Speech	Dysarthria
Neuropathology	Cortical, in the language-dominant hemisphere	Cortical, subcortical in either hemisphere, and/or peripheral
Nonverbal oral movements	Range of movement and strength are typically normal	Range of movement and strength are typically impaired
Speech sounds in error	Consonants; vowels may or may not be affected	Typically, consonants and vowels are affected
Types of articulation errors	Distorted sound substitutions, omissions, and transpositions	Distortions and omissions of speech sounds
Consistency of articulation errors	Variable with periods of error-free speech production	Consistent and predictable with no periods of error-free speech production
Automatic versus volitional speech	Automatic speech can be error free	Automatic and volitional speech are equally affected
Effects of utterance complexity	Utterances with greater complexity usually elicit more errors	Errors occur regardless of utterance complexity
Oral/nasal resonance	Resonance is rarely affected	With involvement of the velum, there will likely be improper balance between oral and nasal resonance
Phonation	Phonation is rarely affected	Phonation is often affected
Respiration	Respiration is rarely affected	Respiration may be affected

based. In the majority of cases of dysarthria, several cranial nerves may be involved or the damage may be more diffuse as the site of lesion tends to be more central.

To the untrained observer, AOS and dysarthria may appear to be very similar disorders. However, to a speech–language pathologist, the difference between the two is more obvious. Table 11-4 provides a summary of some of the differences between AOS and dysarthria. First and foremost, the site of lesion is different between the two. AOS is a central nervous system disorder with damage originating in the language-dominant cerebral hemisphere (for most people, the left hemisphere). In some cases of dysarthria, damage also occurs at the level of the cerebral cortex, but in most cases, the damage is subcortical, bulbar (i.e., brainstem), cerebellar, and/or peripheral. Another noteworthy difference between the two is the fact that AOS tends to be confined to the articulatory system, whereas dysarthria tends to affect every aspect of speech production including respiration, phonation, articulation, and resonance. In the case of dysarthria, the patient *looks* like he has a motor disorder. Finally, differences exist between the two types of motor speech disorder in terms of (1) the speech sounds that tend to be in error; (2) the types of articulation errors that are exhibited; (3) the consistency of articulation errors; and (4) the effect of increasing linguistic context on the patient's speech. These differences in speech production will become more apparent in the follow-

ing sections. You should realize, however, that within each of the two motor speech disorders, there tends to be quite a bit of variability from person to person. Two persons having a diagnosis of AOS or dysarthria may exhibit a different set of articulation errors. Because of this, the discussion below will not focus on specific articulation errors but on generalities.

As a final note, it should be mentioned that the speech–language pathologist tends to see a large number of persons who have had a stroke who exhibit a motor speech disorder along with swallowing difficulties. Estimates of the prevalence of dysphagia among persons who have had a stroke range from 25% to 70% (Howden, 2004; Mann, Hankey, & Cameron, 2000; Marik & Kaplan, 2003; Martino, Foley, Bhogal, et al., 2005; Paciaroni, Mazzotta, Corea, et al., 2004; Schelp, Cola, Gatto, Goncalves da Silva, et al., 2004). Disturbances in any or all of the phases of the swallow can occur (e.g., aspiration, ejection of food outside the mouth or into the nasopharynx, inability to form the bolus or transport it to the oropharynx, pocketing of the bolus in the pyriform sinuses). Because of the high prevalence of dysphagia in persons who have had a stroke, swallowing therapy is likely to be a component of a comprehensive intervention plan.

Apraxia of Speech

AOS is a central nervous system disorder. As was previously mentioned, the focus of neuropathology is in the language-dominant cerebral hemisphere. Rarely would you see a case of isolated AOS. Instead, you are more likely to observe a patient with AOS also having **aphasia**. In terms of speech production, one could think of AOS as a "short circuit" in the brain's ability to program the articulators for correct speech sound production. Think of a lamp that has an electrical short. Sometimes the electrical circuit gets completed so that the light comes on, while at other times the circuit is disrupted and the light goes off. You are not able to predict when the light will come on and when it will go off. Such is AOS; a person with this disorder tends to have periods of fluent, easily understandable speech but other periods of effortful groping to find the correct articulatory postures for speech sounds with numerous speech sound errors.

For a person with AOS, speech sound errors primarily involve the consonants, but in some cases may involve the vowels as well. Errors typically involve distorted sound substitutions, omissions of sounds, and to a lesser degree sound transpositions. Errors occur most often during volitional speech while "automatic" speech (e.g., reciting the days of the week or giving social greetings) tends to remain intact. A patient with AOS will have relatively few articulatory errors when producing utterances of low linguistic complexity, but errors tend to increase considerably as the linguistic context gets more complex (e.g., producing longer sentences or saying words of increasing syllable length). **Prosody** tends to be adversely affected in AOS. Finally, an individual with AOS will likely not exhibit disturbances in respiration, phonation, or resonance as the disorder is primarily an impairment of the articulatory system alone.

Dysarthria

The site of lesion for dysarthria can be the cerebral cortex, the subcortical region of either hemisphere, the cerebellum, the brainstem, and/or the periphery (i.e., the cranial and/or spinal nerves)—quite a wide range of possibilities! There could be damage to the UMNs, LMNs, or both. In Chapter 5, you learned that there are seven types of dysarthria: ataxic, flaccid, hyperkinetic, hypokinetic, spastic, unilateral UMN (UUMN), and mixed. Ataxic dysarthria is associated with cerebellar damage. Flaccid dysarthria involves LMN damage, while spastic dysarthria involves bilateral UMN damage. The site of lesion for UUMN dysarthria is fairly self-explanatory. The site of lesion for the hyperkinetic and hypokinetic types is the basal ganglia. Finally, mixed dysarthria incorporates two or more of the single types; the site of lesion depends on which single types are involved. With such a wide range of possibilities, you can well imagine that the

symptoms you'd observe depend on the specific type of dysarthria. Because of this, it is beyond the scope of this textbook to discuss characteristics of speech production in specific terms.

Perhaps, the most striking difference you'd note between AOS and dysarthria is how widespread dysarthria is by comparison. Dysarthria typically involves every component of speech production—respiration, phonation, articulation, resonance, and prosody. Another difference between the two involves nonverbal oral movements (e.g., sticking out the tongue, moving the tongue from side to side, pursing the lips). In AOS, range of movement and strength of the articulators tends to be intact, while these tend to be impaired in dysarthria. Speech production errors also tend to be different for dysarthria. For example, both consonants and vowels are typically affected in dysarthria. Articulation errors include distortions and omissions of speech sounds. In many cases, the patient exhibits imprecise productions of consonants. Speech may be slow and slurred. By contrast to AOS, there tend to be no periods of error-free speech in dysarthria. Although many speech–language pathologists are realizing that speech sound errors are more consistent in AOS than was originally thought, speech sound errors in dysarthria are *highly* consistent and predictable. In dysarthria, automatic and volitional speech tend to be equally affected, and speech sound errors tend to be consistent regardless of linguistic complexity.

Other Neurological Disorders

There are a whole host of central and/or peripheral nervous system disorders that may affect the speech production mechanism in some way. These remaining disorders have been classified as either progressive or nonprogressive neurological disorders. The term "progressive" refers to the fact that the pathology will worsen over time, and in many cases prove to be fatal. Naturally, nonprogressive disorders do not get worse over time. The patient develops the disorder at some point but symptoms remain pretty much constant across the life span. The progressive neurological disorders that will be presented here include amyotrophic lateral sclerosis (ALS), multiple sclerosis (MS), and Parkinson's disease. These will be discussed to show you the wide range of symptoms and pathological signs that accompany these disorders, including the wide range of speech impairment that exists from disorder to disorder. One nonprogressive disorder will be presented here—cerebral palsy (CP). As you read the sections that follow, you will note almost immediately that when it comes to speech production, these neuropathies include some type of dysarthria. Indeed, the disorders described and discussed in this section are the neurological disorders; the speech disorder (i.e., dysarthria) is just one characteristic of the broader neurological disorder.

Progressive Neurological Disorders

To see the wide range of symptoms and signs that exist from disorder to disorder, we will compare three well-known progressive neurological disorders: ALS, MS, and Parkinson's disease. The three differ in terms of neurological involvement, symptoms, and the speech characteristics that are typically exhibited.

ALS, or Lou Gehrig's disease, is a fatal neuropathy in which the motor neurons—both upper and lower—degenerate, resulting in diminished or lost voluntary muscle activity. As the disease progresses, muscles no longer receive neural impulses, so they become paralyzed and wither away (see Figure 11-8). The etiology is unknown. ALS is slightly more common in men than in women, usually occurring between the ages of 40 and 60 years. In the United States, approximately one person per 250,000 will develop ALS. Early symptoms of ALS include general weakness followed by twitching, cramping, or stiffening of affected muscles usually in an arm or leg. In the later stages of the disease, the muscles of the respiratory system are affected to the point that the individual will likely die of respiratory failure or pneumonia. Because both the upper and lower motor neurons are affected, ALS is a central *and* peripheral nervous system disease. In Chapter 5, you learned that an outcome of UMN damage is spasticity, whereas an outcome of LMN damage is flaccidity. If you think about this in relation to the speech mechanism, you may correctly surmise that ALS results in mixed dysarthria of the flaccid and spastic types. Aberrations in activity for the muscles of the speech production mechanism will result in speech that exhibits the following signs: hypernasality with nasal air emission, imprecise articulation of consonants, slow speaking rate, and vowel distortions. Problems in swallowing are also common, especially in the later stages of the disease. There is, however, a wide range of specific symptoms from person to person (Duffy, 2005).

MS is an autoimmune disorder in which the person's immune system attacks the central nervous system. The myelinated axons of neurons lose their myelination; this process prevents neurons in the brain and spinal cord from communicating with each other by interrupting a neuron's ability to conduct neural impulses to other neurons (see Figure 11-9). The breakdown of myelin creates scar tissue (i.e., sclerosis)

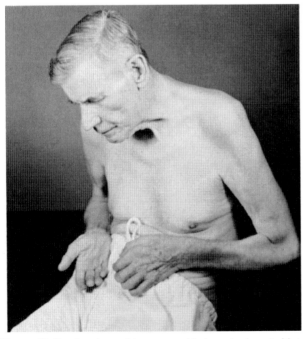

Figure 11-8 A patient with amyotrophic lateral sclerosis. Note the atrophy of muscles in his arms. (Modified with permission from Campbell, W.W. (2005). *DeJong's the neurologic examination* (6th ed.). Philadelphia, PA: Lippincott Williams & Wilkins.)

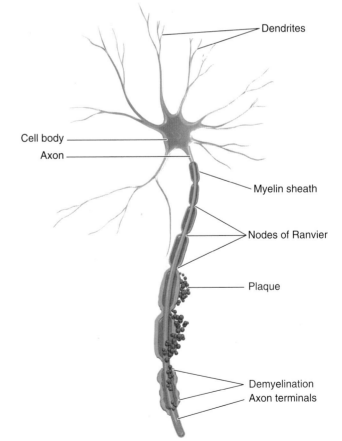

Figure 11-9 Illustration of the demyelination and scarring that occur in multiple sclerosis. (Anatomical Chart Company.)

along the axon. "Multiple" refers to the fact that demyelination can occur in several places within the central nervous system—brainstem, cerebellum, cerebrum, and spinal cord. MS occurs more often in women than in men. Its onset is usually between the ages of 20 and 40 years, although cases have been known to occur in persons older than 40 years. Approximately 140 to 150 persons per 100,000 develop the disease. The specific etiology is unknown, but some believe that its origin may be viral. Symptoms of this disease include chronic fatigue, sensory disturbances (e.g., burning, itching, numbness, and tingling), and visual problems (e.g., double vision, decreased color perception, and reduced visual acuity). Because demyelination can occur in several places within the central nervous system, the resulting dysarthria can be difficult to predict. In many cases, there is no dysarthria at all. For those cases where dysarthria is present, the most common type is mixed with characteristics of the ataxic and spastic types (which would seem to indicate that the cerebellum and UMNs are affected). If the cerebellar system is involved, the distinguishing speech characteristic is imprecise articulation resulting in slurred speech due to poor motor coordination. The person will sound as if she is intoxicated. "Overshooting" of the tongue (possibly due to the spasticity) as it attempts to make articulatory contacts is also fairly common in persons who have MS.

Similar to MS, Parkinson's disease is also a central nervous system neuropathy. The site of lesion is within the basal ganglia in the subcortical regions of the cerebral hemispheres. Diminished production of the neurotransmitter dopamine results in decreased stimulation of the motor cortex by the basal ganglia, which results in the following symptoms: **bradykinesia, masked facies**, muscle rigidity with diminished range of motion, shuffling gait, stooped posture, and tremors (see Figure 11-10). By comparison with other progressive neurological diseases, Parkinson's disease is fairly common, occurring in approximately 350 to 400 persons per 100,000. In the United States, there are nearly twice as many men than women with Parkinson's disease. Toxins and head trauma (such as what a boxer like Muhammad Ali might experience in his career) are thought to be two etiologies. For many persons with Parkinson's disease, the etiology is **idiopathic**. Primarily because of the bradykinesia, the most common articulation and resonance problems are imprecise consonants (due to articulatory undershooting) and hypernasality. Verbal output is also characterized by difficulty in initiating speech, quick rushes of unintelligible speech (usually mumbled), and **palilalia**. Swallowing problems are also common in persons with Parkinson's disease.

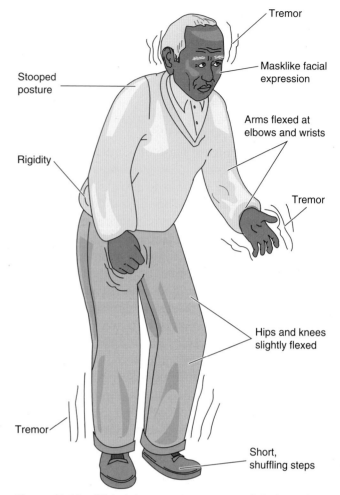

Figure 11-10 Clinical signs seen in a patient with Parkinson's disease. (Modified with permission from Timby, B.K., Smith, N.E. (2003). *Introductory medical–surgical nursing* (8th ed., p. 626). Philadelphia, PA: Lippincott Williams & Wilkins.)

Why You Need to Know

One pathological condition worth noting here is muscular dystrophy (MD). It was not included in the main discussion because technically it is not a neurological disorder. Instead, it is a muscular disorder that affects approximately 15 to 20 persons per 100,000. There are several forms of muscular dystrophy; some affect both males and females while others (e.g., Duchenne MD) affect males almost exclusively. Muscular dystrophy can occur at almost any age, and the severity of symptoms varies across type of MD. Symptoms, however, are chronic, diffuse, and progressive. Although the nervous system typically is not affected by MD, the signs and symptoms of the disorder are similar to what you'd see in many of the degenerative disorders that affect the nervous system. If the structures of the vocal tract are affected, you can expect to see speech (i.e., dysarthria) and swallowing difficulties.

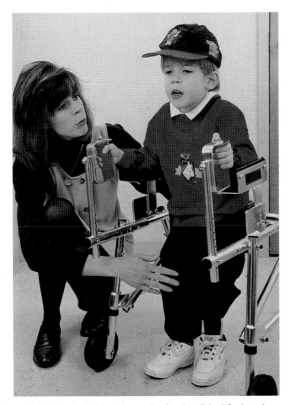

Figure 11-11 A child with cerebral palsy. (Modified with permission from Weber, J., Kelley, J. (2003). *Health assessment in nursing* (2nd ed.). Philadelphia, PA: Lippincott Williams & Wilkins.)

Nonprogressive Neurological Disorders

Cerebral palsy (CP) (see Figure 11-11) is one of the most common nonprogressive neurological disorders and is the most common developmental motor impairment (Best, Bigge, & Sirvis, 1994; Love, 2000). Cerebral palsy is a result of injury to the central nervous system (i.e., the brain) before, during, or soon after birth (Dillow, Dzienkowski, Smith, & Yucha, 1996; Hardy, 1994; Love, 2000). The annual incidence of the disorder is approximately 2 to 2.5 per 1000 live births. There are several types of cerebral palsy. The most common is **spastic** CP, with approximately 50% of all cases being of this type. The **athetoid** type makes up approximately 20% of cases, and the **ataxic** type occurs in approximately 10% of cases. The remaining 20% of cases involve mixed types of cerebral palsy.

Disturbances in speech production may involve the respiratory, phonatory, articulatory, and resonance systems (Bishop, Brown, & Robson, 1990; Dillow et al., 1996; Hardy, 1994; Love, 2000). Persons who have spastic CP may exhibit reduced vital capacity that results in inadequate breath support for speech (in terms of both phonation and articulation). They may also have a degree of hypernasality due to velopharyngeal incompetence. Speech production tends to be slow and laborious, with imprecise articulation especially

for the affricates and fricatives (Love, 2000). Persons with CP of the athetoid variety may exhibit rapid and irregular breathing, and some may even engage in **reverse breathing**. The effect of athetosis on phonation can be quite severe, rendering the person aphonic in the worst cases, and in less severe cases, phonation may be strained and strangled. Poor mobility of the soft palate will result in hypernasality. During articulation, you may observe a person with athetoid CP engaging in exaggerated jaw movements but severely limited tongue movements. These processes will likely result in distortions of the consonants and vowels (in the case of the latter, tongue height is usually not affected but tongue advancement is). Finally, speech characteristics of persons with ataxic CP are similar to what you would expect for ataxic dysarthria due to the incoordination of muscle activity. These include shallow inspiration and lack of expiratory control; imprecise consonants and vowels; inconsistent sound substitutions and omissions; and poor rhythm and reduced prosody of speech. Oral–nasal resonance, on the other hand, tends to be unaffected.

SENSORY DISORDERS THAT MAY AFFECT ARTICULATION AND RESONANCE

There are several sensory impairments that may have an adverse affect on articulation and/or resonance. These include auditory, kinesthetic, and tactile disorders. Of these, only auditory disorders (i.e., hearing impairment) will be presented as an example of how sensory disorders may affect the processes of articulation and resonance.

Hearing Impairment

A final anatomical/physiological correlate to speech sound disorders is hearing impairment. In Chapters 12 and 13, you will learn more about the auditory system and disorders that have an impact upon a person's ability to perceive sound. For this section, you will see the connection between the auditory and speech production systems.

The relationship between hearing impairment and articulatory and resonance disorders cannot be overstated. For persons without hearing impairment, speech production is monitored through several modalities, including the auditory, tactile, and kinesthetic modalities. The auditory channel is the primary means by which we monitor our speech. For those of us who have normal hearing, we are keenly aware of what our voices sound like. To illustrate this, record your voice as you speak. As you are speaking, make note of what your voice sounds like. Then, play back the recording. No doubt you will notice that it does not sound quite the same as when you hear your voice "live." This is because when we speak, our voices are fed back to us through two auditory channels—**air conduction** and **bone conduction**. As your voice leaves your lips, it is transmitted through the air back to your ears (just like it does for anyone else who is near you). However, in addition to receiving feedback in this channel, you are also hearing your own voice through the forced vibrations of your skull as you speak (of course, other people around you do not hear your voice in this manner). When you listen to your voice on a recording, you are only hearing it through air conduction; you lose the bone conduction channel. In other words, when you listen to your voice on a recording, you are essentially hearing it the same way everyone else does. The point in mentioning this is that proper operation of our auditory system is critical to our ability to monitor our speech. You can well imagine that a hearing loss, if severe enough, prevents an individual from monitoring his voice. If he cannot monitor his voice, how is he going to know whether the speech sounds he is producing are accurate? There is still tactile and kinesthetic feedback, but these modalities are secondary to the auditory modality. Loss of the auditory modality will likely have a significant negative impact on the speech production system.

Hearing impairment is described in terms of its type, configuration, and severity. Of particular interest are four types of hearing impairment: central, conductive, mixed, and **sensorineural**. A conductive loss involves the outer and/or middle ears. For some reason, acoustic energy is not being transmitted effectively to the inner ear. This type of hearing loss is reversible. For example, if the etiology is otitis media, it is a relatively simple matter to clear up the infection by a course of antibiotics. Once the infection is cleared, hearing returns to normal. Similarly, if there is damage to the tiny bones of the middle ear (i.e., the ossicles), this can also be addressed through reconstructive surgery. Hearing will then return to normal, essentially. A sensorineural hearing loss, on the other hand, is permanent. In this case, the hair cells within the cochlea (which are necessary to convert mechanical energy from the middle ear into a neural impulse to be sent to the brain via the acoustic nerve) are irreversibly damaged, or the acoustic nerve has some form of pathology. A mixed hearing loss has both a conductive and a sensorineural component. The conductive loss can be corrected, but the sensorineural loss will remain. Finally, a central hearing loss refers to poor auditory reception as a result of central nervous system dam-

age. The hearing mechanism (i.e., outer ear, middle ear, inner ear, and acoustic nerve) is essentially intact, but the neural signal does not make its way to the auditory cortex because of brain damage.

Hearing loss is also described according to its level of severity. Terms such as "mild," "moderate," "severe," and "profound" are often used to describe how severe the hearing loss is. Configuration refers to the extent of the hearing loss in terms of the sound frequencies that are most affected by the loss. For example, a person could have a high frequency hearing loss, a low frequency hearing loss, or a sloping hearing loss (which means that the severity is worse as the frequencies get higher). When it comes to hearing impairment and its effect on speech production, the more severe the loss, the more likely the speech sound system will be adversely affected. Also, you can expect that a hearing loss in the mid-frequencies (i.e., 500, 1000, 2000, and 4000 Hz) will have a greater affect on speech production than other frequencies because the vocal tone consists of these mid-frequencies.

The speech production system may be affected by a hearing loss alone or by a hearing loss that is a component of another anomaly that affects speech. In a previous section of this chapter, you learned that conductive hearing loss is often associated with cleft palate. Because the hard and/or soft palate is compromised, food or drink is susceptible to being injected into the nasopharynx, and from there, bacteria may develop and pass from the Eustachian tube into the middle ear cavity. Otitis media may be the final outcome. In fact, children with cleft palate (or other disorders where the velopharyngeal mechanism is compromised) tend to have recurring bouts of otitis media. You should be able to imagine how these recurring infections and the conductive loss they bring can affect a child's speech sound system, especially if the infections occur often during the speech development period (approximately the first 6 to 8 years of life).

Approximately 1450 persons per 100,000 are deaf. Each year, approximately 1 infant in 1000 will be born with a profound hearing loss. The term "deaf" is used to denote a person whose sense of hearing is essentially nonfunctional. In other words, the hearing loss is likely to be sensorineural (or central), profound, and pervasive across the entire frequency range. Deafness can be congenital or acquired. Some of the most common etiologies are infections, metabolic disorders, neurological disorders, prematurity, toxins, trauma, tumors, and vascular disorders. If the impairment is acquired after the period of speech development, there may be some deterioration of speech sound production and oral–nasal resonance, but for the most part the speech production system will be minimally affected. On the other hand, if the impairment is congenital or acquired before or during the period of speech development, you can expect a greater negative impact on the speech production system. In this case, there may be numerous speech sound errors involving the consonants, diphthongs, and vowels (in fact, the child may have a phonological disorder). Speech sound errors are typically substitutions and omissions (the latter typically occurring for final consonants in words; Abraham, 1989). Other errors may include (1) an inability to distinguish between oral and nasal consonants; (2) frequent substitutions of plosives for fricatives and liquids; (3) an inability to distinguish between voiced and unvoiced consonants; and (4) neutralization of vowels (i.e., the front and back vowels tend to be produced more centrally like the schwa /ə/).

Oral–nasal resonance will also be affected. Persons with profound hearing impairment tend to exhibit a vocal quality known as **cul-de-sac resonance**. The voice of a person who exhibits cul-de-sac resonance will sound "flat" or "muffled." Denasality is also common in persons with profound hearing impairment. There may also be poor coordination between respiration and phonation, resulting in diminished vocal intensity, aberrant stress and intonational patterns, and unusual syntactic phrasing.

Summary

In this chapter, you learned the effect that pathologies of the vocal tract have on the speech production system (i.e., the processes of articulation and resonance). A wide range of pathologies may affect speech sound production and oral–nasal resonance. These include structural disorders, neurological disorders, and sensory disorders. Structural disorders include cleft lip and palate, other craniofacial anomalies such as Apert syndrome, and other structural anomalies such as velopharyngeal incompetence and glossectomy. Neurological disorders were further classified into three groups: cranial nerve damage, motor speech disorders, and other neurological disorders. Motor speech disorders include AOS and dysarthria. You learned that other neurological disorders can be classified as either progressive or nonprogressive. Progressive disorders include ALS, MS, and Parkinson's disease. Cerebral palsy was discussed as an example of a nonprogressive neurological disorder. Finally, hearing impairment was presented as an exemplar of sensory disorders. These disorders have varying effects on an individual's ability to produce speech sounds (consonants, diphthongs, and vowels) and/or to regulate proper oral–nasal resonance. The purpose of this chapter was to instill within you an appreciation of the importance of knowing the anatomy and physiology of the articulatory/resonance system and how pathological conditions may affect speech production and swallowing.

Clinical Teaser—Follow-Up

In Chapter 11, you learned some of the characteristics of Pierre Robin syndrome. You know that it is classified as a craniofacial anomaly. Of primary interest to you are the signs you observed during your evaluation: micrognathia, cleft palate, and glossoptosis. You know that micrognathia means an abnormally small jaw and you also know that glossoptosis is an abnormal downward or backward placement of the tongue. With your knowledge of the articulatory/resonance system and articulatory phonetics, you know there is a strong likelihood that Aidan's untreated cleft palate will adversely affect oral–nasal resonance. Your observations indicate that he does indeed have hypernasality with nasal air emission. The micrognathia and glossoptosis together may have a negative impact on Aidan's ability to produce certain speech sounds. As you know that his habitual tongue placement is too far back, you suspect that he will have difficulty in using the tongue to produce the anterior speech sounds. Aidan's cleft palate is also going to have a negative impact on his speech production, as the excessively diverted air into the nasal cavity will prevent Aidan from generating sufficient intraoral air pressure to produce the pressure consonants—plosives, fricatives, and affricates. Upon administering the *Goldman-Fristoe Test of Articulation*, your suspicions are supported. Aidan exhibited numerous articulation errors, especially in regard to the pressure consonants. Although the *Goldman-Fristoe* does not specifically test vowel sounds, you informally observed that Aidan's productions of the vowels were characterized by pervasive, heavy nasalization; you also noted that he experienced great difficulty in producing the front vowels. Aidan's medical history noted that he had frequent bouts of otitis media. You suspect that the middle ear infections were coming from bacteria that were created by food and drink being injected into the nasopharynx during swallowing.

The primary focus of intervention should be to repair the cleft palate. You predict that by having his cleft palate repaired, several positive outcomes will result: (1) the hypernasality of his voice will decrease or possibly even be eliminated; (2) intraoral air pressure will be restored so that Aidan can produce the pressure consonants; and (3) the ear infections and the conductive hearing loss they create will be dramatically reduced in frequency and number. Once the cleft has been repaired, your focus will be to assist Aidan in acquiring the correct productions of the speech sounds he had in error.

PART 5 SUMMARY

This part provided a thorough description and discussion of the articulatory and resonance system and the pathologies that may affect the integrity of this system. In Chapter 10, you learned that the articulatory/resonance system is composed of the vocal tract, which includes the oral, nasal, and pharyngeal cavities and the structures found within them. These include the lips, teeth, tongue, mandible, alveolar ridge, hard palate, velum, nasal cavity, and pharynx. You learned about the velopharyngeal mechanism and how its function is very important in swallowing and regulating oral-nasal resonance. Finally, you were introduced to the Source-Filter Theory that describes how the vocal tone that is produced by the vocal folds is shaped and formed into speech sounds.

Chapter 11 provided you a thorough discussion of structural, neurological, and sensory pathologies and how they may affect swallowing and speech sound production and/or resonance. Structural problems such as cleft lip and palate or glossectomy can adversely affect the production of many speech sounds and can also affect oral-nasal resonance in a negative manner. Neuropathies also affect an individual's ability to accurately produce speech sounds or to regulate oral-nasal resonance by paralyzing muscles that are necessary for articulation and resonance. Finally, you learned that hearing impairment can also affect articulation and resonance. In general, the more severe the hearing impairment, the more adversely the speech production system will be affected. This is because as hearing impairment becomes more severe, the individual receives even less feedback from the auditory system to allow her to monitor the accuracy and quality of her speech output.

PART 5 REVIEW QUESTIONS

1. Describe the bones of the skull (facial and cranial) and recall as many of the primary landmarks as you can for each bone.
2. What is meant by the term "muscular hydrostat" as a descriptor of the architecture and function of the tongue?
3. Describe the architecture of the velum. How is the architecture of the velum similar to the architecture of the pharynx? List the muscles of the velum and pharynx and explain what they do when they contract.
4. Discuss how the mandibular depressor and elevator muscles can mediate anteroposterior and lateral movements of the jaw.
5. What are the four phases of mastication and deglutition? Describe each phase in as much detail as you can.
6. Explain how Source-Filter Theory accounts for the production of English vowel sounds.
7. How are English vowel sounds classified? What terms are used to describe tongue advancement and tongue height?
8. How are consonants classified? Explain what the terms "place" and "manner" mean.
9. What is velopharyngeal incompetence? Name three pathological conditions in which velopharyngeal incompetence may be an issue.
10. Compare and contrast apraxia of speech and dysarthria.

11. Explain how damage to each of the following muscles can have an adverse effect on speech production: trigeminal; facial; glossopharyngeal; vagus, spinal accessory; hypoglossal.

12. Define "progressive" and "nonprogressive" neurological disorders. Give an example of each one and describe how the disorder may affect speech production.

13. How might a sensory disorder like hearing impairment affect speech production? What would likely result in a more severe articulation disorder—congenital impairment or acquired impairment after the developmental years? Why?

PART 6

Anatomy, Physiology, and Pathology of the Auditory/ Vestibular System

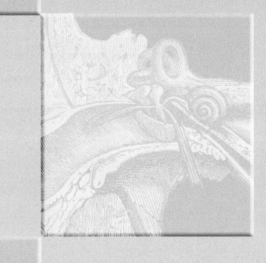

CHAPTER 12

Anatomy and Physiology of the Auditory/Vestibular System

Knowledge Outcomes for ASHA Certification for Chapter 12

- Demonstrate knowledge of the biological basis of the basic human communication processes (III-B)
- Demonstrate knowledge of the neurological basis of the basic human communication processes (III-B)
- Demonstrate knowledge of the acoustic basis of the basic human communication processes (III-B)

Learning Objectives

- You will be able to generalize the anatomical terms used in the study of aural anatomy and physiology.
- You will list and describe the anatomical structures of the conductive auditory mechanism.
- You will list and describe the anatomical structures of the inner auditory mechanism.
- You will list and describe the anatomical structures of the vestibular mechanism.
- You will be able to explain the physiological function of the conductive auditory mechanism.
- You will be able to explain the physiological function of the inner ear in terms of audition and balance.

AFFIX AND PART-WORD BOX

TERM	MEANING	EXAMPLE
audio-	related to hearing	**audio**gram
aur-/auri-	pertaining to the ear	**aur**al; **auri**cular
bi-/bin-	two	**bi**lateral; **bin**aural
contra-	opposite side	**contra**lateral
dB	decibels	60 **dB**
deci-	one-tenth	**deci**bel
Hz	hertz, cycles per second	1000 **Hz**
inter-	between	**inter**aural
intra-	within	**intra**cellular
ipsi-	same side	**ipsi**lateral
mV	millivolts	+80 **mV**
ohms	unit of resistance	41.5 **ohms**
os-/osseo-/osteo-	bone	**osseo**us labyrinth

TERM	MEANING	EXAMPLE
oto-	relating to the ear	**oto**scope
retro-	beyond	**retro**cochlear
-scopy	to look into	oto**scopy**
uni-	one	**uni**lateral
μPa	micropascals	20 **μPa**

Clinical Teaser—Introduction

A 50-year-old father of three, ages 15, 12, and 9, was recently seen by an audiologist for a diagnostic evaluation having been referred by his physician for some very disturbing episodes of dizziness. The first incident took him somewhat by surprise in that he was driving and looking over his shoulder to change lanes. When he turned his head back to center he became so vertiginous that he had to pull over and just sit quietly until the sensation passed, approximately 30 minutes later. He proceeded to drive home but continued to suffer from nausea and lightheadedness upon head turning for the rest of the evening. He reported unsteadiness for the following several days. The next incident was even more eventful and his symptoms seemed to localize to his right ear. Approximately 30 minutes prior to the initiation of the dizziness, his right ear "just closed off" and started roaring. Then the vertigo and nausea began, this time to the point that he actually vomited. By the next morning, he was feeling better. His ear had stopped roaring and it seemed to "open up" but again he had some residual unsteadiness for several days. He did note though that when he goes to sleep at night he can hear a slight noise in his right ear he had not noticed before.

The patient's overall medical condition is good except for some spring hay fever symptoms and the need to lose approximately 40 pounds. The patient states that cola, pizza, and popcorn with lots of butter and salt are his downfall.

His initial audiometric evaluation was unremarkable except for a slight low-frequency hearing loss in his right ear. He was counseled to return for a repeat test when he is having ear symptoms to document any measurable changes.

The patient did return one week later with the presence of a roaring in his right ear and residual unsteadiness from a vertiginous episode the day prior. His right ear hearing thresholds had dropped further in the low frequencies to a mild-moderate level. In light of the progression of his loss and continued symptoms, it was recommended that he be referred to an otologist for a medical evaluation and treatment and return to the audiologist for balance testing.

Are there any terms or concepts in the above case study that are unfamiliar to you? As you read the first chapter in this unit, pay attention to the anatomy and physiology that may be pertinent to this case. You will revisit this case at the end of the second chapter in this part.

Introduction

This unit on the anatomy and pathology of the ear was written by a clinical **audiologist** who has worked for years with physicians identifying hearing disorders. However, it took the labor of teaching students the subject of anatomy, physiology, and pathology to really appreciate the effect one has on the other. This effect is so significant that instruction on the physiology of the auditory system has been blended into the instruction on anatomy in this chapter, as opposed to separating the two topics as has been done in the other chapters in this book. Also within this chapter are Why You Need to Know boxes that contain brief discussions on relevant pathologies, although a more thorough discussion of pathologies will follow in Chapter 13.

You may be interested in the anatomy of the ear from the perspective of a future **speech-language pathologist (SLP)** or audiologist. Not only will the hearing mechanism be discussed in this chapter, but information will also be provided on the primary, basic function of the human inner ear—the balance system. The hearing function of our ear gets the most attention and has a critical purpose for us humans; however, the balance system provides the necessary information to keep us upright and oriented in relation to gravitational forces. Hearing is critical to humans in that it is necessary for the acquisition of our oral communication. We still lack complete understanding of both functions of the ear. This chapter will provide you with the basics of both hearing and balance.

An impairment of the hearing mechanism whether from injury, disease or genetics, often causes a communication problem. Failure to identify hearing loss early in life, no matter the etiology, can have detrimental effects. These effects are seen as delays in speech and language acquisition, difficulties in academic performance, and maladjustment in social emotional development.

INCIDENCE AND PREVALENCE

Knowles Electronics has conducted six MarkeTrak surveys of the United States hearing loss population. The MarkeTrak surveys are then published by the Better Hearing Institute (BHI). The BHI is an independent, not-for-profit corporation that educates the public about the neglected problem of hearing loss and what can be done about it. As summarized by Kochkin (2005), executive director of BHI, the hearing loss population has grown to 31.5 million with continued major increases in the "baby boomers" (persons born between the years 1944 and 1964) and elderly (75+ years of age) brackets. This places the total incidence of hearing loss at approximately 10.4% of the U.S. population. Of the total 31.5 million, there are approximately one million school-aged children in the United States with hearing loss. A little over six million people between 18 and 44 suffer hearing loss from a myriad of either acquired pathologies (e.g., **Ménière's disease**, **otosclerosis**) or hereditary factors (e.g., genetic predisposition). Approximately 12 million baby boomers have some degree of hearing impairment. The incidence of hearing loss for this population is approximately 15%. The incidence of hearing loss increases to 30% to 40% for *all* people over 65 years of age. Using the figures from the MarkeTrak report, the incidence for persons 65 to 74 years of age is approximately 28% and the incidence rises to 29% for persons in the 75 to 84 year age group. Not surprising is the 70% incidence for the 85+ age group. According to the National Institute on Deafness and Other Communication Disorders (1999), approximately 15% of Americans between 20 and 69 years of age suffer from hearing loss as a result of occupational and recreational noise exposure. The high incidence of noise-induced hearing loss is unfortunate as this cause of hearing loss is entirely preventable.

The onset of many hearing disorders is at birth but onset can also be extended into infancy. The cause is split fairly equally between genetic factors and acquired environmental issues (e.g., complications during pregnancy and/or delivery, or **teratogenic** causes). The prevalence of hearing loss is estimated to be 1 to 6 per 1000 newborns and infants (Kemper & Downs, 2000; Northern & Hayes, 1994). Northern and Hayes developed a theoretical model to estimate the overall prevalence of sensorineural hearing loss. Their model includes hearing loss ranging in severity from mild to profoundly deaf and also includes infants with developmental disabilities. The researchers combined the estimate of 3 per 1000 (0.3%) deaf and hard of hearing "well-babies" with the estimate of 30 per 1000 (3.0%) infants "at risk" for developmental disabilities and concomitant hearing loss. (Note that the prevalence of hearing loss in the "at

risk" population is ten times greater than the well-baby population). These indices yield an overall prevalence of hearing loss in newborns and infants of approximately 5.7 per 1000 (0.57%). However, if screening is limited to only the "at risk" population, then almost half of the well-baby nursery population will go unidentified. It was research such as the study discussed above that provided strong evidence for **universal newborn hearing screening** (i.e., screening all newborn babies and infants whether well or at risk). Universal newborn hearing screening programs allow for early identification of hearing loss. The objective of such a program is not only screening by one month of age but also diagnosis of the loss by three months of age *and* enrollment in an appropriate intervention program by six months of age. There is supportive evidence that infants meeting this goal avoid the many delays and difficulties that can be a consequence of hearing loss (Yoshinaga-Itano, Sedey, Coulter, & Mehl, 1998). The clinician should be well versed in the anatomy and physiology of the hearing and balance system to be effective in the assessment and intervention of individuals of all ages with hearing loss.

THE RANGE OF HUMAN HEARING

Study of the etiology of hearing loss consumes a large part of education for audiologists and SLPs. There is a very strong relationship between hearing loss and speech and language problems. Audiologists work to identify hearing loss and SLPs assist in the habilitation of persons with hearing impairment. Both audiologists and speech pathologists must be able to speak a common language and much of the language of communication disorders is derived from the anatomical bases.

The human ear has an incredible ability to detect a wide range of sounds both in terms of frequency (i.e., pitch) and intensity (i.e., loudness). The average frequency range of hearing is from 20 to 20,000 **Hertz (Hz)**; in other words, our ears can detect objects vibrating as few as 20 times per second or as many as 20,000 times per second. In regards to intensity, our ears can respond to a sound pressure wave measuring as little as 20 **micropascals (µPa)** but can withstand (just barely) a pressure wave as intense as 200 million µPa. As such, the pressure of a sound that is as loud as a human can withstand is on the magnitude of approximately 10 million times greater than the pressure for a sound that is barely **audible** to the human ear. This range is expressed on a logarithmic scale of 0 to 140 **decibels (dB)** sound pressure level (SPL). Adding more detail to the above information, human hearing sensitivity is not equal for every frequency. A graph of the required SPL across the hearing sensitivity range is called a minimal **audibility** curve. A curve is an accurate description of the plot points on the XY graph as the lower frequencies (below ~500 Hz) and the higher frequencies (above ~5000 Hz) require more sound pressure to become audible to our ears. Amazingly, the frequency range to which the human ear is most sensitive is approximately the same range as many of our speech sounds (i.e., 125 to 8000 Hz). Can one assume that the speech sounds used in spoken language were selected to take advantage of the frequency range over which our ears are most sensitive? Later in this chapter, there will be a detailed discussion of the physiology of the ear that accounts for the increased sensitivity at a select frequency range.

Why You Need to Know

You are at an electronics store, primed to spend your hard earned dollars on a state-of-the-art sound system. The salesperson is touting the various features of each, selling you on the fact that a particular stereo has a frequency response range up to 30,000 Hz. You are not impressed. You know that the salesperson's pitch is nothing but hype.

You read this chapter before going to the electronics store, so you know that the upper end of the stereo's frequency range is beyond the capacity of the typical human ear to perceive. You know that any frequency above 20,000 Hz will be completely lost on humans. You realize that your pet is going to be the only member of your household who will be able to fully appreciate the entire frequency range of your new stereo system (a dog's hearing range extends to 60,000 Hz and a cat's range extends to 85,000 Hz). You are not willing to spend several hundred dollars on a stereo system only an animal can fully appreciate—even if the animal is your beloved pet!

Anatomy and Physiology of the Auditory and Vestibular Systems

Anatomically, the hearing mechanism can be divided into four parts: **outer ear**, **middle ear**, **inner ear**, and **neural pathway** (see Figure 12-1). The primary struc-

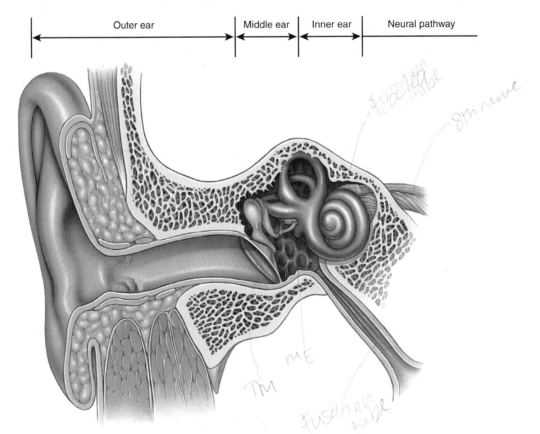

Figure 12-1   Overview of the entire ear with the four anatomical divisions. (1) The outer ear gathers the acoustic pressure wave and directs it to the ear canal. (2) The middle ear acts on the acoustic pressure wave mechanically, contributing by vibrating against the fluid-filled inner ear. (3) The fluid of the inner ear hydromechanically stimulates the specialized structures of hearing transforming the energy to the electrical stimulation received by the neural fibers. (4) The neural pathway carries the electrical energy to the brain, so that the processes of hearing and balance are accomplished. (Reprinted with permission from Anatomical Chart Company.)

tures of the outer ear include the **pinna** (or **auricle**) and the **external auditory meatus** (**EAM**, or **ear canal**). The middle ear consists of the **tympanic membrane** (**TM**; commonly known as the **eardrum**, which forms the boundary between the outer and middle ears), **ossicles** (**malleus, incus**, and **stapes**; collectively known as the **ossicular chain**), **Eustachian** (or **auditory**) **tube**, and the **middle ear cavity** (a space). The inner ear includes the **cochlea**, **vestibule**, and **semicircular canals**. Finally, the neural pathway includes the **vestibulocochlear nerve** (cranial nerve VIII), which consists of the combined cochlear and vestibular branches as it courses through different levels of the brainstem.

The four parts of the auditory system provide their own particular contribution to the pressure wave created by a sound source that is ultimately "heard" by the individual. A pressure wave consists of a repeating pattern of high- and low-pressure regions (relative to atmospheric pressure) moving through a medium. The structures of the ear basically function as an energy transducer converting pressure waves into the electrical energy transmitted to the brain for processing. The outer ear acts on the pressure wave by gathering it into the system. The middle ear then acts on the wave mechanically completing its contribution by vibrating against the fluid-filled inner ear. The fluid within the inner ear hydromechanically stimulates the specialized structures of hearing transforming their energy to the electrical stimulation needed by the neural fibers. The neural fibers carry the electrical energy to the central centers for audition so that hearing can take place.

STRUCTURES OF THE AUDITORY CONDUCTIVE SYSTEM

The anatomical structures of the outer and middle ear are known as the conductive auditory system as they serve to *conduct* the **acoustic** signal to the sensory and neural receptors (i.e., the cochlea and cochlear branch of cranial nerve VIII).

Outer Ear

Pinna and EAM

The pinna or auricle is the most obvious anatomical structure, and is usually what most people think of when a person says the word "ear" (see Figure 12-2). The framework of the pinna is made of cartilage, known as the **auricular cartilage**. There are several muscles that attach the pinna to the head, reverting back to other mammals that turn their ears to localize sound. Most humans have no motor control of these muscles, but there are exceptions. (Every family seems to have one elder relative who likes to entertain small children

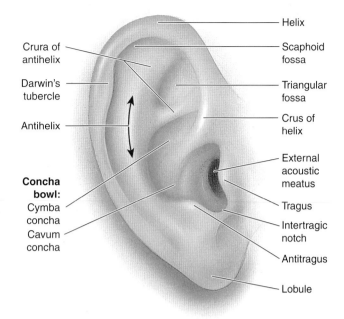

Figure 12-2   Structure of the human pinna (auricle) with pertinent landmarks. (Reprinted with permission from Anatomical Chart Company.)

by voluntarily wiggling their ears.) The **helix** is the outermost portion of the auricular cartilage that curves to form the ear's cupped shape. **Darwin's tubercle** is a cartilaginous protuberance which presents as a thickening on the helix. The tubercle is dominantly inherited but still may or may not be visible. This tubercle is seen as a "throwback" to the higher primates (hence the term Darwin in the name). The helix itself ends inferiorly to form the **lobule** (or **earlobe**). The lobule is the most common site for ear piercing as it is composed of tough connective tissue lacking the firmness and elasticity of cartilage. The lobule has a large blood supply, serving to help warm the ears in cold climates. The earlobe contains many nerve endings and for some people is an erogenous zone. Earlobes elongate slightly with age (and gravity). Human earlobes may be *detached* (*free*) or *attached*. We have our relatives to thank for this characteristic. Free or detached lobes are dominantly inherited and attached earlobes are inherited through recessive gene transmission. The antihelix is another prominent ridge and ends inferiorly to form the **antitragus** which serves to form the lower border of the **concha bowl**. The **tragus** is a flap of cartilage on the anterior wall of the ear canal. Pressing on the tragus serves nicely to close off the canal to dampen unwanted sound. There are no two pinnas alike; even differences exit between the two pinnas of the same individual. It is one part of the aural anatomy that can be easily examined and studied.

The EAM (or ear canal) is continuous with the cartilage of the pinna to about one-third of its depth, but

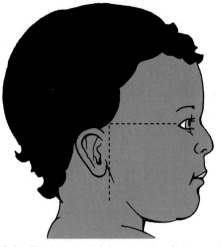

Figure 12-3 The location of the pinna in relation to the other features of the head. Note the alignment of the pinna with the canthus (corner) of the eye. (Reprinted with permission from Nettina, S.M. (2001). *The Lippincott manual of nursing practice* (7th ed.). Baltimore, MD: Lippincott Williams & Wilkins.)

then turns to bone for the remaining two-thirds of its depth (the bone is the temporal bone of the skull). The pinna and EAM reach adult size by about 9 to 12 years of age. The location of the pinna in relation to the other features of the head is very predictable (see Figure 12-3). Moderate deviations of the relationship between the pinna and other facial structures may signal a congenital disorder or syndrome.

The human ear is a paired organ; one benefit of this is in the localization of a sound source. For example, acoustic pressure waves directed toward the right ear will have greater amplitude, contain a broader frequency spectrum, and reach the right ear sooner than the same wave traveling around the head to the left ear opposite from the source. These interaural differences alert the brain and allow humans to locate the source of a sound. The shape of the pinna also acts as a directional microphone. Sounds arriving from behind are dampened slightly compared to sounds that hit the pinna directly from the front. This effect helps us separate the signal from a background sound.

The pinna with the help of the concha bowl (refer back to Figure 12-2) collects and directs the acoustic waves down the EAM. The meatus is basically a tube with the tympanic membrane (TM) being the internal, closed end. Therefore, the ear canal acts as a closed tube resonator having its own **resonant** characteristics. Remembering your high school physics class, certain frequencies will get either enhanced or dampened. The length of the ear canal is approximately 2.5 cm or 25 mm in adults and its diameter of approximately 7 mm will amplify the incoming acoustic wave as much as 20 dB at 2500 Hz. In all, with the addition of the **res-**

onance of the concha bowl, there is a 5 to 20 dB boost of the incoming acoustic wave in the frequency range between 1500 and 7000 Hz.

The pinna and the EAM also have a nonacoustic function. The depth and curvature of the ear canal (a somewhat irregular "S" shape) serves to protect the TM from direct injury. However, small children have been known to place beans, beads, and other various "treasures" down the ear canal.

The ear canal has a self-cleaning function. It is lined with epithelial skin cells. In the ear canal, the skin does not slough off like our other skin cells; instead, the skin migrates along the canal to the entrance from the depth of the eardrum to be sloughed off to the outside. This is called **epithelial migration**. The outer one-third of the canal is also where **cerumen** or ear wax is produced. Cerumen, a yellowish-brown, waxy substance is the normal product of sebaceous glands (i.e., sweat glands) secreting their oily substance onto the cilia, the fine hairs located at the entrance to the canal. Together they protect the canal by repelling water and expelling the dead skin cells. Cerumen is also slightly acidic, which discourages the growth of bacteria and fungi that would otherwise grow in the warm moist environment of the ear canal. For the most part, cerumen build-up is not a problem. The dead skin migrates to the entrance of the ear canal. The action of the cilia, plus the mechanical action of the jaw during talking and chewing, serves to massage the cerumen out of the canal. Impaction of cerumen is typically caused by one's attempt to mechanically clean the canal with a cotton-tip applicator or other ominous tool (your grandmother was correct when she told you not to place anything smaller than your elbow down your ear canal). To inspect for cerumen one performs **otoscopy** using an **otoscope**. The "S" curve of the canal will need to be straightened out. This is accomplished by pulling the helix up and back. This will direct the light of the otoscope down the canal for visualization of its contents and the eardrum.

Middle Ear

Tympanic Membrane

The TM (or eardrum) defines the border between the outer and middle ear (see Figure 12-4). It is a true membrane in that it is very thin, having a very small mass. A healthy TM is a relatively transparent, pearl-gray allowing the observer to identify several structures behind it in the middle ear. Its thinness and small mass make it very mobile, yet it is also very sturdy. The TM resides at an approximate 55° angle at the end of the ear canal. It is slightly taller than it is wide and is concave in shape

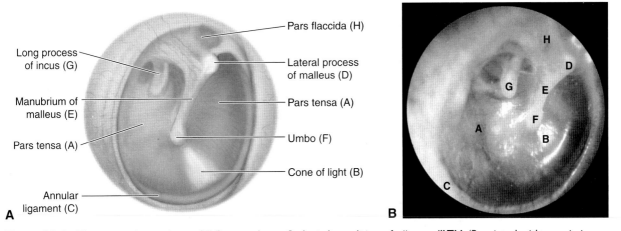

Long process of incus (G)

Pars flaccida (H)

Manubrium of malleus (E)

Lateral process of malleus (D)

Pars tensa (A)

Pars tensa (A)

Umbo (F)

Cone of light (B)

Annular ligament (C)

A

B

Figure 12-4   The tympanic membrane (TM) or eardrum. **A**. Artist's rendition of a "normal" TM. (Reprinted with permission from Tank, P.W., Gest. T.R. (2008). *Lippincott Williams & Wilkins atlas of anatomy*. Baltimore: Lippincott Williams & Wilkins.) **B**. A "normal" TM (*in vivo*) with visible landmarks. Using otoscopy, the observer should be able to identify several structures that lie behind a healthy TM. (Reprinted with permission from Moore, K.L., Agur, A. (2002). *Essential clinical anatomy* (2nd ed.). Philadelphia: Lippincott Williams & Wilkins.)

so that its center is displaced medially, toward the structures of the middle ear cavity. For most of its circumference, the TM fits in a small sulcus in the bony wall of the EAM called the **annular** or **tympanic sulcus**. Since the outer ring of the TM is fixed into the sulcus, not all of the surface of the TM can vibrate. The effective vibrating area of the TM is approximately 55 mm².

The TM consists of three layers. The central fibrous layer of the TM accounts for its sturdiness. This central or intermediate layer is comprised of radial and circular fibers held together by connective tissue, and sandwiched between the two remaining layers. The outermost (i.e., lateral) layer consists of a thin epithelium that is continuous with the lining of the ear canal. The innermost or medial layer is a mucous membrane that is continuous with the lining of the middle ear cavity. The fibers of the intermediate (i.e., middle) layer are found mostly throughout the TM except in a small superior portion. Because of the sparseness of the fibers in this superior region, it is referred to as the **pars flaccida**. The remaining fibrous portion of the TM is known as the **pars tensa**. The pars flaccida is not acoustically active, but serves to equalize pressure by moving outward when the air in the middle ear cavity is compressed by inward movement of the pars tensa, serving in essence as a relief valve.

Otoscopy is the primary means of inspecting the TM. Visualized on a healthy TM are the tiny blood vessels that course its surface. Another landmark seen when performing otoscopy is the **cone of light**, which is the reflection of the otoscope light due to the concavity of the TM. The cone of light will be present at approximately 5 o'clock for the right ear and 7 o'clock for the left. Many physicians use the pres-

ence or absence of the cone of light to aid in their diagnosis of middle ear disease. In cases of disease due to poor ventilation of the middle ear cavity, the TM tends to displace medially or inward due to the negative pressure within the middle ear cavity. This typically causes the cone of light to be absent during otoscopy. When there is an absence of the cone of light, many physicians will report that the eardrum looks "dull."

Why You Need to Know

*Poor ventilation from Eustachian tube dysfunction results in negative pressure within the middle ear cavity. The pars flaccida region of the TM may become displaced inward. When this condition becomes problematic, the physician must attempt to equalize the negative pressure within the middle ear cavity to the more positive atmospheric pressure. This is done by placing a **pressure equalization (PE) tube** in the TM. The pars tensa is the region where these tubes are placed because of its ability to retain the PE tube for a relatively long period of time. The epithelial tissue of the eardrum will eventually grow under the tube and expel it from the surface. The TM can spontaneously perforate from infection or be perforated from trauma. It can usually heal itself from small perforations but when a large perforation typically does not heal on its own, a surgical procedure called a **tympanoplasty** can be performed. The middle ear is naturally sealed off from water exposure, so when a TM perforation allows water (and the bacteria that accompany it) to enter the middle ear space, it can lead to an increased risk of middle ear infection.*

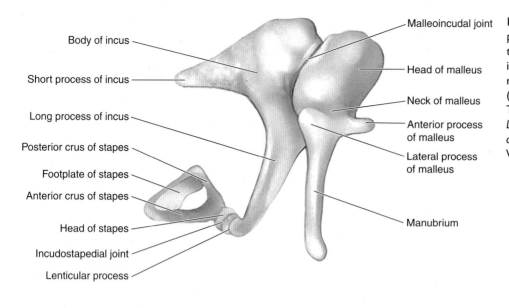

Body of incus

Short process of incus

Long process of incus

Posterior crus of stapes

Footplate of stapes

Anterior crus of stapes

Head of stapes

Incudostapedial joint

Lenticular process

Malleoincudal joint

Head of malleus

Neck of malleus

Anterior process of malleus

Lateral process of malleus

Manubrium

Figure 12-5 The ossicles with pertinent landmarks. Located in the middle ear space, the malleus, incus, and stapes are collectively referred to as the ossicular chain. (Reprinted with permission from Tank, P.W., & Gest, T.R. (2008). *Lippincott Williams & Wilkins atlas of anatomy*. Baltimore: Lippincott Williams & Wilkins.)

Ossicular Chain

Portions of the ossicles can be identified through the transparent TM during otoscopy. The cavity medial to the TM is called the middle ear cavity or space. Located within the space is a chain of three linked bones. Collectively they are referred to as the ossicular chain, or ossicles (see Figure 12-5). These three bones are among the smallest in the entire human body; one can place all three bones on the surface of a dime and still have room to spare! As one proceeds medially from the TM, the first and largest bone in the chain is called the malleus which is approximately 9 mm in length. During otoscopy, one can see the long process of the malleus, called the **manubrium**. The manubrium appears as an opaque whitish streak behind the TM coursing downward at about one o'clock in the right ear and 11 o'clock in the left. The manubrium is firmly attached to the medial surface of the TM. It is the manubrium that draws the TM inward toward the middle ear space giving the TM its concave shape. The most depressed part of this concavity is named the **umbo**. In addition to the manubrium, there are two projections off the malleus called processes. They are the anterior and lateral processes, named for the location of their anatomical directions. The lateral process is in the anterosuperior quadrant of the TM, and appears as if it is "pointing" at the observer when seen through a healthy, transparent TM. The anterior process cannot usually be visualized with otoscopy. The pars tensa and pars flaccida appear to be divided by a fold, known as the **malleolar fold**, running along the upper portion of the TM. This fold is created by an anterior attachment of a ligament band to the anterior process of the manubrium and a posterior attachment of a ligament band to the lateral process of the manubrium.

The second bone in the ossicular chain is the incus. It weighs slightly more than the malleus but is shorter, being approximately 7 mm in length. Using otoscopy, only a portion of the incus, its **long process**, can be visualized through a healthy transparent TM. The long process hangs down parallel to the manubrium and the **short process** of the incus projects posteriorly. The body of the incus and the bulky head of the malleus cannot be seen while performing otoscopy. They are suspended above the level of the TM in the uppermost region of the middle ear cavity called the **epitympanic recess**, or **attic**. The head of the malleus and body of the incus articulate with each other, forming the **malleoincudal joint**. There appears to be only limited range of motion of this joint.

The third and most medial bone in the ossicular chain is the stapes. The stapes is not only the smallest of the three bones that comprise the ossicular chain, but is also the smallest bone in the human body, at a mere 3.5 mm in length. The angle of the stapes, along with its distance medially from the TM, makes it invisible to the otoscope. The head of the stapes articulates with the **lenticular process** of the incus, forming the **incudostapedial joint**.

The neck of the stapes bifurcates to become the **anterior crus** and **posterior crus**. The two **crura** form

> ### Why You Need to Know
> *Chronic middle ear disease or traumatic injury can fairly easily disrupt the incudostapedial joint, causing a disarticulation. This condition results in a moderate loss in the conduction of sound to the inner ear. Surgeons may attempt to repair the integrity of the chain by reconstructing the damaged ossicles.*

an arch in their attachment to the base, which is called the **footplate**. The footplate of the stapes inserts into the **oval window** and is sealed by the elastic **annular ligament** in much the same way as the TM is held in place within the tympanic sulcus. The annular ligament firmly holds the footplate in place while still allowing for efficient vibration within the oval window.

The bones of the ossicular chain are suspended by ligaments attached to strategic places within the walls of the middle ear cavity. These attachments take place in most anatomical directions: lateral, anterior, superior, and posterior. The ligaments are designed to suspend the ossicular chain without interfering with its vibratory efficiency.

Stapedius and Tensor Tympani Muscles

Two important striated muscles attach themselves to two of the three ossicles. The **stapedius tendon** inserts onto the neck of the stapes, hence its name. The body of the **stapedius muscle** is deeply embedded in bone arising from the posterior wall of the middle ear cavity; only its tendon emerges from a bony projection, the **pyramidal eminence**, to attach to the stapes. The stapedius muscle is innervated by its own branch of the facial nerve (cranial nerve VII). The muscle serves to contract in response to sudden loud sounds. Muscle action rotates the stapes in a posterior direction. The **tensor tympani** tendon enters the middle ear cavity from the anterior wall. Similarly to the stapedius muscle, the body of the tensor tympani muscle is housed within a bony canal so that only its tendon enters the middle ear space. The tendon of the tensor tympani muscle attaches to the neck of the malleus. The tensor tympani is innervated by the trigeminal nerve (cranial nerve V). When this muscle contracts, it pulls the malleus in an anteromedial plane reducing the range of motion of the TM. The dual action of stapedius and tensor tympani contraction (termed the **acoustic reflex**) serves to stiffen the ossicular chain, thereby reducing the admittance of the acoustic signal particularly for lower frequency sounds. Therefore, contraction of these muscles is theorized to be a protective mechanism for the cochlea by preventing the stapes from excessively vibrating in the oval window (to be discussed later). However, for most humans the response time for this action is too slow to prevent hearing damage from exposure to sudden, excessive sound (e.g., a shotgun blast or a firecracker exploding).

Why You Need to Know

Audiologists measure the intensity level that triggers the acoustic reflex contraction by monitoring the change in the admittance of the stimulus. On average, it takes 85 dB SPL to elicit a contraction of the stapedius muscle (Gelfand, 1984). The presence or absence of the stapedius reflex contraction is an indirect measure of the integrity of both the cochlear nerve (cranial nerve VIII) and facial nerve (cranial nerve VII) at the level of the lower brainstem (Borg, 1973). The intense acoustic stimulus must travel the reflex arc intact through the cochlear nerve, along the auditory pathway to the level of the superior olivary complex *to communicate with the nuclei of the facial nerve, so that the stimulus will trigger a response from the stapedius muscle. There are several pathological lesions that can interrupt the normal acoustic reflex circuit. For example, a lesion on cranial nerve VII or VIII can elevate the intensity level necessary for contraction or eliminate the muscle contraction altogether. Audiologists utilize a special instrument for testing the acoustic reflex, called an* immittance meter.

Middle Ear Cavity

The middle ear cavity is an air-filled space lined with a mucous membrane. It is located in the petrous portion of the temporal bone of the skull and is approximately two cubic centimeters (2 cm³) in volume. The middle ear cavity is surrounded on all sides by bone except its lateral wall, which houses the TM. It is best known for housing the ossicles but has numerous other significant landmarks. The space as a whole is more hourglass-shaped than cube-shaped as shown in Figure 12-6. It is taller than it is wide, with a narrowing in the middle and a wider space inferiorly and superiorly. The wide upper space of the cavity is known as the epitympanic recess or attic. As mentioned earlier, the epitympanic recess is where the head of the malleus and the body of the incus reside.

For the purpose of examination, the middle ear cavity will be referenced by its walls in the various anatomical directions. The entire lateral wall of the cavity is occupied by the TM. By removing the lateral wall, the remaining contents of the middle ear cavity can be examined. Along the posterior wall in the area of the epitympanic recess is the **aditus**. The aditus is the passageway that leads to the air cells within the mastoid process of the temporal bone of the skull. The air in the middle ear cavity communicates through this passageway with the mastoid air cells. The purpose of the air cells is simply to lessen the weight of the head, since the temporal bone is not solid. If the petrous portion of the temporal bone was solid, the human head would weigh several ounces more than

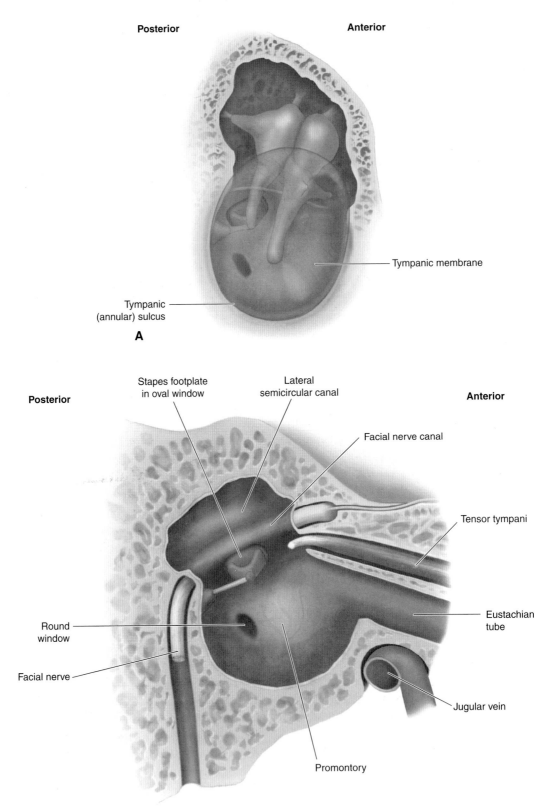

Figure 12-6 The middle ear cavity. Its contents are referenced by its walls in the various anatomical directions. Illustrated are four views of the middle ear cavity. **A.** The tympanic membrane (TM) comprises the lateral wall. Looking into the ear canal, some structures of the middle ear cavity can be viewed through the transparent TM. (Reprinted with permission from Tank, P.W., Gest, T.R. (2008). *Lippincott Williams & Wilkins atlas of anatomy.* Baltimore: Lippincott Williams & Wilkins.) **B.** A view of the medial wall of the cavity with the TM, malleus, and incus removed. (Reprinted with permission from Tank, P.W., Gest, T.R. (2008). *Lippincott Williams & Wilkins atlas of anatomy.* Baltimore: Lippincott Williams & Wilkins.) *(continued)*

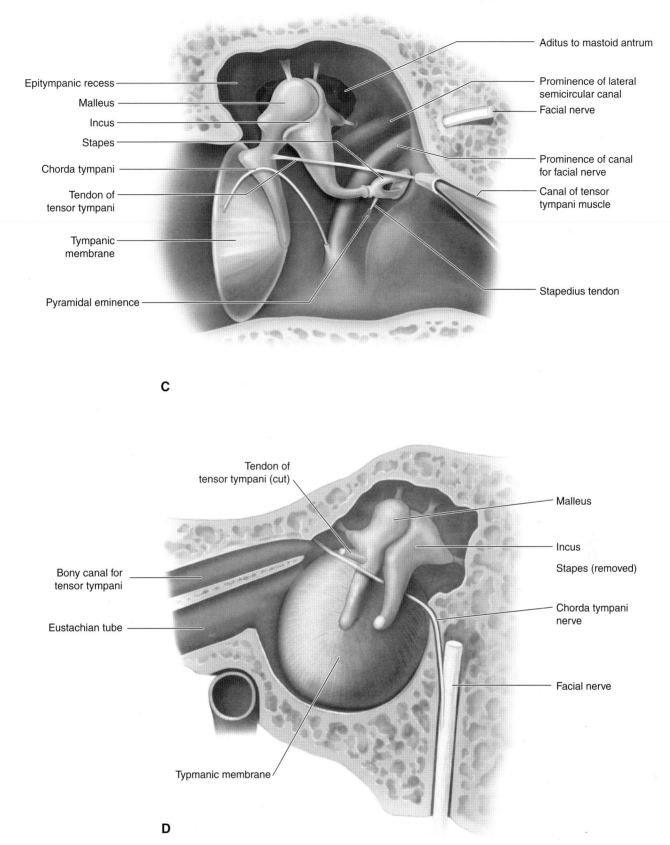

Figure 12-6 (*Continued*) **C**. Coronal section of the cavity facing the posterior mastoid wall. (Modified with permission from Moore, K.L., Dalley, 0A.F., Agur, A.M. (2009). *Clinically oriented anatomy* (6th ed.). Baltimore: Lippincott Williams & Wilkins.) **D**. Inside the middle ear cavity looking laterally at the tympanic membrane. (Reprinted with permission from Tank, P.W., Gest, T.R. (2008). *Lippincott Williams & Wilkins atlas of anatomy.* Baltimore: Lippincott Williams & Wilkins.)

it does. Another significant landmark on the posterior wall just below the level of the aditus is the pyramidal eminence of the stapedius muscle.

The inferior or jugular wall (i.e., the floor) of the middle ear cavity is relatively unremarkable. It consists of a thin plate of bone which separates the tympanic cavity from the **jugular bulb** that lies just beneath its surface. The superior wall, also called the **tegmental wall** or roof, is not known for any specific landmark but is significant in that only a thin plate of bone separates the middle ear cavity from the cranial cavity where the brain resides. Severe or chronic infection in the middle ear space could lead to an abscess in this wall resulting in an infection invading the brain. From studying the areas surrounding the middle ear cavity, it is obvious that complications of recurrent untreated infection can result in mastoiditis or brain abscess.

The remaining walls of the middle ear space have numerous relevant landmarks. The anterior wall is noted for the orifice (i.e., entrance) of the **Eustachian tube (ET)**. The ET orifice is bone that is continuous with the middle ear wall but the ET terminates in the nasopharynx as cartilage. This structure will be examined more thoroughly later. Parallel to the ET runs the tensor tympani muscle. The tensor tympani muscle and the orifice of the ET are separated by a thin curved projection or process of bone called the **cochleariform process**. The tendon of the tensor tympani passes over this process as it exits the anterior wall on its way to attach to the malleus, and in doing so it gains a little leverage when contracting the ossicles. Running along the outside of the anterior wall is a portion of the carotid canal.

Within this area of the middle ear space, the facial nerve is housed in a bony canal. The canal runs from the anterior wall superior to the cochleariform process, then curves across within the medial wall and turns downward to exit deep into bone on the posterior wall. In this immediate area are three branches of the facial nerve. Two of the three deserve mention: the **stapedial branch** and the **chorda tympani** branch. The chorda tympani conveys taste sensation from the anterior two-third of the tongue. It traverses the middle ear cavity between the long process of the incus and the manubrium of the malleus. The stapedial branch innervates the stapedius muscle. When otologists perform ear surgery, they are careful to identify the facial nerve canal as well as the branches of the facial nerve. Surgeons try not to disturb the chorda tympani although it can tolerate being displaced somewhat during a procedure. The patient may experience some odd metallic taste sensations during post-operative recovery. The facial nerve canal is strictly avoided during any surgical procedure. If the facial nerve is disturbed, the patient can suffer permanent facial weakness or paralysis.

The medial wall, also known as the **labyrinthine wall**, contains landmarks related to the inner ear. Most notable is the oval window. The oval window separates the air-filled middle ear cavity from the fluid-filled contents of the inner ear. The footplate of the stapes rests in the oval window in an anteroposterior orientation and is held in place by the annular ligament. There appears to be a greater degree of attachment of the footplate anteriorly than posteriorly. As mentioned previously, although the footplate is held in place by the annular ligament, it does not adversely affect the vibratory action of the ossicular chain onto the oval window. The vibratory action appears to be more like a swinging gate rather than a plunger motion.

Why You Need to Know

*The stapes may become attached or "fixed" to the surrounding bone by abnormal bone growth. The bone growth is not life threatening and often the only symptom is a roaring **tinnitus** and a resultant hearing loss. The condition, known as **otosclerosis**, is typically identified using **audiometry** and **immittance measures**. The bone growth can be removed and a prosthetic device can be used to "replace" the stapes, thereby restoring the integrity of the ossicular chain.*

A second structure leading to the inner ear (specifically the cochlea) is also located along the medial wall of the middle ear cavity. It is the **round window**. The round window separates the middle ear cavity from the **scala tympani**, a duct within the cochlea. The round window is covered by a flexible membrane. Vibration of the stapes in the oval window compresses the fluid within the cochlea, thereby creating a wave. The inward movement of the stapes footplate is allowed because the round window membrane yields to the fluid wave by bulging toward the middle ear cavity. Between the oval and round windows is the **promontory**, a distinctive bulge in the wall created by the first (i.e., basal) turn of the cochlea on the other side.

Superior to the oval window is the bony prominence of the lateral or horizontal semicircular canal of the vestibular system. The prominence is seen as a bulge on the medial wall. The prominence is thin and can be eroded with severe chronic middle ear disease causing infection to invade the vestibular system. The facial nerve canal (discussed earlier) runs across the medial wall to exit on the posterior wall. It runs between the **lateral semicircular canal** prominence and the oval window.

Contained within the middle ear space are all the attachments that serve to suspend and balance the ossicles. There are eight in all. Three ligaments suspend the malleus: superior, anterior, and lateral malleolar ligaments. The tendon of the tensor tympani muscle also serves to suspend the malleus. The malleus is attached laterally to the TM. The incus is suspended in place by the posterior and superior incudal ligaments. The stapes is suspended in the oval window by the annular ligament and is also suspended by the tendon of the stapedius muscle. These attachments balance the ossicles so that the rotational axis is very near to the center of gravity (CoG). This arrangement allows the TM and ossicular chain to operate as a unit. The TM and ossicles initiate and cease vibration synchronously.

Eustachian Tube

The orifice of the ET was mentioned as a landmark within the anterior wall of the middle ear cavity. It was named for the Italian anatomist and physician Eustachius who lived in the mid-1500s. The ET is the passageway leading from the nasopharynx (just above the soft palate in proximity to the uppermost region of the pharynx) to the anterior wall of the middle ear cavity. The ET opens to replenish the air in the middle ear cavity. For the middle ear to function optimally, the ET must equalize the air pressure within the middle ear and the "atmospheric" air pressure that inhabits the ear canal and impinges upon the eardrum. Atmospheric pressure can vary greatly. For example, air pressure is much lower on Pike's Peak in Colorado than in New Orleans, a city that is predominantly below sea level. The ET allows humans to withstand these great variances in air pressure so that the hearing mechanism will function properly.

The middle ear portion of the ET (i.e., the orifice) is open and fixed within the temporal bone. As one proceeds toward the nasopharynx, the bone gives way to cartilage (approximately one-third of its length is bone, with the final two-thirds being cartilage). Where the bone transitions into cartilage, the ET becomes quite narrow in a region called the **isthmus**. The cartilaginous portion of the ET normally remains closed at rest and opens by the action of two muscles—the **levator veli palatini** and the **tensor veli palatini**.

The ET is approximately 35 mm (3.5 cm) in length in adults. The adult ET is angled downward and forward to set at about a 45° angle. In children the tube is in a more horizontal position. As the child's head grows, it elongates and migrates into a more vertical position. The ET terminates in the nasopharynx where it is surrounded by lymphoid tissue known as the **adenoids**.

Why You Need to Know

Based on work by researchers such as Brodsky and Koch (1993), it has been demonstrated that the adenoids can contribute to recurrent or chronic ear disease as they can harbor a chronic infection. The tissue swells as it reacts to bacteria or other pathogens. In children who have suffered multiple upper respiratory infections (URIs), the adenoids are often very large. The enlarged lymphoid tissue may block the nasopharyngeal opening of the Eustachian tube (ET). Since the ET passageway is lined with mucous membrane, a URI can also cause inflammation of the mucosa leading to further obstruction. An inflamed ET cannot open, and therefore cannot equalize the air pressure within the middle ear to outside atmospheric air pressure. The air pressure in the middle ear space then becomes negative by comparison to outside air pressure. The negative air pressure will cause the mucous membrane that lines the middle ear cavity to secrete fluid. The fluid fills the middle ear space, negatively impacting the ossicular chain by adversely affecting its ability to vibrate. A temporary conductive hearing loss is a very likely outcome of this condition.

The levator veli palatini and tensor veli palatini wrap around the cartilaginous portion of the ET. The two muscles serve a dual purpose in that they assist in opening the cartilaginous ET as well as act upon the soft palate (i.e., velum). It is not known exactly how the muscles open the ET but many anatomists believe that the tensor veli palatini is responsible for dilation whereas the levator veli palatini pulls the cartilage in a medial direction along with the uvula.

When the ET opens, atmospheric air rushes through to replenish the middle ear space. The ET can be forced to open by the **valsalva maneuver**, but natural opening of the ET takes place during yawning, swallowing, chewing or talking. At the same time the ET dilates, the soft palate is raised (primarily by the action of the levator veli palatini) to block or separate the nasal cavity from the oral cavity. The raising of the soft palate shields the ET from food or drink in the oral cavity so that they are not injected into the nasal passageway and out of the nose and/or into the middle ear cavity via the ET. The raising of the soft palate closes off ventilation from the oropharynx and ensures that only nasally inhaled air passes through to the middle ear.

Why You Need to Know

Years ago, surgeons looked for a way to surgically repair a poor functioning Eustachian tube. All attempts failed. It did not appear that correction of negative middle ear pressure could be accomplished by surgical intervention. Surgeons then began to examine other ways in which negative middle ear pressure could be alleviated. Pressure equalization (PE) tubes were first developed to assist combat pilots in equalizing middle ear pressure. They are now commonplace for children who suffer from chronic Eustachian tube dysfunction. Complications from middle ear disease occur less frequently now because the surgeon can bypass the dysfunctional ET by placing PE tubes through the tympanic membrane to equalize pressure via the ear canal.

Why You Need to Know

*Chronic **patulous** (i.e., open) Eustachian tubes can cause a patient severe difficulty. The patulous tube acts as a sound conduit, directing our own vocalizations and breathing up into the middle ear cavity. Patients have an awareness of these sounds (known as **autophonia**) as well as an awareness that their tympanic membranes are vibrating with inhalation and exhalation (Mencher, Gerber, & McCombe, 1997). This can be very disconcerting to the patient. This condition may result from dramatic weight loss or chronic use of decongestants. Historically, physicians have not been very successful at relieving patients' symptoms.*

Transformer Action of the TM and Ossicular Chain

It was previously discussed how the ear canal is capable of amplifying an incoming pressure wave. Once again, thanks to physics, we will see how the TM and the ossicular chain work together to further contribute to the amplification of the acoustic signal. The purpose of the TM and ossicular chain is to transform the acoustic pressure waves that hit the TM into mechanical energy that in turn can be used to set up hydraulic pressure waves within the inner ear. When this **transformer action** takes place, the net result is amplification of intensity of the incoming signal of approximately 27 dB. While the middle ear is transforming the acoustic waves to fluid waves, it is overcoming the resistance of the outside air to the fluid-filled inner ear. Because air and fluid have different densities, there is an **impedance mismatch** between the two mediums. Physics teaches us that for energy to flow with the least resistance (i.e., impedance) or the least amount of energy loss, it must flow continuously through a *similar* medium. Air functions at a resistance of 41.5 **ohms** and cochlear fluid at a resistance of 161,000 ohms, representing a differential ratio of 3880:1 (Wever & Lawrence, 1954). Obviously, the impedance properties of these two media are very different. If the ear had no way of matching these resistances (i.e., making the differences smaller), only one-tenth of 1% of the sound carried on the air pressure wave would pass to fluid, whereas the remaining 99.9% would be reflected back through the outer ear. Therefore, one of the primary functions of the ossicular chain is to act as a mechanical transformer. It accomplishes this in three very distinct ways: **area advantage, curved membrane buckling**, and **lever action**.

The area advantage is the largest contributor to the transformer action of the middle ear.

As illustrated in Figure 12-7, one way to increase pressure is to decrease the area that the force is being distributed across (**pressure = force/area**). The effective vibrating area of the TM is 55 mm^2, whereas the area of the oval window by comparison is about 3.2 mm^2. This means that the area of the TM is 17 times larger than the area of the oval window. By focusing all the acoustic energy from the TM to a smaller area

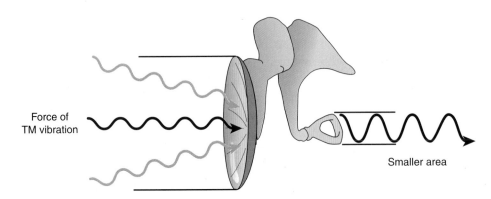

Force of TM vibration

Smaller area

Figure 12-7   The large vibrating area of the tympanic membrane in relation to the smaller vibrating area of the oval window (pressure = force/area). (Modified with permission from Emanuel, D.C., Letowski, T. (2007). *Hearing science.* Philadelphia: Lippincott Williams & Wilkins.)

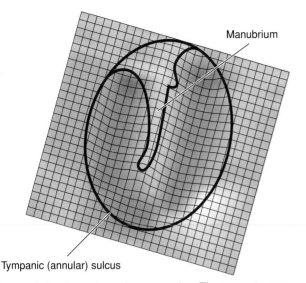

Figure 12-8 Curved membrane coupling. The tympanic membrane vibrates in multiple segments.

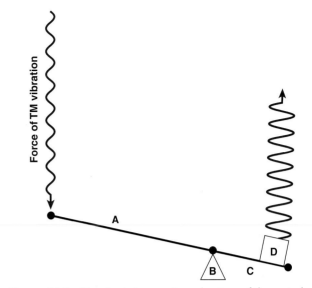

Figure 12-9 The simple lever action advantage of the ossicular chain. **A**. Longer leg (manubrium). **B**. Fulcrum or pivot point (malleoincudal joint). **C**. Shorter leg (long process of incus). **D**. Mass (stapes footplate in the oval window).

(the oval window), pressure is increased considerably. The 17:1 size differential of the TM to the oval window translates into an increase of acoustic pressure of about 25 dB (Bekesy, 1960).

The second variable in transformer action is curved membrane buckling, as illustrated in Figure 12-8. The TM does not vibrate as a whole unit. Instead, it vibrates in segments, with those portions that are least anchored being more readily set into vibration. The segments of the TM closer to the annular sulcus and the manubrium are more resistant to displacement. The force displacing the TM is distributed in multiple segments rather than being displaced in one large segment. This action serves to increase pressure.

The last impedance matching function is accomplished by the ossicular chain acting as a class 1 lever. As Figure 12-9 shows, the efficiency of a lever is increased when the pivot point is placed closer to the load being displaced. In this case the long leg of the lever is the manubrium, the pivot point is the malleoincudal joint, the long process of the incus is the shorter section of our lever, and the load being displaced is the stapes in the oval window. In the end, only a slight amount of pressure placed on the manubrium is necessary to yield an increase in pressure at the oval window. This lever action effect adds an additional gain of 2 dB to the acoustic signal (Wever & Lawrence, 1954). With all three transformer variables acting together, the result is a gain of approximately 27 to 30 dB for the incoming signal. Any disease process or injury that might disrupt even one of these events will result in a significant loss of hearing by adversely affecting the transformer action of the middle ear.

STRUCTURES OF THE INNER EAR LABYRINTH

The inner ear is also referred to as the **labyrinth** because of its maze-like complex structure. It contains the end organs of two sensory systems: the vestibular system and the auditory system.

The inner ear is housed deep in the petrous portion of the temporal bone of the skull. As Figure 12-10 illustrates, the inner ear itself is divided into three sections: (1) the cochlea of the auditory system, (2) the vestibule of the vestibular system, and (3) the semicircular canals

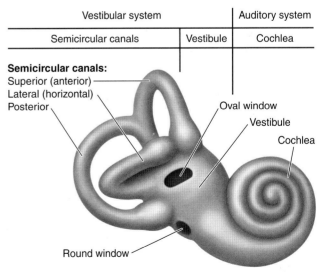

Vestibular system		Auditory system
Semicircular canals	Vestibule	Cochlea

Figure 12-10 The two systems and the three sections of the inner ear. (Reprinted with permission from Tank, P.W., Gest, T.R. (2008). *Lippincott Williams & Wilkins atlas of anatomy*. Baltimore: Lippincott Williams & Wilkins.)

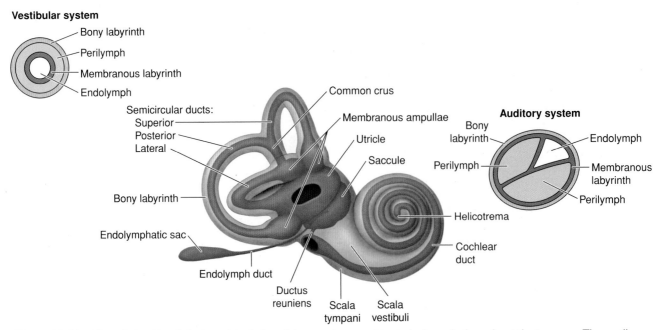

Figure 12-11 The relationship of the bony labyrinth and the membranous labyrinth channels throughout the inner ear. The small views depict how the membranous labyrinth fits within the bony labyrinth of the vestibular system and how within the cochlea the membranous channel is pulled to one side with attachments to the bony labyrinth. These attachments divide the bony labyrinth into two sections, one above and one below the membranous labyrinth. (Reprinted with permission from Tank, P.W., Gest, T.R. (2008). *Lippincott Williams & Wilkins atlas of anatomy.* Baltimore: Lippincott Williams & Wilkins.)

of the vestibular system. The entire inner ear, whether the vestibular system or the auditory system, is housed within a bony (osseous) labyrinth or capsule. Contained within the bony labyrinth is a chambered membranous, epithelium-lined channel. The membranous labyrinth fits within the bony labyrinth and follows its contours. This is mostly true for the vestibular system. However, as seen in Figure 12-11, the channels within the cochlea have a slightly different orientation. All of the channels found within both the bony and membranous labyrinths are filled with fluid.

The two fluids of the inner ear are **perilymph** and **endolymph**. Each fluid has its own distinct chemistry. Perilymph fills the channel formed between the outer wall of the membranous labyrinth and the inner wall of the bony labyrinth. Perilymph resembles the chemistry of extracellular fluid, being high in sodium (Na^+) and calcium (Ca^{++}) and low in potassium (K^+). Endolymph, the fluid within the membranous labyrinth, has a high potassium (K^+) content and low sodium (Na^+) and calcium (Ca^{++}) concentration. The endolymphatic fluids of the membranous labyrinth of the vestibular and auditory systems are interconnected by a series of ducts forming one continuous endolymph filled system—the **ductus reuniens** and another small diversion, the **endolymphatic sac**. The endolymphatic sac lies in a bony niche within the cranium. Nowhere do the endolymph and the perilymph fluids of the two labyrinths communicate with one another.

Structures of the Vestibular System

Vestibule

The vestibule is the central egg-shaped cavity of the inner ear. The vestibule lies medial to the middle ear, having the oval window as its lateral border. Suspended within the perilymph is the vestibule's membranous labyrinth. Within the membranous labyrinth are two end organs known as the **utricle** and **saccule**.

The saccule lies on the medial wall and is continuous with the cochlea. The utricle is the larger of the two and is continuous with the semicircular canals. The semicircular canals open into the utricle by way of five openings. The posterior and anterior semicircular canals share one opening at the **common crus**. Figure 12-12 shows a cutaway of the utricle and saccule exposing the receptor end organ called the **macula**. The two maculae are oriented so that they are at right angles to each other. The macula of the utricle responds to horizontal stimulation and the macula of the saccule responds to vertical stimulation. The major role then of the utricle and saccule is to keep the body vertically oriented with respect to gravity and linear acceleration.

The maculae contain biological sensors called **hair cells**. Each hair cell is innervated by afferent nerve fibers. The hair cells convert the stimulation from gravitational or linear forces into a synapse with the nerve fibers that ultimately make up the vestibular portion of the vestibulocochlear nerve

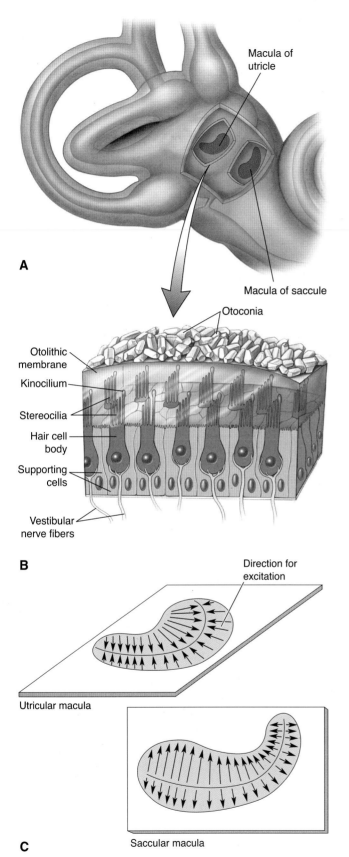

A

B

Otolithic membrane
Kinocilium
Stereocilia
Hair cell body
Supporting cells
Vestibular nerve fibers

Macula of utricle
Macula of saccule
Otoconia

C

Direction for excitation
Utricular macula
Saccular macula

Figure 12-12   Structure of the vestibule of the inner ear. **A.** The bony vestibule cut away to reveal the utricle and saccule. **B.** Structure of the macula. **C.** Orientation of the macula within the utricle and saccule. (Reprinted with permission from Bear, M.F., Connors, B.W., Paradiso, M.A. (2006). *Neuroscience exploring the brain* (3rd ed.). Baltimore: Lippincott Williams & Wilkins.)

(cranial nerve VIII). Hair cells are so named because cilia project from their cell bodies. These **stereocilia** can number between 50 and 100 per hair cell. They project from the cell body and are ordered to angle by height. There is one particularly tall cilium (called the **kinocilium**) located on the perimeter of each hair cell. Whether or not a hair cell is excited depends on which direction its stereocilia are stimulated. When they are bent toward the kinocilium the firing rate increases and bending away from the kinocilium decreases the firing rate to the vestibular nerve. The lineup of hair cells within each macula is arranged so that they lie in different directions. A single sheet of hair cells can detect motion forward and back and side to side. The maculae can therefore cover any motion in a horizontal or vertical plane. The maculae structure consists of a cluster of hair cell bodies with their stereocilia embedded in an epithelial gelatinous membrane called the **otolithic membrane**. Situated on top of the otolithic membrane are tiny calcium carbonate crystals called **otoconia**. The hair cells are stimulated when linear acceleration in any direction causes a weighted shift of the otoconia on the otolithic membrane mass. The otoconia provide the inertia, and the otolithic membrane mass drags on the hair cells. Sudden changes in gravity such as taking a fast elevator ride with a sudden stop at the top or even rapid acceleration in a sports car followed by a sudden stop will cause an individual to experience this reaction. However, once you are moving at a constant speed, again as in a car, the otoliths come to equilibrium and you no longer perceive the motion until you come to a stop.

Semicircular Canals

Arising from the utricle are three loops referred to as the semicircular canals. The three semicircular canals are oriented to different anatomical positions: posterior, anterior (i.e., superior), and lateral (i.e., horizontal). They are oriented spatially at right angles to each other which allow them to respond to angular head motion (e.g., head rotation). Each canal plane is perpendicular to the other canal directions, comparable to the relationship of two right angle sides and the floor of a cube. The canals on each side operate simultaneously as if joined with the canals on the opposite side of the head. The right posterior canal and the left anterior canal, the right and left lateral canals, and the left posterior and right anterior canals respond as a unit. Therefore, head rotation in any direction will stimulate a response from the appropriate paired structure. Each semicircular canal opens into the vestibule by a bulb-like expansion called an **ampulla.** Figure 12-13 shows a cross section of the ampulla and its contents. Housed within the ampulla and lying perpendicular to the long axis of the canal is the receptor end organ called the **crista ampullaris**. The crista contains the vestibular hair cells and supporting cells. The stereocilia of the hair cells extend into a gelatinous mass resembling a semipointed cap, called the **cupula**. When the head rotates in an angular motion, flow of endolymph within the membranous labyrinth lags behind, pushing on the cupula and causing the stereocilia to bend. When the stereocilia bend in the appropriate direction toward the kinocilium, the cell bodies respond and send information via the vestibular branch of the vestibulocochlear nerve to the brain. When the stereocilia are pulled by endolymph flow in a direction away from the kinocilium, there is an abrupt reduction in the information sent to the nerve fibers. Therefore, with head motion, the cupulae of the paired canals (e.g., the right anterior and left posterior) are displaced in a push–pull direction so that one side is always being excited whereas the other is always being inhibited. The push–pull information equals out and the signal is accepted. Dizziness, the inappropriate sensation of motion, is the brain's response from an imbalance of the push–pull system.

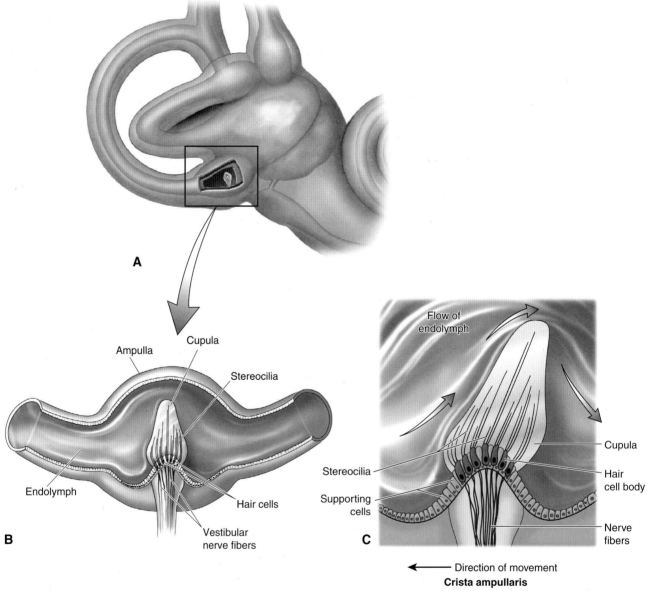

Figure 12-13   Cross section of the ampulla (with the semicircular canals oriented to different anatomical directions). **A**. Each canal opens into the vestibule by a bulb-like expansion called an ampulla. (Reprinted with permission from Anatomical Chart Company.) **B**. Cross section view of the ampulla with the receptor end organ crista ampullaris exposed. (Reprinted with permission from Bear, M.F., Connors. B.W., Paradiso, M.A. (2006). *Neuroscience exploring the brain* (3rd ed.). Baltimore: Lippincott Williams & Wilkins.) **C**. Endolymph flow pushing on the crista. (Reprinted with permission from Anatomical Chart Company.)

Why You Need to Know

Benign paroxysmal positional vertigo *(BPPV) is the most common type of vertigo. Patients report a spinning sensation when lying down, rolling over in bed, bending down or looking up. Estimates indicate that at least 20% of all patients who present to the physician complaining of vertigo have BPPV (Foroehling et al.,1991). The disorder may result from an age-related degeneration of the mechanism. In individuals under the age of 50, it is more often associated with head trauma and is rarely seen in children. For whatever reason, a few of the otoconia from a macula detach from the otolithic membrane and are free to float in the endolymph usually resting in the ampulla of the posterior semicircular canal. A change in head position creates movement of the endolymph and the floating otoconia. Their presence adds to the density of the endolymph flow resulting in stimulation of the cupula which will, in turn, increase the neuronal firing rate of that canal and result in an exaggerated perception of movement. It is believed that the symptoms will subside if the otoconia can be coaxed back to the macula from where they came. This is attempted through a series of positioning maneuvers called canalith repositioning treatment (CRT). For evidence-based practice on BPPV and canalith repositioning treatment, refer to Froehling et al. (2000).*

Vestibular Nerve Pathway

The afferent nerve fibers projecting from the vestibular end organs collect to form **Scarpa's ganglion**. From this ganglion, the vestibular nerve courses through the **internal auditory canal (IAC) (or meatus)** of the temporal bone to enter the brainstem at the **pons-medullary junction**, a deep groove that separates the **pons** from the **medulla**. This is the point of transition from the peripheral vestibular system to the central structures of vestibular input. The central structures consist of four major nuclei: the superior, medial, lateral, and descending. The adaptive process of the central vestibular system takes place in the cerebellum. Its job is to monitor and integrate vestibular, somatosensory and visual sensory input and make conscious and unconscious corrective motor adjustments.

Maintenance of the center of gravity (CoG) is sensed by the integration of three systems—visual, vestibular, and somatosensory—and not one sense is solely responsible for the information. Visual input is responsible for recognizing the horizon, and therefore needs an external reference for its sensations. Vestibular input is the result of an internal reference to the sense of weight (gravity) on the macula during a resting position of the head. The somatosensory input gains information from an internal reference by the orientation of one body part to another through the position and tone of skeletal muscles and the pressure on the soles of the feet from a firm surface. There is no exact combination from the contribution of the three input systems. When there is an absence in either visual or somatosensory information, the vestibular system is utilized. The vestibular system can function independently of the two as its primary interest is controlling head and eye position. The **vestibulo-ocular reflex (VOR)** is a reflexive eye movement that stabilizes vision during head movement by producing an eye movement in the direction opposite to the head movement. (This reflex is what allows us to read while jogging on the treadmill.) The semicircular canals detect the head rotation, which triggers a compensatory movement of the eyes. The VOR does not depend on visual acuity and works in total darkness or when the eyes are closed.

Why You Need to Know

Vestibular rehabilitation therapy (VRT) is balance retraining through physical therapy. As discussed in the text, the maintenance of one's balance involves integration from multiple systems; therefore, successful VRT requires a careful and thorough evaluation to identify the specific area(s) of weakness. The exercises will target the particular deficit(s) and retraining will take advantage of neural mechanisms in the brain for adaptation, plasticity, and compensation. An audiologist will be involved in the evaluation of balance and hearing and maybe even retraining therapy as VRT is within the audiologist's scope of practice (as well as the scope of practice of occupational therapists and physical therapists).

Why You Need to Know

Motion sickness is a result of the visual and somatosensory systems sensing different information. The visual system perceives motion but the somatosensory cannot confirm the motion; therefore, confusion of the integrated signal takes place. When there is confusion in the interpretation, it is the vestibular system that contributes to the maintenance of the center of gravity for balance.

Structures of the Auditory Sensory-Neural System

The anatomical structures of the cochlea and the cochlear nerve are known as the *sensory-neural* system as it houses the fine receptors that must *sense* and change the acoustic signal into the neural information transmitted to the brain for the process we think of as hearing.

Cochlea

The cochlea is the inner ear organ of audition. While the outer and middle ears comprise the mechanism for conducting sound to the cochlea, the cochlea is the mechanism that changes the acoustic signal into the neural impulses that are transmitted to the brain for the process we think of as "hearing."

The cochlea is no larger in size than a pea but is amazing in its function. It is so complex that we do not completely comprehend its physiology and is so embedded in the dense temporal bone that access for the purpose of research is very difficult. The cochlea's position in the head is oriented so that the apex is anterior and slightly lateral within the head pointing toward the cheekbone. The bony labyrinth resembles a snail's shell coiled around itself between 2½ and 2⅝ times before reaching its apex. The cochlea is 5 mm in height; at its base, it is 9 mm in width and tapers toward the apex. Figure 12-14 shows a cross section of the cochlea and its contents. The porous, perforated bony core of the cochlea is called the **modiolus**. The cochlea wraps around the modiolus from base to apex. The perforated modiolus accommodates the blood vessels and nerve fibers leading off from the hair cells. In its design, the modiolus adds protection to the essential blood vessels supplying the cochlea and nerve fibers also coursing through its center.

Housed within the bony labyrinth is its membranous channel known as the **scala media** (also known as the **cochlear duct**). The scala media conforms to the shape of the bony cochlea so that it is also coiled. Uncoiled, the scala media measures approximately 25 to 35 mm in length. In looking at a cross section, the scala media does not float within the perilymph of the bony labyrinth but rather a large section of the scala media is attached to the lateral wall of the bony capsule. There are connections to the medial wall as well, dividing the interior of the cochlea into thirds. The boundaries of the scala media completely separate the bony labyrinth into two channels. Perilymph fills the space above and below the scala media. The two bony channels surrounding the scala media meet at the apical end of the bony labyrinth with a small opening at the apex called the **helicotrema**. This opening allows perilymph to be continuous throughout the bony channel even though there is a division. The upper channel is called the **scala vestibuli** and the oval window forms its point of origination. The lower channel is called the scala tympani and the round window is its point of termination.

There are two, less emphasized, fluid pathways that lead off from the inner ear structures. One leading away from the vestibule is the **vestibular aqueduct (VA)**. Contained within the VA is a membranous sac containing endolymph. The other aqueduct, termed the **cochlear aqueduct (CA)**, leads away from the basal turn of the scala tympani only a few millimeters from the round window to the subarachnoid space of the brain. The CA contains perilymph since it originates at the scala tympani. A commonly accepted view about the CA is that it allows transfer of perilymph to cerebrospinal fluid (CSF). Perilymph has essentially the same chemical composition as CSF.

> ### Why You Need to Know
>
> **Enlarged vestibular aqueduct syndrome (EVAS)** is identified as an inner ear bony malformation causing a bilateral (and usually) progressive sensorineural hearing loss. The specific etiology is unknown, however, it appears to be the result of a gene mutation but environmental factors have also been suspected. The effect is that the membranous sac containing endolymph is much larger than normal. EVAS is diagnosed by high-resolution radiological scans that show the enlarged aqueduct.

The scala media contains the receptor end organ of hearing, the **organ of Corti** (see Figure 12-14). The lateral wall of the scala media is attached to the bony labyrinth by the **spiral ligament**. The medial or modiolar attachment of the scala media is the osseous **spiral lamina**. The spiral lamina consists of two thin plates of bone. There is a space between the two layers of the lamina where the nerve fibers course and is called the **habenula perforata**.

Joining the spiral lamina is the **basilar membrane (BM)** (also known as the **cochlear partition**). The spiral ligament reaches out to meet the BM, completing the floor. The organ of Corti rests on the membrane. The spiral ligament, a band of flexible connective tissue, affixes the BM to the lateral wall of the bony labyrinth. When displaced, the membrane pivots at the point where it attaches to the spiral lamina. Together the BM and the spiral lamina run the entire length of

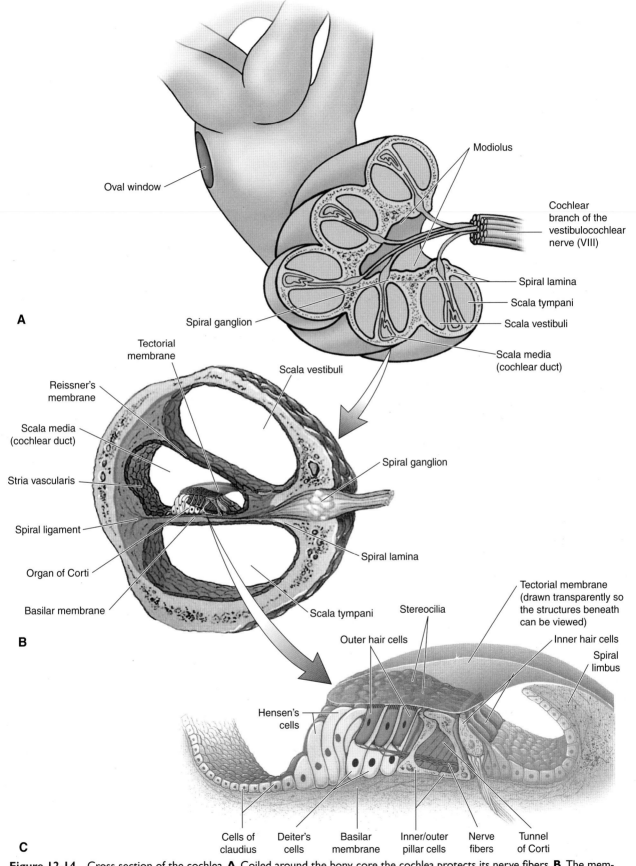

Figure 12-14   Cross section of the cochlea. **A**. Coiled around the bony core the cochlea protects its nerve fibers. **B**. The membranous labyrinth divides the bony labyrinth into two sections: the scala vestibuli above and the scala tympani below. The scala media houses the receptor end organ of hearing. **C**. The structures of the organ of Corti rest on the basilar membrane. (Reprinted with permission from Gartner, L.P., Hiatt, J.L. (2009). *Color atlas of histology* (5th ed.). Baltimore: Lippincott Williams & Wilkins.)

the cochlea, separating the scala media from the scala tympani. The cochlea and spiral lamina are wider at the base than the apex, whereas the BM (cochlear partition) runs just the opposite, being narrower at the base and wider at the apex. Because of this arrangement, the BM is under considerable tension at the base but is relatively flaccid at the apex. The physical characteristics of the BM play a critical role in the process of audition allowing for passive tuning of the high frequencies at the base and low frequencies at the apex.

Reissner's membrane forms the superior wall of the membranous labyrinth. It projects obliquely across the scala media to attach to the lateral wall of the duct. This attachment serves to separate the scala media from the scala vestibuli above. The **stria vascularis** extends along the lateral wall of the scala media from Reissner's membrane to the basilar membrane. The stria vascularis is a highly vascularized layer of epithelium thought to produce and maintain the chemical balance of the ions (in particular potassium) within the endolymph of the scala media.

Organ of Corti

The organ of Corti, named for the Italian anatomist Corti during the mid-1800s, is the end organ for hearing and rests on the BM. Acoustic energy that was transformed into mechanical energy by the middle ear will be further transformed into electrochemical neural information by the organ of Corti. The basic structure includes two types of sensory cells and many supporting cells. Supporting cells include the **inner** and **outer pillar cells**. The arrangement of the pillar cells is in rows which are wide apart at their base and merge together at their apices defining the triangular area called the **tunnel of Corti**, which is filled with its own fluid called **cortilymph**. The base for the pillar cells is on the BM and is broad and supportive.

On the modiolar (i.e., medial) side of the pillar cells is a single row of sensory **inner hair cells (IHCs)**. On the lateral side of the pillar cells are three rows of sensory **outer hair cells (OHCs)**. The IHCs and OHCs are held in place by a complex network of supporting cells. The structure and arrangement of **Deiters' cells** cradle the base of the OHCs and send phalangeal processes to the surface to intermesh forming the roof of the organ of Corti. The tight meshwork is known as the **reticular lamina**. It forms a tight seal to the endolymphatic space. **Hensen's cells** are tall columnar cells adjacent to the last row of Deiters' cells. The Hensen's cells also lend their support to the OHCs and support the **tectorial membrane. Claudius' cells** are cube-shaped cells that rest on the BM and fill the space between Deiters' cells and the base of the stria

vascularis (Claudius, Deiters, and Hensen were 19th century German anatomists). The Claudius cells also add strength to the BM. The **spiral limbus** is a mound of connective tissue that rests on the spiral lamina. It provides the medial attachment for Reissner's membrane and the tectorial membrane.

The tectorial membrane is not really a membrane, but rather a gelatinous flap composed of collagen and proteins (Steel, 1983). The membrane projects radially across the organ of Corti. It has the capability of pivoting from its medial attachment to the spiral limbus. Its function is to provide the mechanical shearing (push or pull) of the stereocilia of the OHCs. The stereocilia of the OHCs, particularly in row 1, are embedded in its inferior surface. It is significant to note that the IHCs are *not* embedded in the tectorial membrane. Endolymph fills the space between the tectorial membrane and the reticular lamina. As seen in Figure 12-15, the different hinge points for the tectorial membrane and the BM lend to the mechanical stimulation of the OHCs. The IHCs are disturbed by the drag imposed on them from the surrounding fluid.

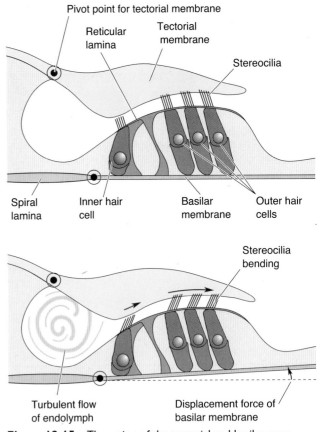

Figure 12-15 The action of the tectorial and basilar membranes on the outer hair cells. The inner hair cells are stimulated by the turbulent flow (i.e., drag) of the endolymph. (Reprinted with permission from Bear, M.F., Connors, B.W., Paradiso, M.A. (2006). *Neuroscience exploring the brain* (3rd ed.). Baltimore: Lippincott Williams & Wilkins.)

The two types of receptor hair cells, inner and outer, are different from each other in several physical ways. The IHCs are "flask" or "tear drop" shaped whereas the OHCs bodies are more cylinder or test tube like in shape. The single row of IHCs numbers approximately 3500 cell bodies and the three to four rows of OHCs number approximately 12,000 to 13,000 cell bodies (Retzius, 1884, as cited in Hudspeth, 1989). Geisler (1998) discovered that the length of the OHCs varies depending on its location along the tuned BM. As one could anticipate, the hair cells are shorter at the base of the BM than the hair cells arranged along the low-frequency tuned apex of the BM. Tilney, Tilney, and DeRosier (1992) reported that the stereocilia projecting from the apical surface of the auditory hair cells are organized into bundles and rows of graded lengths. Both the IHC and OHC bundles lack the tall kinocilium seen with the vestibular hair cells. The pattern of the stereocilia bundle on the IHCs forms a shallow "U" shaped row, whereas the pattern of the stereocilia bundle on the OHCs resembles a "W" or "V." Stereocilia of both cell types are shorter and more numerous at the base of the cochlea than they are at the apex. Maximum numbers seen at the basal end reach approximately 150 per cell body. The number of stereocilia tapers off toward the apical end of the cochlea, where there are approximately 65 to 70 per OHC. The shorter stereocilia are linked laterally ensuring that when they are disturbed, they move more or less as a unit.

The IHCs and OHCs function very differently. The IHCs selectively respond to the various frequencies of an incoming signal. Their shallow U-shaped stereocilia bundle lends itself to stimulation by the flow of endolymph. The OHCs, on the other hand, contain an unusual structural characteristic usually associated with muscle cells and the chemical makeup to change shape. Both factors enable the OHCs to be **motile**, meaning they can shorten or lengthen in response to being stimulated or inhibited (Pickles, 1988). Damage to the hair cells results in a permanent sensory hearing loss. The most likely cause of hair cell death is from excessive noise exposure. Because the cochlea is unable to generate new hair cells, damage is irreversible. It is interesting however that hair cell regeneration is possible in all vertebrates except mammals.

Why You Need to Know

Cotanche (1987) and others discovered in the mid-1980s that mature birds exposed to loud noise or oto-toxic drugs like antibiotics, in as little as 28 days were able to regenerate and replace dead hair cells and return their hearing to near normal levels. Within the avian cochlea at least, the secret seems to be in the supporting cells reentering the cell cycle after injury to regenerate into hair cells complete with stereo-cilia. Researchers Stone and Cotanche (2007) have induced cell division in the inner ear of mice, guinea pigs, and rats using a variety of growth-promoting molecules. They have also discovered one gene (but there are probably more) that is responsible for "turning off" the production. Researchers such as Staecher, Praetorius, Kim, and Douglas (2007) have been most successful in restoring hair cells for the vestibular portions of the inner ear. They know that it is more than knowing how to manipulate the inhibitory genes to control for the appropriate number of cells in the inner ear but also how to keep the cells alive and functional. It is exciting to think that someday (perhaps in the next 10 to 15 years) there may be a treatment for sensory hearing loss in humans.

Experimental evidence demonstrated that Bekesy (1960) was correct in describing the mechanical characteristics of the BM and its passive contribution to the tuning of the incoming acoustic signal. The BM acts like a mechanical resonator, varying in thickness, width, and stiffness. It is thinner, narrower, and stiffer at the base making it more resonant to high-frequency vibration. At the apex, the BM is thicker, wider, and more flaccid, making it more resonant to lower frequencies. The process of audition begins when the fluid within the cochlea is disturbed by the vibrating stapes in the oval window. As illustrated in Figure 12-16, the vibration of the stapes creates a fluid wave that travels from the base to the apex. There is minimal displacement of the membrane until it reaches the point where its physical characteristics are most receptive to the stimulus frequency. In other words, the area of maximum membrane displacement corresponds to the frequency of the stimulus and to the tuning of the hair cells of the organ of Corti.

In addition to the passive mechanical contribution of the BM, researchers beginning with Dallos (1992) described an active contribution the hair cells make in the analysis of the incoming signal. He revealed that they too resonate best at select frequencies. The IHCs and OHCs play different roles in their contribution. The IHCs are necessary for frequency coding. The IHCs are not embedded in the tectorial membrane and therefore must rely on the strong turbulence of endolymph around their stereocilia for their displacement and subsequent excitement. The flow of endolymph alone is not strong enough to disturb the IHCs

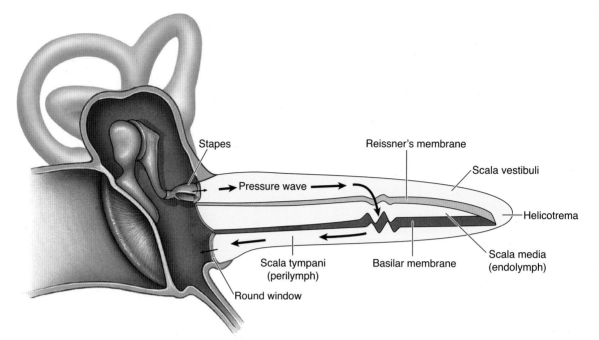

Figure 12-16   The cochlea uncoiled to demonstrate the place of maximum displacement along the basilar membrane for a pure tone.

until the intensity of the stimulus is above approximately 40 dB SPL. The OHCs contribute to hearing sensitivity for less intense sounds. Remember, the difference in the pivot points for the BM and the tectorial membrane contributes to the shearing action of the OHCs. A 40 dB sound is fairly quiet; however, it will still displace the BM so that the OHCs become sheared. The shearing causes the OHCs to react, pulling on the tectorial membrane. The "tightening" of the tectorial membrane modifies the tectorial–reticular lamina spatial relationship. The result is the constriction of the flow of endolymph causing the turbulent flow necessary to stimulate the IHCs. Therefore, the motile activity of the OHCs adjusts the mechanics of the organ of Corti so that the IHCs can react to less intense stimuli, providing the minute frequency coding. The OHCs act as the "cochlear amplifier" providing the necessary sensitivity for humans to hear soft level sounds (Zwislocki, 1990). At the resonate frequency of the hair cell, threshold is easily crossed generating a response. A hair cell can be stimulated at frequencies other than its resonant frequency, but the threshold must be greater than the one required to stimulate the hair cell at its own select frequency.

> ### Why You Need to Know
>
> *Otoacoustic emissions (OAEs) are acoustic signals generated by normal functioning OHCs. The*

> *OHCs spontaneously generate the emission as they expand and contract to incoming acoustic stimulation. These emissions can be detected by inserting a tiny microphone into the ear canal. A mild hearing impairment typically begins as a loss of the motile ability of the OHCs. Consequently,* **evoked** *OAEs provide audiologists with a useful clinical tool in the evaluation of cochlear function.*

Neural Pathways

All cochlear hair cells receive both afferent (i.e., sensory) and efferent (i.e., motor) innervation; however, the majority of fibers are afferent. This section will provide a discussion of the afferent and efferent auditory pathways as they relate to the process of hearing. The central processing of auditory information within and between the two cerebral hemispheres was covered in Chapter 4.

Neurotransmission

The hair cells are innervated by no less than 30,000 nerve fibers. Before joining with the fibers of the IHCs, the nerve fibers that connect to the OHCs course through the tunnel of Corti. Together they move through the habenula perforata. The nerve fibers carry information along their peripheral processes to the **spiral ganglia**. The nerve fibers are unmyelinated in the region between their endings on the hair cells

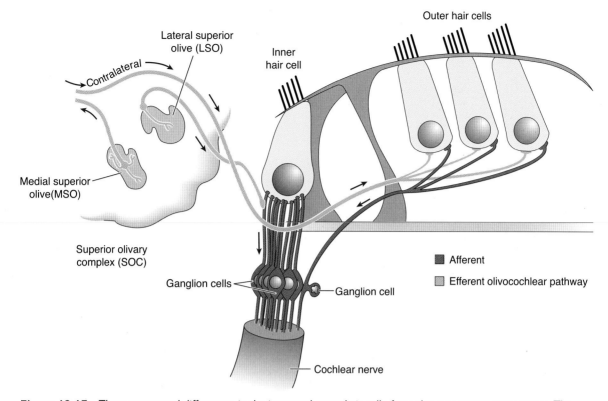

Figure 12-17 There are several differences in the inner and outer hair cells, from shape to innervation pattern. The inner hair cells send 95% afferent information to the cochlear nerve. The outer hair cells receive 95% crossed efferent information from the olivocochlear bundle.

and the habenula perforata but become myelinated as they pass through the internal auditory canal (IAC). For the OHCs, the neural information is a product of the shearing action of the tectorial membrane. For the IHCs, the neural information is a product of the turbulence created in the flow of the endolymph. Although there are approximately three times as many OHCs as IHCs, the OHCs send only 5% of the afferent information along the cochlear nerve. The IHCs send 95% of the afferent information. Each IHC communicates with as many as 10 to 18 ganglion cells (see Figure 12-17). The remaining 5% of peripheral nerve fibers branch with as many as 10 to 50 OHCs (this is a relatively small number of afferent nerve fibers spread out over a relatively large number of OHCs) (Spoendlin, 1974).

The process known as **transduction**, the changing (i.e., transforming) of mechanical vibrations from the BM into neural information, occurs at the level of the hair cells. Endolymph is rich with the positively charged ions potassium and calcium. Endolymph has a resting potential (the voltage potential present with no stimulation) of +100 **millivolts (mV)** to +80 mV (Tasaki & Spiropoulis, 1959). Therefore, the scala media has a strong positive potential called the **endo-**

cochlear potential (EP). Transduction is dependent on the intracellular resting potential of the hair cells, which are about −40 mV for the IHCs and −70 mV for the OHCs (Dallos, Santos-Sacchi, & Flock, 1982). The positive resting potential of endolymph and the negative resting potential of the hair cells yield a very large voltage potential difference of 120 to 150 mV depending on the cell type. As described by Hudspeth (1989), when a stimulus is delivered a mechanical gate on the stereocilia is opened. As seen in Figure 12-18, the **tip links** reach up from the top of the shorter cilia to the side of the adjacent taller cilia. This arrangement allows them to be stretched much like a spring to open a gate (Pickles, Comis, & Osborne, 1984). With the gate now open, a route is provided for the higher concentration of potassium (K^+) in the endolymph to flow toward the lower concentration within the hair cells. As a result of the flow of potassium, the EP shifts negatively from its highly positive charge (the opposite positive and negative charge differences want to balance). The EP shifting of a positive charge is termed **depolarization**. Depolarization activates channel opening along the lateral cell membrane. These channels allow for the influx of calcium and the efflux of potassium from the hair cell. The influx of

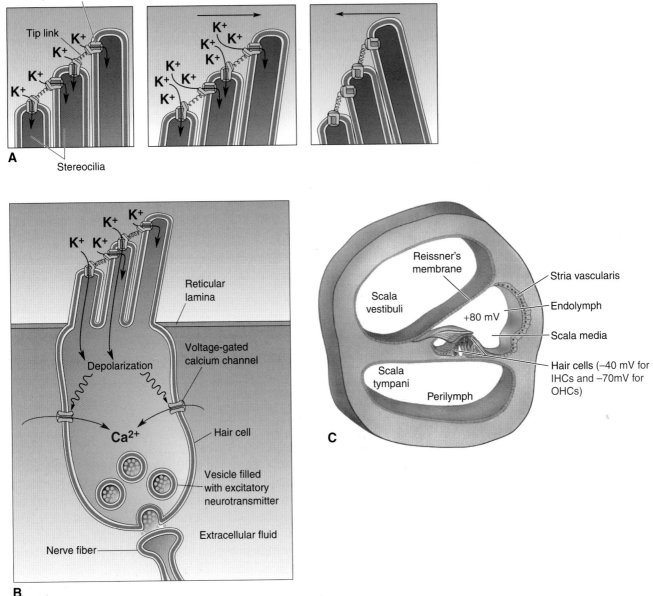

Figure 12-18   Depolarization of a hair cell. **A.** Tip links are stretched to open the potassium (K^+) channels. **B.** Depolarization serves to open the calcium (Ca^{++}) channels, releasing the neurotransmitter. **C.** Endocochlear potential: strong positive potential, negative intracellular resting potential. (Reprinted with permission from Bear, M.F., Connors, B.W., Paradiso, M.A. (2006). *Neuroscience exploring the brain* (3rd ed.). Baltimore: Lippincott Williams & Wilkins.)

calcium triggers the release of the **neurotransmitter** glutamate into the nerve terminals in contact with the hair cell base. The diffusion of the neurotransmitter across the terminal triggers an action potential to be propagated down the nerve fibers. For a split moment, the shifting of the ion concentrations within the hair cells causes the cell to be **hyperpolarized**. When a cell is in a state of hyperpolarization, it is unable to be stimulated. It is not until it regains its resting potential that it is again ready to respond. During the action of transduction, the ion balance within the endolymph is shifted dramatically. It is the func-

tion of the stria vascularis to return the endolymph to its resting (potassium, sodium, and calcium) balance (Pickles, 1988).

The act of transduction is triggered by the frequency of the sound that causes the point of maximum displacement along the passive BM. Researchers have also examined the intensity level necessary to bring about depolarization (Dallos, 1992). The displacement of the membrane increases in magnitude as the stimulus intensity increases. A **tuning curve** (see Figure 12-19) is a graph of the intensity level necessary to trigger (i.e., reach threshold) the hair

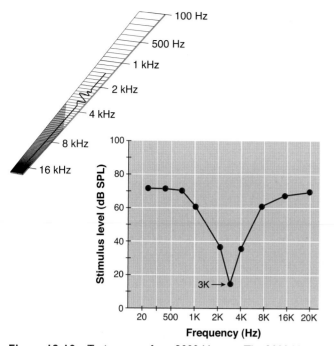

Figure 12-19   Tuning curve for a 3000 Hz tone. The 3000 Hz tone seen along the basilar membrane at the point of maximum displacement.

cell response to an input stimulus. The greater the intensity level, the broader the range of frequencies whose thresholds are crossed (i.e., the broader the shape of the graph). The broadness of the BM response to high intensities decreases the frequency selectivity. The increase number of hair cells that are stimulated creates a greater neural response from the cochlear nerve. In contrast, for less intense stimuli, a response is seen at a limited range of frequencies where threshold is crossed. The magnitude of BM deflection is limited. There is progressively less and less membrane deflection as the intensity of a sound increases.

Once threshold has been crossed and depolarization takes place, impulses (i.e., action potentials) travel down the peripheral processes of the nerve fibers to the spiral ganglion and continue along until they enter the brainstem. As soon as the fibers collect at the exit point from the cochlea's modiolus they form the cochlear branch of the vestibulocochlear nerve (cranial nerve VIII). Yost (2000) reviewed the tonotopic organization of the cochlear branch of cranial nerve VIII. He noted the fibers originating from the apex of the cochlea form the core or center of the branch. The outer layer originates from the basal end of the cochlea and twists around the core, which means that the high-frequency fibers twist around the low-frequency fibers.

> ### Why You Need to Know
>
> *Auditory neuropathy (AN), or to be more exact auditory dys-synchrony (AD), is an unusual hearing disorder that is primarily a timing deficit affecting the normal synchronous activity of the IHCs or the auditory nerve (Zeng et al., 1999). The OHC function is unaffected. The degree of hearing loss is not predictable and may even fluctuate from day to day. The neural dys-synchrony causes speech understanding difficulties that are worse than can be predicted from the pattern of hearing loss. Amplification unfortunately has minimal benefit in improving speech discrimination. Sign language may be necessary for language learning. Identification of auditory dys-sychrony is a diagnosis of exclusion. Otoacoustic emissions are present; however, evoked potential [auditory brainstem response (ABR)] testing of the auditory pathway is abnormal as well as the middle ear muscle reflex. Radiologic evaluations are normal as there is no obvious lesion.*

Afferent Auditory Pathway

The cochlear branch of the vestibulocochlear nerve merges with the vestibular branch that has bundled from the nerve fibers of the ampullae, saccule, and utricle. The two branches maintain their separate identities but combine to become cranial nerve VIII. Cranial nerve VIII meets cranial nerve VII (the facial nerve) to travel through the internal auditory canal (IAC). The cochlear branch occupies a position beneath the facial nerve and to the side of the vestibular nerve.

> ### Why You Need to Know
>
> *The IAC is a site for the growth of a benign Schwannoma neuroma that tends to arise from the vestibular nerve but with time will encroach on the cochlear nerve. The neuroma is contained within the narrow meatus and therefore quickly compresses on the nerve causing unilateral symptoms such as balance disturbances, tinnitus, and hearing loss. Remembering the tonotopic organization of the cochlear nerve, a lesion will initially result in a high-frequency hearing loss. An undiagnosed neuroma may grow large enough to affect the mid to low frequencies and compress on the facial nerve (cranial nerve VII) causing facial paresis.*

Figure 12-20 illustrates the auditory pathway. A lesion along the auditory pathway (e.g., a **Schwannoma** or **acoustic neuroma**) creates a **retrocochlear** hearing loss. Audiometrically, a retrocochlear hear-

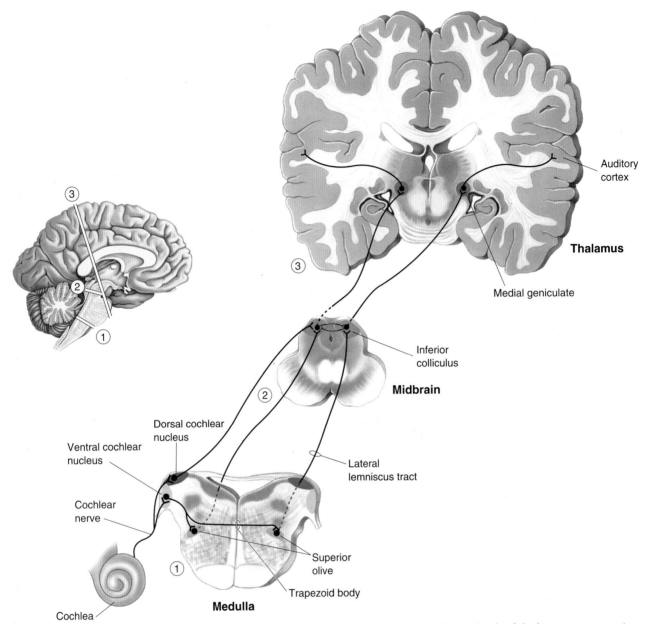

Figure 12-20 Afferent auditory pathway as it leaves the cochlea and travels through the different levels of the brainstem to terminate at the anterior and posterior transverse temporal gyri (i.e., Heschl's gyrus) along the superior temporal gyrus of the cerebrum. (Reprinted with permission from Bear, M.F., Connors, B.W., Paradiso, M.A. (2006). *Neuroscience exploring the brain* (3rd ed.). Baltimore: Lippincott Williams & Wilkins.)

ing loss will look the same as a sensorineural hearing loss (i.e., air and bone conduction loss). A lesion on the cochlear nerve will cause a loss in the detection of sound *and* a loss in the recognition of words.

Cranial nerve VIII enters the brainstem at the junction of the pons and medulla. The cochlear nerve travels through the different levels of the brainstem to terminate at the auditory cortex, **Heschl's gyrus** of the temporal lobe of the cerebrum. The nerve fibers synapse with at least four different nuclei along the way to the cortex. The first-order neurons originate from the cochlear hair cells (mostly the IHCs) and terminate at the **cochlear nuclei**. All fibers terminate at either

the **ventral cochlear nucleus** or the **dorsal cochlear nucleus**, where they synapse with the second-order neurons. It is at this level that the neurons pass through the **trapezoid body** to be distributed to the **ipsilateral** and **contralateral** superior olivary complex. Each superior olivary complex and the nuclei above will have information from both ears. This is referred to as **binaural representation** and is important for localization of a sound source.

Third-order neurons continue upward from the superior olivary complex along a tract called the **lateral lemniscus**. These third-order neurons are joined by some second-order neurons that arose from the cochlear nucleus but bypassed the superior olivary complex. The second- and third-order neurons may terminate at the lateral lemniscus or continue to the **inferior colliculus** at the dorsal midbrain. The majority of neurons will synapse at the inferior colliculus. The inferior colliculus has a large bundle of nerve fibers that cross to communicate with the nucleus on the opposite side. A commissural tract allows the two inferior colliculi to communicate with each other. **Interaural** time and intensity differences occur at this level, playing a role in auditory localization. Fourth-order neurons leave the inferior colliculus to terminate at the **medial geniculate body** of the thalamus. The third-order neurons that bypassed the inferior colliculus will terminate here. In other words, all ascending (i.e., afferent or sensory) neurons will have a final synapse at this subcortical level before proceeding to the auditory cortex. The final destination of afferent fibers is Heschl's gyrus (also referred to as the anterior and posterior transverse gyri), which is found within the superior temporal gyrus along the temporal lobe of the cerebrum (Brodmann areas 41 and 42) in both hemispheres. The frequency organization of the cochlea is preserved along the pathway and in bands across the cortical surface of the superior temporal gyrus. The orderly representation is known as **tonotopic organization**. Researchers (e.g., Troost & Waller, 1998) have demonstrated the tonotopic organization of the medial geniculate body in which low frequencies are represented laterally and high frequencies are located medially in the principal division. The peripheral auditory mechanism is the site for the detection of sound but it is the central cortical level that is the location for conscious processing of sound that we refer to as "hearing."

Why You Need to Know

Auditory brainstem response (ABR) audiometry refers to the measurement of the electrical potential of the auditory pathway as it passes through the different levels of the brainstem. The responses are elicited by an auditory stimulus. Test administration and interpretation are performed by an audiologist. The signal travels along the auditory pathway from the cochlear nucleus to the inferior colliculus. The elicited response can be measured by surface electrodes. The response normally occurs within a 15-millisecond time period after a stimulus is presented. ABR audiometry is considered an effective tool in the evaluation of hearing loss and suspected retrocochlear pathology.

Binaural representation is critical in the processing of acoustic information. It is used for localization as in detecting the origin of a sound. The interaural acoustic information is processed for time, intensity, and frequency characteristics. The differences are conveyed throughout the pathway to the auditory cortex. Damage to the pathway, after the point of binaural representation, usually has no effect on the detection of sound, thanks to the redundancy of information being sent to the brain. Hearing loss (a detection of impaired frequency and intensity of sound) is theoretically only caused by damage to the outer and middle ear, cochlea, or cochlear nerve. Auditory processing is the brain using the frequency, intensity, and pattern of sounds (speech in particular) that our ears detect (the brain using what the ear hears). A lesion along the auditory cortex interferes with the processing of speech creating a central hearing loss. This is most obvious when the speech signal is in competition with or imbedded in background noise. The individual has an inability to filter out competing auditory signals. A **central auditory processing disorder (CAPD)** is the result of a central hearing loss. For the most part, auditory processing works fine in simple face-to-face conversation in a quiet environment. However, when the system is stressed, as when trying to converse in the presence of background noise or listening to instruction while the teacher walks around a large reverberant classroom, a lesion in the system will become apparent and the auditory information will be misunderstood or missed altogether. Many sites can be at fault for a central hearing loss: a deficit in the interpretation of the signal; disruption in the redundant auditory pathway; or lack of communication between the two auditory cortices. The prevalence of CAPD in children is estimated to be between 2% and 3% (Chermak & Musiek, 1997) with it being twice as prevalent in males than females. It often coexists with other disabilities. These include speech and language disorders or delays, learning disabilities or dyslexia, attention deficit disorders with or without hyperactivity, and social and/or emotional problems. Testing for CAPD is complicated and time-consuming. Due to neuromaturation of the central auditory nervous system, assessment of children under age 7 is not recommended due to the high degree of variability in their performance. After an extensive case history and assessment is completed, specific suggestions for management will be shared. Keep in mind this is not a peripheral loss so traditional amplification is not the treatment. CAPD management is usually in the form of an auditory training program and phonological awareness training, therapy for any existing language and/or behavior deficits, and methods for improving the quality of the incoming signal. This can be accomplished with the use of a personal auditory trainer to enhance the signal (e.g., the teacher's voice) over the random background (e.g., other sounds in the classroom), thereby improving the signal-to-noise ratio.

Efferent Auditory Pathway

All the information from the peripheral hearing mechanism is carried along the afferent pathway to the cortex for processing. The efferent pathway is the way the brain communicates information down to the peripheral structures. The **olivocochlear pathway** (refer back to Figure 12-17) carries efferent information from the olivocochlear bundle (OCB) in the superior olivary complex in the brainstem to the hearing mechanism.

Guinan, Warr, and Norris (1983) described two main olivocochlear pathways, one crossed and the other uncrossed. The uncrossed pathway originates from the lateral superior olivary complex (LSOC) and consists of unmyelinated fibers that terminate on the afferent fibers of the IHCs. The OHCs receive few of these same uncrossed fibers. The crossed pathway originates from the medial superior olivary complex (MSOC). These fibers are myelinated and terminate directly on the OHCs. The role of the efferent pathways (both crossed and uncrossed) is believed to be the production of inhibitory effects. Information along the efferent pathway seems to inhibit the OHCs' ability to amplify the BM motion. It is believed that this function further facilitates the active tuning effect of the hair cells.

Middle Ear Muscle Reflex Arc

The auditory pathway described above has been relatively simplified into the major afferent and efferent tracts. There are many lesser tracts that receive stimulation from the cochlear neurons that enter the brainstem. The middle ear muscle reflex arc deserves discussion as its presence or absence is used clinically as an indicator for **site of lesion**. Borg (1973) described the middle ear muscle reflex as being dependent upon contraction of the stapedius muscle in response to loud sounds. An intense sound (e.g., 70 to 110 dB HL) presented to either ear will illicit a contraction of the stapedius muscle in

both ears and therefore can be measured in either an uncrossed (i.e., ipsilateral) or a crossed (i.e., contralateral) condition. The sensory component of the reflex arc is provided by afferents of the cochlear portion of the vestibulocochlear nerve (cranial nerve VIII). The motor component of the reflex is provided by efferent nerve fiber tracts of the facial nerve (cranial nerve VII). The reflex is initiated by a stimulus that is carried to the brainstem by cranial nerve VIII. Once in the brainstem, the afferent fibers travel to the ventral cochlear nucleus, synapse, and then go to the superior olivary nucleus on the ipsilateral side. A portion of the fibers at the superior olivary complex will continue through and cross to the opposite superior olivary nucleus and synapse. Now both the ipsilateral and contralateral superior olivary nuclei have received communication from the stimulus ear. The arc continues from both the ipsilateral and contralateral sides to send efferent information back down to the motor nucleus of the facial nerve (cranial nerve VII). The synapses at the motor facial nucleus will then send an impulse out to elicit a contraction of the stapedius muscles. When measured in healthy, normal-hearing ears, the reflex is roughly symmetrical so that when either ear is stimulated, the reflex will appear on both sides.

Summary

The anatomical ear is easily divided into the two functional systems related to hearing and balance. The anatomical structures of the two systems were identified and the function or physiology of the structures was discussed. The next step in your education is to learn how disease, injury, and genetics can disrupt this normal function to result in a hearing or balance disorder. Proper identification of a disorder is critical in determining what treatment options are available (e.g., surgical vs. medical). Clinicians who specialize in the identification of hearing or balance disorders have a fond appreciation of the anatomy and physiology of the hearing and balance system. In the next chapter, you will learn how diseases and other disorders of the auditory system can negatively impact hearing and balance.

CHAPTER 13

Pathologies Associated with the Auditory/Vestibular System

Knowledge Outcomes for ASHA Certification for Chapter 13

- Demonstrate knowledge of the developmental and life span bases of the basic human communication processes (III-B)
- Demonstrate knowledge of the etiologies of receptive and expressive language disorders (III-C)
- Demonstrate knowledge of the etiologies of hearing disorders (III-C)
- Demonstrate knowledge of the characteristics of hearing disorders (III-C)
- Demonstrate knowledge of the prevention of hearing disorders (III-D)

Learning Objectives

- You will be able to list the five cardinal signs of ear pathology and refer them back to the client's chief complaint.
- You will be able to differentiate the clinical characteristics of common ear pathology.
- You will be able to discuss the communicative impact of ear pathology.
- You will be able to identify genetic and environmental hearing disorders.
- You will be able to recognize the clinical characteristics of congenital syndromic and nonsyndromic hearing disorders.

AFFIX AND PART-WORD BOX

TERM	MEANING	EXAMPLE
dys-	bad, difficult	**dys**function
-gram	a record or picture	audio**gram**
-itis	inflammation	ot**itis** media
-metry	process of measuring	audio**metry**
-oma	tumor	cholesteat**oma**
os-/osseo-/osteo-	bone	**osseo**us labyrinth
oto-	relating to the ear	**oto**scope
-otomy	to cut into	myring**otomy**
-plasty	the surgical formation of	tympano**plasty**
-sclerosis	a hardening of	oto**sclerosis**
-scopy	to look into	oto**scopy**

Introduction

Anatomy can best be learned when the physiology (i.e., function) of the mechanism is taught in parallel. Included in the anatomy section was a smattering of pathology to demonstrate how pathogens, disease, trauma, and genetic aberrations affect the delicate, intricate function of the ear. This chapter will proceed to elaborate on common congenital anomalies and move through acquired pathologies of the outer, middle, and inner ear. There are complete texts on hearing disorders but at the conclusion of this chapter you will be able to demonstrate knowledge of the characteristics and etiologies of some of the more common hearing disorders. Hearing losses are caused by **lesions**, which by definition are changes in either the structures and/or function of the auditory mechanism due to injury or disease. The patient with a hearing loss seeks treatment or assessment from an **otologist** (i.e., ear physician) or **otolaryngologist**, (i.e., ear, nose, and throat physician or ENT). The hearing loss may be the chief complaint or may, as in the case of a draining ear, be a secondary complaint. The clinician (physician or audiologist) will begin the examination by taking a case history. According to Jafek and Barcz (1996), the case history should include questions that are identified as the five "cardinal signs" of ear pathology. The patient's responses will help identify the presence of ear pathology:

1. Is there a presence of hearing loss?
2. Is there a presence of ear pain (i.e., **otalgia**)?
3. Is there a presence of ear discharge (i.e., **otorrhea**)?
4. Is there a presence of ringing, buzzing or humming in the ears (i.e., **tinnitus**)?
5. Is there a presence of dizziness, subjective vertigo (i.e., the patient feels as if he or she is spinning), or objective vertigo (i.e., the patient feels as if the room is spinning)?

When a physician determines the pathology to be **idiopathic** in nature, the specific underlying etiology cannot be identified. Without a known cause, the physician is left to treat the symptoms of the disorder. If the cause is **hereditary** or **familial**, it means the pathology is transmitted by the **genetic** code that one inherits from one or both of their parents. Genetic disorders are often **congenital** meaning they are present at birth or very shortly after. If the disorder should have an impact on speech and language development as in the case of hearing loss, then timing is very important. If the loss is **prelingual**, the timing is prior to the development of speech and language and it will have a greater impact than a **postlingual** loss (i.e., after speech and language patterns have been fairly well established). Disorders that occur after birth and are the result of disease or injury are **acquired**. The pathology can have an effect on one ear (i.e., **unilateral**) or both ears (i.e., **bilateral**). The onset of the pathology can be **sudden** or **gradual**. Much pathology is **acute** (i.e., having a short duration) but some can be very debilitating because of their **chronic** or long-standing nature. Finally, the pathology can be either **temporary** or **permanent**, and can **fluctuate** or be **progressive**. Many disorders, especially syndromes, have a set of characteristics that set them apart. The pathology will not only disrupt the anatomy, but the function (i.e., physiology) as well. If you spend time learning the structures involved in a particular disorder, then you should be able to predict the effect of not having the structures work the way they should.

In order to assess the nature of ear pathology, the clinician (i.e., audiologist) starts by physically examining the outer ear. This process begins with a gross inspection of the outer ear. First, the clinician will note the position of the pinna. In referring back to Figure 12-3, it can be seen that the normal position of the pinna is determined by noting the relationship of the superior border of the helix of the pinna to the outer **canthus** (i.e., corner) of the eye. The two should be in alignment on a horizontal plane. The clinician will look for the presence of malformations such as pits, tags, sinuses, or suture lines in front of or behind the pinna. The clinician will also inspect for any obvious drainage from the ear canal. If there is no drainage, the clinician will perform an otoscopic exam. The presence of cerumen is expected but should not be excessive. A buildup of excessive cerumen may make it difficult to visualize the tympanic membrane. The clinician will note any deviations of the anatomical structures that can be visualized through otoscopy. With a case history completed and otoscopy performed the audiologist then compares the normal function of the mechanism to any abnormal findings observed in the patient. This is accomplished by the audiologist performing a battery of tests that determine hearing acuity, middle ear function, speech recognition, and in some cases, electrophysical measures of the vestibular and auditory mechanism. These tests are collectively referred to as **audiometry**.

The degree of hearing loss affected by injury or pathology can range from slight to profound. The effect may be limited to the high frequencies, low frequencies, or create a flat configuration where a broad range of frequencies are affected. Thresholds are obtained for each ear and each pathway. **Air conduction** scores are

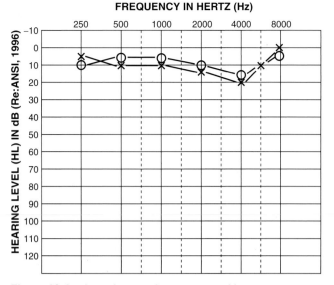

FREQUENCY IN HERTZ (Hz)

Figure 13-1 An audiogram depicting normal hearing sensitivity for both the left and right ear. Note that information regarding frequency (i.e., 250 to 8000 Hz) is plotted horizontally while information regarding intensity (i.e., –10 to 120 dB HL) is plotted vertically.

plotted (right = O and left = X) and **bone conduction** scores are plotted (right = < and left = >) on a graph called an **audiogram** (see Figure 13-1). Audiograms are designed so that the frequencies range from low to high: the frequencies from 250 to 8000 Hz are in octave bands across the top and hearing levels (HLs) in decibels from –10 to 120 dB are down the side. Zero (0) dB HL represents perfect hearing across all the frequencies on an audiogram. The frequencies that are tested represent the frequencies of the phonemes in most languages rather than all the frequencies in one's **audible** range (remember that the audible range for a typical human is between 20 and 20,000 Hz). The remainder of this section is organized to discuss the common congenital and acquired pathologies associated with each of the outer, middle, and inner ear divisions.

An exhaustive description of audiometry is beyond the scope of this text. One audiometric procedure is noteworthy however, because it will be mentioned in subsequent sections of this unit. The procedure involves air and bone conduction audiometry. The audiologist measures the patient's hearing thresholds for both the air conduction pathway and bone conduction pathway. The air conduction pathway is the route taken by sound waves entering the ear canal and making their way through the entire auditory system. Therefore, air conduction testing measures the *total* hearing loss the patient is experiencing. Earphones or foam tip inserts are used in air conduction testing. The bone conduction pathway is the route taken by sound waves with enough acoustic energy to vibrate

the skull bones. Remember the cochlea resides deep in the petrous portion of the temporal bone so that when the skull bones receive auditory vibrations, it sets the cochlear fluids in motion even though the outer and middle ear structures are bypassed. Therefore, bone conduction testing measures the degree of sensory and/or neural hearing loss the patient is experiencing. Bone conduction testing is performed using a bone vibrator held in place on the mastoid process or the forehead. In audiometry, air and bone conduction measures are used in determining the nature of hearing loss. The **air-bone gap** is an index that allows the clinician to determine the extent of the difference between what the total auditory structures are hearing and what the sensory-neural structures (i.e., cochlea and nerve) are capable of hearing. Therefore, the presence or absence of an air-bone gap is used to determine whether a hearing loss is **conductive** (i.e., an air-bone gap is present), **sensorineural** (i.e., no air-bone gap is present), or **mixed** (see Figure 13-2 for an illustration of the air-bone gap).

> ## Why You Need to Know
>
> *The bone conduction pathway has implications for noise damage to the cochlea. In terms of protecting one's hearing, conservation measures are limited to intense air conduction sources (i.e., earplugs, earmuffs, etc.). There is little if any protection afforded the cochlea from bone conducted noise.*

The normal development of the auditory mechanism begins in utero and continues along a predictable timetable with little variation. When there is a disturbance in this developmental sequence, an anomaly is the result. The anomaly may be visible (as with an ear tag) or invisible (as with an ossicular fixation). The anomaly may be benign (i.e., not affecting the hearing mechanism in any appreciable way), or may adversely affect the function of the hearing mechanism. Along the predictable timetable, the embryo develops many separate systems concurrently, and within a single system many structures are also developing concurrently. Therefore, if there is an anomaly within one system, another system may also be affected. A disruption rarely disturbs a single system. For example, maternal rubella may disturb several developing systems, including the circulatory system (heart and blood vessels), the visual system (eyes), and the auditory system (ears).

The severity of the deformity is dependent on the timing of the disruption. Timing is integral to the study of cause and effect. Maternal rubella contracted

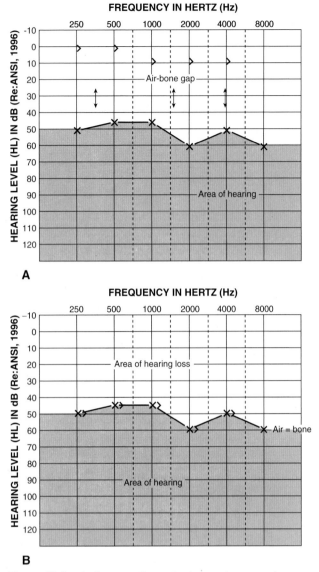

A

B

Figure 13-2 Audiograms illustrating how to interpret the air-bone gap. **A.** This audiogram shows a significant gap between bone (>) and air (X) conduction thresholds for the left ear. This is indicative of a conductive hearing loss because the patient has normal cochlear sensitivity (through the bone conduction pathway, which stimulates the cochlea directly) while having elevated thresholds for the air conduction pathway (where sound must pass through the outer and middle ears before stimulating the cochlea). **B.** This audiogram reveals no air-bone gap. Air and bone conduction thresholds are the same and both are outside the range that is considered "normal" (i.e., 0 to 20 dB). This is indicative of a sensorineural hearing loss because hearing thresholds are beyond normal whether the test signals are stimulating the cochlea directly through the bone conduction pathway or are passing through the outer and middle ears to stimulate the cochlea (i.e., the air conduction pathway).

during the first trimester of pregnancy is devastating, causing cardiac defects, cataracts, mental retardation, **microcephaly**, short stature, and hearing loss. If maternal rubella is contracted during the second or third trimester, hearing loss may be the only result.

Therefore, if one understands timetables relative to prenatal development of the various structures within a system and among the various systems, the suspicion of hearing loss and its subsequent identification and assessment can be accomplished early so that effective intervention can be provided as soon as possible.

At 20 weeks gestation (full term is between 38 and 40 weeks), the pinna reaches its adult-like shape. The pinna is one of the few auditory structures that continues to grow in size after birth. It will continue to grow for approximately 9 to 12 years until its adult size is reached. A "normal" pinna can take a wide variety of shapes and forms as seen in Figure 13-3.

Complete maturation of the entire cochlea is complete at approximately the 20th week (fifth month) of gestation. The inner ear is the only sense organ to reach full adult size by fetal midterm. Thus, the cochlea is susceptible to developmental deviations, malformation, and acquired agents.

Anomalies of the Outer Ear

CONGENITAL ANOMALIES OF THE OUTER EAR

Anotia and Microtia

At birth, the pinna will be either completely formed, partially absent or completely absent. **Anotia** refers to complete absence of the pinna while **microtia** refers to partial development of the pinna. Figure 13-4 illustrates several congenital anomalies of the pinna. A genetic disturbance is the etiology for microtia of the pinna in 5% of the population, whereas microtia is present 50% of the time as part of a syndrome. The remaining 45% of cases of microtia are categorized as idiopathic or of unknown etiology (Mastroiacovo et al., 1995). Authors/physicians Stephen Park and David Chi (2005) in a recent discussion on microtia reported an overall incidence of 1 in 5000 to 1 in 20,000 births. They further reported that the incidence of microtia ranges from 1 in 900 to 1200 births in the Navajo population to 1 in 4000 births in the Japanese population. The male-to-female ratio for microtia is 2.5:1 and is four times more likely to be unilateral than bilateral. The right ear is affected more frequently than the left ear (right-to-left ear ratio of 3:2). Microtia does not cause substantial hearing loss but can cause major cosmetic problems. The wearing of eyeglasses can be especially problematic.

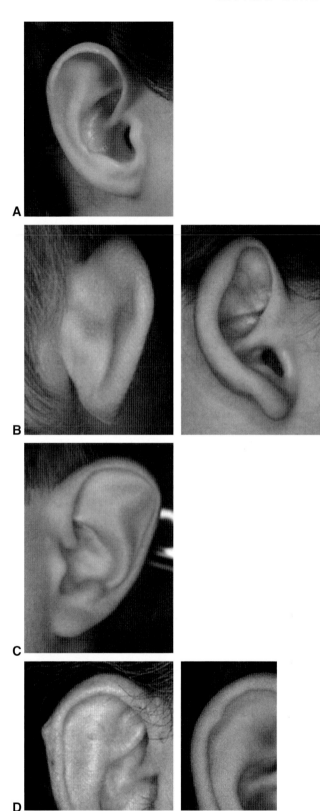

Figure 13-3 Normal variations in size and shape of the pinna (auricle). **A**. Normal pinna. **B**. Prominent ears (normal when occurring bilaterally and having familial characteristics). **C**. Incomplete structures such as an incomplete helix are often seen in premature infants, but they typically become normal as the baby matures. **D**. Darwin's tubercle is a normal variant frequently appearing as a nodule along the posterior segment of the helix. (**B, C,** and **D**. Reprinted with permission from Michael Hawke, MD. Hawke Library, hawkelibrary.com.)

Tags, Pits, and Sinuses

Preauricular tags, pits, and sinuses are probably the most common minor ear malformations with a frequency of 5 to 6 per 1000 live births (Kugelman et al., 1997). Most often they are benign and occur unilaterally but occasionally they will occur bilaterally. In referring to Figure 13-4, it can be seen that a preauricular tag is a mound of epithelial skin that arises near the front of the ear in the area of the tragus. Tags alone do not pose any threat to the structure of the ear and are merely a cosmetic deformity (Kankkunen & Thiringer, 1987). A pit or sinus results from an abnormal connection between the skin and the underlying tissue. They are the result of incomplete closure from an invagination of the embryologic tissue. Ear tags are often seen in isolation; however, pits can be associated with renal anomalies, occurring with a frequency of 5% to 40% (Wang, Earl, Ruder, & Graham, 2001). The incidence of spontaneous formation of ear pits in persons who do not exhibit some type of syndrome is less than 1%.

Atresia and Stenosis

Atresia occurs when the external auditory canal has failed to develop. Atresia of the ear canal often accompanies microtia of the pinna (see Figure 13-4). If the ear canal is present but is abnormally narrow, the condition is referred to as **stenosis**. Atresia of the external auditory canal may occur unilaterally or bilaterally, and is almost always accompanied by ossicular abnormality. The nature and degree of hearing loss should be evaluated for both ears. Because of the differential timing of the development of the inner and outer ears, the inner ear structures may not be affected, thereby limiting the hearing loss to being conductive in nature. The audiometric results will determine the need for amplification in one or both ears and the need for a traditional or a bone conduction aid. If there is unilateral involvement with normal hearing in the uninvolved ear, then surgery is delayed until the child is at least 5 years old. The surgical risk in a young child is in injuring an abnormally situated facial nerve (cranial nerve VII).

> ### Why You Need to Know
> The **Baha**® system utilizes the body's natural bone conduction pathway to conduct sound. For people with hearing loss, this provides another pathway to perceive sound. Typical hearing aids rely on air conduction and a functioning middle ear. In cases where the outer or middle ear function is damaged or occluded, the Baha implant is an alternative device

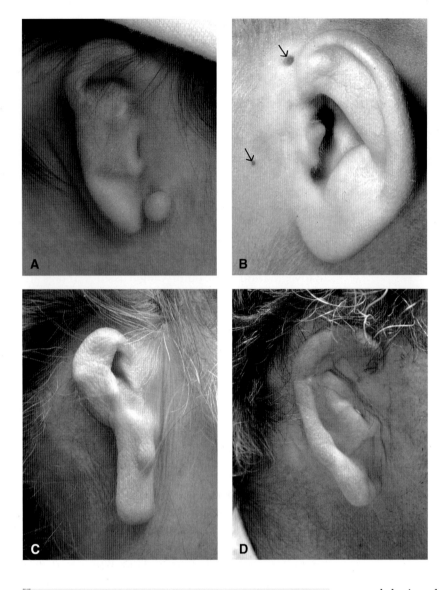

Figure 13-4   Anomalies of the pinna.
A. Microtia with atresia and preauricular tag.
B. Preauricular pits (arrows). **C**. Microtia with atresia. **D**. Atresia.

as it bypasses these structures altogether. Instead, sound is sent around the damaged or problematic area, naturally stimulating the cochlea through bone conduction. Once the cochlea receives these sound vibrations, the organ "hears" in the same manner as through air conduction; the sound is converted into neural signals and is transferred to the brain, allowing a Baha recipient to perceive sound.

ACQUIRED PATHOLOGIES OF THE OUTER EAR

Trauma

Cauliflower ear is an acquired pathology of the pinna resulting from trauma. Wrestlers and prizefighters are at high risk of acquiring this lesion. It is a direct result of the cartilage of the pinna and its connective tissue covering (i.e., **perichondrium**) being sepa-

rated during the trauma. Blood collects in the space, called a **hematoma**, causing the pinna to lose its normal shape, as seen in Figure 13-5. In the acute stage, the pinna will be tender and marked redness will be present. The pinna will not return to its normal shape unless treated. The hematoma will need to be aspirated and direct pressure applied until the tissue can reattach itself to the cartilage. A successful outcome is dependent on early treatment. Hearing loss is not usually a factor unless the opening of the external auditory meatus is occluded.

Neoplasms

Squamous cell carcinoma is a malignant tumor that is commonly seen on the pinna because of its obvious exposure to the sun. Squamous cell carcinoma is characterized by persistent thickening of the skin with red scaling, development of a painless pale outgrowth, and formation of open sores with a raised edge (see

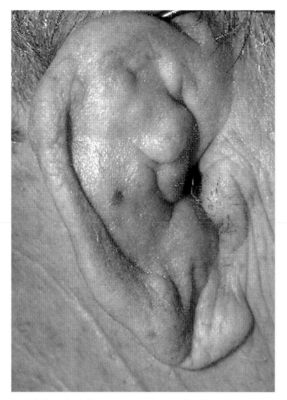

Figure 13-5 Cauliflower ear is the result of trauma to the pinna. Blood collects between the layers of tissue causing the deformity. The ear will not return to its normal shape unless treated.

Figure 13-6). The tumor can increase in size to a large mass and metastasize if not treated early. **Basal cell carcinoma** is a slow growing malignant skin cancer that also is prevalent on the pinna and also is a result of repeated sun exposure. It presents as a flat, painless lesion with the edges becoming slightly raised.

Basal cell carcinoma

Squamous cell carcinoma

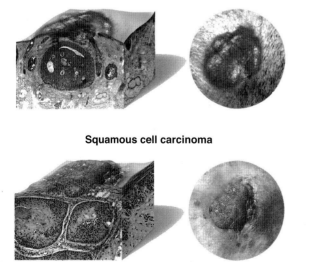

Figure 13-6 Basal cell and squamous cell carcinoma are types of skin cancers commonly seen on the pinna as a result of overexposure to the sun. (Reprinted with permission from Anatomical Chart Company.)

The lesion develops a rolled edge with a penetrating central ulcer that bleeds easily. It typically remains localized but there is a small possibility for metastasis. Although hearing may not be adversely affected, these cancers can be life threatening and should be reported to a physician immediately.

Obstructions

Obstructions of the ear canal are common. The vast majority of objects found in the ears are placed there, usually by children, and are a common reason for emergency room visits. Objects are limited only by the diameter of the ear canal, and might include earring backs, artificial fingernails, beans, beads, or insects. The vast majority of the objects are harmless. Some, however, can be extremely uncomfortable and require an anesthetic to be removed. If medical treatment is delayed, the object can quickly produce an infection.

Excessive cerumen is the most likely natural cause of ear canal obstruction (see Figure 13-7). Cerumen is created when the migrating skin of the canal mixes with the cilia and secretions from the ceruminous glands located in the outer one-third of the canal. Cerumen buildup occurs when the cilia that protect the entrance to the ear canal become matted with the migrating dead skin cells, impeding the natural sloughing process. Impaction is more common in males due to the presence of thicker, courser cilia. Cerumen also tends to become drier with age. Cotton swabs, earplugs, and hearing aids all can impact cerumen. Impaction can cause a temporary mild conductive hearing loss and in some cases discomfort. Removal of excessive cerumen is accomplished by **curette**, suction, or irrigation. However, before clean-

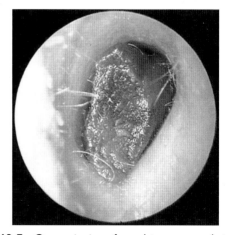

Figure 13-7 Otoscopic view of complete cerumen obstruction. (Reprinted with permission from Weber, J., Kelley, J. (2003). *Health assessment in nursing* (2nd ed.). Philadelphia: Lippincott Williams & Wilkins.)

ing the ear canal by irrigation, the tympanic membrane should be examined for the presence of a perforation or pressure equalization (PE) tube, so that cleaning agents are not forced into the middle ear cavity during the removal process.

Another common obstruction occurring in the ear canal is an **osteoma**. These are smooth, benign bony tumors that reside in the ear canal, most commonly at the isthmus where bone and cartilage meet. They are typically a result from swimming, surfing, or diving in cold water. Upon otoscopic examination, they appear as singular or multiple masses. They are usually not painful unless touched. Osteomas can continue to grow and interfere with the normal process of migration of skin to the outer ear. If large enough, they may block the canal and cause a conductive hearing loss. Osteomas can be surgically removed if necessary.

Inflammation

Figure 13-8 illustrates external otitis (i.e., **otitis externa**), which is an inflammatory condition of the ear canal. The organism that causes the inflammation is either fungi or bacteria that invade breaks in the epithelial lining of the ear canal. The organism resides in water and becomes trapped in the tortuous ear canal when it is repeatedly exposed to the water. Swimmers are prone to external otitis, hence its common name "swimmer's ear." The normally oily lining of the canal becomes inflamed, swollen, and itchy, creating a white discharge. The pinna can be painful to the touch, particularly in the area of the tragus. External otitis can either be acute or chronic. The individual prone to chronic inflammation prevents reoccurrence by protecting the ears from water. This can be accomplished with the use of custom earplugs worn during hair washing or swimming. Hearing aid users must be particularly careful to dry their ears before inserting their

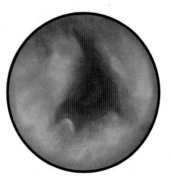

Figure 13-8 Acute external otitis (otitis externa) is an inflammation of the skin lining the ear canal. It is typically very painful and is caused from repeated exposure to water. (Reprinted with permission from Bickley, L.S., Szilagyi, P. (2003). *Bates' guide to physical examination and history taking* (8th ed.). Philadelphia: Lippincott Williams & Wilkins.)

aids. The ear mold or shell can trap moisture in the ear canal exposing the skin to bacteria or fungi.

Anomalies of the Middle Ear

Although anomalies of the middle ear can be congenital in nature, especially if they are part of a genetic syndrome, they tend to be relatively rare. The most common problems associated with the middle ear are acquired. Two acquired anomalies of the middle ear deserve a thorough discussion because of their prevalence in children and adults: **otitis media (OM)** and otosclerosis.

ACQUIRED PATHOLOGIES OF THE MIDDLE EAR

Otitis Media

OM is an inflammation of the lining of the middle ear. It is the most common of childhood infections and one of the most frequent reasons parents take their children to the physician. According to Schappert (1992) from the National Center for Health Statistics, visits to the physician for OM in 1975 totaled 10 million. By 1990, the number had increased to 25 million. As a population, children younger than 2 years of age have the highest rate of office visits for OM. It has been hypothesized that the high rate of OM in children is because they are together in large groups such as daycares and preschools, where exposure to the viruses and bacteria that cause the inflammation is more likely. Grundfast and Carney (1987) offered some additional statistics related to OM. In the United States, 85% to 90% of all children before the age of 6 years will have had at least one ear infection. Half of the children who have one ear infection before the age of one will have six or more episodes in the following 2 years. Therefore, the younger they start having infections, the more likely they are to continue. Nearly 20% of children who suffer ear infections will at some point require surgery to correct the problem. In addition, 25% to 40% of all upper respiratory infections (URIs) are associated with OM.

Howie, Ploussard, and Sloyer (1975) reported that gender and family history play a role in the incidence of OM. In terms of gender, males have a higher incidence of OM than females. In terms of family history, if a parent or parents had many ear infections when they were children, their own children will most likely have several infections. There is no OM gene *per se*, but facial features are inherited. For example, poor function of the structures of the nasopharynx such as the Eustachian tube (ET) can be inherited and can lead to bouts of OM.

There are several contributing factors that place a child at risk for OM. One is the exposure to second-hand cigarette smoke (Ey et al., 1995). The products in cigarette smoke can irritate the nasopharynx and lead to the onset of OM. A child of low socioeconomic status who lives where there are poor sanitary conditions or overcrowding and repeated exposed to chemicals, viruses, and bacteria that cause URI will place the child at greater risk for OM. Climate in and of itself is not a direct contributor to OM, but children who spend most of their time indoors because of poor outdoor weather conditions may be in close contact with many people and therefore may pass around viruses and bacteria that lead to URIs.

OM is nearly always the result of the Eustachian tube (ET) not opening to ventilate the middle ear. It may become blocked by inflammation of surrounding tissue. In particular, adenoid tissue may swell in response to irritants, viruses or bacteria. The inflamed adenoids block the nasopharyngeal opening of the ET. As was discussed in Chapter 12, the ET must be able to open to ventilate the middle ear cavity and thereby equalize air pressure between the middle ear and the atmosphere. In its acute form, OM commonly develops in association with an URI. Children and adults who have a syndrome or disorder whose sequelae include structural or functional abnormalities of the pharyngeal muscles are significantly at risk for middle ear disease.

There are basically three stages of OM: **acute OM**, **OM with effusion** and **OM with tympanic membrane perforation**. Acute OM commonly presents with a sudden onset of otalgia in association with symptoms of URI such as **rhinorrhea**, nasal congestion, cough and fever; however, these symptoms are not always present. Similarly, not all cases of otalgia are caused by OM.

Otoscopy performed on an individual who presents with acute OM reveals a red or yellow tympanic membrane depending on the degree of inflammation and the amount of purulent material in the middle ear cavity. There may be bulging of the pars flaccida or the entire eardrum. The movement of the tympanic membrane may be diminished. If the tympanic membrane is ruptured, ear pain will diminish but cloudy or purulent drainage in the ear canal will be visible. Antibiotic therapy is used to treat the infection and anti-inflammatory medication is used to treat the pain.

OM with effusion is the stage where fluid occupies the normally air-filled middle ear cavity. The fluid may be a remnant from the acute stage or may develop silently without the presence of a bacterial infection. OM with effusion creates a mild conductive hearing loss. On average there is a 27 dB hearing

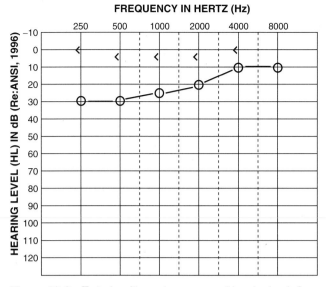

Figure 13-9 Typical audiometric pattern and hearing levels for a right ear with otitis media.

loss based on pure tone air conduction thresholds (see Figure 13-9). The majority of the loss is in the lower frequencies. Long standing, untreated OM can lead to much more complicated and severe ear disease processes, not to mention the concomitant hearing loss causing a delay in speech development of children who are in the critical years for speech and language acquisition.

When the ET does not function properly, it does not allow for ventilation of the middle ear cavity. The air that is normally in the cavity becomes stagnant and is absorbed by the membranous lining of the walls of the cavity. As a result, air pressure within the cavity will decrease (i.e., become negative) relative to atmospheric air pressure outside the cavity. The negative pressure causes the eardrum to be drawn inward or retracted from its normal position. The area of the pars flaccida is more susceptible to this negative pressure. Retraction of the eardrum is what causes the ear pain. Also as a result of the negative air pressure, serous fluid is secreted by the mucous membrane that lines the middle ear cavity. This fluid is thin and watery in consistency. If the ET continues to remain closed or inflamed, the consistency of the middle ear fluid will become thick and mucous-like. Bacteria can cause inflammation at any stage and create a pus-filled space. The term mucoid OM would eventually be applied with continued thickening of the effusion leading to **adhesive OM** or "glue ear." As the middle ear fluid gets thicker in consistency, hearing loss gets progressively worse. At the point where adhesive OM is present, there may be as much as a 40- to 50-dB conductive hearing loss. The hearing loss from serous OM may be the only sign of ear pathology. Middle ear fluid may not be obvious on otoscopic

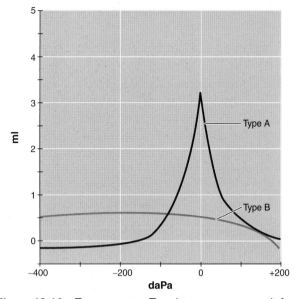

Figure 13-10 Tympanograms: Type A tympanogram result for a normal ventilated middle ear; Type B pattern indicates effusion (lack of ventilation) in the middle ear space.

examination, so detection is aided by the audiologist performing **tympanometry** to measure the immittance (i.e., mobility) of the eardrum. Middle ear fluid is indicated by a lack of movement, which reveals itself as an abnormal (i.e., flat-type B) **tympanogram** (see Figure 13-10).

There are several surgical options for treatment of OM. When OM has been attributed to blockage of the ET by hypertrophic (i.e., enlarged) adenoids, an

adenoidectomy will be recommended. If fluid has filled the middle ear cavity, a **myringotomy** may be performed. A myringotomy is an incision that is made in the tympanic membrane, with suctioning of the fluid from the middle ear cavity being done through the incision. The incision in the eardrum will heal in a matter of days. There is a chance that fluid will form again if whatever is causing the inflammation of the ET is not treated.

A **pressure equalization (PE) tube**, made of silastic material, is placed through a myringotomy incision into the eardrum (see Figure 13-11). The tube acts to ventilate the middle ear cavity by allowing outside atmospheric air to enter through the eardrum, thereby circumventing the function of the ET. The result is that the middle ear space is ventilated, with hearing returning to normal. Insertion of PE tubes buys time for the ET to begin working on its own or the child to outgrow whatever caused the ET to dysfunction in the first place. A PE tube will stay in place for months, until the eardrum heals and the tube is expelled into the ear canal. The normal migration of the ear canal epithelium will carry the tube along until it reaches the entrance of the canal where it will simply be sloughed off or can be reached by the physician's curette. When tubes are in place, there is concern about keeping water out of the ears. Conceivably, bacteria carried in water could enter the middle ear through the patent PE tube and cause an infection. Custom earplugs can be fit for hair washing, bathing, and swimming.

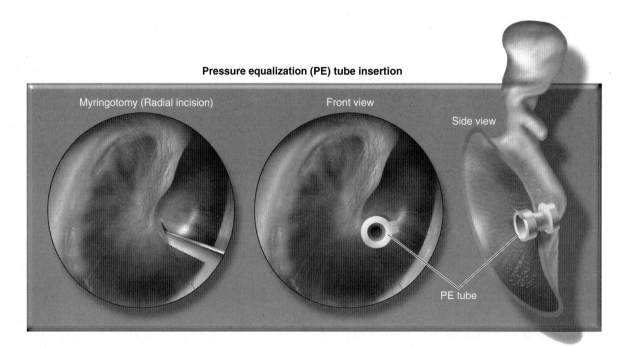

Figure 13-11 Myringotomy and placement of a pressure equalization (PE) tube into the tympanic membrane. (Reprinted with permission from Anatomical Chart Company.)

Complications of OM

Some complications of OM can be very significant and some can be minor. The most common complication is **tympanosclerosis** or scar tissue on the eardrum. It is the result of tissue changes that form on the TM as a result of recurrent ear infections. Tympanosclerosis is often seen as a white calcium plaque or scar tissue on the pars tensa. Fortunately, it has little effect on hearing.

Perforations of the eardrum can be caused by chronic ear infections where the TM ruptures and fails to heal, but can also be caused by trauma such as a puncture or forceful slap to the ear by a cupped hand or loud explosion. A perforation is described by its location on the eardrum: central, attic or marginal. A central perforation is shown in Figure 13-12. Small perforations will usually heal spontaneously. However, larger perforations generally require a surgical repair called a **myringoplasty** or Type I tympanoplasty. The surgeon uses the patient's own tissue (usually taken from the back of the ear) to create a graft that will be inserted underneath the eardrum remnant to close the perforation.

Remember that the middle ear cavity has the ability to communicate with the mastoid air cells; thus, bacterial secretory mucous (i.e., acute OM) can spread into the mastoid cavity, resulting in **mastoiditis**, a potentially life-threatening infection. Infected debris in the mastoid is trapped and can only be removed by surgical cleaning of this space. The surgeon removes the infected debris by drilling out the individual air cells leaving one large cavity (referred to as a **mastoidectomy**). The healthy cavity must then be mechanically cleaned periodically to prevent further disease. Another complication of OM is the formation of a **cholesteatoma**, a cyst made of layers of epithelial debris from the

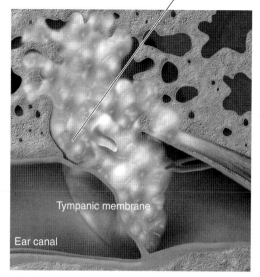

Figure 13-13   A cholesteatoma is a complication from poor Eustachian tube function and otitis media. Debris forms in a retraction pocket in the pars flaccida region of the tympanic membrane. (Reprinted with permission from Anatomical Chart Company.)

tympanic membrane. The cyst contains considerable amounts of keratin, a protein found in cells. Formation of a cholesteatoma is usually associated with poor ET function and chronic OM where the TM has been in a long-standing retracted state. A pocket is formed in the area of the pars flaccida by the continual retraction from negative middle ear pressure. As illustrated in Figure 13-13, the pocket retains sloughed debris. Inflammation causes the pocket to swell and expand. It can eventually invade the epitympanic recess or attic of the middle ear cavity. The expanding cholesteatoma destructively encroaches upon the middle ear cavity and structures. As it continues to grow, it has the potential to erode away portions of the ossicles and invade other structures such as the mastoid air cells, the horizontal semicircular canal, and even the bones of the cranium. Its aggressive capability makes it potentially life threatening. It is also a major cause of a conductive hearing loss. A cholesteatoma should be surgically removed and monitored because of its ability to reform.

Otosclerosis

Otosclerosis is a middle ear disease in which normal bone is progressively reabsorbed and replaced by spongy bone growth. This condition most often takes place around the footplate of the stapes and the oval window. The new growth of bone interferes with the normal vibration of the stapes footplate. It is not painful and the patient does not even know what is happening except for the progression of a hearing

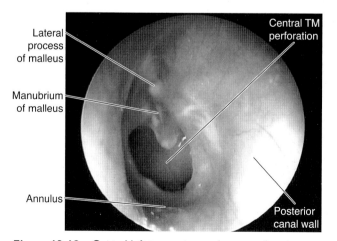

Figure 13-12   Central left tympanic membrane perforation typically caused by chronic ear infections.

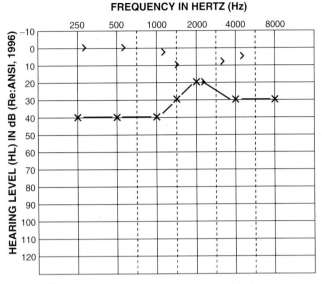

Figure 13-14 Typical audiometric pattern and bone conduction Carhart's notch for a left ear with otosclerosis.

loss. There are often head noises, typically a roaring or seashell-like sound. The progression of the disease is slow and takes place over several years. Otosclerosis is usually bilateral, first seen in one ear and then progressing to the other ear. However, the disease tends to progress at different rates for each ear. The ears are otoscopically normal with the possible exception of **Schwartze's sign**, a reddish or pinkish glow visualized through the tympanic membrane produced by increased vascularity on the promontory.

Otosclerosis impedes the vibration of the footplate of the stapes resulting in a conductive hearing loss. The hearing loss worsens in degree as the disease progresses. Audiometry and immittance measures are performed to aid in the identification of this disease.

As charted in Figure 13-14, the conductive portion of the loss is usually moderate (no greater than a 60-dB loss) depending on the disease progression. Bone conduction thresholds are often elevated at 2000 Hz. This classic pattern is called **Carhart's notch** and is typically only seen with otosclerosis. The notch in the bone conduction threshold for 2000 Hz is thought to be a result of the diminished **resonance** of the ossicular chain.

There are varying estimates of the prevalence of hearing loss as a result of otosclerosis. Pearson (1974) reported the prevalence as high as 10% of the general population. Declau et al. (2001) also studied prevalence and compared it to what was seen clinically. Their estimate of 0.3% (3 per 1000) was much more conservative than Pearson's estimate. Many clinicians would agree that the prevalence reported by Declau et al. (2001) is a more realistic estimate. The cause of otosclerosis is not fully understood. It may begin at any age but there seems to be a relationship between otosclerosis and the timing of hormonal changes typically seen in puberty, pregnancy, or menopause. Otosclerosis tends to be more prevalent in families and more so in Caucasian women.

Otosclerosis cannot be treated medically but surgery is an option. The goal of surgery is to restore the air conduction hearing levels for the patient. Amplification is also an option when surgery is not elected. A good candidate for surgery should exhibit a substantial air-bone gap (greater than 20 dB) with normal or near-normal bone conduction thresholds and good word recognition scores. The surgery, called a **stapedectomy**, involves removal of the stapes superstructure and footplate (see Figure 13-15). Upon removal of the stapes, the oval window is sealed

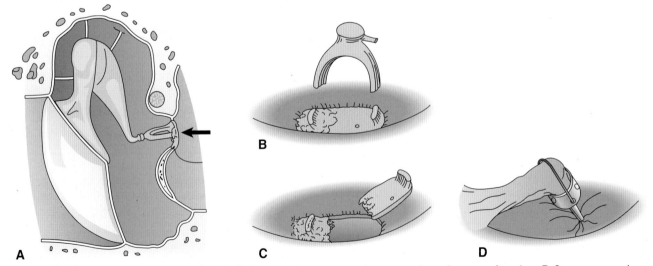

Figure 13-15 Stapedectomy for otosclerosis. **A**. Arrow points to spongy bone growth on the stapes footplate. **B**. Stapes removed. **C**. Footplate is removed. **D**. Prosthesis placed into position. (Reprinted with permission from Smeltzer, S.C., Bare, B.G. (2000). *Textbook of medical-surgical nursing* (9th ed.). Philadelphia: Lippincott Williams & Wilkins.)

with connective fascia tissue. The stapes is then replaced with a prosthetic device made of Teflon and titanium. The head of the prosthesis is crimped to the lenticular process of the incus, thereby reestablishing the ossicular chain. The other end of the prosthesis is articulated with the oval window. The intact chain can once again transmit vibrations to the cochlea. When otosclerosis is bilateral, surgery is performed on one ear at a time; the ear with the larger air-bone gap is usually operated on first. The second ear surgery is delayed a minimum of 6 months to ensure that the initial result is successful. Surgery is considered successful when the preoperative air-bone gap is closed.

Anomalies of the Inner Ear

GENETICS OF HEARING LOSS

Smith, Green, and Van Camp (1999) authored an excellent review of genetics and hearing loss. They reported that genetics account for approximately 50% of the cases of hearing loss. The remaining 50% are acquired (i.e., nongenetic) from environmental causes. There is however, within the acquired environmental group 25% that are idiopathic in nature, meaning that there is no known cause.

Hereditary hearing loss through genetic transmission may be syndromic or nonsyndromic. A syndrome is a consistent pattern of abnormalities and/or symptoms that results from the same underlying cause. The term nonsyndromic refers to a disorder that occurs in isolation of any other genetic features. Seventy percent of genetic hearing losses are nonsyndromic and 30% are syndromic.

The mode of inheritance typically takes one of three forms: **autosomal dominant, autosomal recessive**, or **X-linked recessive**. For autosomal dominant, one parent carries the dominant gene on at least one chromosome and he or she is affected by the trait (in this case, hearing loss). The genetic transmission from one parent is sufficient to produce the disorder. Therefore, each time there is a pregnancy, there is a 50% chance the baby will receive the dominant gene trait (see Table 13-1).

Autosomal recessive trait is illustrated in Table 13-2. The parent carries the gene but does not exhibit the trait (i.e., hearing loss). The parent most likely would not even be aware that they carry the gene. The genetic trait from only one parent is not enough to produce the disorder in the offspring. With autosomal recessive transmission, both carrier parents are needed for the trait to be expressed (i.e., a deaf or hard of hearing offspring). Each time there is a pregnancy, the baby will have a 25% chance of the recessive trait

TABLE 13-1

AUTOSOMAL DOMINANT MODE OF INHERITANCE		
N/n Normal hearing parent *H/h Hearing loss *Dominant gene trait 50% chance for hearing loss 50% chance for normal hearing	N	n
*H	*HN (Hearing loss)	*Hn (Hearing loss)
h	Nh	hn

being expressed, 50% chance of receiving the recessive gene and being a carrier like the parents, and 25% chance of losing the recessive gene altogether.

A genetic (but nonsyndromic) hearing loss is suspected when a child is either born with a hearing loss or acquired it very early in their life. During the period 1996–1997, researchers such as Kumar and Gilula (1996) identified the gene responsible for the majority of recessive inherited sensorineural deafness. The offspring of two (hearing) carrier parents inherits the mutated gene (**GJB2**) located on the 13th chromosome. The gene GJB2 encodes for the **gap junction channel** protein **connexin 26**. Gap junctions are clusters of intercellular channels that allow communication between cells. Without proper cellular communication, the chemical balance of the endolymph and the perilymph within the organ of Corti cannot be maintained.

TABLE 13-2

AUTOSOMAL RECESSIVE MODE OF INHERITANCE		
N/*n Normal hearing but a carrier *Recessive gene trait 50% chance of carrying the gene 25% chance for hearing loss 25% chance to lose the trait	N	*n
N	NN	N*n (Carrier)
*n	N*n (Carrier)	*n*n (Hearing loss)

TABLE 13-3

X-LINKED RECESSIVE MODE OF INHERITANCE		
X/Y Dad X/*x Mom (Carrier) *Recessive gene trait 50% chance a son will have hearing loss 50% chance a daughter will be a carrier	X	Y
X	XX daughter	XY son
*x	X*x daughter (Carrier)	*xY son (Hearing loss)

X-linked recessive trait accounts for only about 2% of the cases of congenital hearing loss. Transmission is always from mother to son as males get either their dominant X or recessive x chromosome from their mother. The mother does not have the hearing loss and she most likely is unaware that she is a carrier. When the gene trait is expressed, the son inherits his mother's recessive x for hearing loss. When that son has children, his daughters will inherit the recessive gene trait making them carriers; his sons will be fine because they will inherit either their X or x from their mother. X-linked recessive trait is illustrated in Table 13-3.

CONGENITAL DISORDERS OF THE INNER EAR

Anomalies of the inner ear may be associated with genetic syndromes or may occur alone. The most extreme and rare form of an inner ear anomaly is called **Michel dysplasia**. The term dysplasia means a malformation of the bone that may occur in any part of the body. Michel dysplasia results when cochlear development is arrested early during the embryonic period. With extreme dysplasia, there are no definitive cochlear or vestibular structures (Kavanagh & Magill, 1989). A common cavity may occur and in some cases the entire auditory nerve may also be absent. Michel dysplasia may affect only the cochlea and the vestibule, with the semicircular canals being essentially normal. Michel dysplasia is seen in 1% of individuals with profound hearing loss.

Mondini dysplasia involves the normal development of the first 1½ turns of the cochlea. The remaining turn will be either absent or markedly malformed in that there is no separation between the osseous and membranous labyrinth. The vestibule and semicircular canals may or may not be normally developed. Mondini dysplasia may be present at birth or develop later in adult life. Since the basal end of the cochlea is essentially missing, the loss in the high frequencies will be profound.

Scheibe dysplasia is the most common form of congenital malformation of the inner ear. The bony labyrinth is typically complete and intact. However, the membranous labyrinth is intact for the semicircular canals and utricle but the saccule and **cochlear duct** (scala media) are poorly defined with atrophy of the organ of Corti. The degree of hearing loss is of course profound.

Alexander aplasia is typically limited to the absence of the basal turn of the cochlear duct, organ of Corti, and ganglion cells. Absence of the basal portion of the cochlea will result in high-frequency hearing loss while low-frequency hearing remains relatively intact.

Associated Anomalies

Syndromes present themselves from a genetic origin 30% of the time. Hearing loss is but one of the associated anomalies. The other anomalies that are frequently seen in syndromes with hearing loss are classified as:

- integumentary (pertaining to the skin)
- skeletal
- ocular (visual impairment)
- other (commonly, renal or cardiac).

When an error in the genetic message interrupts the embryologic developmental process in one area (such as skin), another area (such as skeletal formation) may also be disrupted. Integumentary anomalies pertain to pigmentation changes of the skin. Integumentary anomalies and congenital sensorineural hearing loss are the chief sequelae of many syndromes. Both skin and portions of the cochlea have the same embryological origin. The genetic message that results in the abnormal patterns of pigmentation such as **albinism** (i.e., a lack of pigmentation) or **piebaldism** (i.e., strips of too much or too little

TABLE 13-4

GENETIC SYNDROMES AND SEQUELAE TO IDENTIFY ASSOCIATED ANOMALIES

Syndrome	Associated Sequelae
Alport	Kidney problems
Brachio-Oto-Renal (BOR)	Neck cysts and kidney problems
Jervell and Lange-Nielsen	Cardiac problems
Pendred	Thyroid enlargement or low thyroid function
Stickler	Unusual facial features, cleft palate, eye problems (e.g., nearsightedness, cataracts, or retinal detachment), arthritis, cardiac problems
Usher	Progressive blindness
Waardenburg	White patch of hair or light-colored skin patches; eyes of two different colors, or bright blue eyes, or widely spaced eyes

pigmentation) may also result in a severe congenital sensorineural hearing loss. **Waardenburg syndrome** is an example of a syndrome with multiple associated anomalies.

A syndrome characterized by a skeletal defect is **Klippel-Feil syndrome**. Persons with this syndrome exhibit a shortened neck, curvature of the spine, and within the middle ear a poorly shaped stapes. The origin of skeletal and ossicular malformations can often be traced back to the same embryologic beginnings. Poor fusion of the cranial structures is sometimes associated with atresia of the ear canal.

Ocular anomalies are commonly associated with hearing loss. A variety of ocular anomalies are seen with **Crouzon syndrome**. These anomalies can range from complete absence of the eyes, to widely separated eyes, to bulging of the eyes. **Usher's syndrome** is associated with a slow progressive loss of vision resulting from **retinitis pigmentosa** (i.e., atrophy of the retina) and a gradual loss of hearing. Visual impairment is one of the three most common disorders associated with hearing loss. Table 13-4 presents a brief chart of genetic syndromes associated with hearing loss. Note the associated anomalies that often accompany the hearing loss.

ACQUIRED ETIOLOGY OF CONGENITAL HEARING LOSS

The TORCH Complex

Twenty-five percent of the cases of congenital hearing loss are acquired from various etiologies. From the third to ninth week of gestation, the developing embryo is extremely susceptible to **teratogenic** agents. It is during this period that the fetal organs are formed from the primitive **germ cell layers**; therefore, it is the timing of fetal exposure that determines the severity of the problem. When present in the fetal environment, a teratogenic agent may cause disorders that affect the baby's development and/or learning. Maternal infections are of primary concern; in particular, the major teratogenic agents that cross the pregnant mother's placenta to infect the fetus are referred to by the acronym **TORCH**: <u>T</u>oxoplasmosis, <u>O</u>ther (including syphilis), <u>R</u>ubella, <u>C</u>ytomegalovirus, and <u>H</u>erpes. Some of the TORCH infections, such as toxoplasmosis and syphilis, can be effectively treated with antibiotics if the mother is diagnosed early in her pregnancy. Many of the viral TORCH infections have no effective treatment, but some, notably Rubella, can be prevented by vaccinating the mother prior to pregnancy. If the mother has active herpes simplex, delivery by Caesarean section can prevent the newborn from contact and consequent infection with this virus.

Toxoplasmosis is a parasitic infection contracted by consumption of contaminated raw meats and eggs as well as from improper handling of cat feces. The parasite called *Toxoplasma gondii* multiplies in the intestine of cats and is shed in cat feces, mainly into litter boxes and garden soil. Healthy mothers usually do not suffer ill effects from toxoplasmosis; at most they may feel like they have the flu. The disease is transmitted to the developing fetus through the placenta. Infected babies may not develop the disease or they may become very ill. The exposed newborn often has low birth weight, jaundice, an enlarged liver, inflammation of the retina, and hearing loss which may be moderate to severe and progressive. Toxoplasmosis is preventable by avoiding exposure to the agents that carry the parasite. If you have been infected previously (at least 6 to 9 months before your pregnancy) with toxoplasma, you will develop immunity to it. The infection will not be active when you become pregnant, and so there is rarely a risk to the baby.

Congenital **syphilis** is a sexually transmitted bacterial infection (*Treponema pallidum*) that is passed from the mother to her fetus. The infection affects many of the baby's systems and early signs include skin lesions, meningitis, mental retardation, seizures, and hearing loss to list just a few. The disease was dubbed the "great imitator" because so many of its signs and symptoms are indistinguishable from those of other diseases. The sensorineural hearing loss is typically delayed in onset, developing at any time during childhood or adulthood. The loss may have a sudden onset or may progress slowly, and may be unilateral or bilateral. Early identification and prompt treatment with high doses of antibiotics improves the potential for reversibility.

Congenital rubella is a viral infection passed from the mother to her baby through the placenta. Infection spreads through direct contact with discharge from the nose or throat of an affected individual. If the infection is contracted within the first trimester of pregnancy, it poses the greatest risk to the developing fetus. Rubella syndrome in the newborn results in a consistent pattern of physical abnormalities characterized by rash, low birth weight, small head size (i.e., microcephaly), cardiac abnormalities, hearing loss, visual problems, and bulging fontanelle. Since it is a viral infection, there is no cure; only treatment of the symptoms is possible. An epidemic of rubella occurred in the 1960s; however, the development of a vaccine in 1968 has greatly reduced the incidence of this disease.

Cytomegalovirus (CMV), a virus of the herpes group, can be transmitted sexually or by close contact with infected secretions. It is a virus most humans are exposed to at some time in their life, but typically only individuals with a weakened immune system become ill from CMV infection. By 40 years of age, between 50% and 80% of adults in the United States have been infected with CMV. Adults acquire CMV through sexual contact with an infected partner who is shedding the virus in blood, semen or vaginal fluids. Adults and children can acquire it from contact with infected children shedding the virus in blood, saliva, and urine as might be the case in a daycare environment. An infected mother may even transmit the virus to her infant through contact with breast milk. Pass, Hutto, Reynolds, and Polhill (1984) tested a cohort of children less than 12 months of age at a typical daycare center. Less than 10% of the children were shedding the virus at the time they enrolled in the daycare but 6 to 12 months later 78% were shedding the virus. Once an individual is infected with the virus, it remains for life. Eventually, the virus goes dormant and the individual's immune system develops antibodies to fight it. Therefore, for the majority of people, it is "silent" and not a serious problem. However, a primary (or first) CMV infection in a pregnant woman can cause serious harm to the developing fetus. About 1% to 4% of pregnant women experience a primary CMV infection. Thirty-three percent of these women pass the virus to their unborn babies. High levels of stress can also reactivate the dormant virus in a pregnant woman but this happens less than 1% of the time.

A baby infected *in utero* (i.e., congenital CMV) may be symptomatic or asymptomatic at birth. Five percent of infected newborns are symptomatic and present with symptoms ranging from mild to severe. The mild symptoms may include being small for gestation age (SGA), having an enlarged spleen or liver, exhibiting jaundice, and having a distinctive purplish rash. Up to 10% of symptomatic infants die shortly after birth; of the survivors, many suffer from serious impairments such as mental retardation, hearing loss, and visual impairment. Sensorineural hearing loss is present in approximately 40% of these symptomatic infants. Infants with the more severe effects from primary CMV are born to women who contracted the infection in the first trimester of pregnancy.

Approximately 95% of babies who are infected with the virus *in utero* are asymptomatic at birth (Oshiro, 1999). There is approximately a 5% chance of these babies developing a complication. Hearing loss is the most common complication (in 7% to 15% of cases) and very often is delayed in its onset, with 4 years of age being the average age of onset. Researchers such as Foulon et al. (2008) have seen the onset of hearing loss attributed to congenital CMV up to the age of 15. Once the hearing loss presents itself, it is always progressive and usually severe to profound in degree. To summarize the incidence of congenital CMV, one child out of 150 births is infected. Approximately one child out of 750 born with the infection develops permanent disabilities; this equates to 6000 children each year. Congenital CMV is as common a cause of serious disability as Down syndrome and fetal alcohol syndrome. Being a common cause of hearing loss in childhood, regular audiometric evaluations should be conducted in children with known congenital CMV.

Neonatal herpes is a sexually transmitted viral disease that can be passed from the infected mother to her fetus either during pregnancy or during delivery if the disease is active. One of every 3000 newborns delivered is infected with neonatal herpes. Over 70% of infants infected with the herpes simplex virus are from mothers with a primary infection who have asymptomatic viral shedding during labor. Infected infants even with immediate treatment may have central nervous system involvement and sensorineural hearing loss.

Bacterial Meningitis

Bacterial meningitis is an acquired pathology that is spread by direct contact with nasal secretions, saliva or sputum from an infected individual. It can also be a major complication from an untreated ear or sinus infection. It is seen almost exclusively in children less than 5 years of age. Contracting the infection places the individual at significant risk for hearing loss. The bacteria enter the blood stream and spread to the meninges covering the brain and the spinal cord (in particular the subarachnoid space). The extent the infection spreads explains the symptoms including high fever, vomiting, a stiff neck, and malaise. Several bacterial strains can be responsible for meningitis but 70% of the infections are from the **haemophilus influenzae Type b (Hib)**. Although Hib is the most common bacteria to cause meningitis, fortunately it is the least likely to result in hearing loss (in only 3% to 16% of cases). Other causes of bacterial meningitis include the **pneumococcal** and **meningococcal** strains. These have a much lower incidence of causing meningitis but a higher incidence of causing hearing loss (24% to 36% of cases). Treatment for meningitis is with antibiotics delivered intravenously. Successful treatment depends on prompt diagnosis. A lumbar puncture is often necessary to check for the presence of the bacteria in the cerebrospinal fluid. The haemophilus influenzae Type b bacteria can be safely and effectively prevented from causing meningitis with the use of the Hib vaccine that was introduced in 1990.

Severe to profound sensorineural hearing loss occurs when the cochlea is invaded by the bacterial infection. Any episode of meningitis warrants a hearing evaluation even before the patient is discharged from the hospital. It is recommended that any finding of hearing loss be followed with monthly reevaluation until the hearing loss stabilizes. The major complication of an infection invading the cochlea is the ossification of the bony labyrinth. The ossification process begins to appear within 3 months of the onset of meningitis and may be complete by 1 year. The ossification is often bilateral. If the hearing loss is profound and a **cochlear implant (CI)** is considered (see Figure 13-16), the presence of ossification within the cochlea can create problems with placement of the electrode array (refer to the Why You Need to Know box on the CI); therefore, the typical waiting period is waived to expedite the surgery before ossification can become too advanced and reduce the likelihood of successful implantation.

Other Risk Factors

There are several other birth complications that place an infant at risk for an acquired hearing loss. Prior to the advent of universal newborn hearing screening, the presence of "risk factors" were used to aid in early identification efforts. It is now accepted that screening children based on risk factors alone is not enough.

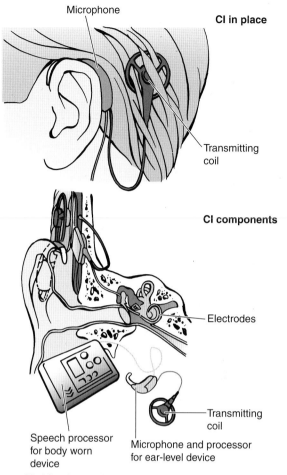

Figure 13-16 A typical cochlear implant (CI) system. Sounds are picked up by the small directional microphone located in the headset at the ear. A thin cord carries the sound from the microphone to the speech processor which, in turn, filters, analyzes, and digitizes the sound into coded signals that are sent from the processor to the transmitting coil. The transmitting coil sends the coded signals (RF signals) to the CI located under the person's skin. The implant delivers the appropriate electrical signals to an array of electrodes that have been inserted into the cochlea. The electrodes within the cochlea stimulate the remaining fibers of the cochlear portion of the vestibulocochlear nerve (cranial nerve VIII). These fibers then send the sound information to the auditory cortex for interpretation. (Reprinted with permission from Nettina, S. M. (2001). *The Lippincott manual of nursing practice* (7th ed.). Philadelphia: Lippincott Williams & Wilkins.)

Recall that 25% of cases of hearing loss are idiopathic in origin. Additionally, there might not be an obvious family history of hearing loss. As previously discussed, 70% of the cases of nonsyndromic hearing loss are due to autosomal recessive gene transmission where the individual is unaware of the genetic link. With that said, the 2007 Joint Committee on Infant Hearing (JCIH) established a position statement outlining principles and guidelines for Early Hearing Detection and Intervention (EHDI) programs.

The JCIH endorses early detection of and intervention for infants with hearing loss. The goal of EHDI is to maximize linguistic competence and literacy development for children who are deaf or hard of hearing. Without appropriate opportunities to learn language, these children will fall behind their hearing peers in communication, cognition, reading, and social–emotional development. Such delays may result in lower educational and employment levels in adulthood. To maximize the outcome for infants who are deaf or hard of hearing, the hearing of all infants should be screened at no later than 1 month of age. Those who do not pass screening should have a comprehensive audiological evaluation at no later than 3 months of age. Infants with confirmed hearing loss should receive appropriate intervention at no later than 6 months of age from health care and education professionals with expertise in hearing loss and deafness in infants and young children. Regardless of previous hearing–screening outcomes, all infants with or without risk factors should receive ongoing surveillance of communicative development beginning at 2 months of age during well-child visits in the **medical home** [boldface added]. EHDI systems should guarantee seamless transitions for infants and their families through this process (Joint Committee on Infant Hearing, 2007, p. 898).

The position statement does establish several criteria for identifying children at risk for congenital, delayed-onset, permanent, or progressive hearing loss during childhood (several of these criteria have been discussed in this chapter). These criteria include:

- caregiver concern regarding hearing, speech, language, or developmental delay

- a family history of permanent childhood hearing loss

- a stay in the neonatal intensive care unit (NICU) of more than 5 days

- *in utero* infections, such as CMV, herpes, rubella, syphilis and toxoplasmosis

- syndromes known to be associated with hearing loss or progressive or late-onset hearing loss

- physical findings that are associated with a syndrome known to include a sensorineural or permanent conductive hearing loss

- the presence of craniofacial anomalies, including those that involve the pinna, ear canal, ear tags, ear pits, and temporal bone anomalies

- culture positive postnatal infections associated with sensorineural hearing loss including confirmed bacterial meningitis

- neurodegenerative disorders or sensory motor neuropathies

- head trauma, especially basal skull/temporal bone fractures that require hospitalization

- chemotherapy.

The position statement recommends that the hospital-based EHDI screening program provides the parents with information about hearing, speech, and language milestones. The screening results will be sent to the medical home for management and any need for referral and follow-up. The primary care provider will refer to an audiologist any patient for whom there are concerns or findings consistent with hearing loss. Therefore, for infants with a risk factor which may be considered low risk, at least one audiology assessment by 24 to 30 months is the recommendation. In contrast, for an infant with risk factors known to be associated with late onset or progressive hearing loss (such as CMV or family history), early and more frequent assessment is appropriate. Early and more frequent can be interpreted as every 6 months or more, depending on the clinical findings and concerns.

Why You Need to Know

The cochlear implant (CI) is a management tool for deafness, not a treatment for deafness. In fact, the CI relies on the functioning structures of the auditory mechanism. The implant provides electrical stimulation to the cochlear nerve fibers by bypassing the missing or damaged hair cells. In most cases of deafness, the cochlear nerve remains functional. Sounds are picked up by the implant's external microphone and sent to a processor. The processor converts the acoustic signal into a digital signal. The transmitter, held in place by a magnet, sends the signal via radio waves to the implanted receiver to be delivered by the electrode array hugging the modiolus. The receiver is surgically placed in a well drilled into the mastoid process. The electrode array is inserted through a hole drilled into the promontory (basal turn of the cochlea). The processor takes advantage of the tonotopic organization of the cochlea, delivering high-frequency information to electrodes hugging the basal end of the cochlea and low-frequency information to electrodes hugging the apex. The main indication for CI candidacy (adults and children) is limited speech recognition with amplification. Also paramount is for adults who are prelingually deafened and parents of children with severe-to-profound hearing loss to have a strong desire for oral communication. The Federal Drug Administration has approved CIs for children at age 12 months with enrollment in an educational environment that stresses oral communication.

ACQUIRED DISORDERS OF LATER ONSET

Ménière's Disease

Ménière's disease was first described in 1861 by the French physician, Prosper Ménière. Classic Ménière's syndrome is characterized by vertigo, fluctuating hearing loss, ear noise, and a pressure sensation in the ear. **Episodic vertigo** is often accompanied by nausea and vomiting. The hearing loss is sensorineural in nature. In the initial stages, the typical configuration involves low-frequency hearing loss, but as the disease progresses the higher frequencies will decline as well, flattening out the audiometric pattern. The hearing loss often fluctuates, worsening just prior to an attack and usually improving as the other symptoms subside. The individual may experience an unusual intolerance to loud sounds known as **recruitment**. The involved ear will likely be afflicted by low-pitch seashell or roaring tinnitus. The tinnitus usually gets more intense just prior to an attack. A full, plugged or pressure sensation may be experienced in the involved ear. This may be a constant symptom or one that is only present just prior to an attack. Many sufferers experience an aura or premonition of an impending attack. The disease usually affects one ear but there may be bilateral involvement. Males under the age of 50 are more prone to the disease.

The symptoms of Ménière's are associated with disturbances that affect the entire inner ear. The disease, therefore, involves the structures related to both the vestibular and auditory systems. Recall the one structure that is common to both is the membranous labyrinth. The disease causes a change in the endolymphatic fluid volume within the labyrinth. It is not clear if the cause is related to excessive production of endolymph or the inefficient reabsorption of excessive endolymph.

Many experts believe that endolymphatic fluid volume builds within the labyrinth to the point that Reissner's membrane will bulge and eventually rupture. Recall, Reissner's membrane separates endolymph in the scala media from perilymph in the scala vestibuli. When Reissner's membrane ruptures there is a mixing of the two fluids. The abrupt chemical disruption accounts for the sudden severe attack of vertigo with nausea and vomiting. After the acute attack of vertigo subsides, hearing will improve and the ear noise will alleviate. Attacks vary in their frequency but the patient experiences vertigo for several hours and may experience unsteadiness for days. This process may repeat itself in as little as several days or may not occur again for several months. Hence, the episodic nature of the disease is very unpredictable.

Ménière's disease has been attributed to many different causes: allergic reaction, trauma, viral infection, syphilis, and genetic origin. However, the primary etiology of Ménière's disease is idiopathic, meaning the underlying cause is unknown. There is no cure for Ménière's disease, but medical intervention is often helpful in managing the symptoms. Treatment involves controlling the dizziness with medication that suppresses the central nervous system's reaction to the unequal information from the vestibular structures. Treatment also focuses on prevention of future attacks by diet and lifestyle changes. It is recommended that the sufferer avoid factors known to exacerbate the symptoms such as alcohol, caffeine, tobacco, foods high in sodium, and to the extent possible, stress. Diuretics may be prescribed to control symptoms by reducing fluid retention and antihistamines may be used to control allergies.

Ménière's syndrome is diagnosed by an extensive case history and audiometric evaluation to document the hearing loss by configuration and degree. Serial audiometric evaluations are performed to document the fluctuation of hearing levels. The integrity of the vestibular system may be measured and monitored with **electronystagmography (ENG)**. The physician will use nuclear imaging techniques to rule out the presence of a tumor on the vestibulocochlear nerve.

Surgical procedures are usually attempted only when medical treatment has been exhausted and the patient is incapacitated by the disease. The least invasive procedure involves the placement of a shunt to reestablish the function of the endolymphatic sac. In theory, the shunt should decompress the excessive fluid in the sac and allow the inner ear to reequilibrate, taking pressure off the nerve endings of hearing and balance. The fluctuating hearing levels should stabilize. When there is residual hearing worth preserving a vestibular **neurectomy** is the procedure of choice (Mattox, 2000). The vestibular branch of the vestibulocochlear nerve is sectioned. Control of vertigo is successful in 90% of patients as it insures that the diseased vestibular system can no longer send signals to the brain. In individuals who have very little functional hearing and very poor discrimination, where preservation is not the goal, a **labyrinthectomy** can be performed. This is a procedure where the entire diseased inner ear is surgically removed or chemically poisoned with ototoxic drugs (i.e., drugs that are toxic only to the hearing mechanism).

Following surgery, there is usually a period of severe vertigo. This can be controlled with medication and should be temporary as the opposite (i.e., healthy) ear takes over the command of the entire balance function and assumes full control. If one vestibular system is sending damaged signs to the brain, the brain has trouble adapting since it is intermittently getting wrong signals mixed with correct ones. However, if the inner ear balance nerve is completely shut off on one side and the damaged system removed, the brain will adapt to this new situation since it now receives only correct signals from the one remaining healthy system which will control the entire balance function. Sadly, about 20% of people with Meniere's disease will also develop the illness in their opposite ear later in their lifetime.

Autoimmune Inner Ear Disease

The immune system is very complex and is the first line of defense against infectious organisms and foreign substances that invade our body and cause disease. The immune system is made up of a network of cells and proteins that work together to fight the invaders. For the most part the immune system functions without a problem. However, when dysfunction occurs, the result can be relatively minor or can result in major disease. Certain lifestyle issues (i.e., poor diet, cigarette smoking) and even some prescription medications can trigger an improper response from the immune system. Some diseases, such as rheumatoid arthritis, are believed to be caused by an overactive immune system. How the immune system works is not completely understood. A healthy immune system recognizes "invaders" such as viruses, bacteria or anything foreign that is not a normal part of the body and destroys it. Inflammation is a major function of the immune system, yet sometimes this works against us. **Autoimmune inner ear disease (AIED)** is the result of an improper response from the immune system that affects the auditory and balance system. This is a syndrome characterized by progressive hearing loss and/or dizziness which is caused by antibodies that attack and cause damage to the inner ear. The classic set of symptoms (and hence the term syndrome) are: bilateral progressive hearing loss accompanied with tinnitus (i.e., ringing, buzzing or humming in the ears), spells of dizziness, and abnormal blood tests for general autoimmune diseases. The diagnosis is based on history, physical examination, blood tests, and hearing and balance tests. AIED may resemble other inner ear disorders such as those seen in Meniere's disease, auditory neuropathy, and even syphilis. In general, autoimmune disorders occur more frequently in women than men and less frequently in children and

the elderly. There are several theories as to what causes AIED. One theory is *bystander damage*. In this theory, damage to the inner ear causes cytokines (involved in the regulation of various inflammatory responses) to be released which provoke, after a delay, additional immune reactions. This theory might explain the occasional cyclical nature of the disease.

> ### Why You Need to Know
>
> *Cytokines* *are a class of proteins that are secreted by cells into the circulation or directly into the tissue. The cytokine proteins locate the target immune cells and act by binding with them. The result is inflammation. A certain amount of inflammation is necessary for healing; however, overproduction or inappropriate production of certain cytokines by the body can result in disease. For example, in many types of arthritis, the body's inflammatory response is misdirected.*

Another theory is *cross-reaction*. Antibodies created to fight a virus or bacteria that are attacking the body can mistakenly attack the inner ear too as they can share common **antigens** (Boulassel, Tornasi, Deggoui, & Gersdorff, 2001). It is also common for antigens to be released following surgery, so the body may wrongly mount an attack on the "foreign" antigen residing in the inner ear.

An early diagnosis is important in the treatment of AIED. With proper treatment, the hearing loss may be reversed or at least the progression arrested. The standard treatment for an autoimmune reaction is often the same antirejection medications used for transplant patients. Chemotherapy is an option sometimes delivered as long-term therapy. Unfortunately, the side effects of these medications can be numerous or dramatic and can affect the entire body.

Presbycusis

An acquired hearing disorder that is the result of aging is referred to as **presbycusis**. This term has been used to describe the "deafness of aging." Not surprisingly, the prevalence of presbycusis increases as age increases. The incidence of hearing loss is approximately 30% to 40% for all individuals over 65 years of age, increasing to 40% to 66% for individuals older than 75 years, and more than 80% for individuals older than 85 years (American Speech-Language-Hearing Association, 2008). As an overall health concern for the elderly, hearing loss is the third most prevalent chronic health concern ranking just behind arthritis and hypertension.

Presbycusis is difficult to study as an isolated hearing disorder. By the time an individual's life extends into the 70s through 90s, their auditory mechanism has been exposed to many agents (e.g., medications, noise, and trauma) that could contribute to a loss of hearing sensitivity. The loss of sensitivity is gradual and the affected person notices that they have increasing difficulty understanding conversation.

There are many peripheral changes that occur to the outer and middle ear structures with advancing age. The tissue of the pinna loses elasticity and the skin becomes scaly and dry, appearing translucent with pigmentation spots. Males experience an increase in hair growth within the folds of the pinna. The changes in the appearance of the pinna do not directly affect hearing sensitivity. The epithelial lining of the ear canal becomes thin and dry. The skin has difficulty migrating to the external meatus, which can result in obstruction or impaction that can then result in a temporary conductive hearing loss.

Changes that occur in the middle ear affect the conduction of sound into the inner ear. The middle ear muscles and tendons atrophy with advanced age. There may be a loss of elasticity in the ossicular joints, rigidity of the ossicular chain, and a loss of elasticity of the tympanic membrane. These structural changes may add a slight conductive component to the hearing loss.

The majority of the changes related to advanced age occur within the structures of the cochlea or cochlear nerve. Degeneration of the hair cells and basilar membrane will take place initially at the basal end of the cochlea. The cochlear branch of the vestibulocochlear nerve (cranial nerve VIII) may partially atrophy as well as the spiral ganglion. Degeneration of the stria vascularis causes a disruption in the ion balance necessary for cellular function for the entire cochlea.

Schuknecht (1974) described specific audiometric configurations that are predictable from the structural changes. The type of hearing loss is sensorineural in nature but as seen in Figure 13-17, the patterns vary. The changes within the cochlea and cochlear nerve exhibit a sloping high-frequency loss due to the changes along the basal end of the basilar membrane. Audiometrically, the stria vascularis changes will also produce a sensorineural hearing loss but exhibit a more flat configuration since the stria vascularis degeneration affects the physiology of the entire cochlea.

Peripheral structures may deteriorate, but there is also apparent involvement in the central auditory system. Recall this system allows for interpretation or processing of what the peripheral system detects. As a

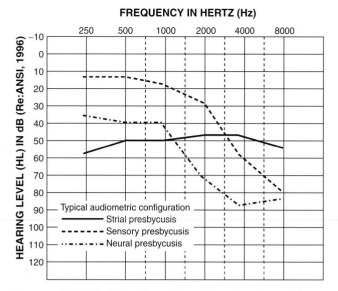

Figure 13-17 Typical audiometric configurations for specific causes of presbycusis.

person ages, the ascending auditory pathway from the cochlea through the various levels of the brainstem will typically experience a reduction in the number of functioning neurons, especially at the level of the superior olivary complex. The outcome of this central structural change is a disproportionate difficulty in understanding speech, greater than one would expect from audiometric results. This condition is termed **phonemic regression**.

Many structural changes do not occur in isolation. Depending on the degree of outer or middle ear involvement, a conductive component yielding a slight air-bone gap may also be seen. Speech discrimination may be fair to poor depending on the degree of central involvement.

The longevity of the auditory mechanism varies greatly from person to person. The high-frequency information affected by the aging process makes it difficult for the individual to hear conversations clearly. The aging listener will complain that most speakers sound as if they are mumbling. Appropriately fit amplification will help the individual be more aware of conversational speech but may not aid in clarifying speech if the person is experiencing central processing changes.

Noise-Induced Hearing Loss

Noise-induced hearing loss (NIHL) is the most common form of acquired hearing disorder. It is completely preventable and yet 10 million Americans suffer its effects. The National Institute for Occupational Safety and Health (1998) has designated NIHL as one of the ten leading occupational diseases and injuries. Elevated recreational noise will also permanently damage the cochlea. It is not the source of the noise that is damaging but rather the level of the noise and time of exposure that causes the damage.

There are two types of noise-induced damage: (1) acoustic trauma resulting in permanent damage from a single exposure to very high noise levels and (2) continuous exposure to repeated moderately intense levels resulting in a gradual hearing loss. Continuous exposure initially affects thresholds for high frequencies (3000 to 6000 Hz) with a typical "notch" at 4000 Hz (Clark & Bohne, 1999). As exposure continues, the mid to lower frequencies become affected. Both forms of NIHL can be prevented by the regular use of hearing protection such as earplugs or earmuffs.

Tinnitus (e.g., ringing, buzzing or humming in the ears) or difficulty understanding conversation is often the first symptom of an NIHL. Hearing loss and tinnitus may be experienced in one or both ears, and tinnitus may be constant or just occasional after noise exposure.

Sound intensity is measured on a logarithmic scale known as the decibel (dB) scale. Noise exposure measurements are often expressed as dB (A). The A scale is weighted toward the higher frequency sounds to which the human ear is most sensitive. Unprotected exposure to impulse or continuous noise levels in excess of 90 dB (A) for an 8-hour period will cause a shift in an individual's hearing thresholds. This shift in threshold is referred to as a **temporary threshold shift (TTS)**. In most instances, the TTS largely subsides 16 to 48 hours after exposure (Clark, Bohne, & Boettcher, 1987). However, with repeated exposure and repeated TTS, damage occurs, and hence the insidious nature of noise. As the decibel level of a sound increases, the exposure time before there is permanent damage decreases. Decibel values are based on a logarithmic scale, so what seems like a slight increase in decibels—say from 80 dB IL to 90 dB IL—is actually a *ten-fold increase* in intensity. OSHA's table of permissible noise exposure outlines a worker's duration per day in hours against the decibel level. Basically, for every 5 dB increase in noise level, the exposure time is cut in half. Therefore, a 4-hour exposure to noise at 95 dB (A) is considered to provide the same noise "dose" as 8 hours of exposure to noise at 90 dB (A). Think about this: a single gunshot of approximately 140 dB (A) has the same sound energy as 40 hours of 90 dB (A) noise! Gradual NIHL typically affects both ears equally creating a symmetric audiometric pattern. By comparison, noise from such sources as tractors or firearms expose one ear more than the other producing an asymmetric hearing loss.

In today's noisy world, young adults are exposed to many sources of loud noise that place them at risk for hearing loss. Most high school industrial arts programs must include education on hearing conservation. The simplest solution is to simply turn down the volume or, if possible, wear appropriate hearing protection. The following signs are an indication that the noise level around you is too loud and could cause damage if exposure is continued:

- You have to shout to be heard above the noise.
- You cannot understand someone who is speaking to you from less than 2 feet away.
- A person standing near you can hear the sound from your stereo headset while it is on your head.

Noise causes permanent changes to the cochlea resulting in a sensorineural hearing loss. The physical structures of the cochlea literally get beat to death by the insidious pounding of acoustic pressure waves. The stereocilia of the cochlea's hair cells are damaged, bent or broken. When stereocilia are damaged, the corresponding hair cell body dies and the neurons that synapse with the hair cell degenerate.

Why You Need to Know

Loud rock concerts have contributed to hearing loss in the baby boomer generation but iPod and similar players are much worse for the present generation. The problem begins with the headphones resting directly in the ear canal (concha bowl). This allows the user to easily overcome any background noise such as the noise of the school lunch room or lawn mower. As a result, they easily desensitize the user to dangerously high sound levels. Portable CD players do too, but iPods pose an additional danger because they hold thousands of songs and can play for hours without recharging so users tend to listen continuously for hours at a time. The user does not have to stop to change a CD or a tape. Damage to hearing caused by high volume is determined by its duration; continuous listening even at a seemingly reasonable level can damage the hair cells in the inner ear resulting in permanent hearing loss. Denying the danger of noise-induced hearing loss would not be so easy if loud music made the ears bleed, but the early symptoms tend to come on gradually. It typically starts with ringing in the ears. The problem often times becomes advanced before people realize they are having serious difficulty hearing. Adapted from a CBS News interview August 25, 2005, by Lloyd de Vries, MP3s May Threaten Hearing Loss: Experts Discuss Risk to Hearing from Listening to Music Devices.

Avoiding noise exposure or using appropriate hearing protection stops further progression of the damage. In the future, the use of chemoprotective agents such as antioxidants as well as identification of possible risk factors for susceptibility to NIHL may enhance prevention and treatment efforts. Risk factors include but are not limited to cigarette smoking, excessive caffeine consumption, and concurrent exposure to ototoxic substances such as solvents and heavy metals (Morata et al., 1993).

The characteristic audiometric pattern indicating NIHL is a notch in the high frequencies. Figure 13-18 illustrates the classic research by Taylor, Pearson, Mair, and Burns (1965) which demonstrates the effect of long-term exposure to noise on hearing levels. The figure demonstrates the hearing threshold levels of workers comprised over many years of exposure. The hearing loss continues to get more severe as the years of exposure continue. The purpose of the study was to demonstrate the detrimental effect of chronic noise exposure on hearing.

Noise Exposure Regulations

An employer must provide for his workers a place of employment that is free from recognized hazards. The Occupational Safety and Health Administration (2002) requires employers to provide hearing conservation programs for employees where an 8-hour exposure exceeds an 85-dB weighted average. An occupational hearing conservation program includes:

- engineering and administrative controls to reduce noise exposures

- monitoring of noise levels
- annual audiometric testing for the purpose of monitoring for significant threshold shifts (defined as a shift of 10 dB or more in the worse threshold of 2000, 3000 or 4000 Hz)
- use of hearing protectors (i.e., the employer must provide a reasonable choice of adequate hearing protectors free to all employees)
- employee training on the use of hearing protection
- adequate record keeping.

Claims for occupational hearing loss are typically handled through state Labor and Industry Workman's Compensation. A mathematical formula is used to convert the worker's degree of hearing loss into a percentage of impairment. Only certain frequencies are considered compensable and a minimum amount of hearing loss must be present. The American Medical Association (1979) uses the average thresholds of 500, 1000, 2000, and 3000 Hz to determine the amount of hearing loss. A 25 dB threshold fence is then subtracted and that figure is multiplied by a constant (1.5) to obtain the percentage of monaural hearing loss.

Noise exposure, whether occupational or recreational, is the leading cause of a preventable acquired hearing disorder. Occupational hearing loss is minimized by well fitting hearing protection and worker compliance. Recreational NIHL can be reduced by public education of the harmful effect of noise on the delicate auditory mechanism.

Summary

A good clinician will begin patient evaluation by taking a thorough case history. The case history will include questions that are identified as the five "cardinal signs" of ear pathology. The patient's responses will help identify the presence of ear pathology. A clinician often times feels like a detective, asking several specific questions to get more and more detail. Is the loss in one ear or both? Is there any pain or pressure present, and if so, when did it start? As a student you will learn to recognize the classic signs and symptoms for a particular pathology. For example, a patient suffering from Ménière's disease will experience low-pitch tinnitus and a low-frequency hearing loss. On the other hand, a person suffering from an NIHL will suffer from high-pitch tinnitus and a high-frequency hearing loss. Genetics and environmental agents are equally responsible for the cause of most hearing disorders and the

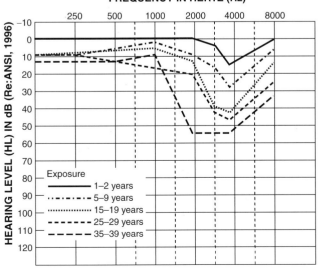

Figure 13-18 Audiometric configuration illustrates the long-term effect of noise on hearing levels compromised over many years of exposure.

patient is simply at their mercy. What *is* unfortunate is when a hearing loss is preventable as is often the case with hearing loss from exposure to excessive levels of noise. Part of our job as a speech or hearing specialist is to inform the public about the dangers of exposure to high levels of noise in one's daily life.

Clinical Teaser—Follow-Up

At the beginning of this part, you were asked to note any terms and concepts in the case study that were unfamiliar to you. As you read Chapter 12, you were to pay particular attention to the anatomy and physiology pertinent to this case. Now we return to the case for further discussion.

We can interpret this case regarding etiology and pathology. The gentleman did not report a head injury or trauma or a family history of ear disease or hearing loss. The etiology of the disease is unknown (i.e., idiopathic). The gentleman suffered from both auditory and vestibular symptoms, thereby leading us to conclude that the entire inner ear must be involved. The perilymph and endolymph fluids are common to both the auditory and vestibular systems. There are several diseases that can have this effect on the entire inner ear. The results of a battery of audiometric and vestibular tests lead us to the conclusion that this patient evidences Ménière's disease in his right ear. What pertinent information from the case history assisted you in drawing this conclusion? What pertinent (though limited) information from the audiometric evaluation assisted you in drawing this conclusion? Lastly, using the information about Ménière's in this chapter, explain a treatment option for this patient paying particular attention to the anatomy that would be affected by the disease.

PART 6 SUMMARY

The ear, organ of hearing and balance, is mostly invisible with the pinnae being the only visible structures. We recognize that they are similar in shape among individuals, but when we closely examine each one, there are many differences. Even the right and left pinna within the same person can be very different. The remaining structures of the outer, middle, and inner ear have some uniqueness as well but must not deviate far from the intended design. Injury, disease, and genetics can produce an acquired or congenital hearing or balance disorder. Timing is the key to the overall effect on the structures involved.

The mechanical role of the outer ear may not be as dramatic as that of the electro-chemical role of the inner ear but is still very necessary. The ear canal resonance boosts an incoming signal by a significant amount at a very specific and useful frequency range (20 dB in the range from 1500 to 7000 Hz). The curvature of the ear canal serves to protect the fine structures of the tympanic membrane and middle ear. The tympanic membrane and ossicular chain obey the laws of physics. The transformer action of the structures boosts the signal by approximately 27 dB to overcome the impedance mismatch of the air-filled middle ear to the fluid-filled inner ear.

The inner ear vestibular system is the primary organ for allowing independent and precise head and eye control in the execution of many complex motor activities such as running. Vestibular input is critical for balance when there is misleading information from the other senses (e.g., visual and somatosensory).

The inner ear auditory system is remarkable. The structure and function of the cochlea is so intricate that we have yet to completely understand how it all works. The outer hair cells embedded in the tectorial membrane mechanically amplify the soft sounds so that the inner hair cells may respond. The endolymph flow displaces the stereocilia of the hair cells. The tip links attached to the stereocilia act as mechanical gates opening channels for ion (i.e., potassium and calcium) exchange. The ion exchange depolarizes the hair cell stimulating the release of a neurotransmitter. The stria vascularis then recycles the cochlear fluids so that the process can then be repeated over and over again at a mind-boggling rate.

Once the cochlear nerve enters the brainstem, we begin the discussion of the auditory pathway. The reflex arc of the middle ear muscles relies on the auditory pathway. The processing of the acoustic information along the pathway facilitates the localization of a sound source. The redundancy of the auditory pathway as it travels to Heschl's gyrus preserves and protects the acoustic information that was sensed by the peripheral structure.

The moment an acoustic pressure wave is directed by the pinna down the ear canal, the reaction of the ear structures is set in motion. Many influences, natural or otherwise, disrupt the function of the aural anatomy and cause a hearing disorder. The hearing impairment that accompanies the hearing disorder may cause a communication problem. Timing is everything. The earlier in life and the more severe the impairment, the more detrimental the effect will likely be on both aural (i.e., listening) and oral (i.e., speaking) communication.

PART 6 REVIEW QUESTIONS

1. Describe how the anatomical structures of the outer, middle, and inner ear each contributes to the physiology of the auditory and/or vestibular systems.

2. Discuss the similarities and differences between the sensory receptors of the semicircular canals (crista ampullaris) and the vestibule (macula). Draw a simple illustration of each identifying the landmarks.

3. Discuss the differences and similarities between the inner and outer hair cells and draw a simple illustration of each identifying the landmarks.

4. Choose and describe one of the three ways the conductive mechanism overcomes the impedance mismatch between the air-filled middle ear and the fluid-filled inner ear.

5. Choose an ear pathology; identify a chief complaint for that pathology. Answer the "five cardinal signs of pathology" as if you were the patient suffering from the pathology you chose.

6. Choose a syndromic hearing disorder of genetic origin. Identify the systems that are affected in addition to the auditory system and identify the syndrome's mode of inheritance. List the possible transmission probabilities (i.e., percentages) if you marry someone without any trace of the disorder. List the possible transmission percentages if you marry someone with the exact same syndrome.

7. Choose an ear pathology that is typically seen within each of the following age groups: 0 to 18, 18 to 50, 50 to 64, and 65+. Discuss the etiology of each pathology.

APPENDIX

Terms and Affixes to Assist You in Learning the Meanings of Anatomical and Physiological Words

TABLE A-1

TERMS AND PREFIXES USED TO DESCRIBE MOVEMENT

Term	Definition
Abduction	Movement away from the median plane; separation of two structures (e.g., the vocal folds)
Adduction	Movement toward the median plane; bringing together of two structures (e.g., the vocal folds)
Circumduction	Movement in a circular direction (e.g., rotating the eyeballs)
Deglutition	The process of swallowing
Depressor	The process of lowering a structure (e.g., depressor anguli oris—a muscle that lowers the corner of the mouth)
Eversion	Turning outward (e.g., turning the sole of the foot laterally)
Extension	Stretching out (e.g., straightening the arm by extending it outward)
Flexion	Bending (e.g., bending the forearm toward the shoulder by contracting the biceps)
Hyper-	Excessive (e.g., hyperkinesis—excessive, uncontrollable movements)
Hypo-	Diminished or deficient (e.g., hypokinesis—diminished or slow movement)
Inversion	Turning inward (e.g., turning the sole of the foot medially)
Levator	The process of raising a structure (e.g., levator veli palatini—a muscle that raises the soft palate)
Mastication	The process of chewing
Opposition	Moving a structure toward another structure (e.g., contacting the thumb and index finger)
Tachy-	Rapid movement (e.g., tachycardia—an unusually fast heart rate)
Tensor	The process of tensing a structure (e.g., tensor veli palatini—a muscle that tenses the soft palate)

TABLE A-2

TERMS AND AFFIXES USED TO DENOTE ANATOMICAL STRUCTURES OR THEIR PARTS

Term	Definition	Example
Ary-	Pertaining to the arytenoid cartilage	*Ary*epiglottic fold—the fold of tissue that runs from the lateral aspect of the epiglottis to the arytenoid cartilages
Clavius	Pertaining to the clavicle	Sub*clavius*—a muscle found immediately below, and running parallel to, the clavicle
Cleido-		Sterno*cleido*mastoid—a muscle that has three attachments, to the sternum, clavicle, and mastoid process
Costal	Pertaining to the ribs	*Costal* pleura—a layer of connective tissue that adheres to the inner rib cage
Costalis		Lateral ilio*costalis*—a muscle that runs from the ilium to the lower ribs, assisting in depressing them
Costarum		Levator *costarum* brevis—short muscles just lateral to the spinal column along the rib cage that assist in elevating the ribs

Continued on following page

353

TABLE A-2

TERMS AND AFFIXES USED TO DENOTE ANATOMICAL STRUCTURES OR THEIR PARTS (Continued)

Term	Definition	Example
Crico-	Pertaining to the cricoid cartilage	*Crico*arytenoid—the joint formed by the articulation of the cricoid cartilage with each of the arytenoid cartilages
-dontia	Pertaining to the teeth	Ano*dontia*—any number of missing teeth
Genio-	Pertaining to the chin	*Genio*glossus—a muscle that runs from the inside of the chin to the tongue
Glosso-	Pertaining to the tongue	*Glosso*pharyngeal—cranial nerve IX that provides motor fibers to parts of the tongue and pharynx
-glossus		Genio*glossus*—a muscle that runs from the inside of the chin to the tongue
-gnathia	Pertaining to the jaw	Micro*gnathia*—an unusually small mandible
Hyo-	Pertaining to the hyoid bone	*Hyo*thyroid—a membrane that fills the space between the hyoid bone and the thyroid cartilage
Iliac	Pertaining to the ilium	*Iliac* crest—the prominent ridge of the ilium, more commonly referred to as the hip bone
Ilio-		Lateral *ilio*costalis—a muscle that runs from the ilium to the lower ribs, assisting in depressing them
Labio-	Pertaining to the lips	*Labio*version—any number of anterior teeth that are tilted toward the lips
Laryngo-	Pertaining to the larynx	*Laryngo*pharynx—the lowermost part of the pharynx in the general region of the larynx, immediately above the esophagus
Lingua-	Pertaining to the tongue	*Lingua* nigra—a tongue disease caused by excessive use of antibiotics; also known as "black hairy tongue"
Linguo-		*Linguo*version—any number of teeth that are tilted toward the tongue
Lingual		*Lingual* frenulum—a fold of mucous membrane extending from the floor of the mouth to the undersurface of the anterior tongue
Lumbo-	Pertaining to the lumbar vertebrae or the lower back	*Lumbo*costal ligament—connective tissue that binds the twelfth rib to the first two lumbar vertebrae
Lumborum		Quadratus *lumborum*—a rectangular-shaped muscle deep within the abdomen in the region of the lower back
Mandibular	Pertaining to the mandible (jaw)	Temporo*mandibular* joint—the joint formed by the condyle of the mandible and the mandibular fossa of the temporal bone of the skull
Mental	Pertaining to the protruding part of the chin (mentum)	*Mental* foramen—a small opening in the mandible in the region of the chin
Mylo-	Pertaining to the lower jaw, more specifically the molar teeth	*Mylo*hyoid—a muscle that runs from the mylohyoid line (a prominent ridge along the inner aspect of the lower jaw) to the hyoid bone
Naso-	Pertaining to the nasal cavity	*Naso*pharynx—the uppermost region of the pharynx in the general region of the posterior nasal cavity
Oculo-	Pertaining to the eyes	*Oculo*motor—cranial nerve III, responsible for movements of the eyeball
Omo-	Pertaining to the shoulder region	*Omo*hyoid—a two-bellied muscle that runs from the hyoid bone to the scapula (shoulder blade)
Oro-	Pertaining to the oral cavity	*Oro*pharynx—the middle region of the pharynx in the general region of the back of the oral cavity
Palatine	Pertaining to the palate, either hard or soft	*Palatine* processes—the bony shelves of the maxilla that help form the hard palate
Palatini	Pertaining to the palate, more often the soft palate	Tensor veli *palatini*—a muscle that makes up the bulk of the body of the soft palate; its function is to tense the soft palate
Palato-		*Palato*glossus—a muscle that runs from the sides of the soft palate, around the sides of the posterior oral cavity, and into the sides of the posterior tongue

TABLE A-2

TERMS AND AFFIXES USED TO DENOTE ANATOMICAL STRUCTURES OR THEIR PARTS (Continued)

Term	Definition	Example
Pharyngeal ⎤ Pharyngo- ⎦	Pertaining to the pharynx	*Pharyngeal* aponeurosis—the broad, flat, funnel-shaped tube of connective tissue that forms the skeleton of the pharynx *Pharyngo*palatine—a muscle that runs from the pharynx to the soft palate
Pterygo-	Pertaining to the pterygoid process of the sphenoid bone of the skull	*Pterygo*mandibular ligament—a ligament that connects the mandible to the pterygoid process
Sacro-	Pertaining to the sacrum	*Sacro*spinalis—muscle that runs from the sacrum to the lower spinal column
Spheno-	Pertaining to the sphenoid bone of the skull	*Spheno*-occipital—pertaining to the sphenoid bone and the basilar process of the occipital bone
Sternal ⎤ Sterni ⎟ Sterno- ⎦	Pertaining to the sternum (breastbone)	*Sternal* notch—the indentation along the superior border of the manubrium of the sternum Manubrium *sterni*—the upper part of the sternum *Sterno*thyroid—a muscle that runs from the sternum to the thyroid cartilage
Stylo-	Pertaining to the styloid process	*Stylo*hyoid—a muscle that runs from the styloid process (on the inferior surface of the temporal bone of the skull) to the hyoid bone
Thyro-	Pertaining to the thyroid cartilage	*Thyro*epiglottic ligament—a ligament that attaches the petiolus of the epiglottis to the thyroid cartilage
Tracheo- ⎤ Tracheal ⎦	Pertaining to the trachea (windpipe)	*Tracheo*-esophageal puncture—a surgical procedure where an airway is established between the trachea and esophagus, so that a person who has undergone a laryngectomy can produce voicing Crico*tracheal* ligament—the ligament that anchors the cricoid cartilage onto the superior border of the trachea
Veli ⎤ Velo- ⎦	Pertaining to the velum (soft palate)	Levator *veli* palatini—a muscle whose purpose is to raise the soft palate *Velo*pharyngeal port—the variable-sized opening between the soft palate and the posterior pharyngeal wall
Vertebro-	Pertaining to the spinal column	*Vertebro*sternal—the articulation between the true ribs and the sternum; in this case, *vertebro-* comes from the fact that all the ribs have a posterior attachment to the vertebral column

TABLE A-3

TERMS AND PREFIXES USED TO DESCRIBE COLOR, FORM, GENERAL LOCATION, RELATIVE SIZE, OR SHAPE

Term	Definition	Example
Abdominus	Pertaining to the abdomen (belly)	Transversus *abdominus*—a muscle of the abdominal wall whose fibers run from side to side
Alba	White	Linea *alba*—"white line"; a white line of connective tissue running vertically down the midline of the belly
Apical	Toward the apex or tip	*Apical* foramen—an opening at the tip of the roots of the teeth where blood vessels and nerve fibers pass into the interior of the tooth
Bifid	Separated or split	*Bifid* uvula—a uvula that is split into two parts
Brevis	Muscle fibers of relatively short length	Levator costarum *brevis*—short muscles just lateral to the spinal column along the rib cage that assist in elevating the ribs
Buccal	Pertaining to the cheeks	*Buccal* cavity—the space between the inside of the cheeks and the premolar and molar teeth
Cyan-	Blue	*Cyan*osis—the condition of turning blue because of a lack of oxygen
Di-	Two	*Di*gastricus—a muscle having two bellies

Continued on following page

TABLE A-3

TERMS AND PREFIXES USED TO DESCRIBE COLOR, FORM, GENERAL LOCATION, RELATIVE SIZE, OR SHAPE (Continued)

Term	Definition	Example
-gastricus	Pertaining to the belly or stomach	Di*gastricus*—a muscle having two bellies
Jaun-	Yellow	*Jaun*dice—a yellow pigmentation of the skin and eyeballs due to the presence of bile
Latissimus	Pertaining to a lateral direction	*Latissimus* dorsi—a muscle whose fibers swing laterally from the lower spinal region and sacrum to the humerus of the arm
Leuko-	White	*Leuko*cyte—a white blood cell
Linea	A line	*Linea* alba—the line of connective tissue running longitudinally down the midline of the belly, separating the abdominal muscles into pairs, left and right
Longissimus	Pertaining to a longitudinal direction	*Longissimus* dorsi—a back muscle whose fibers run longitudinally from the sacrum to the uppermost ribs, traversing the entire length of the rib cage
Longus	Muscle fibers of relatively greater length	Levator costarum *longus*—muscles confined to the lower ribs, just lateral to the spinal column and approximately twice the length of the levator costarum brevis muscles
Macro-	Large, long	*Macro*dontia—any number of disproportionately large teeth
Major	Of relatively larger size	Pectoralis *major*—a muscle of the lateral upper chest, larger in size than the pectoralis minor
Micro-	Small, short	*Micro*dontia—any number of proportionately small teeth
Minor	Of relatively smaller size	Psoas *minor*—a muscle deep within the abdomen in the region of the pelvic girdle, smaller in size to the psoas major
Nigra	Black	Substantia *nigra*—darkly pigmented nerve cell bodies in the midbrain
Oblonga	Having an oblong, somewhat oval appearance	Fovea *oblonga*—an oblong depression along the anterolateral base of the arytenoid cartilages
Petrous	Dense, hard (like a rock)	*Petrous* portion of the temporal bone—the denser portion of the temporal bone where the hearing mechanism is housed
Quadrate	Somewhat square or rectangular shaped	Posterior *quadrate* lamina—the somewhat square-shaped posterior wall of the cricoid cartilage
Quadratus		*Quadratus* lumborum—a somewhat rectangular-shaped muscle in the deep abdomen in the region of the pelvic girdle
Rubro-	Red	*Rubro*spinal tract—a part of the extrapyramidal motor system that originates in the red nucleus and proceeds down the spinal cord along with the corticospinal tract
Serratus	Jagged or sawtooth shaped	*Serratus* anterior—a muscle of the anterolateral rib cage that inserts into the ribs from a somewhat oblique direction, giving the muscle a jagged appearance
Thoracis	Pertaining to the thorax (chest)	Transversus *thoracis*—a muscle of the inner rib cage that extends transversely from the sternum to the ribs
Torus	A rounded bulge or ridge	*Torus* palatinus—a rounded bulge on the midline of the hard palate in some people
Trapezius	Having a somewhat trapezoidal shape	*Trapezius*—a muscle that is shaped somewhat like a trapezoid, running from the spinal column of the neck and thorax to the clavicle (collar bone) and scapula (shoulder blade)

TABLE A-4

TERMS AND AFFIXES USED IN REFERENCE TO BONES, CARTILAGES, CAVITIES, MEMBRANES, OR SPACES

Term	Definition	Example
Aditus	An inlet or opening	*Aditus* laryngis—the opening into the interior of the larynx
Alveolus	A small cavity or socket	Dental *alveolus*—a tooth socket
Arcuate	Arched or bow shaped	*Arcuate* ridge—a bow-shaped ridge on the anterolateral surface of the arytenoid cartilage
Cecum	A cul-de-sac	Foramen *cecum*—a small cul-de-sac depression at the sulcus terminalis of the tongue
Cerato-	Pertaining to a horn	*Cerato*glossus—the posterior portion of the hyoglossus muscle whose origin is the greater horn of the hyoid bone
Chondro-	Pertaining to cartilage	*Chondro*blasts—cells that allow for growth of cartilage
Concha	A structure that is somewhat shell shaped	Nasal *concha*—a turbinate bone within the lateral wall of the nasal cavity that is somewhat shell shaped
Condyle	A rounded articular surface at the end of a bone or bony process	Mandibular *condyle*—the rounded surface at the superior margin of the ramus of the mandible that articulates with the temporal bone of the skull
Corpus	Body	*Corpus* of the hyoid—the body of the hyoid bone
Crest	A bony ridge	Palatine *crest*—a bony ridge on the inferior surface of the horizontal plate of the palatine bone
Cribriform	A plate of bone containing many perforations	*Cribriform* plate—the horizontally directed plate of the ethmoid bone of the skull containing many perforations through which nerve fibers from the olfactory nerve pass as they enter the nasal cavity
Crus	A structure that is somewhat shaped like a leg	*Crus* cerebri—the mass of nerve fibers resembling a leg that passes through the ventral surface of the midbrain
Fossa	A longitudinally directed depression in bone	Glenoid *fossa*—the depression in the head of the scapula that receives the head of the humerus
Fovea	A somewhat shallow depression or pit	*Fovea* oblonga—a shallow depression along the base of the anterolateral surface of the arytenoid cartilage
Fronto-	Pertaining to the frontal bone of the skull	*Fronto*parietal—the joint between the frontal and parietal bones of the skull
Glottic	Pertaining to the glottis	Sub*glottic* space—the space immediately below the level of the glottis
Lamina	A thin plate or flat layer (usually in reference to bone or cartilage)	Posterior quadrate *lamina*—the somewhat flat, square-shaped posterior portion of the cricoid cartilage
Meatus	A channel or passageway	External auditory *meatus*—the channel that runs from the pinna on the outer surface of the head to the eardrum within the temporal bone
Musculo- Myo-	Pertaining to muscles	*Musculo*skeletal—the attachments of muscles to the skeleton *Myo*fascial pain dysfunction syndrome—a condition where the muscles of mastication spasm, causing great pain to the sufferer
Nuchal	Pertaining to the back of the neck	Superior *nuchal* line—a small ridge running horizontally across the occipital bone of the skull where some posterior neck muscles attach
Occipito-	Pertaining to the occipital bone of the skull	*Occipito*mastoid—the region of the mastoid process of the occipital bone
Orbital	Pertaining to the eye sockets	Infra*orbital* foramen—a small opening just below the orbit of the eye
-osseo- Osteo-	Pertaining to bone	Chondro-*osseo*us union—a junction between cartilage and bone *Osteo*blasts—bone-forming cells
Parieto-	Pertaining to the parietal bones of the skull	*Parieto*-occipital—the joint between the parietal and occipital bones of the skull

Continued on following page

TABLE A-4

TERMS AND AFFIXES USED IN REFERENCE TO BONES, CARTILAGES, CAVITIES, MEMBRANES, OR SPACES (Continued)

Term	Definition	Example
Pars	A part or portion	*Pars* oblique—a bundle of diagonally directed fibers of the cricothyroid muscle
Pectoral	Pertaining to the chest	*Pectoral* girdle—the bones, ligaments, and muscles that form the shoulder region
Pectoralis		*Pectoralis* major—a large fan-shaped muscle of the upper lateral chest
Pelvic	Pertaining to the lower region of the abdomen and the hips	*Pelvic* girdle—the bones, ligaments, and muscles that make up the lower abdominal and hip region
Process	A projection or outgrowth on bone or cartilage	Vocal *process*—the projection at the base of the arytenoid cartilage where the medial and anterolateral surfaces meet that serves as the posterior point of attachment of the vocal fold
Salpingo-	Referring to a tube	*Salpingo*pharyngeus—a muscle that makes up the medial wall of the cartilaginous portion of the Eustachian tube
Spine	A short thorn-like process of a bone	*Spine* of the scapula—the sharp process of the scapula where the trapezius muscle attaches
Symphysis	The union of two structures	Pubic *symphysis*—the fibrocartilaginous joint between the two pubic bones
Temporo-	Pertaining to the temporal bone of the skull	*Temporo*mandibular joint—the joint formed between the mandibular fossa of the temporal bone and the condyle of the mandible
Ventricular	Pertaining to the ventricular (false) folds	*Ventricular* ligament—the skeleton of connective tissue on which a ventricular fold attaches
Vocal	Pertaining to the vocal folds	*Vocal* ligament—the skeleton of connective tissue on which a vocal fold attaches

TABLE A-5

TERMS AND AFFIXES USED IN REFERENCE TO THE NERVOUS SYSTEM

Term	Definition	Example
Afferent	Inflowing or toward the center	*Afferent* nerves—nerves that send impulses toward the central nervous system, that is, sensory nerves
Amygdaloid	Almond shaped	*Amygdaloid* nucleus—an almond-shaped collection of nerve cell bodies in the temporal lobe of the cerebrum, immediately anterior to the inferior horn of the lateral ventricle
Arachnoid	Resembling a spider's web	*Arachnoid*—the intermediate (middle) layer of the meninges
Arbor vitae	Literally, "tree of life"	*Arbor vitae*—the white matter of the cerebellum; upon sagittal sectioning, its appearance is similar to a tree with branches
Bulbar	Pertaining to the brainstem	*Bulbar* palsy—progressive muscular paralysis that results from degeneration of the cell bodies of the cranial nerves in the brainstem
Callosum	Huge, massive	Corpus *callosum*—a massive bundle of myelinated fibers connecting the two cerebral hemispheres
Cauda equina	Literally, "horse tail"	*Cauda equina*—the roots of all of the spinal nerves below the first lumbar spinal nerves, somewhat resembling a horse's tail due to their arrangement
Caudate	Pertaining to a tail	*Caudate* nucleus—a mass of nerve cell bodies that consists of a head with a long curved tail

TABLE A-5

TERMS AND AFFIXES USED IN REFERENCE TO THE NERVOUS SYSTEM (Continued)

Term	Definition	Example
Cerebellar	Pertaining to the cerebellum	*Cerebellar* gait—a wide-based gait with unsteadiness evident upon lateral movement
Cerebelli		Tentorium *cerebelli*—a strong fold of the dura mater that separates the cerebellum from the occipital region of the cerebrum
Cerebello-		*Cerebello*pontine angle—a recessed area where the cerebellum, pons, and medulla converge
Cerebral	Pertaining to the cerebrum	*Cerebral* palsy—a neurological condition affecting motor ability and coordination due to damage to the primary and/or secondary motor pathways
Cerebri		Crus *cerebri*—the tightly compacted nerve fibers passing through the ventral midbrain
Cerebro-		*Cerebro*vascular accident—a stroke, caused by damage to the vascular system of the cerebrum
Cingulate	To surround	*Cingulate* gyrus—a long curved convolution of the medial cerebral hemisphere immediately above the corpus callosum and surrounding it to a certain degree
Colliculus	A small mound or elevation	Inferior *colliculus*—one of two paired swellings in the dorsal midbrain that are part of the auditory pathway
Corona	A crown	*Corona* radiata—widely radiating fibers of the internal capsule that somewhat resemble a crown
Corpora	A body	*Corpora* quadrigemina—four oval masses (superior and inferior colliculi) found in the dorsal midbrain that are part of the visual and auditory pathways
Cortical	Pertaining to the cerebral cortex	*Cortical* blindness—a loss of vision as a result of damage to the visual areas of the cerebral cortex
Cortico-		*Cortico*spinal tract—the primary motor pathway that originates in the precentral gyrus of the cerebral cortex and provides input to the spinal nerves
Cranial	Pertaining to the cranium or head	*Cranial* nerves—the nerves originating in the brainstem that primarily supply the muscles and viscera of the head and neck
Dural	Pertaining to the dura mater	Sub*dural* hematoma—a hemorrhage into the space immediately below the dura mater
Efferent	Outflowing or away from the center	*Efferent* nerves—nerves that send impulses away from the central nervous system, that is, motor nerves
Encephalon	Pertaining to the brain	Mes*encephalon*—the midbrain
Fasciculus	A bundle, usually in reference to nerve fibers	Arcuate *fasciculus*—a bowed bundle of nerve fibers in the cerebrum connecting Broca's area with Wernicke's area
Fissure	A deep furrow or cleft	Longitudinal *fissure*—the deep cleft that separates the two cerebral hemispheres
Flocculo-	Pertaining to the flocculus (a part of the cerebellum)	*Flocculo*nodular lobe—a small lobe of the cerebellum that is part of the vestibular system
Geniculate	Bent sharply, like a knee	Medial *geniculate* body—one of a pair of bodies on the posterior and inferior surface of the thalamus that are part of the auditory pathway
Lemniscus	Ribbon-like	Lateral *lemniscus*—a thin tract of fibers in the brainstem that sends auditory information to the inferior colliculus in the midbrain
Lenticular	Bi-convex or lentil shaped	*Lenticular* nucleus—a bi-convex lens-shaped nucleus consisting of the putamen and globus pallidus
Meningeal	Pertaining to the meninges covering the brain and spinal cord	*Meningeal* vessel grooves—a series of depressions on the inner surface of the bones of the cranium where the blood vessels covering the brain reside
-neurium	Pertaining to nerve tissue or nerves	Epi*neurium*—the outermost layer of connective tissue surrounding peripheral nerve trunks

Continued on following page

TABLE A-5

TERMS AND AFFIXES USED IN REFERENCE TO THE NERVOUS SYSTEM (Continued)

Term	Definition	Example
Neuro-	Pertaining to the nervous system or nerves	*Neuro*muscular junction—the point where nerve fibers innervate muscle fibers to create a contraction
Nodular	Pertaining to the nodulus (a part of the vermis of the cerebellum)	Flocculo*nodular* lobe—a small lobe of the cerebellum that is part of the vestibular system
Olivo-	Pertaining to the olivary nucleus	*Olivo*cerebellar—nerve fibers that pass from the olivary nucleus in the medulla to the opposite hemisphere of the cerebellum
Pontine	Pertaining to the pons	Cerebello*pontine* angle—a recessed area where the cerebellum, pons, and medulla converge
Pyramidal	Pertaining to the pyramids on the anterior surface of the medulla	*Pyramidal* motor tract—the primary motor pathway that originates in the precentral gyrus of the cerebral cortex and eventually decussates at the pyramids before traveling down the spinal cord
Quadrigemina	Fourfold	Corpora *quadrigemina*—four oval masses (superior and inferior colliculi) found in the posterior midbrain that are part of the visual and auditory pathways
Spinal	Pertaining to the spinal column	Cortico*spinal* tract—the primary motor pathway that originates in the precentral gyrus of the cerebral cortex and provides input to the spinal nerves
Striatum	Striped	Corpus *striatum*—a subcortical mass of gray matter just anterior to the thalamus, consisting of the caudate and putamen
Sulcus	A slight groove or depression, not quite as deep as a fissure	Central *sulcus*—an obliquely directed groove in each cerebral hemisphere that separates the frontal from parietal lobes
Thalamic	Pertaining to the thalamus	Sub*thalamic* nucleus—a subcortical mass of nerve cell bodies within proximity to the substantia nigra
Thalamo-		*Thalamo*cortical tract—an efferent nerve tract running from the thalamus to the cerebral cortex
Uncinate	Hook shaped	*Uncinate* fasciculus—nerve fibers that hook around the lateral sulcus to connect the orbital cortex with the anterior temporal cortex

TABLE A-6

TERMS AND PREFIXES USED IN REFERENCE TO THE AUDITORY / VESTIBULAR SYSTEM

Term	Definition	Example
Audio-	Pertaining to hearing	*Audio*meter—an electronic instrument for the measurement of hearing thresholds
Auricular	Pertaining to the ear	*Auricular* cartilage—the cartilage that makes up the skeleton of the auricle or pinna
Cochlear	Pertaining to the cochlea	*Cochlear* nerve—the portion of cranial nerve VIII that sends sensory information regarding hearing to the brain, originating in the cochlea
Incudis	Pertaining to the incus	Fossa *incudis*—a hollow within the middle ear cavity where the short process of the incus resides
Incudal		*Incudal* ligament—a singular ligament that suspends the incus in place
Incudo-		*Incudo*stapedial joint—the point of articulation between the incus and stapes
Malleo-	Pertaining to the malleus	*Malleo*incudal joint—the point of articulation between the malleus and incus
Malleolar		*Malleolar* ligaments—a series of three ligaments that suspend the malleus in place

TABLE A-6

TERMS AND PREFIXES USED IN REFERENCE TO THE AUDITORY / VESTIBULAR SYSTEM (Continued)

Term	Definition	Example
Ot-	Pertaining to the ear	*Ot*itis media—inflammation of the middle ear
Otic		*Otic* capsule—the hollow area of the inner ear in which the cochlea, vestibule, and semicircular canals reside
Oto-		*Oto*sclerosis—a condition in which spongy bone forms around the stapes, preventing it from functioning properly
Scala	A cavity or chamber	*Scala* tympani—the lower chamber within the cochlea below the spiral lamina
Spiral	Coiled (usually in reference to structures within the cochlea)	*Spiral* ligament—the connective tissue within the cochlea that forms the outer wall of the scala media and anchors it to the spiral lamina
Stapedial	Pertaining to the stapes	Incudo*stapedial* joint—the point of articulation between the incus and stapes
Stapedius		*Stapedius* muscle—a tiny muscle in the middle ear that tenses the stapes so that the stapes does not excessively drive the oval window
Tympani	Pertaining to the eardrum	Tensor *tympani*—a tiny muscle in the middle ear that tenses the eardrum and malleus to dampen vibration of the ossicular chain
Tympanic		*Tympanic* membrane—the eardrum, which forms the lateral wall of the middle ear cavity
Vestibular	Pertaining to the balance portion of the inner ear	*Vestibular* nerve—the portion of cranial nerve VIII that sends sensory information regarding head position and movement to the brain, originating in the vestibule and semicircular canals
Vestibulo-		*Vestibulo*cochlear nerve—cranial nerve VIII that sends sensory information (hearing and balance) from the inner ear to the brain

TABLE A-7

MISCELLANEOUS TERMS AND AFFIXES USED IN ANATOMY, PHYSIOLOGY, AND PATHOLOGY

Term	Definition	Example
A-	Without, absence of, inability	*A*phonia—absence or loss of voice
An-		*An*oxia—without oxygen
Amelo-	Enamel	*Amelo*genesis imperfecta—poorly formed enamel on the teeth
-arthria	Articulation (speech)	Dys*arthria*—a disturbance in the ability to speak
-blast	A germ or cell (usually in an immature form)	Chondro*blast*—a cell that assists in the growth of cartilage
Cemento-	Cementum	*Cemento*enamel junction—the point where the cementum and enamel of a tooth meet
-clast	A germ or cell that breaks down tissue	Osteo*clast*s—cells that break down bone tissue so that it can be absorbed
-cyte	A cell	Leuko*cyte*—a white blood cell
Deci-	One-tenth	*Deci*bel—unit of measure for expressing the relative loudness of a sound on a logarithmic scale; literally one-tenth of a bel
Deciduous	Nonpermanent	*Deciduous* teeth—the primary set of teeth that are shed during childhood and replaced by permanent teeth
Dentino-	Dentin	*Dentino*genesis imperfecta—poorly formed dentin, the substance comprising the bulk of a tooth
Dys-	Difficulty, distress, or abnormal	*Dys*pnea—difficulty breathing
-ectomy	Removal of an anatomical part	Laryng*ectomy*—surgical removal of the larynx
Edema	An accumulation of fluid in the cells, tissues, or cavities	Reinke's *edema*—swelling of the vocal folds due to an accumulation of fluid within them
Eu-	Well, good, or normal	*Eu*pnea—normal breathing
-graphia	Writing	A*graphia*—impaired ability to write

Continued on following page

TABLE A-7

MISCELLANEOUS TERMS AND AFFIXES USED IN ANATOMY, PHYSIOLOGY, AND PATHOLOGY (Continued)

Term	Definition	Example
Hema-	Pertaining to the blood	*Hema*toma—a localized mass of blood that collects within tissue, organs, or in cavities or spaces
Hemi-	One-half	*Hemi*anopsia—loss of half of the visual field
Incisive	Pertaining to the incisors	*Incisive* foramen—a small opening in the alveolar ridge immediately posterior to the central incisors
-itis	Inflammation	Ot*itis* media—inflammation of the middle ear
-kinesia	Pertaining to motion or movement	Dys*kinesia*—difficulty in performing voluntary movements
-lexia	Reading	Dys*lexia*—Difficulty in the ability to read
Malacia	A softening or loss of consistency of tissues or organs	Chondro*malacia*—cartilage that is too soft
-oma	A tumor	Carcin*oma*—a malignant tumor
-opia / -opsia	Pertaining to vision	Presby*opia*—diminished sight as a result of aging Hemian*opsia*—loss of half of the visual field
-osis	A process, condition, or state	Cyan*osis*—the condition of turning blue because of a lack of oxygen
-otomy	An operation involving cutting	Trache*otomy*—an operation in which a small opening is cut into the anterior trachea to assist the patient in breathing
-phagia	Eating (usually in reference to swallowing)	Dys*phagia*—disruption of the ability to swallow properly
-phonia	Pertaining to the voice	A*phonia*—absence (loss) of voice
-plasia	Growth	Dys*plasia*—abnormal development or growth of cells, tissues, or organs
-plasty	A surgical procedure to mold or shape a structure	Rhino*plasty*—plastic surgery to repair a defect of the nose
-pnea	Pertaining to respiration (breathing)	A*pnea*—cessation of breathing
Pneumo-	Presence of air or gas; the lungs; breathing	*Pneumo*thorax—the presence of air or gas in the pleural cavity
Presby-	Pertaining to the aging process or old age	*Presby*cusis—a gradual loss of hearing that tends to occur as a person gets older
-sclerosis	The hardening of a structure	Oto*sclerosis*—a condition in which spongy bone forms around the stapes, hardening and preventing it from functioning properly
-scopy	Viewing (usually by means of some type of instrument)	Oto*scopy*—visual inspection of the ear through the use of a special instrument called an otoscope
-tonia	Pertaining to muscle tone	Dys*tonia*—a state of abnormal muscle tone
Vaso-	Pertaining to blood vessels	*Vaso*constriction—narrowing of a blood vessel's interior due to smooth muscle contraction

GLOSSARY

abducens: cranial nerve VI, involved with lateral eye movement.

abduction: movement of the vocal folds away from the median position, thereby opening the glottis.

absolute refractory period: the time immediately following an action potential when a neuron cannot fire.

acetabulum: the crater-shaped depression on the lateral aspect of the ischium where the head of the femur articulates.

acoustic: pertaining to sound and its perception.

acoustic neuroma: see *Schwannoma neuroma*.

acoustic reflex: middle ear muscle (i.e., stapedius and tensor tympani) contraction in response to the direction of loud sound; muscle contraction serves to stiffen the ossicular chain for the presumed purpose of protecting the inner ear from loud noises.

acquired: obtained after birth.

acrocephalosyndactyly: also known as Apert syndrome; a craniofacial anomaly affecting primarily the head, face, hands, and feet.

acromion: the process of the scapula where the clavicle articulates.

acute: of immediate concern; medically the stage where a patient presents with severe symptoms and short duration of immediate illness.

acute otitis media: quick onset of middle ear inflammation, lasting fewer than 21 days.

adduct: to close (adduction); movement of the vocal folds toward midline.

adduction: movement of the vocal folds toward midline, thereby bringing them together and closing the glottis.

adenoidectomy: surgical removal of the adenoid tissue in the nasopharynx.

adenoids: the mass of lymphoid tissue at the back of the pharynx, above the soft palate.

adhesive otitis media: prolonged inflammation of the middle ear with a retracted opaque, immobile tympanic membrane.

adipose: loose connective tissue with a high number of fat storing cells.

aditus: opening that connects the epitympanic recess of the middle ear cavity to the mastoid antrum.

aditus laryngis: the entrance to the larynx, formed by the superior border of the epiglottis anteriorly, the aryepiglottic folds laterally, and the arytenoid cartilages posteriorly.

afferent: the conduction of nerve impulses toward the central nervous system (i.e., sensory).

agnosia: a perceptual impairment related to the inability to recognize stimuli despite an intact sensory system; it can occur in any sensory modality— vision, audition, touch, etc.

agrammatism: a term meaning without grammar; a characteristic of nonfluent aphasia manifested by the omission of function words (e.g., articles, conjunctions, prepositions) in verbal expression.

air-bone gap: the difference between bone conduction thresholds and air conduction thresholds, reported in decibels for each ear at each frequency; used to determine type of hearing loss.

air conduction: in reference to audiometric testing, a method that is typically used to evaluate hearing threshold levels for a wide range of frequencies; the stimuli (pure tones) are delivered through a set of earphones in an attempt to evaluate the entire auditory system so that what is measured is what is "heard" through the air as opposed to what is heard through vibrations of the bones of the skull; the transmission of sound to the inner ear through the structures of the ear canal and middle ear cavity.

alar plate: dorsal region of the spinal cord during neurodevelopment that develops into nervous tissue serving sensory purposes.

albinism: condition of a person who is congenitally deficient in pigment. The individual typically has milky or translucent skin, white or colorless hair, and eyes with a pink or blue iris and a deep-red pupil.

Alexander aplasia: incomplete or faulty development of the membranous labyrinth of the cochlea; the organ of Corti and the spiral ganglion at the basal turn are most affected, resulting in a high-frequency hearing loss, while low-frequency hearing is relatively preserved.

alveoli pulmoni: tiny pouches along the alveolar sacs, alveolar ducts, and terminal bronchioles where the exchange of oxygen and carbon dioxide takes place.

Alzheimer's disease: the most common type of dementing disease resulting in progressive cognitive decline.

amphiarthrodial: pertaining to joints that yield.

ampulla: bulbous portion of the semicircular canal that communicates with the utricle and contains the receptor end organ, the crista ampullaris; plural: ampullae.

amygdala: almond-shaped subcortical nuclei deep to the uncus in the anterior temporal lobe, part of the limbic system and involved in emotion.

amyotrophic lateral sclerosis (ALS): a degenerative disorder of the upper and lower motor neurons; commonly referred to as "Lou Gehrig's disease."

anastomoses: the communication between two arteries.

anatomical position: the general position of a cadaver used as a reference point in describing position and spatial orientation of various parts of the body; the cadaver is upright facing the observer with arms extended to the sides, and head, eyes, and palms of the hands facing forward.

anatomy: the scientific study of the structure and organization of living organisms.

aneurysm: the bulging out of weak blood vessel walls, a precursor to hemorrhage.

annular ligament: the ligament that holds a membrane in place within a cartilaginous ring or sulcus, for example, the tympanic membrane in the tympanic sulcus and the footplate of the stapes in the oval window.

annular sulcus: the ringlike structure in which the tympanic membrane resides, held in place by the annular ligament; also referred to as the tympanic sulcus.

anosognosia: denial of illness; associated with right hemisphere syndrome.

anotia: a congenital absence of the pinna.

anterior arch: the narrower, anterior portion of the cricoid cartilage.

anterior cranial fossa: two forward-most depressions in the base of the interior cranium where the frontal lobes of the brain reside.

anterior cricoarytenoid ligament: connective tissue anchoring the anterior base of the arytenoid cartilage to the posterior quadrate lamina of the cricoid cartilage, thereby restricting the posterior rocking movement of the arytenoid.

anterior crus: anatomical structure resembling a leg; this crus and the posterior crus of the stapes connect to the footplate.

antigens: substances that trigger the immune system to produce antibodies.

antitragus: a cartilaginous prominence on the inferior concha ridge of the pinna opposite the tragus.

aperiodic sounds: complex sounds whose waveforms have no discernible repetitive pattern.

aphasia: a central nervous system disorder in which there is partial or complete impairment of language comprehension and/or production typically affecting several modalities (e.g., gesturing, listening, reading, speaking, writing).

aphonia: absence of phonation; a lack of sound produced by vocal fold vibration; no voice.

apical foramen: a small opening at the tip of the root of a tooth where nerve fibers and blood vessels enter the interior of the tooth.

apneustic area: the respiratory area in the pons that promotes inspiration.

aponeuroses: broad, tendinous sheets of connective tissue.

apraxia of speech (AOS): a sensorimotor disorder of articulation originating in the central nervous system characterized by impaired ability to volitionally program the position and sequencing of muscles involved in speech.

aprosodia: decreased use of the prosodic features of language including pitch, intensity, and timing to signal intonation; associated with right hemisphere syndrome.

arachnoid granulations: projections of arachnoid mater into dural sinuses for cerebrospinal fluid diffusion into the venous blood supply.

arachnoid mater: the middle meningeal layer that envelopes the central nervous system.

arcuate fasciculus: an association tract connecting the frontal lobe speech and language centers with the temporal lobe language centers; also known as the superior longitudinal fasciculus.

arcuate ridge: the horizontally directed ridge along the anterolateral surface of the arytenoid cartilage that separates the triangular fovea from the fovea oblonga.

area advantage: the large area of the tympanic membrane (TM) being focused down to the smaller area of the oval window serving to increase the pressure placed upon the fluids of the inner ear.

areolar: loose connective tissue that forms the bed for skin.

arteriosclerosis: the accumulation of plaque (e.g., fats and cholesterol) in blood vessels resulting in a narrowing of the arterial lumen.

arteriovenous malformation (AVM): congenital abnormality of capillary beds in brain tissue.

arthro-ophthalmopathy: also known as Stickler syndrome; a craniofacial anomaly affecting primarily the joints and eyes.

articulation: the process of forming and producing the speech sounds of a language; the process of speech production produced by movements of the structures of the vocal tract.

articulation disorder: an impairment in the ability to produce the speech sounds that make up a language.

aryepiglottic folds: folds of tissue that begin at the lateral-superior borders of the epiglottis and proceed posteriorly to the arytenoid cartilages along the inner surface of the thyroid cartilage; these folds form the superior border of the quadrangular membrane.

arytenoid articular facets: small projections on the sloping borders of the posterior quadrate lamina of the cricoid cartilage where the arytenoid cartilages articulate with the cricoid.

arytenoids: two somewhat pyramid-shaped cartilages that rest upon the sloping borders of the posterior quadrate lamina of the cricoid cartilage; the posterior attachment of the vocal folds is on the vocal processes at the base of these cartilages.

aspiration: the penetration of liquid or food below the true vocal folds into the lower airway.

association areas: cortical regions of the cerebral hemispheres involved in elaboration of respective primary areas (unimodal) or involved in higher cortical functions (multimodal).

association fiber tracts: bundles of axons that run in the cerebral hemispheres; these can be short or long.

asthma: a disease characterized by muscular spasms of the bronchial tubes and subsequent mucous membrane edema resulting in wheezing, difficulty breathing, and cough; often triggered by allergens.

astigmatism: irregular curvature of the cornea of the eye resulting in blurred vision.

astrocytes: a type of glial cell that supports neurons and contributes to the blood–brain barrier.

astrocytomas: benign tumors of the central nervous system; a type of glioma.

ataxic: a type of cerebral palsy or dysarthria characterized by poor coordination of motor movement.

atherosclerosis: the buildup of fatty deposits (i.e., plaque) within arterial walls.

athetoid: a type of cerebral palsy characterized by slow, writhing, involuntary movements of the hands, feet, and other body parts.

atmospheric pressure: the force that air exerts upon objects within the external environment.

atresia: absent formation of the external auditory meatus (ear canal).

atrophy: the withering away of a body part due to lack of use.

attack phase: that part of vocal fold vibration from the point where the vocal folds have adducted to the first cycles of vibration.

attic: upper portion of the middle ear cavity where the heads of the ossicles reside; also referred to as the epitympanic recess.

audibility: state of being audible.

audible: capable of being heard.

audiogram: the output of audiometry; a graph that shows hearing thresholds through air and bone conduction for each ear at various frequencies.

audiologist: as stated in the American Academy of Audiology (AAA) Scope of Practice, an audiologist is a professional who diagnoses, treats, and manages individuals with hearing loss or balance problems. Audiologists have received a master's or doctoral degree from an accredited university graduate program. Their academic and clinical training provides the foundation for patient management from birth through adulthood. Audiologists determine appropriate patient treatment of hearing and balance problems by combining a complete history with a variety of specialized auditory and vestibular assessments. Based upon the diagnosis, the audiologist presents a variety of treatment options to patients with hearing impairment or balance problems. Audiologists dispense and fit hearing aids as part of a comprehensive habilitative program. Audiologists may be found working in medical centers and hospitals, private practice settings, schools, government health facilities and agencies, and colleges and universities. As a primary hearing health provider, audiologists refer patients to physicians when the hearing or balance problem requires medical or surgical evaluation or treatment.

audiometry: hearing measures such as pure tone thresholds and speech discrimination performed with an audiometer.

auditory radiations: the final component of the auditory pathway carrying auditory information from the medial geniculate nucleus to the primary auditory cortex.

auditory tube: structure connecting the middle ear cavity to the nasopharynx; responsible for the equalization of air in the middle ear space with that of atmospheric pressure; also referred to as the Eustachian tube (ET).

augmentative and alternative communication (AAC): a specialty of speech–language pathology and other disciplines (such as medicine, occupational therapy, physical therapy) that has an emphasis in providing systems of communication for persons who have no speech ability or whose speech is not sufficient to meet their daily communication needs.

auricle: the visible portion of the outer ear used for the collection of sound; also referred to as the pinna.

auricular cartilage: cartilaginous framework of the pinna.

autoimmune inner ear disease (AIED): a syndrome characterized by progressive hearing loss, tinnitus, and/or dizziness which is caused by immune cells that attack and cause damage to the inner ear.

autonomic nervous system (ANS): also referred to as the visceral nervous system; the division of the nervous system that innervates smooth muscles, glands, cardiovascular function, and internal organs; the parasympathetic and sympathetic branches are further divisions of the ANS.

autophonia: abnormal resonance of one's own voice heard inside their head.

autosomal dominant: a pattern of genetic transmission from one parent to offspring where only one gene of a pair is necessary to express the trait; not related to the sex chromosomes.

autosomal recessive: a pattern of genetic transmission from both parents to offspring where two copies of a gene are necessary to express the trait; not related to the sex chromosomes.

axon: the part of the neuron specialized to transmit impulses away from the cell body and toward the terminal.

axon hillock: the enlarged junction of the axon with the cell body; it has a lower threshold for the initiation of an action potential than the rest of the cell.

bacterial meningitis: a bacterial inflammation of the meninges of the brain, labyrinth, or lining of cranial nerve VIII (the vestibulocochlear nerve).

Baha®: a commercially available system that utilizes a surgically implanted bone-conduction device. The receiver is implanted and is designed to communicate with an external amplifier bypassing air-conducted delivery. This allows the bone to transfer sound to a functioning cochlea, thereby bypassing the outer and middle ear. Once the cochlea receives these sound vibrations, the sound is converted into neural signals and is transferred to the brain, allowing a Baha recipient to perceive sound.

basal cell carcinoma: slow-growing malignant skin cancer with a raised or rolled border and a central ulcer; usually a result of chronic sun exposure.

basal ganglia: a collection of subcortical nuclei including the telencephalic caudate nucleus, globus pallidus, putamen, and subthalamic nucleus; functionally, the mesencephalic substantia nigra is also included.

basal plate: ventral region of the spinal cord during neurodevelopment that develops into nervous tissue serving motor purposes.

basilar artery: a major supply of blood to the brain; begins at the foramen magnum where the vertebral arteries converge on it and feed into the circle of Willis.

basilar membrane (BM): along with the spiral lamina, it forms the floor of the scala media running the length of the cochlea and supporting the organ of Corti.

benign paroxysmal positional vertigo (BPPV): brief episodes of vertigo that occur with changes in head position with respect to gravity; results from loose otoconia from the utricle floating into the posterior semicircular canal and adhering to its cupula.

Bernoulli effect: an increase in the velocity of a fluid (e.g., air) results in a decrease in its pressure.

bilateral: both sides; both ears.

binaural representation: reception of information from both ears to one location.

biology: the scientific study of life and living organisms.

blood–brain barrier: specialized barrier to the transport of noxious substances to the extracellular fluid of the brain due to the unique anatomical configuration of brain capillaries.

bolus: a small, soft, cohesive mass of food formed through mastication prior to a swallow.

bone conduction: in reference to audiometric testing, the transmission of test signals to the cochlea by vibrations of the skull; the transmission of sound to the inner ear through forced vibrations of the bones of the skull.

Boyle's law: the principle that states: with temperature being constant, volume and pressure are inversely related to each other.

bradykinesia: slow movement; difficulty initiating and regulating movement once begun; associated with Parkinson's disease.

brainstem: area of the brain located between the spinal cord and diencephalon; composed of the midbrain (i.e., mesencephalon), pons (i.e., part of the metencephalon), and medulla (i.e., myelencephalon).

breath groups: verbal utterances spoken on a single breath.

breathy attack: vocal fold vibration characterized by expired air escaping through the glottis before the vocal folds have fully adducted, thereby creating a breathy vocal quality.

Broca's area: frontal lobe premotor region involved in expressive speech and language function.

Brodmann areas: numbered regions of the cerebral cortex reflecting its cytoarchitecture.

buccae: the cheeks.

cadaver: from the Latin phrase "caro data vermibus," meaning "flesh given to worms"; a deceased human body donated for the advancement of science.

calcarine sulcus: the furrow that divides the medial aspect of the occipital lobe.

callosal sulcus: the furrow that surrounds the superior border of the corpus callosum.

calvaria: the skullcap which is formed by the vaulted frontal, parietal, and occipital bones.

canthus: either of the angles formed by the meeting of the eye's upper and lower eyelids.

capsular ligaments: a general term used to denote the ceratocricoid ligaments collectively.

cardiac impression: the indentation along the medial wall of the left lung where the heart resides.

Carhart's notch: audiometric pattern of bone conduction thresholds typically at 2,000 Hz; associated with otosclerosis.

carina: the keel-shaped landmark formed by the bifurcation of the last tracheal ring into the two main stem bronchi.

cartilaginous joint: the anatomical classification of joints that yield but do not freely move.

cataracts: clouding of the lens of the eye, resulting in opacity and visual impairment.

cauda equina: the collection of spinal nerves caudal to lumbar vertebra number one (L1); literally, horse's tail.

caudate nucleus: one of the telencephalic basal ganglia; involved with higher order motor functions.

cauliflower ear: caused by trauma to the pinna; separation of skin from underlying connective tissue with swelling, thickening, and malformation; related to trauma from the sport of wrestling or boxing.

cementoenamel junction: the part of the outer surface of a tooth where the cementum ends and the enamel begins, located approximately at the gum line.

cementum: the calcified covering of the root of a tooth.

central auditory processing disorder (CAPD): a disorder resulting from lesions along the higher levels of the auditory pathway or auditory cortex; the lesion interferes with the processing of auditory information fed to the brain by the peripheral ear.

central canal: narrow lumen within and running the length of the spinal cord; part of the ventricular system.

central chemoreceptors: sensory receptors responding to alterations in carbon dioxide in cerebral spinal fluid; located at the medulla.

central sulcus: furrow separating the frontal lobe from the parietal lobe.

central tendon: the three-lobed connective tissue core on which the fibers of the diaphragm insert.

centriole: an organelle that assists with nuclear and cell division.

ceratocricoid ligaments: a series of three ligaments (anterior, posterior, and lateral) that hold in place the articulation between the inferior cornua (horns) of the thyroid and the cricoid.

cerebellar peduncles: three major pairs of tracts—the superior, middle, and inferior—running from the brainstem to the cerebellum.

cerebellopontine (CP) angle: the anatomical angle created by the junction of the pons with the cerebellum where the facial (VII) and vestibulocochlear (VIII) nerves enter the brainstem.

cerebral aqueduct: the canal that joins the third and fourth ventricles.

cerebral peduncles: major motor tracts running in the ventral midbrain.

cerebrospinal fluid: a thin, watery substance produced by the choroid plexus that circulates throughout the ventricles and the subarachnoid space to cushion and provide nourishment to the central nervous system.

cerebrovascular accident (CVA): see *stroke*.

cerumen: substance created by a mixture of sloughed skin cells and secretions from the sebaceous glands located in the ear canal; also referred to as ear wax.

cervical segment: the most superior of the five parts of the spinal cord corresponding to the neck region.

checking mechanism: the action of the external intercostal muscles upon the rib cage during expiration; these muscles relax gradually during expiration to prevent the rib cage from recoiling too quickly.

choanae: the posterior openings of the nasal cavity into the region of the nasopharynx.

cholesteatoma: a pearl-like epithelial mass invading the middle ear space, usually secondary to prolonged retraction of the pars flaccida of the tympanic membrane from chronic Eustachian tube dysfunction.

chondro-osseous juncture: any juncture between cartilage and bone, for example, the juncture where the bony ribs terminate at cartilages that articulate with the sternum.

chorda tympani: a branch of the facial (VII) nerve that passes through the middle ear space; conveys taste sensation from the anterior two-thirds of the tongue.

choroid plexus: the delicate tissue composed of pia mater, capillaries, and ependymal cells that produces cerebrospinal fluid (CSF); found in the walls of the ventricles.

chronic: a longstanding condition.

chronic bronchitis: a longstanding and persistent inflammation of the mucous membranes of the bronchi.

chronic obstructive pulmonary disease (COPD): various diseases of the lower airways; often referring to emphysema and chronic bronchitis.

cilia: short, hairlike structures protruding from some epithelial tissue types.

cingulate sulcus: the furrow surrounding the superior border of the cingulate gyrus.

cisterna magna: a large subarachnoid space also referred to as the cerebellomedullary cistern for its location; contains cerebrospinal fluid (CSF).

Claudius' cells: lateral support cells for the organ of Corti, in particular the outer hair cells.

clavicle: commonly referred to as the collarbone, it runs in a horizontal plane from the sternum (breastbone) to the scapula (shoulder blade).

coarticulation: the simultaneous or overlapping articulation of two phonemes; for example, in the word "sweet," the lips round for the /w/ sound even as the /s/ sound is being produced (which by itself does not require lip rounding).

coccygeal segment: the most inferior of the five parts of the spinal cord; corresponding to the tailbone.

cochlea: contains the sensory organ of hearing (the organ of Corti); found within the inner ear labyrinth, within the petrous portion of the temporal bone.

cochlear aqueduct (CA): the canal or passage leading away from the cochlea to terminate within the subarachnoid space of the brain; it contains perilymph because it originates at the scala tympani.

cochlear duct: the membranous labyrinth of the cochlea where the organ of Corti resides; filled with endolymph, it is bordered by the basilar membrane, spiral lamina, spiral ligament, and Reissner's membrane; also referred to as the scala media.

cochlear implant (CI): surgically implanted receiver that when coupled with its external processor offers direct electrical stimulation of the cochlear nerve fibers for the purpose of hearing.

cochlear nuclei: the first large collection of nerve cells within the brainstem along the auditory pathway, at the level of the caudal pons.

cochlear partition: the anatomical structure made up of the osseous spiral lamina, basilar membrane, and the spiral ligament that separates the scala media from the scala tympani.

cochleariform process: bony process projecting into the middle ear space from the anterior wall; the tendon of the tensor tympani angles over the process to attach to the manubrium of the malleus.

cognate pair: two speech sounds that have the same place and manner of articulation, but differ only in the fact that vocal fold vibration occurs for one sound but not the other.

cognitive–communicative disorder: a communication impairment that results from underlying cognitive deficits.

commissural fiber tracts: bundles of axons that run from one cerebral hemisphere to the other; the corpus callosum is the largest of these.

common carotid arteries: large arteries ascending the neck to supply blood to the head; they have external and internal branches.

common crus: the point where the legs of the posterior and superior semicircular canals meet and merge.

complex tone: any sound composed of two or more individual (pure) tones blended together; most sounds in the environment are complex tones, including the human voice.

concha bowl: deep bowl-like portion of the pinna just above the lobule that leads to the external auditory meatus.

conductive: in reference to diminished hearing acuity, a reversible hearing loss due to pathology of the outer and/or middle ear; treating the pathology usually results in a reversal of the loss.

conductive hearing loss: a correctible hearing loss originating in the outer or middle ear, caused by a breakdown in the eardrum's and/or ossicular chain's ability to transform acoustic energy into mechanical energy, or to transmit mechanical energy to the inner ear.

condylar process: the posterior rounded process on the ramus of the mandible that articulates with the temporal bone of the skull, forming the temporomandibular joint (TMJ).

cone of light: the reflection of otoscopic light that appears on the surface of the tympanic membrane (TM) as a bright streak of light when the TM is resting at its normal 55-degree angle.

cones: one type of photoreceptor found in the retina; they code color and shape for visual acuity.

congenital: present at the time of birth.

congenital rubella: rubella (German measles) present in the pregnant mother that may cause developmental anomalies in the fetus.

congestive heart failure (CHF): inadequate pumping of blood by the heart, resulting in poor circulation.

connective tissue: tissue that combines body structures, supports the body, and aids in body maintenance.

connective tissue cell: any cell involved with connecting, anchoring, and supporting body structures;

specialized for the formation of various types of extracellular connecting and supporting elements.

connexin 26: transmembrane proteins that facilitate rapid transport of ions or small molecules between cells.

constructional impairments: marked by decreased ability to draw or put together objects using visuospatial skills; associated with right hemisphere syndrome.

contralateral: pertaining to the opposite side of the body.

contrecoup: focal area of lesion opposite the initial site of impact in a closed head injury.

conus elasticus: the lower portion of the elastic membrane that extends from the anterior arch of the cricoid cartilage inferiorly to the vocal ligaments superiorly.

conus medullaris: the inferior, terminal point of the spinal cord.

corium: a dense, feltlike network of connective tissue lying beneath the mucous membrane of the tongue, in essence forming the skeleton for the tongue.

corniculate tubercles: the medial bumps or swellings in the posterior aryepiglottic folds created by the corniculate cartilages lying within.

corniculates: two tiny cone-shaped cartilages that rest upon the apices of the arytenoid cartilages and are embedded within the aryepiglottic folds.

coronal suture: the seam running transversely across the anterior part of the skull that serves as the joint between the frontal bone and two parietal bones.

coronoid process: the flat, anterior process on the ramus of the mandible that serves as the insertion for the temporalis and masseter muscles.

corpora quadrigemina: the collection of four nuclei—two superior and two inferior colliculi—found in the dorsal midbrain.

corpus callosum: the large commissural tract connecting the right and left cerebral hemispheres.

corticobulbar tract: bundles of axons carrying motor information from the cortex to the brainstem; part of the pyramidal tracts.

corticospinal tract: bundles of axons carrying motor information from the cortex to the spinal cord; part of the pyramidal tracts.

cortilymph: fluid within the tunnel of Corti that is similar in composition to perilymph.

costal pleura: the connective tissue membrane that lines the interior of the rib cage; also known as the parietal pleura.

coup: focal area of lesion at the site of impact in a closed head injury.

cranial nerves: bundles of axons carrying a combination of motor, sensory, and autonomic nervous system (ANS) information in the peripheral nervous system; there are 12 pairs of cranial nerves.

craniofacial anomaly: a disorder or syndrome affecting the structures of the skull and/or face.

craniofacial dysostosis: also known as Crouzon syndrome; a craniofacial anomaly that is similar to Apert syndrome but less severe, affecting the bones of the face and skull.

cranium: the rounded part of the skull posterior to the face that houses the brain.

cribriform plate: the perforated central part of the ethmoid bone through which fibers of the olfactory nerve (I) pass from the nasal cavity to the olfactory bulbs.

cricoarytenoid joint: the articulation between each arytenoid cartilage and the posterior quadrate lamina of the cricoid cartilage.

cricoid: the ring-shaped cartilage forming the base of the larynx; it articulates with the thyroid cartilage and the arytenoid cartilages.

cricoid articular facets: two small projections on the superior sloping border of the posterior quadrate lamina of the cricoid cartilage that serve as the point of articulation for the arytenoid cartilages.

cricothyroid joint: the articulation between the cricoid and thyroid cartilages; there are two of these joints, each formed by an inferior cornu of the thyroid and the lateral surface of the cricoid in the region where the anterior arch ends and the posterior quadrate lamina begins.

cricothyroid ligaments: the inferior portions of the conus elasticus that bind the cricoid and thyroid cartilages.

cricotracheal ligament: connective tissue that binds the cricoid cartilage to the trachea at the first tracheal ring.

crista ampullaris: receptor end organ for balance (specifically angular acceleration) found in the ampulla of the semicircular canals; plural: cristae ampullares.

crista galli: literally "cock's comb"; the vertically oriented process of the ethmoid bone on which a portion of the dura mater of the brain anchors.

Crouzon syndrome: congenital autosomal dominant disorder with manifestations related to premature fusion of the cranial sutures including atresia; conductive or mixed hearing loss may be a component.

crura: plural of crus.

crus: anatomical structure resembling a leg; the anterior and posterior crura of the stapes connect to the footplate.

cul-de-sac resonance: an aberration of oral–nasal resonance in which the vocal tone resonates excessively within the pharynx and/or nasal cavity instead of within the oral cavity.

cuneiform: two tiny wedge-shaped cartilages that are embedded within the aryepiglottic folds somewhat lateral and anterior to the corniculate cartilages.

cuneiform tubercles: the lateral bumps or swellings in the posterior aryepiglottic folds created by the cuneiform cartilages lying within.

cupid's bow: the superior border of the upper lip that resembles an archer's bow due to the impression of the philtrum upon the medial part of the upper lip.

cupula: gelatinous membrane covering the stereocilia of the crista within the ampullae of the semicircular canals.

curette: a surgical instrument that has a scoop, wire loop, or ring at its tip and is used to clean the ear canal of debris.

curved membrane buckling: the eardrum vibrates in segments rather than as a whole unit serving to increase the pressure propagated to the ossicles.

cytoarchitecture: the structure and arrangement of cell bodies in different regions of the cerebral cortex.

cytokines: proteins secreted by cells especially of the immune system that are involved in the regulation of inflammatory responses.

cytomegalovirus (CMV): a herpes virus; a prenatal intrauterine infection which can cause central nervous system disorders, brain damage, hearing loss, vision loss, and seizures in the infant.

cytoplasm: the fluid interior of the cell outside of the nucleus.

Darwin's tubercle: anatomical feature of the pinna that is present in approximately 10.4% of the population; it presents as a thickening on the helix at the junction of the upper and middle thirds; the gene for Darwin's tubercle is inherited in an autosomal dominant pattern, but has incomplete penetrance, meaning not all who possess the gene will necessarily possess the ear tubercle; it is thought to be a sign of wisdom.

decibels (dB): one-tenth of a bel; the unit of sound intensity based on the logarithmic relationship of an observed intensity or pressure to a reference intensity or pressure.

declarative memory: explicit and conscious recall of facts.

deglutition: referring to the process of swallowing.

Deiter's cells: supporting cell group for the outer hair cells, resting on the basilar membrane residing in the organ of Corti; cradles the bases of the outer hair cells.

dementia: a progressive brain disease resulting in cognitive decline over time.

dendrites: multiple branches off the cell body of a neuron that transmit neural information toward the cell body.

dens: a toothlike, vertically oriented projection on the axis (C2) upon which the atlas (C1) rotates; also referred to as the odontoid process.

dentate nucleus: the most laterally located of the deep cerebellar nuclei.

dentin: the body of a tooth overlying the pulp cavity and covered by the enamel and cementum of the tooth.

depolarization: positive change in neuronal membrane potential moving it from resting membrane potential (i.e., −70 mV) to a less negative value (e.g., −15 mV); this allows for membrane channels to open so that calcium may infuse the cell causing the release of a neurotransmitter.

desaturation: decreased levels of oxygen in the arterial blood.

developmental articulation disorder: a term used to denote an articulation disorder that occurs during childhood, usually functional in nature.

diarthrodial: freely moving joints.

diencephalon: centrally located region of the brain that develops from the prosencephalon; includes the thalamus, hypothalamus, and epithalamus.

differentiation: one of the stages of neurodevelopment during which neurons become further specialized making their functional connections.

diphthongs: vowel sounds that have two articulatory positions during production, resulting in a shifting acoustic spectrum.

diplophonia: the simultaneous perception of two pitches during phonation; a phenomenon frequently associated with dysphonia.

diplopia: double vision (one object seen as two) due to disrupted innervation to the muscles of the eyes.

distoversion: malposition of a tooth away from the midline of the dental arch.

dorsal cochlear nucleus: the dorsal portion of the cochlear nucleus; the first central synapse for the cochlear nerve as it travels the pathway to the auditory cortex.

dorsal fasciculus: the dorsal or posterior region of spinal cord white matter where ascending bundles of nerve fibers are found.

dorsal root ganglion: a cluster of neuronal cell bodies for sensory functions found in the dorsal root of the spinal cord.

dowagers hump: colloquial term for hyperkyphosis describing excessive posterior curvature of the thoracic vertebrae; usually seen in elderly women.

ductus reunions: a small tube of the membranous labyrinth where the cochlea and the saccule meet; it carries endolymph between the auditory and vestibular systems.

dura mater: the most superficial and toughest layer of the meninges; cranial dura is double layered (periosteal outer layer and meningeal inner layer), spinal dura is single layered.

dysarthria: a motor speech disorder due to muscle paresis, paralysis, incoordination, or altered tone affecting speech processes of respiration, phonation, articulation, resonance, and prosody.

dysphagia: any difficulty, discomfort, or pain associated with swallowing; a swallowing disorder.

dysphonia: disordered phonation; phonation that brings negative attention to the speaker; often described by such terms as hoarse, breathy, tense, harsh, weak, strident or thin, among others.

dyspnea: general term for difficult or labored breathing.

ear canal: the tubular portion of the outer ear leading from the pinna to the tympanic membrane; also referred to as the external auditory meatus (EAM); part of the canal is bone and part of it is cartilage.

eardrum: also referred to as the tympanic membrane (TM), the thin membrane that forms the border between the outer and middle ear; the TM vibrates in response to acoustic pressure waves and transmits the resulting mechanical vibrations to the structures of the middle ear (i.e., ossicles).

earlobe: see *lobule.*

ectrodactyly–ectodermal dysplasia-clefting syndrome: also known as EEC syndrome; a craniofacial anomaly affecting the hands, feet, skin, nails, hair, and oral structures.

edema: swelling of tissues.

edematous: swollen with an accumulation of fluid.

efferent: the conduction of nerve impulses away from the central nervous system (i.e., motor).

elastic cartilage: specialized connective tissue that provides some structural support and is extremely flexible.

elastic membrane: a thin, broad sheet of connective tissue that binds the laryngeal cartilages together from within; it is composed of the quadrangular membrane superiorly and the conus elasticus inferiorly.

electronystagmography (ENG): electrical measurement of involuntary eye movements (i.e., nystagmus) to assess the integrity of the vestibular mechanism.

eleidin: a gel-like, translucent substance in the second layer of the skin of the lips that exposes the underlying vascular tissue, giving the lips a darker hue than the rest of the skin of the face.

embolic: a type of stroke due to an embolus—a traveling clot or plug that occludes an artery.

emboliform nucleus: medially located deep cerebellar nuclei.

emphysema: chronic and irreversible lung disease characterized by enlargement of the alveoli due to breakdown of their walls and loss of elasticity; often associated with smoking.

enamel: the calcified covering of the crown of a tooth.

encephalitis: inflammation of the brain.

endocochlear potential (EP): the differentiated potential between voltages of the endolymph within the scala media and the perilymph of the scala tympani.

endolymph: fluid of the membranous labyrinth; its composition has a high concentration of potassium and calcium and a low concentration of sodium.

endolymphatic sac: saclike portion of the membranous labyrinth connected to the endolymphatic duct, believed to play a role in absorption of endolymph.

endomysium: the connective tissue covering a muscle fiber.

endoneurium: the connective tissue covering a nerve cell fiber.

endoplasmic reticulum: an organelle that synthesizes, stores, and releases various substances within the cell.

endothelial tissue: a type of epithelial tissue that makes up the vessel linings for the circulatory and lymph systems.

endotracheal: within or passing through the trachea.

enlarged vestibular aqueduct syndrome (EVAS): a collection of symptoms that results from an already enlarged vestibular aqueduct becoming traumatized such as in the case of a head injury or sudden change in barometric pressure; the collection of symptoms typically comes on suddenly—a flat or sloping hearing loss and vertigo or symptoms of disequilibrium. The hearing loss is not present at birth and can fluctuate with each traumatic incident to the ear.

ependymal cells: a type of glial cell that lines the ventricular cavities and is part of the choroid plexus.

epiglottis: the leaf- or shoehorn-shaped cartilage lying immediately behind the hyoid bone and thyroid cartilage. It moves backward and downward to cover the opening of the larynx during swallow.

epimysium: the connective tissue covering a group of muscle fasciculi.

epineurium: the connective tissue covering a group of nerve fascicles.

episodic memory: a subtype of declarative memory regarding events that are time and place specific.

episodic vertigo: recurring spells of vertigo (dizziness) lasting for several minutes at a time.

epithalamus: part of the thalamus, involved in autonomic and limbic system functions.

epithelial cell: cells that cover surfaces and form selective barriers; specialized for selective secretion and absorption of molecules and ions.

epithelial migration: the natural migration of the dead skin of the ear canal from the level of the tympanic membrane to the outside.

epithelial tissue: tissue that lines the outer surface of the body as well as the internal passageways and body cavities.

epithelial tissue proper: a type of epithelial tissue that forms the skin and the internal membranes that are continuous with the skin.

epitympanic recess: see *attic.*

esophageal stage: the stage of the swallow from the bolus entering the esophagus to the bolus entering the stomach.

ethmoid bone: a central bone of the skull that forms part of the anterior cranial floor as well as the ceiling of the nasal cavities.

ethmoid paranasal sinuses: hollow chambers found within the ethmoid bone formed by the ethmoid labyrinths, opening into the nasal cavity.

ethmoidal labyrinths: a paired series of three (anterior, middle, and posterior) thin-walled cavities within the ethmoid bone.

etiology: the cause of a disorder.

Eustachian tube (ET): see *auditory tube.*

evoked: an event that occurs in response to stimulation.

excitatory postsynaptic potentials (EPSP): depolarizing graded potentials at the postsynaptic cell making the cell more likely to fire.

executive function: an integrative cognitive process directing initiation, planning, organizing, self monitoring, and control to achieve a goal.

exocytosis: the process of neurotransmitters being released from the synaptic vesicle into the synaptic cleft.

expiratory reserve volume (ERV): the volume of air that can be forcibly expired from the lungs at the end of a normal tidal exhalation.

external auditory meatus (EAM): see *ear canal.*

external carotid artery: a division off the common carotid artery supplying blood to the extracranial head and face.

extracellular: the area external to the cell.

extrinsic: a membrane or muscle whose origin, insertion, or both resides outside an anatomical structure such as the larynx or tongue.

facial: cranial nerve VII; innervates facial muscles, eyelid depressor muscles, the stapedius muscle, and some taste receptors.

falsetto: the loft register; phonation in a higher than normal pitch range characterized by unique free margin vibration of the anterior two-thirds of the vocal folds.

falx cerebelli: the sickle-shaped extension of the dura mater found between the cerebellar hemispheres.

falx cerebri: the sickle-shaped, arched fold of the dura mater of the brain that occupies the longitudinal fissure and anchors anteriorly onto the crista galli; it separates the two cerebral hemispheres.

familial: occurring in members of the same family but not necessarily being genetic.

fascia: a sheet of fibrous tissue found below the surface of the skin that encloses muscles and groups of muscles.

fascicle: a bundle of nerve fibers.

fasciculations: involuntary contractions or twitching of muscle fibers.

fasciculus: a bundle of muscle fibers.

fastigial nucleus: the most medially located of the deep cerebellar nuclei.

faucial pillars: two pairs of lateral folds at the posterior limit of the oral cavity formed by the palatoglossus and palatopharyngeus muscles which serve as the passage between the oral and pharyngeal cavities.

fibrous cartilage: specialized connective tissue that provides strong structural support and is slightly compressible.

fibrous joint: the anatomical classification of joints that are only slightly movable or immovable.

fibrous midline septum: the vertically oriented cavity within the interior of the tongue; its presence means that the intrinsic muscles of the tongue are paired.

filiform: cone-shaped papillae on the outer surface of the tongue; these are more numerous than any of the other types of papillae of the tongue.

filter: in acoustics, any structure (e.g., a cavity or chamber) that resonates certain frequencies while damping others.

flaccid dysphonia: the dysphonia of muscular hypotonia; the disordered voice associated with vocal fold paralysis or reduced muscle tension.

flaccid paralysis: a loss of voluntary movement associated with a reduction in muscle tone.

flexibility: in speech, the perception of frequency and intensity variation; the complexity of pitch and loudness for linguistic effectiveness and appropriate cultural affect.

flocculonodular lobe: the oldest part of the cerebellum on its inferior surface.

fluctuate: to alternately increase and decrease in severity.

fluent aphasias: a classification of language disorders due to brain lesion characterized by relatively effortless speech production and average utterance length of more than three words.

footplate: the base of the stapes bone to which the crura are attached; the portion of the stapes that fits into the oval window.

foramen cecum: a small depression in the middle of the sulcus terminalis at the root of the tongue.

foramen magnum: the large opening at the base of the occipital bone through which the spinal cord passes on its way down the spinal column.

formants: peaks of resonance in the vocal tract, that is, bands of frequencies with relatively high energy or amplitude.

Fourier analysis: a process by which a complex tone can be analyzed into its individual pure tone components.

fourth ventricle: part of the ventricular system; the space located at the dorsal surface of the brainstem between the pons and medulla (anterior) and the cerebellum (posterior).

fovea: the retinal depression in the eye where light rays are focused for the best acuity.

fovea oblonga: a depression along the base of the anterolateral surface of the arytenoid cartilage where the bulk of the posterior vocal fold attaches.

frequency: a physical measure of the number of times an object vibrates per second; frequency is perceived by humans as the pitch of a sound; the unit of measure for frequency is Hertz (Hz).

frons: the forehead.

frontal paranasal sinuses: a pair of cavities within the frontal bone that open into the nasal cavity.

frontotemporal dementias: subtypes of dementia that have primary degeneration of nervous tissue in the frontal and temporal lobes; includes Pick's disease and primary progressive aphasia.

functional disorder: an impairment that exists in the absence of a known or observable etiology.

functional residual capacity (FRC): the amount of air that remains in the lungs after a normal tidal expiration; it includes expiratory reserve volume and residual volume.

fundamental frequency: the lowest individual frequency (i.e., pure tone) in a complex tone.

fungiform: approximately 100 mushroom-shaped papillae on each side of the anterior tongue, each one housing approximately two to four taste buds.

gap junction channel: intercellular passages that open to allow certain chemicals to pass.

genetic: related to the inheritance from one's immediate family.

genetic mutation: a permanent change in one specific gene; associated with single-gene hereditary disorders such as Huntington's disease.

genetic variants: changes in a gene that act as genetic risk factors.

germ cell layers: primal embryologic source of organs.

gingivae: the gums; the mucous membrane that surrounds the teeth.

GJB2: the gene on chromosome 13 that codes for the development of connexin 26, a gap junction protein.

glabella: the portion of the frontal bone between the eyebrows and immediately superior to the nasal bones.

glenoid fossa: the crater-shaped depression on the scapula where the head of the humerus articulates.

glial cell: support cells of the nervous system.

gliomas: tumors of the central nervous system of glial cell origin.

globose nucleus: medially located deep cerebellar nuclei.

globus pallidus: a telencephalic nucleus of the basal ganglia involved in higher order motor control.

glossectomy: surgical removal of the tongue, either in part or totally.

glossoepiglottic folds: slips of mucous membrane that extend from the posterior base of the tongue to the lingual (anterior) surface of the epiglottis.

glossopharyngeal: cranial nerve IX; innervates some pharyngeal and lingual muscles, transmits taste and sensation from the throat.

glottal attack: vocal fold vibration characterized by complete adduction of the vocal folds before expired air reaches the larynx; the result is often an initiation of phonation that is explosive in nature.

glottal chink: any opening of the vocal folds while they are adducted in the median position; a posterior glottal chink is typically seen during whisper.

glottal fry: phonation of excessively low frequency due to maximum mass and minimum tension of the vocal folds; vocal fold vibration composed of the lowest frequencies in the vocal range—the voice typically sounds creaky when the vocal folds vibrate in glottal fry; also known as vocal fry.

glottal stop: an unvoiced glottal plosive seen in some languages and used in certain contexts in English; sometimes used as a compensatory strategy when the individual exhibits insufficient intraoral air pressure for the production of pressure consonants (e.g., affricates, fricatives, and plosives).

glottis: the variable-sized opening between the vocal folds at their superior edge.

goblet cells: specialized epithelial cells in the mucous membrane of the respiratory passageway that secrete mucous.

golgi apparatus: an organelle that packages and stores intracellular materials.

gomphosis: the virtually immovable joint formed by a tooth and its articulation with an alveolus (tooth socket).

graded potentials: small, localized, electrical changes from resting membrane potential on postsynaptic neurons; may be hyperpolarizing or depolarizing in effect.

gradual: proceeding by steps or degrees.

gustatory cortex: cortical region of the insula and overlying frontal operculum involved with the processing of neural information regarding taste.

habenula perforata: the space between the bony layers of the spiral lamina where the nerve fibers pass as they lead into the modiolus.

habitual pitch: the pitch range typically used by an individual for most vocal activity; the modal pitch range.

haemophilus influenzae Type B (Hib): responsible for a wide range of clinical diseases; one of the known bacteria to cause meningitis; vaccination with Hib conjugate vaccine is effective in preventing infection, and several vaccines are now available for routine use.

hair cells: inner ear sensory receptor cells with stereocilia projecting from the cell bodies, typically embedded in a gelatinous membrane that provides mechanical stimulation.

hamulus: the hook-like terminus of the medial pterygoid lamina of the sphenoid bone which serves as the pulley for the tendon of the tensor veli palatini muscle.

harmonic: any individual frequency that is a multiple integer of the lowest tone in a complex tone (i.e., fundamental frequency); for example, for a fundamental frequency of 200 Hz, the third harmonic would be three times the fundamental frequency, or 600 Hz.

hay fever: allergic response to environmental allergens.

helicotrema: apical portion of the cochlear duct where the perilymph of the scala vestibuli and the scala tympani is continuous.

helix: an anatomical structure of pinna; the outermost prominent curved rim or ridge.

hematoma: a clot of blood that forms in a tissue, organ, or body space as a result of a broken blood vessel.

hemispatial neglect: a lack of awareness of the environment opposite the site of lesion.

Hensen's cells: supporting cells of the organ of Corti that serve as an attachment for the tectorial membrane.

hereditary: result of genetic transmission; familial inheritance.

Hertz (Hz): the unit of measurement for frequency, representing vibration in cycles per second.

Heschl's gyrus: the transverse temporal gyrus that houses the auditory cortex for the central processing of speech.

hilum: the point where the main stem bronchi enter the lungs.

hippocampus: a subcortical nucleus found deep to the temporal lobe in each cerebral hemisphere; part of the limbic system and involved in memory, especially for new learning.

homeostasis: the physiological balance of the body's internal environment.

horizontal processes: the horizontally oriented plates of the palatine bones that make up the posterior part of the hard palate.

Huntington's disease: a hereditary degenerative disease of the telencephalic basal ganglion resulting in chorea.

hyaline cartilage: specialized connective tissue that provides strong structural support with some flexibility.

hydrocephalus: a pathological accumulation of cerebrospinal fluid (CSF) casually referred to as "water on the brain"; caused by blockage in CSF drainage or malfunction of absorption of CSF into the blood stream.

hydrostat: an anatomical structure (e.g., the tongue) that has the ability to move with little or no skeletal support for the muscles that comprise it; the structure makes hydraulic movements in the absence of fluid, and these movements do not diminish the structure's volume.

hyoepiglottic ligament: connective tissue that binds the superior, lingual (anterior) surface of the epiglottis to the posterior surface of the corpus of the hyoid bone.

hyoid: a U- or horseshoe-shaped bone in the superior region of the neck that is suspended in place by a series of muscles attaching to it from structures above and below; the hyoid primarily serves as the base of the tongue, but it is also bound to the larynx by the hyothyroid membrane.

hyothyroid membrane: a thin sheath of connective tissue that binds the inferior surface of the hyoid bone to the superior surface of the thyroid cartilage, thereby binding the hyoid bone and larynx together.

hypercapnia: elevated carbon dioxide levels in the blood.

hypernasality: abnormal, excessive nasal resonance that affects the proper production of nonnasal speech sounds.

hyperpolarization: a negative change in the neuronal membrane potential moving it from resting membrane potential (i.e., –70 mV) to a more negative number (i.e., –90 mV).

hyperpolarized: denoting an increase in the electrical potential difference across a cell membrane; neural impulses cannot be created during this state.

hypoglossal: cranial nerve XII, responsible for innervating muscles of the tongue.

hypoglossal canal: a small opening anterolateral to the foramen magnum where the hypoglossal nerve (XII) passes from the region of the medulla oblongata to the oral cavity.

hypopharynx: most inferior portion of the pharynx posterior to the laryngeal opening (aditus), also called the laryngopharynx.

hypothalamus: diencephalic region inferior to the thalamus, composed of a set of nuclei involved in autonomic and endocrine nervous system functions.

hypoxemia: low blood oxygen levels.

idiopathic: having an unknown cause.

ilium: the superiormost and largest of the three bones that make up the pelvis (the other two being the ischium and pubis).

immittance measures: measurement of the flow of energy through a medium; energy flow through the middle ear for the purpose of assessing its static condition, Eustachian tube function and the acoustic reflex.

immittance meter: a device used to measure immittance, usually of the middle ear.

impedance mismatch: a condition in which media have dissimilar impedances; therefore, when a stimulus travels from one medium to another, there is a loss of energy.

incisive foramen: a small opening in the maxillae immediately behind and between the two upper central incisors.

incudostapedial joint: the articulated joint between the incus and stapes.

incus: the second bone in the ossicular chain attached to the malleus and the stapes; consists of a body and a short and long process.

induction: refers to the interaction of ectoderm with the underlying mesoderm around the 18th day of gestation causing a commitment of tissue to become neural tissue.

infarct: a localized area of dead tissue.

inferior colliculi: see *inferior colliculus.*

inferior colliculus: auditory nucleus located in the midbrain; relays information from the superior olivary nucleus to the medial geniculate body; also plays a part in the startle reflex in reaction to a sudden, loud noise. Plural: inferior colliculi.

inferior cornua: two short, narrow legs of cartilage extending inferiorly from the posteriormost regions of the thyroid laminae; they articulate with the cricoid cartilage on each side.

inferior frontal gyrus: the cortical region of the frontal lobe housing Broca's area.

infrahyoid: a term used to denote any muscle that has an origin on a structure that is below the hyoid bone and then rises to insert onto the inferior surface of the hyoid.

infraorbital foramen: a small opening in the maxilla immediately below the orbit of the eye.

infraversion: malposition of a tooth so that it does not rest at the line of occlusion, that is, the tooth is "lower" than adjacent teeth.

infundibulum: connects the pituitary gland to the hypothalamus; also referred to as the pituitary stalk.

inguinal ligaments: bands of fibrous connective tissue formed by the aponeurosis of the external oblique muscle running from the iliac spine to the pubis; they separate the contents of the lower abdomen from the lower extremities.

inhalatory laryngeal stridor: an audible, noisy sound produced by an obstruction within the larynx (usually the adducted vocal folds) during inhalation.

inhalatory stridor: see *inhalatory laryngeal stridor.*

inhibitory postsynaptic potentials (IPSP): hyperpolarizing graded potentials at postsynaptic cells making the cells less likely to fire.

inner ear: houses the sensory organs of hearing and balance including the cochlea, vestibule, and semicircular canals.

inner hair cells (IHC): receptor sensory hair cells located in the organ of Corti within the cochlea of the auditory system of the inner ear.

inner pillar cells: supporting cells for the organ of Corti that stabilize the inner hair cells; they form the tunnel of Corti.

inspiratory capacity (IC): an individual's maximum capacity to inspire air; it includes tidal volume and inspiratory reserve volume.

inspiratory reserve volume (IRV): the volume of air that can be further inhaled after a normal tidal inhalation.

insula: region of the cerebral cortex deep to the lateral fissure involved with speech functions, the limbic system, and visceral function.

intensity: a physical measure of the amount of pressure that is generated within a medium by a vibrating object; intensity is perceived by humans as the loudness of a sound; the unit of measure for intensity is the decibel (dB).

interarytenoid muscles: a term used to denote the transverse and oblique arytenoid muscles collectively.

interaural: between the two ears.

intermaxillary suture: the seam or joint between the two maxillae.

intermediate tendon: a short inscription of tendon that connects two bellies of the same muscle; the omohyoid and digastricus muscles each have two bodies that are bound together by an intermediate tendon.

internal auditory canal (IAC): the bony pathway in the petrous portion of the temporal bone in which the vestibulocochlear (VIII) and facial (VII) nerves pass; blood vessels that supply the inner ear also pass through this canal.

internal auditory meatus: see *internal auditory canal (IAC).*

internal capsule: large projection pathway connecting higher (e.g., telencephalon) with lower (e.g., diencephalon) central nervous system regions.

internal carotid artery: a pair of arteries ascending on the superior anterior lateral neck that runs through the carotid foramen of the petrous portion of the temporal bone to join the circle of Willis at the base of the brain.

interthalamic adhesion: loose fibrous tissue connecting the two halves of the thalamus; also called the massa intermedia.

interventricular foramen: the paired set of canals joining the lateral ventricle to the third ventricle; a passageway for cerebrospinal fluid (CSF); sometimes referred to as the foramen of Monro.

intervertebral discs: cartilaginous discs between adjacent vertebrae in the spinal column.

intonation: a feature of spoken language in which pitch and stress are varied for phonemic and affective purposes; the rising and falling modulation of vocal pitch during speech production.

intracellular: originating or occurring within a cell.

intraoral air pressure: air pressure that is generated in the oral cavity for the production of speech sounds; the pressure is generated by the obstruction (e.g., plosives) or constriction (e.g., fricatives) of expired air by the articulation of various oral structures such as the lips, teeth, tongue, palate, etc.

intratracheal membrane: a connective tissue membrane that lines the interior of the trachea; muscle fibers and mucous membrane are superimposed upon it.

intrinsic: a membrane or muscle whose origin and insertion reside within an anatomical structure such as the larynx or tongue.

ipsilateral: on the same side.

ischemia: decreased oxygen to the brain.

ischium: the middle of the three bones that comprise the pelvis (the other two being the ilium and pubis).

isthmus: anatomical part or passage where bone and cartilage meet.

jargon: a series of fluently spoken neologisms and inappropriately used real words that make little or no sense to the listener.

jugular bulb: bulbous protrusion of the floor of the middle ear to accommodate the jugular vein.

kinesthetic: pertaining to the unconscious sense that detects position, weight, or movement of the muscles, tendons, and joints; also referred to as proprioception.

kinocilium: the tallest cilium of a bundle projecting from a cell body in the receptor end organs for balance.

Klippel–Feil syndrome: a craniofacial disorder with cleft palate and skeletal anomalies characterized by a short neck, scoliosis (abnormal curvature of the spine), kidney problems, and malformed stapes.

kyphoscoliosis: referring to scoliosis.

kyphosis: an abnormal anterior curvature of the spine; also known as "swayback."

labioversion: malposition of an anterior tooth (incisor or cuspid) so that it is tilted toward the lips.

labyrinth: the name for the mazelike structures of the inner ear; includes the cochlea, vestibule, and the semicircular canals.

labyrinthectomy: surgical destruction of the inner ear.

labyrinthine arteries: paired arteries arising from the basilar artery to supply blood to the inner ear.

labyrinthine wall: the most medial wall of the middle ear space.

lambdoidal suture: the seam or joint between the occipital bone and the two parietal and temporal bones.

lamina papyracea: the thin plate forming the lateral surface of the labyrinths of the ethmoid and forming a large part of the medial wall of the orbit of the eye.

laryngectomee: a person who has had his or her larynx surgically removed because of cancer or trauma.

laryngopharynx: a division of the pharynx that extends from the level of the hyoid bone to the esophagus, found immediately posterior to the larynx; also referred to as the hypopharynx.

larynx: a singular, musculocartilaginous structure within the neck that serves two purposes: (a) a protective device for the lower respiratory passageway; (b) the source of phonation for vocal activity.

lateral fasciculus: lateral region of spinal cord white matter where ascending and descending bundles of nerve fibers are found.

lateral geniculate nucleus (LGN): a point of synapse in the thalamus for primary visual system fibers; also referred to as the lateral geniculate body.

lateral glossoepiglottic folds: two folds of connective tissue that extend from the lingual (anterior) surface of the epiglottis to the base of the tongue; they are separated from each other by the median glossoepiglottic fold and valleculae.

lateral hyothyroid ligaments: somewhat thicker portions of the hyothyroid membrane that bind the superior cornua of the thyroid cartilage to the greater cornua of the hyoid bone; in many individuals, tiny cartilages (triticial cartilages) are embedded within these ligaments.

lateral lemniscus: the auditory tract or nerve bundle located on the lateral edge of the pons between the superior olivary nucleus and the inferior colliculus.

lateral semicircular canal: one of the three canals of the vestibular system; contains the sensory receptors for angular acceleration; also referred to as the horizontal semicircular canal.

lateral sulcus: the dividing fissure between the frontal and temporal lobes of the cerebrum, also referred to as the Sylvian fissure.

lateral ventricles: telencephalic brain cavities that produce cerebrospinal fluid.

left hemispatial neglect: the failure to report, respond, or orient to novel or meaningful stimuli to the left hemispace following damage to the right cerebral hemisphere.

lenticular process: small bony knob at the end of the long process of the incus that articulates with the head of the stapes.

lenticulostriate arteries: small arterial branches from the middle cerebral arteries that supply blood to portions of the basal ganglia and internal capsule.

leptomeninges: the collective name for the pia mater and arachnoid meningeal layers.

lesion(s): pathological changes to tissue structure or function due to injury or disease.

levator veli palatini: along with the tensor tympani, one of the two muscles responsible for opening the Eustachian tube; this muscle also elevates the soft palate during swallowing.

lever action: the ossicles work together as a lever to increase the pressure placed on the fluids of the inner ear.

lexical memory: a type of declarative memory specific to word meaning, spelling, and pronunciation.

ligament: dense connective tissue found at joints that attaches bone to bone, bone to cartilage, or cartilage to cartilage.

limbic areas: cortical regions (e.g., cingulate gyrus) and subcortical nuclei (e.g., hippocampi) involved in the limbic system functions of emotion and memory.

linea alba: a tight band of connective tissue extending from the xiphoid process to the pubis, formed by the aponeuroses of the external oblique, internal oblique, and transversus abdominus muscles; this vertical line separates the abdominal muscles into left and right mirror-image pairs.

lingual frenulum: a fold of mucous membrane that extends from the gingivae of the mandible and floor of the mouth to the anterior undersurface of the tongue.

Lissauer's tract: dorsolateral white matter region of the spinal cord involved with transmitting pain and temperature sensations.

literal (phonemic) paraphasias: unintentional errors of word retrieval in aphasia where wrong sounds are substituted for the correct sounds.

lobule: literally means small lobe, the anatomical structure hanging at the base of the pinna; the lobule is devoid of cartilage but is composed of adipose (i.e., fatty) connective tissue; also known as the earlobe.

loft register: the range of vocal pitches that is associated with falsetto, that is, the highest pitches of the vocal range.

logorrhea: excessive language output with little or no self-monitoring; can be seen with fluent aphasia; also known as press of speech.

long process: the prominent bony structure of the incus that terminates at the lenticular process which articulates with the head of the stapes.

longitudinal fissure: large furrow that divides the right cerebral hemisphere from the left.

longitudinal median sulcus: a depression on the midline superior surface of the tongue that runs along its length.

longitudinal tension: the force that is created by lengthening and shortening of the vocal folds; when the vocal folds are lengthened, longitudinal tension increases and when the vocal folds are shortened, longitudinal tension decreases; the laryngeal adjustment that regulates frequency of the vocal tone.

longitudinal wave: a wave that propagates (i.e., spreads out) in the same direction as the movement of the air molecules being displaced; that is, when an object vibrates, the air molecules are displaced by to-and-fro movements and the wave that is generated by the displacement also spreads out in the same direction (i.e., along the same plane as the molecules). Contrast this to a transverse wave which is seen when a rock is thrown into a pond. The water molecules move up and down but the wave spreads out horizontally from the point where the rock entered the water, creating a ripple effect. With a transverse wave, propagation is perpendicular to the movement of the molecules.

long-term memories: see *retrospective memories.*

lordosis: an abnormal posterior curvature of the spine; also known as "roundback."

loudness: the perceptual correlate of sound intensity.

lower motor neuron (LMN): a nerve cell whose body is located in the spinal cord or in the brainstem and whose axon passes by way of a peripheral nerve to innervate skeletal muscle.

lumbar cistern: enlarged subarachnoid space surrounding the inferior end of the spinal cord; contains cerebrospinal fluid (CSF).

lumbar segment: one of the five segments of the spinal cord corresponding to the lower back region.

lysosome: an organelle that is responsible for the digestion of bacterial and cellular debris.

macula: receptor end organ of the utricle and saccule housed in the vestibule; sensitive to linear and gravitational stimulation; plural: maculae.

macula flava anterior: the region immediately below the thyroid notch, somewhat yellowish in color, where the two vocal folds converge anteriorly.

main sensory nucleus: brainstem nucleus found in the pons that receives sensory information from the trigeminal (V) nerve regarding touch.

malleoincudal joint: articulated joint between the malleus and incus.

malleolar fold: a ridge along the tympanic membrane formed by ligament attachments to the anterior process of the malleus.

malleus: the largest and most lateral bone in the ossicular chain; articulates with the tympanic membrane and the incus.

mandible: the jaw bone.

mandibular fossa: also known as the glenoid fossa; a depression in the temporal bone immediately anterior to the external auditory meatus where the condylar process of the mandible articulates with the skull, thereby forming the temporomandibular joint (TMJ).

manubrium: the long process of the malleus that articulates with the tympanic membrane (TM) or eardrum.

masked facies: an expressionless face typically seen in Parkinson's disease.

mass effect: the resulting compression of surrounding nervous tissue by a lesion such as a hemorrhage or tumor.

mass lesions: foreign masses on the vocal folds that affect their ability to phonate properly, such as nodules, papillomae, or polyps.

mastication: the process of chewing food through mandibular and tongue movements to form a bolus.

mastoid air cells: the labyrinth of variable-sized cavities within the mastoid bone.

mastoid process: the rounded, posterior part of the temporal bone immediately behind the external auditory meatus and lateral to the styloid process; it serves as an attachment for several muscles.

mastoidectomy: the surgical removal of the bony partition of the mastoid air cells for mechanical cleaning of infection within the mastoid process of the temporal bone.

mastoiditis: inflammation of the mastoid air cells within the mastoid bone.

matrix: extracellular material that is part of connective tissue.

maxillary paranasal sinuses: spaces within the maxillae that open into the nasal cavity.

maximum minute volume: the amount of air that can be forcibly and maximally inspired and expired over the course of one minute.

mechanoreceptors: sensory receptors that respond to mechanical deformation of tissue such as compressing, stretching, etc.; for the respiratory system, these are found in the pulmonary apparatus and chest wall.

medial compression: the force of vocal fold adduction; as medial compression increases, the vocal folds become more resistant to subglottic air pressure; the laryngeal adjustment that regulates vocal intensity.

medial cranial fossa: two middle depressions at the base of the interior cranium where the temporal lobes of the brain reside.

medial geniculate body: the auditory nucleus within the thalamus that receives primary ascending fibers from the inferior colliculus and then relays them to the auditory cortex.

medial geniculate nucleus (MGN): see *medial geniculate body.*

medial lemniscus: a sensory tract traveling from the nuclei gracilis and nuclei cuneatus (dorsal column nuclei) in the medulla to the thalamus.

medial longitudinal fasciculus: ascending brainstem tract carrying information from the vestibular nuclei to the motor nuclei that control eye movement.

median glossoepiglottic fold: a single midline fold of connective tissue that courses from the lingual (anterior) surface of the epiglottis to the base of the tongue.

mediastinum: the cavity between the pleurae of the lungs containing the heart and thoracic viscera.

medical home: an approach to providing comprehensive primary medical care that facilitates a partnership between an individual patient and their personal physician; a medical home allows better access to health care and increased satisfaction with care by insuring the patient's continuity of care; also known as Patient-Centered Medical Home (PCMH).

medulla: see *medulla oblongata.*

medulla oblongata: referred to as the medulla, it is the most caudal component of the brainstem and is continuous with the spinal cord.

medullaris: the lower, tapering part of the spinal cord at the level of the first lumbar segment (L1); also known as the conus medullaris.

medullary centers: large volume of white matter fibers found in the cerebral hemispheres; the three types of fibers comprising the medullary centers are association, projection, and commissural fibers.

medullary rhythmicity center: the part of the medulla oblongata that controls the rate, depth, and rhythm of breathing.

Ménière's disease: a disease of idiopathic etiology that results from the excessive accumulation of endolymph within the membranous labyrinth; syndromes include episodic vertigo, fluctuating sensory hearing loss, and a sensation of fullness in the affected ear.

meninges: connective tissue coverings of the central nervous system (CNS); there are three meningeal coverings: the dura mater, the arachnoid, and the pia mater.

meningiomas: central nervous system tumors arising from meningeal connective tissue.

meningitis: an inflammation of the meninges from bacterial or viral causes.

meningococcal: referring to an organism that is one cause of bacterial cerebrospinal meningitis.

mental symphysis: the fibrocartilaginous juncture at midline of the two halves of the mandible that ossifies during the first year of life; the chin.

mesencephalic nucleus: a brainstem sensory nucleus receiving information regarding proprioception from the trigeminal (V) nerve.

mesencephalon: the midbrain, found caudal to the diencephalon.

mesioversion: malposition of a tooth toward the midline of the dental arch.

mesothelial tissue: a type of epithelial tissue that lines the internal body cavities.

metamemory: a higher level cognitive function denoting the ability to know and predict recall; memory about memory.

metencephalon: developed from the rhombencephalon; consists of the pons and cerebellum.

metopic suture: the seam that divides the two halves of the frontal bone in infants and children that usually disappears by the age of 6 so that the frontal bone is a singular unit.

Michel dysplasia: a malformation of the inner ear characterized by its failure to develop, resulting in complete unilateral or bilateral deafness.

microcephaly: abnormal smallness of the head.

microfilament: an organelle that assists with cell movement and transport of substances within the cell.

microglia: a type of glial cell with many small, fine processes; involved in phagocytosis following neuronal death.

micropascals (μPa): unit of measurement of pressure representing one-millionth of a pascal.

microtia: malformation of the pinna.

microtubule: an organelle that assists with cell movement and transport of substances within the cell.

middle ear: portion of the hearing mechanism medial to the tympanic membrane and lateral to the vestibule of the inner ear.

middle ear cavity: air-filled space in the temporal bone where the contents of the middle ear reside; also referred to as the middle ear space.

midline raphe: the midline seam where the two mylohyoid muscles (left and right) meet as their fibers course to insert onto the hyoid bone.

migration: one of the stages of neurodevelopment during which neurons move to their destined locations.

millivolts (mV): one-thousandth of a volt; a unit of measure for electrical current.

minute volume: the amount of air that is exchanged during quiet, tidal breathing over the course of one minute.

mitochondria: an organelle that provides the energy source for the cell.

mixed: in reference to diminished hearing acuity, a hearing loss that has both conductive and sensorineural components; the conductive component can be treated but the sensorineural component is permanent.

modal register: the range of frequencies associated with the vocal midrange; it is associated with habitual pitch.

modiolus: the bony central core of the cochlea that houses the nerve fiber ganglia of cranial nerve VIII as well as blood vessels.

Mondini dysplasia: a specific malformation of the cochlea where only the basal turn is developed, thereby restricting the bony cochlea to 1.5 turns.

monophthongs: vowel sounds that have only one articulatory position throughout their production; also known as pure vowels.

motile: capable of movement.

motor homunculus: the topographical map of the precentral gyrus indicating body representation regarding motor function.

motor speech disorder: a disorder in which the planning, initiation, timing, coordination, or strength of voluntary muscle movements for speech is adversely affected; includes apraxia of speech (AOS) and dysarthria.

mucoperiosteum: the lining of the interior paranasal sinuses (as well as other parts of the body such as the auditory structure) formed by the intimate union of the periosteum and a mucous membrane.

mucosal wave: the repetitive, undulating vibration of the mucous membrane covering of the vocal folds during phonation; aberrations of the mucosal wave may indicate vocal fold pathology.

multiple sclerosis: an acquired, degenerative, demyelinating disease of the central nervous system.

muscle cell: synonymous with muscle fiber; specialized for the production of mechanical force.

muscular dystrophy: a genetic disease characterized by progressive muscle deterioration and weakness.

muscular process: the rounded projection at the base of each arytenoid cartilage where the posterior and anterolateral surfaces meet; the muscular processes are the insertion point for the lateral and posterior cricoarytenoid muscles.

musculocartilaginous: referring to an anatomical structure that is composed primarily of cartilages and muscles; the larynx is a musculocartilaginous structure.

myelencephalon: develops from the rhombencephalon; consists of the medulla.

myelin: axonal covering necessary for rapid impulse conduction; oligodendroglia make up myelin in the central nervous system (CNS) and Schwann cells make up myelin in the peripheral nervous system (PNS).

mylohyoid line: a ridge running transversely along the interior surface of the corpus of the mandible; it is the point of origin for the mylohyoid and other muscles.

Myoelastic Aerodynamic Theory: a theory that describes how the vocal folds vibrate according to principles of aerodynamics (e.g., airflow, Bernoulli effect, pressure); the explanation of the phonatory process that accounts for the vibratory capacity of the vocal folds based on their mass and elasticity (myoelastic) and the movement of air (aerodynamic) through the glottis.

myopia: nearsightedness.

myringoplasty: a surgical procedure to close a tympanic membrane perforation.

myringotomy: surgical incision of the tympanic membrane to remove effusion of the middle ear.

nasal cannulae: tubes inserted into the nasal openings to deliver oxygen.

nasal murmur: an additional resonance below 500 Hz for the nasal consonants.

nasal septum: the midline division between the two halves of the nasal cavity which is formed by bone (the perpendicular plate of the ethmoid and the vomer) posteriorly and cartilage (septal cartilage) anteriorly.

nasopharynx: a division of the pharynx which extends from the base of skull to the level of the velum; the pharyngeal region posterior to the nasal cavity.

natural resonant frequency: the frequency at which a system vibrates with greatest amplitude when driven by an external force.

nebulizer: a mechanical device used to administer medication to individuals with respiratory disease via a liquid mist to the airways.

neocortex: the newest cortex from an evolutionary perspective; it is six-layered and makes up the cerebral cortex.

neologisms: made-up words that are not found in the patient's language.

neonatal herpes: herpes infection in the newborn baby.

neoplasm(s): tumors, whether benign or malignant.

nerve cell: synonymous with neuron; specialized for the initiation and conduction of impulses.

neural arch: the bony arch on the dorsal side of a vertebra formed by the pedicles and laminae extending from the corpus.

neural crest: neuroectodermal tissue that separates from the neural tube and develops into structures of the peripheral nervous system.

neural pathway: the nerve cells and pathways of the auditory and vestibular systems.

neural plate: early stage of neurodevelopment following induction; neuroectoderm thickening that develops into the neural tube.

neural tube: neuroectodermal tissue that folds in upon itself to form a tube and later develops into the central nervous system.

neuralgia: pain associated with a nerve.

neurectomy: the surgical excision of part of a nerve.

neurogenic dysphagia: a swallowing disorder with a neurological etiology.

neurological disorder: any disorder whose etiology can be traced to the central or peripheral nervous system.

neuromas: tumors of the nervous system, whether benign or malignant.

neuromuscular junction: the point of synapse between a neuron and the muscle fibers it innervates; also referred to as the myoneural junction.

neuropathy: a disease or abnormality of the nervous system.

neurotransmitter(s): chemical agents at synaptic junctions that allow neural impulses to propagate.

nodes of Ranvier: intervening spaces between myelin segments on an axon where the axon communicates directly with the extracellular space.

noise-induced hearing loss (NIHL): hearing loss due to exposure to excessive noise levels; the loss is sensorineural and permanent in nature.

nonfluent aphasias: a classification of language disorders due to a brain lesion characterized by effortful speech production and average utterance length of less than three words.

nucleus: the control center of a cell which houses genetic material.

oblique line: a somewhat ill-defined ridge running diagonally along each thyroid lamina.

occipital condyles: two processes on either side of the foramen magnum that serve as the point of articulation between the base of the skull and the first cervical vertebra (C1 or the atlas).

occipitomastoid suture: the seam or joint between the occipital bone and the mastoid process of the temporal bone which is continuous with the lambdoidal suture.

occiput: the back of the cranium.

octave: in speech science, a doubling of frequency usually in reference to the fundamental frequency; for example, if the fundamental frequency is 150 Hz, the first octave is 300 Hz.

oculomotor: cranial nerve III, innervates multiple muscles for eye movement.

odontoid process: a toothlike, vertically oriented projection on the axis (C2) upon which the atlas (C1) rotates; also referred to as the dens.

ohms: unit of measure of resistance for electrical or other forms of energy.

olfactory: cranial nerve I, projects from the nasal cavity to the olfactory bulb transmitting sensory information regarding smell.

oligodendroglia: a type of glial cell responsible for producing myelin in the central nervous system.

olivocochlear pathway: efferent pathway projecting from the medial and lateral superior olivary complex and coursing down to the inner and outer hair cells for the purpose of inhibition.

operculum: area of the cerebral cortex that overlies the insula; includes the frontal opercula, temporal opercula, and parietal opercula.

optic: cranial nerve II, transmits visual information from the retina exiting the optic disc and traveling caudally on the ventral surface of the frontal lobes.

optic canals: two short openings in the lesser wings of the sphenoid bone where the optic nerves (cranial nerve II) and ophthalmic arteries pass from the orbits of the eye into the cranial cavity.

optic chiasm: partial crossing point of the optic nerve and part of the primary visual pathway.

optic radiations: part of the primary visual pathway carrying fibers from the lateral geniculate nucleus of the thalamus to the primary visual cortex in the occipital lobe.

optic tract: part of the primary visual pathway carrying fibers from the optic chiasm to synapse at the lateral geniculate nucleus of the thalamus.

optimal pitch: natural pitch; the voice fundamental achieved at maximum phonatory efficiency in the modal register.

oral preparatory stage: the first stage of swallow, including removing food from a cup or utensil and chewing (i.e., mastication) to form the bolus.

oral stage: the second stage of the swallow where the bolus is propelled toward the pharynx to initiate a swallow reflex.

oral transit time (OTT): the amount of time it takes to move the bolus toward the pharynx and initiate a swallow.

orbit: the large opening in the facial part of the skull where an eyeball resides.

organ of Corti: organ within the scala media of the cochlea where the receptor hair cells and supporting cells reside resting on the basilar membrane.

organelles: structures inside a cell that perform vital functions for the life of the cell.

organic: relating to the structure, function, or health of living things; see also organic disorder.

organic disorder: an impairment that can be traced back to an observable structural or physiological etiology.

oropharynx: a division of the pharynx that extends from the level of the velum to the level of the hyoid bone; the pharyngeal region posterior to the oral cavity.

ossicles: the bones of the middle ear: malleus, incus, and stapes.

ossicular chain: the collection of the articulated bones of the middle ear: malleus, incus, and stapes.

osteoblasts: specialized cells that are responsible for forming or reforming bone.

osteoclasts: specialized cells that are responsible for the resorption of bone.

osteoma: benign slow growing bony mass in the ear canal usually located at the junction of the cartilaginous portion and the bony portion; exposure to cold water is thought to stimulate their growth.

osteoporosis: significant loss of bone density.

otalgia: ear pain.

otitis externa: an inflammation of the skin lining of the external auditory meatus or ear canal.

otitis media (OM): inflammation of the middle ear resulting primarily from poor Eustachian tube function.

otitis media with effusion: inflammation of the middle ear with the development of fluid in the middle ear space.

otitis media with tympanic membrane perforation: inflammation of the middle ear with a secondary perforation of the tympanic membrane (TM) or eardrum.

otoconia: calcium crystals that add mass to the structure of the maculae of the utricle and saccule; they are located on the gelatinous (i.e., otolithic) membrane in which the stereocilia of the hair cells are embedded.

otolaryngologist: a physician who specializes in the diagnosis, management, and treatment of ear, nose, and throat conditions; also known as an ENT.

otolithic membrane: the gelatinous membrane that the otoconia rest upon that provides for the stimulation of the embedded stereocilia hair cells of the maculae.

otologist: a physician who specializes in the diagnosis, management, and treatment of ear disease.

otorrhea: drainage from the ear.

otosclerosis: formation of new spongy bone growth around the stapes footplate and oval window resulting in stapes fixation and a concomitant conductive hearing loss.

otoscopy: inspection of the external auditory meatus and tympanic membrane through use of an otoscope.

outer ear: the outermost portion of the hearing mechanism, beginning with the pinna, that functions to gather and conduct sound waves down to the level of the tympanic membrane.

outer hair cells (OHC): motile cells within the organ of Corti that seem to be responsible for enhancing tectorial membrane movement at low intensity levels to facilitate stimulation of the inner hair cells.

outer pillar cells: supporting cells for the organ of Corti that stabilize the outer hair cells; they form the tunnel of Corti.

oval window: the opening on the medial wall of the middle ear leading into the scala vestibuli of the inner ear; the footplate of the stapes fits in this window.

palatal aponeurosis: a broad, flat sheet of connective tissue that serves as the skeleton for the velum (soft palate).

palatine processes: the horizontally directed processes of the maxillae that form the anterior portion of the hard palate.

palatoglossal arches: also known as the anterior faucial pillars; two folds on either side of the posterior oral cavity that are formed by the palatoglossus muscles.

palilalia: a pathological condition in which words are rapidly and involuntarily repeated.

palliative care: care that is focused on the comfort of the individual through the prevention and relief of suffering to improve quality of life.

palsy: partial or complete paralysis of muscles, often accompanied by loss of sensation and uncontrollable body movements such as tremors.

papilloma: also known as juvenile papillomatosis; benign tumors of the larynx in children.

paradoxical vocal fold movement (PVFM): adductory rather than normal abductory vocal fold movement during inspiration resulting in constriction or complete occlusion of the airway.

paragrammatism: language errors in the use of grammatical markings seen in persons exhibiting fluent aphasia.

parahippocampal gyrus: cortical region inferior to the cingulate gyrus at the medial surface of the temporal lobe.

paramedian position: the somewhat halfway abducted position that the vocal folds take at rest; the vocal folds can either adduct from this position or more fully abduct.

parasympathetic division: a division of the autonomic nervous system; serves to conserve body energy and maintain the internal balance of body systems.

parenchyma: organ tissue.

parenchymal: deep to the cerebral cortex; also referred to as intracerebral.

parietal pleura: see *costal pleura.*

parietal–temporal–occipital (P-T-O) region: the multimodal association cortex at the convergence of the parietal, temporal, and occipital lobes.

Parkinson's disease: a degenerative disease of the mesencephalic basal ganglia, specifically the substantia nigra.

pars flaccida: the superior region of the tympanic membrane (TM) having less support from the central fibrous layers.

pars oblique: a bundle of fibers from the cricothyroid muscle that course in a somewhat diagonal direction; the lateral bundles of the cricothyroid muscles.

pars recta: a bundle of fibers from the cricothyroid muscle that course in a somewhat vertical direction; the medial bundles of the cricothyroid muscles.

pars tensa: make up the body of the tympanic membrane (TM); consisting of three sturdy fibrous layers.

Passavant's pad: a bulging of the posterior wall of the nasopharynx created by contraction of the muscles that comprise the superior pharyngeal constrictors.

pathology: the scientific study of the nature of diseases and of the structural and functional changes that occur to the living organism due to disease processes.

patulous: abnormally open.

pericardial cavity: internal body cavity that houses the heart.

pericardium: the membranous sac that contains the heart.

perichondrium: fibrous membrane surrounding the outer surface of cartilage.

perilymph: cochlear fluid found in the scala vestibuli and scala tympani; it is high in concentrations of sodium and calcium and low in concentration of potassium.

perimysium: connective tissue covering each muscle fasciculus.

perineurium: connective tissue covering each nerve fascicle.

periodic sounds: sounds whose waveforms repeat themselves at equal intervals over time.

periodontal ligament: the connective tissue that holds a tooth within its alveolus, thereby forming a joint called a gomphosis.

periosteum: fibrous membrane surrounding the outer surface of bone.

peripheral chemoreceptors: sensory receptors responding to changes in oxygen levels in the blood; located at the bifurcation of the common carotid arteries.

peristalsis: the unidirectional wavelike muscular contractions in the pharynx and esophagus that force food and drink down toward the stomach.

peristaltic: referring to a wavelike action.

peritoneal cavity: internal body cavity that houses the abdominal viscera.

permanent: continuing indefinitely without fundamental change.

perpendicular plate of the ethmoid: a vertically oriented lamina of the ethmoid bone that extends below and perpendicular to the cribriform plate, forming the superior part of the bony nasal septum.

petiolus: the narrow stalk at the inferior end of the epiglottis that is bound to the thyroid cartilage just behind the thyroid notch by way of the thyroepiglottic ligament.

phagocytic cells: cells that capture and absorb waste material, harmful microorganisms, and other foreign bodies.

phagocytosis: the process of ingesting cellular debris.

pharyngeal aponeurosis: a broad, flat sheet of connective tissue that serves as the skeleton for the pharynx.

pharyngeal fricative: an unvoiced sound occurring naturally in some languages (but not English) that is produced by creating turbulence within the pharynx; in speakers for whom the sound doesn't occur naturally, this sound is sometimes used as a compensatory strategy when intraoral air pressure is insufficient to produce the oral fricatives.

pharyngeal stage: third stage of the swallow that is initiated with the swallow reflex and ends with the bolus entering the esophagus.

pharyngeal transit time (PTT): the time it takes for the bolus to pass through the pharynx and into the esophagus.

pharyngeal tubercle: the region immediately anterior to the foramen magnum on the basilar part of the occipital bone where the pharyngeal raphe attaches (the pharyngeal raphe, in turn, serves as the point of origin and insertion for the pharyngeal constrictor muscles).

pharynx: the upper end of the alimentary canal that extends from the oral and nasal cavities to the esophagus; also known as the throat.

philtrum: the vertically oriented groove or depression located midline between the nose and the upper lip bordered on either side by the columellae nasi.

phonation: the physiological process by which vocal fold vibration results in a vocal tone; the process of producing a voice by way of vocal fold vibration.

phonation breaks: phonatory discontinuity; phonation is interrupted with brief periods of aphonia.

phonemic paraphasias: see *literal (phonemic) paraphasias.*

phonemic regression: age-related reduction in the ability to recognize words greater than expected from the amount of documented hearing loss.

phonological disorder: a speech disorder characterized by speech sound errors that are cognitively or linguistically based, as opposed to simple errors in motor production.

photoreceptors: sensory receptors for vision; these include the rods and cones of the retina.

phrenic nerve: the nerve created by combined branches of spinal nerves C3, C4, and C5 that innervates the diaphragm.

phrenology: the correlation of the structure of the head with personality and intellect proposed by Franz Joseph Gall in 1809.

physiology: the scientific study of the function of the living organism and its parts.

pia mater: the innermost of the three meningeal layers; very delicate and transparent.

piebaldism: an autosomal dominant genetic disorder of pigmentation characterized by congenital patches of white skin and hair.

pinna: visible portion of the outer ear for the collection of sound; also referred to as the auricle.

pitch: the perceptual correlate of sound frequency.

pitch breaks: a sudden, noticeable, often unexpected shift from one pitch to another during phonation; commonly an upward shift of an octave or more from the modal register to the loft register (falsetto).

plane of reference: the vertical, horizontal, or other direction in which an anatomical structure is being viewed by the observer; these include the coronal, sagittal, and transverse planes.

plasma membrane: double-layered outer membrane of a cell.

plethysmograph: a device that allows one to study movements of the chest and abdomen by observing changes in thoracic and abdominal volumes.

pleurae: the serous membrane that surrounds the lungs and interior of the thorax consisting of two layers: the costal pleura and the visceral pleura.

pleural cavities: internal body cavities that house the lungs.

pleural linkage: the binding of the lungs to the interior of the rib cage by way of the airtight adhesion of the visceral pleura of the lungs to the costal pleura of the rib cage, and of the lungs to the superior surface of the diaphragm by way of the visceral pleura they both share.

pneumococcal: referring to an organism that is one cause of bacterial cerebrospinal meningitis.

pneumonia: lung inflammation that is secondary to infection or other causes such as aspiration.

pneumotachometer: a device that allows one to study changes in air pressure and air flow.

pneumotaxic area: the respiratory area in the pons that inhibits inspiration to prevent overinflation of the lungs.

pneumothorax: the presence of gas in the pleural cavity which results in a collapsed lung.

polyps: nonmalignant growths or tumors protruding from the mucous membrane of a structure such as the nasal cavity or vocal folds.

pons: a broad mass of chiefly transverse nerve fibers in the brainstem lying ventral to the cerebellum at the anterior end of the medulla oblongata; the bridge between the brainstem and the structures of the midbrain.

pons-medullary junction: the junction on the ventral aspect of the brainstem that demarcates the pons from the medulla oblongata; cranial nerve VIII emerges here.

pontine cisterns: enlarged subarachnoid spaces that are ventral to the pons; contains cerebrospinal fluid (CSF).

posterior cranial fossa: the two rear-most depressions in the base of the interior cranium where the two lobes of the cerebellum of the brain reside.

posterior cricoarytenoid ligament: connective tissue anchoring the posterior base of the arytenoid cartilage to the posterior quadrate lamina of the cricoid cartilage, thereby restricting the anterior rocking movement of the arytenoid.

posterior crus: anatomical structure resembling a leg; this crus along with the anterior crus of the stapes connect to its footplate.

posterior faucial pillars: bands of tissue running from the soft palate to the pharynx, overlying the palatopharyngeus muscles.

posterior quadrate lamina: the broader posterior portion of the cricoid cartilage that projects superiorly to occupy some of the open space in the posterior inner region of the thyroid cartilage.

postlingual: after speech and language skills have been developed.

precentral gyrus: convoluted gray matter anterior to the central sulcus; involved in volitional movement.

prefrontal cortex: the multimodal association area of the most rostral region of the frontal lobes.

prelingual: prior to the development of speech and language skills.

premaxilla: the triangular part of the anterior hard palate that is formed by two tiny sutures originating bilaterally between the lateral incisors and cuspids and coursing back to terminate at the incisive foramen; this region is typically fused in humans.

prephonation phase: that part of the vibratory cycle where the vocal folds move from the paramedian position to the median position by means of adduction.

presbycusis: age-related progressive hearing loss most often sensorineural and bilateral in nature.

presbylaryngis: progressive voice degeneration attributed to the aging process.

press of speech: see *logorrhea*.

pressure = force/area: a law of physics that states that pressure change occurs as a force is displaced over a change in area; with force being constant, pressure increases as area decreases and vice versa.

pressure consonants: consonant sounds that require a degree of intraoral air pressure to be produced; includes the plosives and affricates primarily but can include the fricatives.

pressure equalization (PE) tube: a silastic tube or grommet surgically placed in the tympanic membrane to provide passive ventilation of the middle ear space.

primary areas: regions of the cerebral cortex that have single functions.

primary auditory cortex: receives projections from the auditory pathway, also called Heschl's gyrus; Brodmann areas 41 and 42.

primary motor cortex: the precentral gyrus in the frontal lobe; gives off projections for volitional motor movement; Brodmann area 4.

primary progressive aphasia (PPA): a subtype of dementia with the primary symptom of progressive deterioration of language abilities.

primary somatosensory cortex: the postcentral gyrus in the parietal lobe that receives sensory projections; Brodmann areas 3, 1, 2.

primary visual cortex: the cuneus and lingual occipital gyri regions surrounding the calcarine fissure where the sense of sight is interpreted; Broadmann area 17.

primary visual pathway: the axonal fibers and nuclei involved in transmitting visual neural information from the retina to the primary visual cortex in the occipital lobe.

progressive: advancing in degree or severity.

progressive neurological disorder: a pathological condition arising from the central and/or peripheral nervous system that gets progressively worse over time and is often fatal.

projection fiber tracts: bundles of axons that transmit neural information from higher to lower (and vice versa) centers of the central nervous system (CNS).

proliferation: one of the stages of neurodevelopment during which neurons multiply.

promontory: the bony prominence in the medial wall of the middle ear cavity created by the basal turn of the cochlea.

propagation: the transmitting of an action potential down an axon toward the terminal.

proprioceptive: pertaining to the sense of body position, posture, and movement.

prosencephalon: a term signifying the rostral vesicle of the neural tube early in neurodevelopment; further differentiates to form the telencephalon and diencephalon.

prosody: the intonation and stress that overlies the production of speech sounds during conversational speech, signaled by modifications in vocal pitch, intensity, and duration.

prosopagnosia: an inability to recognize familiar faces; a type of perceptual impairment.

prospective memory: memory for future events and information; remembering to remember.

protoplasm: the basic living substance of cells.

pseudobulbar palsy: a condition resulting in dysarthria as a result of lesions occurring above the level of the brainstem.

psychogenic: of psychological origin; from the mind; often used to mean functional or in the absence of an organic etiology.

ptosis: droopy eyelid(s) secondary to oculomotor (III) nerve involvement.

puberphonia: also known as mutational falsetto; use of a high pitch, often falsetto, usually in postpubescent and young adult males such that age and gender identity may be lost and/or negative attention results.

pubic symphysis: the joint formed by the union of the medial aspects of the two pubic bones.

pubis: the inferiormost of the three bones that comprise the pelvis (the other two being the ilium and ischium).

pulmonary edema: abnormal buildup of fluid in the lungs.

pulmonary pressure: the force that air exerts upon the alveoli pulmoni within the lungs; also referred to as alveolar pressure.

pulmonologist: a medical doctor who specializes in diseases of the lungs and respiratory tract.

pulp cavity: the central cavity of a tooth that contains soft tissue pulp.

pulse oximeter: a medical device used to measured heart rate or pulse as well as to estimate blood oxygen levels.

pulse register: the range of vocal pitches that is associated with glottal fry, that is, the lowest pitches of the vocal range.

pure tone: an individual, discrete sound frequency; tones produced by audiometers and tuning forks are pure tones.

putamen: one of the nuclei of the basal ganglia found in the telencephalon lateral to the globus pallidus; involved in higher-order motor control.

pyramidal eminence: pyramid-shaped bony projection lying on the posterior wall of the middle ear cavity that houses the stapedius muscle.

pyramids: bulges on the ventral aspect of the rostral medulla; corticospinal and remaining corticobulbar tracts underlie the pyramids.

quadrangular membrane: the superior portion of the elastic membrane that extends from the aditus laryngis superiorly to the ventricular ligaments inferiorly.

recruitment: an abnormal sensitivity to loud stimuli associated with sensorineural hearing loss.

recurrent laryngeal nerve: a peripheral branch of the vagus nerve (cranial nerve X) that innervates all intrinsic muscles of the larynx except for the cricothyroid muscles; it is given the name "recurrent" because it takes an indirect route to the larynx by first descending into the upper thorax.

Reissner's membrane: membrane within the cochlear duct separating the scala vestibuli and the scala media; projects obliquely from the osseous spiral lamina and the outer wall of the cochlea; also referred to as the vestibular membrane.

relative refractory period: brief period of time following the firing of an action potential when the neuron will only fire if more depolarization than normally required is generated.

residual volume (RV): the volume of air that remains in the lungs and cannot be forcibly expelled; its purpose is to prevent the lungs from collapsing completely.

resonance: selective amplification of certain sound frequencies due to the natural resonant characteristics of a cavity; the enhancement of certain tones within the vocal tone as it passes through the vocal tract; those tones that are tuned to the shape and configuration of the vocal tract will resonate.

resonant: pertaining to the rate at which a mass will vibrate most effectively when set into free motion.

resonator: any object or entity that is set into vibration by the action of an outside force.

respiration: the exchange of oxygen for carbon dioxide at the level of the alveoli in the lungs.

resting membrane potential (RMP): the voltage charge maintained across a neuronal membrane when no action potential is being generated; RMPs are approximately −70 mV.

resting volume: the volume of air that is in the lungs when they are at their resting state between breaths.

reticular lamina: the netlike structure forming the upper surface of the organ of Corti; formed from the phalangeal processes of the supporting cells.

retinitis pigmentosa: a disease caused by overactivity of the pigmented retinal epithelial cells; leads to damage and occlusion of the photoreceptors resulting in blindness.

retrocochlear: the structures of the auditory system beyond the level of the cochlea, especially cranial nerve VIII and the brainstem.

retrospective memories: memories for past events and information; also known as long-term memories.

reverse breathing: a respiratory anomaly seen in some cases of athetoid cerebral palsy that is characterized by depression of the sternum during inspiration instead of elevation.

rhinorrhea: excessive secretion of mucous from the nose; also referred to as a runny nose.

rhombencephalon: term signifying the caudal vesicle of the neural tube early in neurodevelopment; further differentiates to form the metencephalon and myelencephalon.

rima glottis: the technical name for the glottis, the variable-sized opening between the vocal folds when they are in varying degrees of abduction.

rima oris: the mouth; the entrance into the oral cavity.

rods: one type of photoreceptor found in the retina specialized for sensing light.

round window: the membrane-covered window leading to the scala tympani, located within the medial wall of the middle ear space.

saccule: the structure housed in the vestibule of the inner ear closest to the cochlea that contains the end organ (macula) sensitive to linear acceleration and gravity.

sacral foramina: a series of four paired holes or openings within the sacrum where nerves and blood vessels pass from the lower abdomen to the lower extremities.

sacral segment: one of the five segments of the spinal cord corresponding to the hip region.

sagittal suture: the seam running longitudinally down the center of the skull that serves as the joint between the two parietal bones.

saltatory conduction: the high-speed impulse conduction of myelinated axons; propagation occurs between nodes of Ranvier.

sarcoidosis: an autoimmune disease in which granulomatous substances are deposited into the tissues of organs, including the nervous system.

scala media: see *cochlear duct.*

scala tympani: the lower chamber of the cochlea, filled with perilymph fluid; it terminates at the round window and the helicotrema.

scala vestibuli: the upper chamber of the cochlea, filled with perilymph fluid; it terminates at the oval window and the helicotrema.

scapula: known more commonly as the shoulder blade, the somewhat triangularly shaped bone that is attached to the axial skeleton by way of the clavicle; it serves as the point of articulation for the humerus.

Scarpa's ganglion: a ganglion of the vestibular nerve leading into the internal auditory canal within the vestibular branch of cranial nerve VIII; two ganglia consisting of the bodies of the primary vestibular neurons which separate into a superior and an inferior group.

Scheibe dysplasia: the most common form of congenital dysplasia of the inner ear; the bony labyrinth and membranous utricle and semicircular canals are fully formed, but the saccule and scala media are poorly differentiated; resulting from an autosomal recessive inheritance.

Schwann cell: a type of glial cell that produces myelin to insulate the axons in the peripheral nervous system (PNS).

Schwannoma neuroma: a benign neoplasm composed of Schwann cells arising from the vestibular portion of cranial nerve VIII; also referred to as an acoustic neuroma.

Schwartze's sign: a reddish glow seen on the promontory produced by increased vascularity; it can be visualized through the tympanic membrane during otoscopy; considered an early sign of otosclerosis.

scoliosis: a lateral spinal curvature or "sideways" bending of the spine.

selective permeability: the ability of a neuron to let certain ions in to the cell and keep other ions out of the cell given certain conditions.

sella turcica: a saddle-shaped depression in the sphenoid bone at the base of the skull that contains the hypophyseal fossa which in turn holds the pituitary gland.

semantic memory: a type of declarative memory specific to conceptual or world knowledge.

semantic paraphasias: see *verbal (semantic) paraphasias.*

semicircular canals: a part of the vestibular system of the inner ear, consists of three looped canals of bony labyrinth oriented to anatomical directions: anterior, lateral, and posterior; contain sensory receptor end organs that are sensitive to angular acceleration.

sensorineural: in reference to diminished hearing acuity, an irreversible hearing loss due to pathology of the inner ear; damage to the inner ear (e.g., the hair cells within the cochlea) cannot be alleviated.

sensory disorder: an impairment of any of the senses such as feeling, hearing, seeing, smelling, or tasting.

sensory homunculus: the topographical map of the postcentral gyrus indicating body representation regarding sensation.

septal cartilage: the anterior, cartilaginous part of the nasal septum.

septum pellucidum: the thin, membranous covering of the medial aspect of the lateral ventricles.

short process: the process of the incus that arises from the bulky body portion of the ossicles.

silent aspiration: penetration of the airway by saliva, food, or drink that does not produce a cough reflex.

simple: minute papillae found along the sides of the tongue approximately two-thirds of the way between the tip and root forming parallel grooves, each groove housing several hundred taste buds.

simultaneous attack: vocal fold vibration in which expired air reaches the vocal folds at the same time they reach adduction; the result is relatively effortless and smooth phonation.

site of lesion: the source or location of pathological change in the structure of an organ due to injury or disease.

SOAP notes: a method of documentation employed by health care providers to write out notes in a patient's medical chart; SOAP is an acronym for subjective, objective, assessment, and plan.

sodium–potassium pump (SPP): an ion pump in the plasma membrane of the neuron that exchanges intracellular sodium (Na^+) for extracellular potassium (K^+) to assist in restoring and maintaining the resting membrane potential.

somatic nervous system: a division of the peripheral nervous system; provides motor and sensory innervation to the joints, skin, and skeletal muscles.

spasmodic dysphonia: a voice disorder characterized by spasmodic functioning of the larynx that results in extreme phonatory tension; the vocal folds can spasm shut resulting in the more common adductor type or can spasm open resulting in abductor spasmodic dysphonia.

spastic: a type of cerebral palsy or dysarthria characterized by involuntary jerky muscular contractions resembling spasms.

spatial summation: the addition of multiple postsynaptic potentials occurring at more than one synapse site on the same cell.

spectrum: a graphic depiction of the frequencies of a complex tone (represented along the horizontal axis of the graph) along with their amplitudes (represented along the vertical axis).

speech–language pathologist (SLP): health care professional who is credentialed in the practice of speech–language pathology to provide a comprehensive array of services related to prevention, evaluation, and rehabilitation of speech, language, and swallowing disorders.

sphenoid paranasal sinuses: a pair of cavities within the sphenoid bone that open into the nasal cavity.

spinal accessory: cranial nerve XI, having a cranial and spinal branch; the cranial branch assists the glossopharyngeal and vagus nerves in innervating muscles of the velum and pharynx while the spinal branch innervates some muscles of the neck and shoulder.

spinal nerves: mixed (i.e., sensory and motor) nerves from the spinal cord that innervate the body (e.g., muscles, glands, mucous membranes, joints).

spinal trigeminal nucleus: a brainstem sensory nucleus receiving information regarding pain and temperature from the trigeminal (V) nerve.

spinous process: the posteriorly directed spine on a vertebra; in some vertebrae, this process is horizontally oriented, and in others, it is more obliquely oriented.

spiral ganglia: see *spiral ganglion.*

spiral ganglion: the location of the cell bodies for the auditory nerve fibers of the cochlea located in the modiolus; plural: spiral ganglia.

spiral lamina: two thin shelves of bone arising from the modiolar side of the cochlea between which courses the afferent and efferent nerve fibers from the inner and outer hair cells.

spiral ligament: a band of connective tissue that anchors the basilar membrane to the outer bony wall of the cochlear labyrinth.

spiral limbus: a mound of connective tissue in the scala media that provides the medial attachment for the tectorial membrane.

spirometer: a device that measures the amount of air that enters and leaves the lungs; it is typically used clinically to measure vital capacity.

squamous cell carcinoma: a form of skin cancer, the most common malignant tumor of the pinna, seen as a slow growing scaly patch of skin with a thickening outgrowth; a result of chronic sun exposure.

stapedectomy: a surgical procedure to remove the stapes footplate after it has been fixed in the oval window due to otosclerosis; a prosthesis is used in place of the stapes to restore the integrity of the ossicular chain.

stapedial branch: a branch of cranial nerve VII (facial nerve) that innervates the stapedius muscle.

stapedius muscle: striated muscle of the middle ear that attaches to the neck of the stapes and contracts in response to loud incoming sounds; innervated by the cranial nerve VII (facial nerve).

stapedius tendon: a tendon of the stapedius muscle that projects from the pyramidal eminence of the middle ear to insert onto the head of the stapes bone.

stapes: the most medial bone in the ossicular chain; the head of the stapes articulates with the lenticular process of the incus and the footplate resides in the oval window.

stenosis: a narrowing of a tube or passageway.

stereocilia: hairlike projections from the cell body of a hair cell; actin filaments provide support for the cilia; disturbance of the stereocilia opens the channels that allow for depolarization which results in a neural impulse.

sternum: also referred to as the breastbone, the elongated bone situated at midline of the ventral thorax that serves as a point of articulation for most of the ribs as well as the clavicle.

stoma: a surgical opening into the body from the outside.

strabismus: the misalignment of one eyeball with the other; sometimes referred to as "lazy eye."

stria vascularis: a highly vascularized collection of cells located on the lateral surface of the scala media; responsible for the recycling of endolymphatic fluids.

striatum: term indicating both the caudate nucleus and the putamen nucleus of the basal ganglia.

stroke: a sudden interruption of the blood supply to the brain; also referred to as a cerebrovascular accident.

structural disorder: an impairment whose etiology involves anatomical deviation.

stylohyoid ligament: fibrous connective tissue that originates at the styloid process of the temporal bone of the skull and terminates at the hyoid bone; the hyoid bone is suspended in place by two of these ligaments, one coming from each side.

styloid process: a pencil tip–shaped projection at the base of the temporal bone that serves as a point of attachment for the stylohyoid and stylopharyngeus muscles.

subarachnoid space: the area immediately below the arachnoid layer of the meninges; blood vessels and cerebrospinal fluid (CSF) are found in this space.

subclavian arteries: major arterial blood supply arising superiorly off the aortic arch.

subglottic pressure: the force that expired air exerts upon the inferior surfaces of the vocal folds when they adduct and occlude the breath stream; this pressure is necessary to initiate and maintain phonation.

subglottic space: the region immediately below the level of the vocal folds, that is, the inner cricoid cartilage and uppermost part of the trachea.

subthalamus: the nuclei that are inferior to the thalamus; part of the basal ganglia system.

sudden: acute with rapid onset.

sulci: grooves or furrows in the cerebral cortex running between adjacent gyri; singular: sulcus.

sulcus limitans: the separation point in spinal cord neurodevelopment of the alar plate from the basal plate; cells that develop into autonomic nervous system functions are located near the sulcus limitans.

sulcus terminalis: the transversely oriented groove along the posterior dorsum of the tongue, shaped like a chevron or inverted letter "V."

superior colliculi: paired nuclei in the dorsal midbrain where secondary fibers from the visual pathway synapse; involved in visual reflexes.

superior cornua: two long, narrow legs of cartilage extending superiorly from the posteriormost regions of the thyroid laminae; they articulate with the greater cornua of the hyoid bone on each side.

superior laryngeal nerve: a branch of the vagus nerve (cranial nerve X) that innervates the cricothyroid muscles; these nerves take a more direct path to the larynx than the recurrent laryngeal nerves.

superior olivary complex: the auditory nucleus located in the hindbrain that relays information from the cochlear nucleus to the lateral lemniscus.

superior olivary nucleus: a nucleus in the caudal pons and a point of synapse for the auditory pathway transmitting neural signals from the cochlear nuclei on to the inferior colliculi.

superior orbital fissures: clefts between the greater and lesser wings of the sphenoid bone through which all or part of four cranial nerves (III, IV, V, and VI) as well as blood vessels pass from the cranial cavity into the orbits of the eyes.

superior sagittal sinus: a space found between the dural layers of the falx cerebri; venous blood drains here and cerebrospinal fluid (CSF) diffuses into this sinus.

suprahyoid: a term used to denote any muscle that has an origin on a structure that is above the hyoid bone, and then descends to insert onto the superior surface of the hyoid.

suprasegmental: a feature that overlays the actual production of speech sounds during conversational speech such as intonation, stress, or juncture.

supratonsillar fossa: the part of the tonsillar fossa immediately above the palatine tonsil.

supraversion: malposition of a tooth so that it extends beyond the line of occlusion, that is, the tooth is "higher" than adjacent teeth.

sympathetic division: a division of the autonomic nervous system; serves to prepare the body for "fight or flight" situations.

symptoms: deviations from normal function.

synarthrodial: referring to immovable joints.

synchondrosis: a cartilaginous or amphiarthrodial joint involving hyaline cartilage.

syndrome: a collection of symptoms.

synovial: pertaining to the secretion of fluid associated with diarthrodial joints.

synovial joint: anatomical classification of joints that are freely movable.

syphilis: an acquired or congenital venereal disease which may result in secondary auditory or vestibular disturbances of the membranous labyrinth.

tactile: pertaining to the conscious sense of touch or contact.

tectorial membrane: the gelatinous membrane of the organ of Corti projecting radially and overlying the reticular lamina in which the cilia of the outer hair cells are embedded.

tegmen tympani: the roof of the middle ear cavity that is created by the very thin anterior surface of the petrous portion of the temporal bone.

tegmental wall: the superior wall or roof of the middle ear cavity.

telencephalon: anteriormost area of the brain that includes the cerebral hemispheres; developed from the prosencephalon.

telodendria: the projections extending from an axon's terminal.

temporae: the temples.

temporal summation: the addition of multiple postsynaptic potentials occurring in rapid succession at one synapse site on a postsynaptic cell.

temporary: of short duration and eventually returning to a baseline.

temporary threshold shift (TTS): a temporary reversible hearing loss as a result of exposure to elevated noise levels; can result in permanent loss with repeated incidences of exposure.

temporomandibular joint (TMJ): the joint formed by the articulation of the condylar process of the mandible and the mandibular fossa of the temporal bone; although there are actually two joints, they act as a single unit.

tendon: dense connective tissue that connects muscle to bone, cartilage, or another muscle.

tensor tympani: the striated middle ear muscle attached to the manubrium of the malleus that contracts in response to a loud stimulus; innervated by the trigeminal nerve (V).

tensor veli palatini: a muscle found in the nasopharynx that serves to tense the soft palate upon elevation and facilitates opening of the Eustachian tube.

tentorium cerebelli: the tentlike fold of dura mater that separates the occipital lobes from the cerebellum.

teratogenic: an agent that negatively influences embryologic development resulting in an anomaly or malformation.

terminal boutons: end points of axon terminals that make synaptic contact with other cells.

thalamus: diencephalic structure composed of separate nuclei associated with sensory, motor, and cognitive functions having multiple reciprocal connections with the neocortex.

third ventricle: a diencephalic cavity located in the center of the thalamus that provides a conduit for cerebrospinal fluid (CSF).

thoracic segment: one of the five segments of the spinal cord corresponding to the thoracic (i.e., rib cage) region.

threshold(s): (1) the lowest levels of sound intensity that will yield a response 50% of the time; (2) the lowest millivolt depolarization that causes an action potential to occur.

thrombotic: a type of stroke due to a thrombus; a gradual accumulation of material (i.e., plaque) within arterial walls to the point of occlusion.

thyroepiglottic ligament: a band of connective tissue that binds the petiolus of the epiglottis to the inner aspect of the thyroid cartilage immediately below the thyroid notch.

thyroid: the largest of the laryngeal cartilages, it articulates with and is immediately superior to the cricoid cartilage.

thyroid angle: the angle formed by the nearly complete union of the two lamina of the thyroid cartilage; in adult males, this angle is approximately 90 degrees and in adult females, it is approximately 120 degrees.

thyroid laminae: the two prominent walls of the thyroid cartilage that meet anteriorly at midline and fuse almost completely except superiorly where the thyroid notch is formed.

thyroid notch: a prominent indentation in the anterior midline of the thyroid cartilage, formed by the incomplete fusion of the two thyroid laminae.

thyroid prominence: a prominent protrusion of the thyroid cartilage anteriorly, immediately below the thyroid notch; also known as the Adam's apple.

tidal volume (TV): the volume of air that is typically exchanged during a cycle of quiet, vegetative breathing.

tinnitus: a sensation of noise within the ears (perceived typically as a ringing, buzzing, or humming sound) without an external cause.

tip links: extracellular linking proteins that run between the tips of the stereocilia; their function is to open the cell membrane channels for the process of transduction.

tonotopic organization: peripheral and central auditory nervous system maintenance of the frequency organization that originated along the basilar membrane within the cochlea.

tonsillar fossa: the cavity or space between the palatoglossal and palatopharyngeal arches (i.e., anterior and posterior faucial pillars).

TORCH: an acronym for a small group of viral agents (toxoplasmosis, rubella, cytomegalovirus, herpes simplex, and "other" agents) that can cross the placental barrier and cause similar symptoms in newborns—one of which is hearing loss.

torsiversion: malposition of a tooth so that it is twisted upon its own vertical axis; for example, in 180-degree torsiversion, the back of the tooth is facing the front and vice versa.

torus tubarius: a comma-shaped ridge in the region of the nasopharynx that is formed by the salpingopalatine and salpingopharyngeus muscles; the opening of the Eustachian tube is located beneath the curved part of this structure.

total lung capacity (TLC): the sum of all lung volumes, including inspiratory reserve volume, tidal volume, expiratory reserve volume, and residual volume.

toxoplasmosis: an infection caused by a single cell parasite (*toxoplasma gondii*) that invades the tissues and may seriously damage the central nervous system, especially in infants.

tragus: the cartilaginous part of the pinna that projects outward from the face toward the external auditory meatus; pressing down on it will effectively close off the meatus to block incoming sound.

transduction: the conversion of mechanical energy to chemical to electrical energy; carried out in the inner ear by the sensory receptor cells.

transformer action: function of the structures of the middle ear to overcome the impedance mismatch of the air-filled middle ear cavity to the fluid-filled cavity of the inner ear.

transient ischemic attack (TIA): a brief interruption of blood supply to the brain without lasting effects; a warning sign for stroke.

transverse foramina: the small holes or openings typically found in the region of the transverse processes of the cervical vertebrae where nerves and blood vessels pass along the length of the neck.

transverse processes: the two projections of bone extending laterally from a vertebra at the juncture of its corpus and neural arch.

trapezoid body: fiber tract of the auditory pathway leading from the cochlear nucleus to the superior olivary complex.

traumatic brain injury (TBI): brain damage due to external forces; can be due to penetrating (i.e., open) head injury or nonpenetrating (i.e., closed) head injury.

triangular fovea: a small depression toward the apex of the arytenoid cartilage on its anterolateral surface, immediately superior to the arcuate ridge.

trigeminal: cranial nerve V, innervates muscles of mastication and carries sensory information from the head (including the dura mater) and mouth.

trisomy-21: a chromosomal disorder in which there are three instead of two 21st chromosomes; the result is Down syndrome.

trochlear: cranial nerve IV, innervates eye muscles for movement.

tuberculosis: a bacterial infectious disease characterized by ulcerations and the formation of cavities in the lungs; accompanied by cough and fever.

tuning curve: a plot showing the lowest intensity at which a nerve fiber will respond as a function of frequency.

tunnel of Corti: within the organ of Corti, the triangular space created by the inner and outer pillar cells.

turbinates: also known as conchae; three long, thin scrolls of bone that extend into the nasal cavity from its lateral walls.

tympanic antrum: a cavity within the petrous portion of the temporal bone that communicates posteriorly with the mastoid air cells and anteriorly with the epitympanic recess of the middle ear cavity.

tympanic membrane (TM): see *eardrum.*

tympanic sulcus: see *annular sulcus.*

tympanogram: a graph of tympanic membrane admittance across a positive to negative pressure gradient, for the purpose of assessing the function of the Eustachian tube and the contents of the middle ear cavity.

tympanometry: the procedure used to determine function of the middle ear; the output of this procedure is called a tympanogram.

tympanoplasty: the surgical repair of the tympanic membrane and contents of the middle ear; classified by types (Type I, II) according to the magnitude of repair.

tympanosclerosis: the formation of a whitish plaque on the tympanic membrane usually as a result of chronic otitis media.

umbo: the center of the tympanic membrane where the tip of the manubrium of the malleus is attached.

uncinate fasciculus: an association tract connecting the rostral temporal lobe with the orbital gyri of the frontal lobe.

uncus: gyrus found at the anterior end of the parahippocampal gyrus of the medial temporal lobe; the amygdala nucleus underlies the uncus.

unilateral: pertaining to one side only.

universal newborn hearing screening: screening for hearing loss in the newborn population, prior to the age of one month, typically hospital based, using otoacoustic emissions or automated auditory brainstem response measures.

unvoiced: a term used to describe some consonant sounds that are produced without vocal fold vibration.

upper esophageal sphincter (UES): the most superior aspect of the esophagus which includes the cricopharyngeus muscle; the valve that prevents acid from refluxing into the esophagus from the stomach.

upper motor neuron (UMN): a nerve cell whose body is located in the motor area of the cerebral cortex and whose processes connect with motor nuclei in the brainstem or in the anterior horn of the spinal cord prior to exiting the central nervous system toward the periphery.

Usher's syndrome: an inherited condition characterized by congenital sensorineural hearing loss and progressive loss of vision due to retinitis pigmentosa.

utricle: the structure housed in the vestibule of the inner ear closest to the semicircular canals that contains the end organ (macula) sensitive to linear acceleration and gravity.

uvula: the small, midline terminal of the velum created by the mucous membrane–covered musculus uvulae muscle.

vagus: cranial nerve X, which has multiple branches involved in autonomic functions as well as skeletal movement and sensation; it is involved with innervating the intrinsic muscles of the larynx and some muscles of the velum and pharynx in addition to transmitting sensation.

vallate: also referred to as circumvallate papillae; large button-shaped papillae arranged in a row resembling an inverted letter "V" immediately anterior to the sulcus terminalis, housing several hundred taste buds.

valleculae: small furrows or pits at the base of the tongue immediately anterior to the lingual surface of the epiglottis and found between the median and lateral glossoepiglottic folds.

Valsalva maneuver: a procedure that manually forces the opening of the Eustachian tube to ventilate the middle ear space, performed by blowing while holding the nostrils and mouth closed; it also generates greater subglottic pressure.

velocardiofacial syndrome: a craniofacial anomaly affecting the velum, heart, and face.

velopharyngeal incompetence (VPI): a condition, either functional or organic in etiology, in which the soft palate does not make a sufficient seal with the posterior pharyngeal wall, resulting in improper balance between oral and nasal resonance.

velopharyngeal mechanism: the mechanism created by the soft palate and posterior pharyngeal wall that mediates oral–nasal resonance; when the soft palate meets the posterior pharyngeal wall, nasal resonance is diminished; when the soft palate is lowered, some of the vocal tone passes into the nasal cavity to resonate there.

velum: the soft palate.

ventilation: the movement of air in and out of the lungs.

ventilator: a device that mechanically assists the patient in exchanging oxygen and carbon dioxide; also referred to as an artificial respirator.

ventral cochlear nucleus: portion of the cochlear nucleus for the first central synapse for the cochlear nerve as it travels through the levels of the brainstem to the auditory cortex.

ventral fasciculus: the ventral or anterior region of spinal cord white matter where descending bundles of nerve fibers are found.

ventral posterior medial (VPM) nucleus: the medial part of the ventral posterior nucleus receiving sensory input from the face and tongue.

ventricle: the space between the ventricular (or false) folds and the vocal folds, running horizontally along the length of the two sets of folds.

ventricular folds: the technical name for the false vocal folds, found immediately superior to the true vocal folds and separated from them by the ventricle.

ventricular ligaments: bands of connective tissue forming the inferior border of the quadrangular membrane and serving as the skeleton for the ventricular folds.

verbal (semantic) paraphasias: unintentional errors of word retrieval in aphasia where wrong words are substituted for the correct words.

vermilion zone: the part of the upper and lower lips that is darker in hue due to the visualization of vascular tissue below the translucent eleidin.

vermis: the central gray matter of the cerebellum.

vertebral: a term used to describe R11 and R12, which only have an articulation with the vertebral column; these ribs are more commonly referred to as "floating" ribs.

vertebral arteries: supply blood to the brain; arise from the subclavian artery and ascend via the transverse foramen of the cervical vertebrae entering through the foramen magnum to converge on the basilar artery.

vertebral canal: the central space formed by the vertical orientation of the vertebrae; houses the spinal cord.

vertebrochondral: a term used to describe R8, R9, and R10 because the cartilages for these three ribs merge to form a single piece that articulates with the sternum; these ribs are more commonly referred to as "false" ribs.

vertebrosternal: a term used to describe R1 through R7 because each of these ribs has its own cartilage that directly articulates with the sternum; these ribs are more commonly referred to as "true" ribs.

vertex: the uppermost part of the skull.

vestibular aqueduct (VA): a narrow bony canal that courses from the vestibule of the inner ear to the cranial cavity; thought to regulate endolymphatic pressure within the inner ear.

vestibule: (1) the egg-shaped central portion of the inner ear that houses the balance receptors sensitive to linear acceleration and gravity—the utricle and saccule are housed within; (2) the wide space within the cavity of the larynx immediately superior to the ventricular folds and inferior to the aditus laryngis.

vestibulocochlear (nerve): cranial nerve XIII, involved in hearing and balance; the vestibular nerve and cochlear nerve branches combined.

vestibulo-ocular reflex (VOR): a reflexive eye movement that stabilizes vision during head movement (eye movement is in the opposite direction of the head movement); the semicircular canals detect rotation of the head and send a signal to the oculomotor nuclei of the brainstem, which in turn innervate the eye muscles.

vestibulospinal tracts: tracts originating from the vestibular nuclei in the medulla to the spinal cord; involved in motor reflexes and balance.

videostroboscopy: an imaging technique that combines flexible endoscopy with a strobe light; the endoscope is used to view the vocal folds and the strobe light is used to make the vocal folds appear as if they're vibrating slowly so that one can view their vibratory pattern.

visceral nervous system: a division of the peripheral nervous system; innervates glands, internal organs (i.e., viscera), and blood vessels; also called the autonomic nervous system.

visceral pleura: the connective tissue membrane that covers the surface of each lung as well as the superior surface of the diaphragm.

vital capacity (VC): the amount of air that can be forcibly expelled from the lungs after a maximal inspiration; it includes inspiratory reserve volume, tidal volume, and expiratory reserve volume.

vocal fry: see *glottal fry*.

vocal ligaments: the thickened, free superior border of the conus elasticus extending from the macula flava anterior to the vocal processes of the arytenoids, forming the point of attachment of the thyroarytenoid muscles (i.e., the true vocal folds).

vocal nodules: benign callous-like bumps on the edges of the vocal folds, usually bilateral at the juncture of the middle and anterior third of the vocal folds.

vocal process: a projection at the base of the arytenoid cartilage where the anterolateral and medial surfaces meet that serves as the posterior attachment of the vocal ligament.

vocal registers: modes of vocal fold vibration that have distinct physical, acoustic, and perceptual characteristics; see also *loft register, modal register, pulse register.*

voice disorders: pathological conditions where the voice is different enough in pitch, loudness, quality, and/or flexibility that it calls negative attention to the speaker and/or interferes with communication; also referred to as dysphonia.

voice fundamental: the basic laryngeal tone; the lowest vibratory frequency produced by the vocal folds during phonation; also referred to as the fundamental frequency.

voiced: a term that is used to describe vocal fold vibration during the production of speech sounds; all vowels and most consonants are voiced.

Waardenburg syndrome: a dominantly inherited syndrome characterized by widely spaced eyes, broad nose, multicolored irises, white forelock, and a sensorineural hearing loss.

Waldeyer's ring: a circle of lymphoid tissue formed by the adenoids superiorly, lingual tonsil inferiorly, and palatine tonsils laterally.

watershed area: the region of overlapping blood supply from the anterior, middle, and posterior cerebral artery distributions.

Wernicke's area: the superior temporal lobe region involved in language comprehension.

working memory: a short-term memory process where sensory input is compared to long-term memory stores for decision making; a component of executive functioning.

X-linked recessive: a pattern of inheritance on the X chromosome; the trait is linked from mother to son; 50% chance of son inheriting trait; 50% chance of a daughter being a carrier; an affected father will pass the carrier status to 100% of his daughters.

zygomatic arch: the cheekbone, which is formed by contributions of the frontal, maxillary, temporal, and zygomatic bones.

REFERENCES

Abraham, S. (1989). Using a phonological framework to describe speech errors of orally trained, hearing-impaired school-agers. *Journal of Speech and Hearing Disorders, 54,* 600–609.

Adams, J.H., Graham, D.I., Murray, L.S., & Scott, G. (1982). Diffuse axonal injury due to nonmissile head injury in humans: An analysis of 45 cases. *Annals of Neurology, 12,* 557–563.

Agur, A.M.R., & Dalley, A.F. (2005). *Grant's atlas of anatomy* (11th ed.). Baltimore, MD: Lippincott Williams & Wilkins.

American Cancer Society. (2004). *Cancer facts and figures.* Atlanta, GA: Author.

American Cleft Palate-Craniofacial Association and Cleft Palate Foundation. (1997). *About cleft lip and cleft palate.* Chapel Hill, NC: Author.

American Heart Association. (2007). Atherosclerosis. Accessed March 16, 2007, from http://www.americanheart.org/presenter.jhtml?identifier+4440.

American Lung Association (2007). *Trends in tobacco use.* Epidemiology and Statistics Unit Research and Program Services. Accessed December 28, 2007, from http://www.lungusa.org.

American Medical Association. (1979). Guide for the evaluation of hearing handicap. *Journal of the American Medical Association, 241,* 2055–2059.

American Psychiatric Association. (1994). *Diagnostic and statistical manual of mental disorders (DSM-IV)* (4th ed.). Washington, DC: Author.

American Speech-Language-Hearing Association (ASHA). (2005a). *Paradoxical vocal fold movement (PVFM): Causes and numbers.* Accessed September 22, 2009, from http://www.asha.org/public/speech/disorders/PVFMcauses.htm.

American Speech-Language-Hearing Association (ASHA). (2005b). Roles of the speech-language pathologist in the identification, diagnosis, and treatment of individuals with cognitive-communicative disorders: Position statement. Available at www.asha.org/policy.

American Speech-Language-Hearing Association (ASHA). (2008). *The incidence and prevalence of hearing loss and hearing aid use in the United States.* Accessed June 1, 2009, from http://www.asha.org.

Angle, E.H. (1899). Classification of malocclusion. *Dental Cosmos, 41,* 248–264, 350–357.

Aronson, A.E. (1990). *Clinical voice disorders* (3rd ed.). New York: Thieme Publishers, Inc.

Baijens, L.W.J., Speyer, R., Roodenburg, N., & Manni, J.J. (2008). The effects of neuromuscular electrical stimulation for dysphagia in opercular syndrome: A case study. *European Archives of Otorhinolaryngology, 265,* 825–830.

Barsoumian, R., Kuehn, D., Moon, J., & Canady, J. (1998). An anatomic study of the tensor veli palatini muscle and dilator tubae muscles in relation to Eustachian tube and velar function. *Cleft Palate-Craniofacial Journal, 35,* 101–110.

Bayles, K. (2006, June). *Science based clinical strategies for facilitating cognitive-linguistic functioning in adults with brain injury and disease.* Presentation given at Evergreen Hospital Medical Center, Kirkland, WA.

Baynes, R.A. (1966). An incident study of chronic hoarseness among children. *Journal of Speech and Hearing Disorders, 31,* 172–176.

Bear, M.F., Connors, B.W., & Paradiso, M.A. (2007). *Neuroscience: Exploring the brain* (3rd ed.). Baltimore, MD: Lippincott Williams & Wilkins.

Bekesy, G. (1960). *Experiments in hearing.* New York: McGraw-Hill.

Benson, D.F. (1989). Disorders of visual gnosis. In J.W. Brown (Ed.), *Neuropsychology of visual perception.* Hillsdale, NJ: Lawrence Erlbaum.

Berke, G., & Gerratt, B. (1993). Laryngeal biomechanics: An overview of mucosal wave mechanics. *Journal of Voice, 7,* 123–128.

Best, S., Bigge, J., & Sirvis, B. (1994). Physical and health impairments. In N. Haring, L. McCormick, & T. Haring (Eds.), *Exceptional children and youth: An introduction to special education* (pp. 300–341). New York: Merrill.

Bhatnager, S.C. (2008). *Neuroscience for the study of communicative disorders* (3rd ed.). Baltimore, MD: Lippincott Williams & Wilkins.

Bishop, D., Brown, B., & Robson, J. (1990). The relationship between phoneme discrimination, speech production, and language comprehension in cerebral-palsied individuals. *Journal of Speech and Hearing Research, 33,* 210–219.

Boone, D.R., McFarlane, S.L., Von Berg, S.L., & Zraick, R. (2010). *The voice and voice therapy* (8th ed.). Needham Heights, MA: Allyn & Bacon.

Boorman, J., & Sommerlad, B. (1985). Levator palati and palatal dimples: Their anatomy, relationship and clinical significance. *British Journal of Plastic Surgery, 38,* 326–332.

Borg, E. (1973). On the neuronal organization of the acoustic middle ear reflex: A physiological and anatomical study. *Brain Research, 49,* 101–123.

Boulassel, M.R., Tornasi, J.P., Deggoui, N., & Gersdorff, M. (2001). COCHB5 B2 is a target antigen of anti-inner ear antibodies in autoimmune inner ear diseases. *Otology and Neurotology, 22,* 614–618.

Bourgeios, M., & Hopper, T. (2005, February). *Evaluation and treatment planning for individuals with dementia.* Presentation at the ASHA Health Care Conference 2005: Dementia, vocal pathologies, and pediatric dysphagia: Clinical approaches for SLPs in health care settings, Palm Springs, CA.

Bradley, W.G. (2002). Cerebrospinal fluid dynamics and shunt responsiveness in patients with normal pressure hydrocephalus. *Mayo Clinic Proceedings, 7*(6), 507–508.

Brodsky, L., & Koch, R.J. (1993). Bacteriology and immunology of normal and diseased adenoids in children. *Archives of Otolaryngology—Head and Neck Surgery, 119,* 821–829.

Bromberg, M. (1999). Accelerating the diagnosis of amyotrophic lateral sclerosis. *Neurologist, 5*(2), 63–74.

Brookshire, R. (2003). *Introduction to neurogenic communication disorders* (6th ed.). St. Louis, MO: Elsevier Mosby.

Burns, M. (1985). Language without communication: The pragmatics of right hemisphere damage. In M.S. Burns, A.S. Halper, & S.I. Mogil (Eds.), *Clinical management of right hemisphere dysfunction* (pp. 17–28). Rockville, MD: Aspen Publications.

Centers for Disease Control (CDC). (2005). Annual smoking-attributable mortality, years of potential life lost, and productivity losses—United States. *Morbidity and Mortality Weekly Report, 54*(25), 625–628.

Centers for Disease Control and Prevention. (2007). *More information on vaccines.* Accessed September 16, 2010, from http://www.cdc.gov/meningitis/vaccine-info.html.

Chermak, G.D., & Musiek, F.E. (1997). *Central auditory processing disorders: New perspectives.* San Diego: Singular Publishing Group.

Chiara, T., Martin, D., & Sapienza, C. (2007). Expiratory muscle strength training: Speech production outcomes in patients with multiple sclerosis. *Neurorehabilitation and Neural Repair, 21*(3), 239–249.

Clark, W.W., & Bohne, B.A. (1999). Effects of noise on hearing. *Journal of the American Medical Association, 281,* 1658–1659.

Clark, W.W., Bohne, B.A., & Boettcher, F.B. (1987). Effect of periodic rest on hearing loss and cochlear damage following exposure to noise. *Journal of the Acoustical Society of America, 82,* 1253–1264.

Cohen, M.M. Jr., & Bankier, A. (1991). Syndrome delineation involving orofacial clefting. *Cleft Palate-Craniofacial Journal, 28,* 119–120.

Corbin-Lewis, K., Liss, J.M., & Sciortino, K.L. (2005). *Clinical anatomy and physiology of the swallow mechanism.* New York: Thomson Delmar Learning.

Cotanche, D.A. (1987). Regeneration of hair cell stereociliary bundles in the chick cochlea following severe acoustic trauma. *Hearing Research, 30,* 181–196.

Crary, M.A., & Groher, M.E. (2003). *Introduction to adult swallowing disorders.* St. Louis, MO: Butterworth Heinemann.

Cummings, J.L., Vinters, H.V., Cole, G.M., & Khachaturian, Z.S. (1998). Alzheimer's disease: Etiologies, pathophysiology, cognitive reserve, and treatment opportunities. *Neurology, 51,* S2–S17.

Dallos, P. (1992). The active cochlea. *The Journal of Neuroscience, 12,* 4578–4585.

Dallos, P., Santos-Sacchi, J., & Flock, A. (1982). Intracellular recordings from cochlear outer hair cells. *Science, 218,* 582–584.

Darley, F.L., Aronson, A.E., & Brown, J.R. (1975). *Motor speech disorders.* Philadelphia, PA: W.B. Saunders.

Darley, F.L., Brown, A.E., & Goldstein, N.P. (1972). Dysarthria in multiple sclerosis. *Journal of Speech and Hearing Research, 15,* 229–245.

Declau, F., Van Spaendonck, M., Timmermans, J.P., Michaels, L., Liang, J., Qiu, J.P., & Van de Heyning, P. (2001). Prevalence of otosclerosis in an unselected series of temporal bones. *Otology and Neurotology, 22,* 596–602.

Deem, J.F., & Miller, L. (2000). *Manual of voice therapy* (2nd ed.). Austin, TX: Pro-Ed.

Dillow, K.A., Dzienkowski, R.C., Smith, K.K., & Yucha, C.B. (1996). Cerebral palsy: A comprehensive review. *The Nurse Practitioner, 21,* 45–61.

Draper, M., Ladefoged, P., & Whitteridge, D. (1959). Respiratory muscles in speech. *Journal of Speech and Hearing Research, 2,* 16–27.

Duffy, J.R. (2005). *Motor speech disorders: Substrates, differential diagnosis, and management* (2nd ed.). St. Louis, MO: Elsevier Mosby.

Dworkin, J.P., & Meleca, R.J. (1997). *Vocal pathologies: Diagnosis, treatment, and case studies.* San Diego, CA: Singular Publishing Group, Inc.

Ey, J.L., Holberg, C.J., Aldous, M.B., Wright, A.L., Martinez, F.D., & Taussig, L.M. (1995). Group health medical associates: Passive smoke exposure and otitis media in the first year of life. *Pediatrics, 95,* 670–677.

Fant, G. (1960). *Acoustic theory of speech production.* The Hague, The Netherlands: Mouton.

Finucane, T., Christmas, C., & Travis, K. (1999). Tube feeding in patients with advanced dementia: A review of the evidence. *Journal of the American Medical Association, 282,* 1365–1370.

Firlik, K. (2006). *Another day in the frontal lobe: A brain surgeon exposes life on the inside.* New York: Random House.

Foulon, I., Naessens, A., Foulon, W., Casteels, A., & Gordts, F. (2008). A 10-year prospective study of sensorineural hearing loss in children with congenital cytomegalovirus infection. *Journal of Pediatrics, 153,* 84–88.

Fox, M.J. (2002). *Lucky man: A memoir.* New York: Hyperion.

Froehling, D.A., Bowen, J.M., Mohr, D.N., Brey, R.H., Beatty, C.W., Wollan, P.C., & Silverstein, M.D. (2000). The canalith repositioning procedure for the treatment of benign paroxysmal positional vertigo: A randomized controlled trial. *Mayo Clinic Proceedings, 75,* 695–700.

Froehling, D.A., Silverstein, M.D., Mohr, D.N., Beatty, C.W., Offord, K.P., & Ballard, D.J. (1991). Benign positional vertigo: Incidence and prognosis in a population-based study in Olmsted County, Minnesota. *Mayo Clinic Proceedings, 66,* 596–601.

Gazzaniga, M.S., Ivry, R.B., & Mangun, G.R. (1998). *Cognitive neuroscience: The biology of the mind.* New York: W.W. Norton & Company, Inc.

Geisler, C.D. (1998). *From sound to synapse: Physiology of the mammalian ear.* New York: Oxford University Press.

Gelfand, S.A. (1984). The contralateral acoustic reflex threshold. In S. Silman (Ed.), *The acoustic reflex: Basic principles and clinical applications* (pp. 137–186). Orlando, FL: Academic Press.

Goodglass, H. (1993). *Understanding aphasia.* San Diego, CA: Academic Press.

Goodglass, H., Kaplan, E., & Barresi, B. (2001). *The assessment of aphasia and related disorders* (3rd ed.). Baltimore, MD: Lippincott Williams & Wilkins.

Goodman, A. (2003). *Understanding the human body: An introduction to anatomy and physiology, Part 1* (video lectures). Chantilly, VA: The Teaching Company. www.TEACH12.com.

Gordon-Brannan, M.E., & Weiss, C.E. (2006). *Clinical management of articulatory and phonologic disorders* (3rd ed.). Baltimore, MD: Lippincott Williams & Wilkins.

Gorlin, R.J., Cohen, M.M. Jr., & Levin, L.S. (1990). Syndromes of the head and neck. *Oxford Monographs on Medical Genetics,* No. 19. New York: Oxford University Press.

Grundfast, K., & Carney, C.J. (1987). *Ear infection in your child.* Hollywood, FL: Compact Books.

Guinan, J., Warr, W., & Norris, B. (1983). Differential olivocochlear projections from lateral versus medial zones of the superior olivary complex. *Journal of Comparative Neurology, 221,* 358–370.

Hagen, C. (1998). *The Rancho levels of cognitive functioning: The revised levels* (3rd ed.). Retrieved August 27, 2010 from www.rancho.org/patient_education/cognitive_levels.pdf.

Halpern, H. (2000). *Language and motor speech disorders in adults* (2nd ed.). Austin, TX: Pro-Ed.

Hardy, J.C. (1994). Cerebral palsy. In W.A. Secord, G.H. Shames, & E. Wiig (Eds.), *Human communication disorders: An introduction* (4th ed., pp. 562–604). New York: Merrill.

Harold, C. (Ed.) (2009). *Professional guide to diseases* (9th ed.). Baltimore, MD: Lippincott Williams & Wilkins.

Hirano, M. (1974). Morphological structure of the vocal cord as a vibrator and its variations. *Folia Phoniatrica, 26,* 89–94.

Hirano, M. (1981). *Clinical examination of voice.* New York: Springer-Verlag.

Hirano, M., Kakita, Y., Kawasaki, H., Gould, W., & Lambiase, A. (1981). Data from high-speed motion picture studies. In K. Stevens & M. Hirano (Eds.), *Vocal fold physiology* (pp. 85–93). Tokyo, Japan: University of Tokyo Press.

Hirano, M., Yoshida, T., & Tanaka, S. (1991). Vibratory behavior of human vocal folds viewed from below. In J. Gauffin & B. Hammarberg (Eds.), *Vocal fold physiology: Acoustic, perceptual, and physiological aspects of voice mechanisms* (pp. 1–6). San Diego, CA: Singular Publishing, Inc.

Hixon, T.J. (1973). Respiratory function in speech. In F.D. Minifie, T.J. Hixon, & F. Williams (Eds.), *Normal aspects of speech, hearing, and language.* Englewood Cliffs, NJ: Prentice-Hall, Inc.

Hixon, T.J., & Hoit, J.D. (2005). *Evaluation and management of speech breathing disorders: Principles and methods.* Tucson, AZ: Redington Brown LLC.

Hixon, T.J., Mead, J., & Goldman, M. (1976). Dynamics of the chest wall during speech production: Function of the thorax, rib cage, diaphragm, and abdomen. *Journal of Speech and Hearing Research, 19,* 297–356.

Hixon, T.J., Weismer, G., & Hoit, J.D. (2008). *Preclinical speech science: Anatomy, physiology, acoustics, perception.* San Diego, CA: Plural Publishing.

Hoit, J.D., & Shea, S.A. (1996). Speech production and speech with a phrenic nerve pacer. *American Journal of Speech-Language Pathology, 5,* 53–60.

Hollien, H. (1972). Three major vocal registers: A proposal. In A. Rigault & R. Charbonneau (Eds.), *Proceedings of the Seventh International Congress of Phonetic Sciences* (pp. 320–331). The Hague, The Netherlands: Mouton.

Hollien, H. (1974). On vocal registers. *Journal of Phonetics, 2,* 25–43.

Howden, C.W. (2004). Management of acid-related disorders in patients with dysphagia. *American Journal of Medicine, 117,* 44S–48S.

Howie, V.M., Ploussard, J.H., & Sloyer, J. (1975). The "otitis-prone" condition. *American Journal of Diseases of Children, 129,* 676–678.

Hudspeth, A.J. (1989). How the ear's works work. *Nature, 341,* 397–404.

Jafek, B.W., & Barcz, D.V. (1996). The otologic evaluation. In J. Northern (Ed.), *Hearing disorders* (pp. 33–34). Needham Heights, MA: Allyn & Bacon.

Johnson, A.F., & Jacobson, B.H. (2007). *Medical speech-language pathology: A practitioner's guide* (2nd ed.). New York: Thieme Publishers.

Joint Committee on Infant Hearing. (2007). Position statement: Principles and guidelines for early hearing detection and intervention programs. *Pediatrics, 120,* 898–921.

Kankkunen, A., & Thiringer, K. (1987). Hearing impairment in connection with preauricular tags. *Acta Paediatrica Scandinavia, 76,* 143–146.

Katzman, R., & Bick, K. (Eds.) (2000). *Alzheimer disease—The changing view.* Orlando, FL: Academic Press.

Kavanagh, K.T., & Magill, H.L. (1989). Michel dysplasia: Common cavity inner ear deformity. *Pediatric Radiology, 19,* 343–345.

Kemper, A.R., & Downs, S.M. (2000). A cost-effective analysis of newborn hearing screening strategies. *Archives of Pediatric and Adolescent Medicine, 154,* 484–488.

Kennedy, M., Strand, E., Burton, W., & Peterson, C. (1994). Analysis of first-encounter conversations of right-hemisphere-damaged adults. *Clinical Aphasiology, 22,* 67–80.

Kersten, L. (1989). *Comprehensive respiratory nursing: A decision making approach.* Philadelphia, PA: W.B. Saunders.

Kier, W., & Smith, K. (1985). Tongues, tentacles, and trunks: The biomechanics of movement in muscular-hydrostats. *Zoological Journal of the Linnean Society, 83,* 307–324.

Kirkpatrick, J.B., & DiMaio, V. (1978). Civilian gunshot wounds of the brain. *Journal of Neurosurgery, 49,* 185–198.

Kochkin, S. (2005). MarkeTrak VII. *Hearing Review, 12,* 16–29.

Kreiborg, S. (1981). Crouzon syndrome. *Scandinavian Journal of Plastic and Reconstructive Surgery* (Suppl. 18), 1–198.

Kuehn, D., & Kahane, J. (1990). Histologic study of the normal human adult soft palate. *Cleft Palate Journal, 27,* 26–34.

Kuehn, D., & Moon, J. (2005). Histologic study of intravelar structures in normal human adult specimens. *Cleft Palate-Craniofacial Journal, 42,* 481–489.

Kuehn, D., Templeton, P.J., & Maynard, J.A. (1990). Muscle spindles in the velopharyngeal musculature of humans. *Journal of Speech and Hearing Research, 33,* 488–493.

Kugelman, A., Hadad, B., Ben-David, J., Podoshin, L., Borochowitz, Z., & Bader, D. (1997). Preauricular tags and pits in the newborn: The role of hearing tests. *Acta Paediatrica Scandinavia, 86,* 170–172.

Kumar, N.M., & Gilula, N.B. (1996). The gap junction communication channel. *Cell, 84,* 381–388.

Kumin, L. (1998). Speech and language skills in children with Down syndrome. *Mental Retardation and Developmental Disabilities Research Reviews, 2,* 109–115.

LaPointe, L.L. (1994). Neurogenic disorders of communication. In F.D. Minifie (Ed.), *Introduction to communication sciences and disorders.* San Diego, CA: Singular Publishing.

Lehman-Blake, M., Duffy, J.R., Myers, P.S., & Tompkins, C.A. (2002). Prevalence and patterns of right hemisphere cognitive/communicative deficits: Retrospective data from an inpatient rehabilitation unit. *Aphasiology, 16,* 537–547.

Liss, J. (1990). Muscle spindles in the human levator veli palatini and palatoglossus muscles. *Journal of Speech and Hearing Research, 33,* 736–746.

Logemann, J.A. (1998). *Evaluation and treatment of swallowing disorders* (2nd ed.). Austin, TX: Pro-Ed.

Love, R.J. (2000). *Childhood motor speech disability* (2nd ed.). Boston, MA: Allyn & Bacon.

Lubinski, R. (2005, February). *Basics of aging and dementia*. Presentation at the ASHA Health Care Conference: Dementia: Clinical Approaches for SLPs in Health Care Settings, Palm Springs, CA.

Mann, G., Hankey, G.J., & Cameron, D. (2000). Swallowing disorders following acute stroke: Prevalence and diagnostic accuracy. *Cerebrovascular Disease, 10*, 380–386.

Marik, P.E., & Kaplan, D. (2003). Aspiration pneumonia and dysphagia in the elderly. *Chest, 124*, 328–336.

Martino, R., Foley, N., Bhogal, S., Diamant, N., Speechley, M., & Teasell, R. (2005). Dysphagia after stroke: Incidence, diagnosis, and pulmonary complications. *Stroke: A Journal of Cerebral Circulation, 36*, 2756–2763.

Massey, A.J. (2005, February). *Medication-related issues associated with managing dementia*. Presentation at the ASHA Health Care Conference: Dementia: Clinical Approaches for SLPs in Health Care Settings, Palm Springs, CA.

Mastroiacovo, P., Corchia, C., Botto, L.D., Lanni, R., Zampino, G., & Fusco, D. (1995). Epidemiology and genetics of microtia-anotia: A registry based study on over one million births. *Journal of Medical Genetics, 32*, 453–457.

Mateer, C.A., & Ojemann, G.A. (1983). Thalamic mechanisms in language and memory. In J. Segalowitz (Ed.), *Language functions and brain organization* (pp. 171–191). New York: Academic Press.

Mathers-Schmidt, B. (2001). Paradoxical vocal fold motion: A tutorial. *American Journal of Speech-Language Pathology, 10*, 111–125.

Mattox, D.E. (2000). Surgical management of vestibular disorders. In S. Herdman (Ed.), *Vestibular rehabilitation* (pp. 251–262). Philadelphia, PA: F. A. Davis Company.

Mencher, G.T., Gerber, S.E., & McCombe, A. (1997). *Audiology and auditory dysfunction*. Needham Heights, MA: Allyn & Bacon.

Mesulam, M.-M. (1981). A cortical network for directed attention and unilateral neglect. *Annals of Neurology, 10*, 309–325.

Miller, J.L., Watkin, K.L., & Chen, M.F. (2002). Muscle, adipose, and connective tissue variations in intrinsic musculature of the adult human tongue. *Journal of Speech, Language and Hearing Science, 45*, 51–65.

Miller, N. (2002). The neurological basis of apraxia of speech. *Seminars in Speech and Language, 23*, 223–230.

Moll, K.L. (1962). Velopharyngeal closure on vowels. *Journal of Speech and Hearing Research, 5*, 30–37.

Monoson, P., & Zemlin, W. (1984). Quantitative study of whisper. *Folia Phoniatrica, 36*, 53–65.

Moon, J., & Kuehn, D. (2004). Anatomy and physiology of normal and disordered velopharyngeal function for speech. In K. Bzoch (Ed.), *Communicative disorders related to cleft lip and palate* (5th ed., pp. 67–98). Austin, TX: Pro-Ed.

Morata, T.C., Dunn, D.E., Kretschmer, L.W., Lemasters, G.K., & Keith, R.W. (1993). Effects of occupational exposures to organic solvents and noise on hearing. *Scandinavian Journal of Work and Environmental Health, 19*, 245–254.

Muscular Dystrophy Association. (n.d.) *MDA is knowledge: Diseases*. Retrieved December 30, 2007, from http://www.mdausa.org/disease/.

Myers, P. (1999). *Right hemisphere damage: Disorders of communication and cognition*. San Diego, CA: Singular Publishing.

Myers, P. (2005). CAC classics: Profile of communicative deficits in patients with right cerebral hemisphere damage: Implications for diagnosis and treatment. *Aphasiology, 19*, 1147–1160.

National Institute for Occupational Safety and Health. (1998). *Revised criteria for a recommended standard—Occupational noise exposure*. U.S. Department of Health and Human Services, Public Health Service, Centers for Disease Control and Prevention, National Institute for Occupational Safety and Health, DHHS (NIOSH) Publication 98–126.

National Institute of Neurological Disorders and Stroke (NINDS). (n.d.). *Muscular dystrophy information page*. Retrieved December 30, 2007, from http://www.ninds.nih.gov/disorders/md/md.htm.

National Institute on Deafness and Other Communication Disorders. (1999). *Noise-induced hearing loss* (Publication No. 97-4233), National Institutes of Health.

National Scoliosis Foundation. (n.d.a). *Information and support*. Retrieved February 26, 2008, from http://www.scoliosis.org/info.php.

National Scoliosis Foundation. (n.d.b). *Medical updates: Understanding kyphosis*. Retrieved February 26, 2008, from http://www.scoliosis.org/resources/medicalupdates/kyphosis.php.

National Scoliosis Foundation. (n.d.c). *Medical updates: Understanding lordosis*. Retrieved February 26, 2008, from http://www.scoliosis.org/resources/medicalupdates/lordosis.php.

National Spinal Cord Injury Statistical Center. (n.d.). *Facts and figures at a glance—updated June 2006*. Retrieved December 20, 2007, from http://www.spinalcord.uab.edu/show.asp?durki=19775.

Netsell, R. (1973). Speech physiology. In F.D. Minifie, T.J. Hixon, & F. Williams (Eds.), *Normal aspects of speech, hearing and language* (pp. 211–234). Englewood Cliffs, NJ: Prentice-Hall, Inc.

Nicolosi, L., Harryman, E., & Kresheck, J. (2004). *Terminology of communication disorders: Speech-language-hearing* (5th ed.). Baltimore, MD: Lippincott Williams & Wilkins.

Nolte, J. (1999). *The human brain: An introduction to its functional anatomy* (4th ed.). Baltimore, MD: Mosby.

Northern, J., & Hayes, D. (1994). Universal screening for infant hearing impairment. *Audiology Today, 6*, 10–13.

Occupational Safety and Health Administration. (2002). Occupational noise exposure standard. 29 CFR, Part 1910.95. *Hearing Conservation (revised)*, 1–32.

Orlikoff, R., & Kahane, J. (1996). Structure and function of the larynx. In N. Lass (Ed.), *Principles of experimental phonetics* (pp. 112–181). St. Louis, MO: Mosby.

Oshiro, B.T. (1999). Cytomegalovirus infections in pregnancy. *Contemporary Obstetrics/Gynecology, November*, 16–24.

Paciaroni, M., Mazzotta, G., Corea, F., Caso, V., Venti, M., Milia, P., Silvestrelli, G., Palmerini, F., Parnetti, L., & Gallai, V. (2004). Dysphagia following stroke. *European Neurology, 51*, 162–167.

Pandya, A., Arnos, K.S., Xia, X.J., Welch, K.O., Blanton, S.H., Friedman, T.B., Garcia Sanchez, G., Liu, X.Z., Morell, R., & Nance, W.E. (2003). Frequency and distribution of GJB2 (connexin 26) and GJB6 (connexin 30) mutations in a large North American repository of deaf probands. *Genetics in Medicine, 5*, 295–303.

Pannbacker, M. (1992). Some common myths about voice therapy. *Language, Speech, and Hearing Services in Schools, 23*, 12–19.

Park, S.S., & Chi, D.H. (2005). *External ear, aural atresia.* Accessed March 13, 2008, from http://www.emedicine.com/ent/topic 329.htm.

Pass, R.F., Hutto, S.C., Reynolds, D.W., & Polhill, R.B. (1984). Increased frequency of cytomegalovirus infection in children in group day care. *Pediatrics, 74*, 121–126.

Pearson, R. (1974). Incidence of diagnosed otosclerosis. *Archives of Otolaryngology, 99*, 288.

Peterson-Falzone, S.J., Hardin-Jones, M.A., & Karnell, M. (2001). *Cleft palate speech* (3rd ed.). St. Louis, MO: Mosby.

Pickles, J. (1988). *An introduction to the physiology of hearing* (2nd ed). London: Academic Press.

Pickles, J., Comis, S., & Osborne, M. (1984). Cross-links between stereocilia in the guinea pig organ of Corti, and their possible relation to sensory transduction. *Hearing Research, 15*, 103–112.

Prutting, C.A., & Kirchner, D.M. (1987). A clinical appraisal of the pragmatic aspects of language. *Journal of Speech and Hearing Disorders, 52*, 105–119.

Raphael, L.J., Borden, G.J., & Harris, K.S. (2007). *Speech science primer: Physiology, acoustics, and perception of speech* (5th ed.). Baltimore, MD: Lippincott Williams & Wilkins.

Reinmuth, O. (1994, February). *Stroke: New frontiers in diagnosis and management.* Telerounds video presentation, National Center for Neurogenic Communication Disorders, University of Arizona, Tucson, AZ.

Reisberg, B., Ferris, S., de Leon, M.J., & Crook, T. (1982). The global deterioration scale for assessment of primary degenerative dementia. *American Journal of Psychiatry, 139*, 1136–1139.

Retzius, G. (1884). *Das gehororgan der wirbeltheire* (Vol. 2). Stockholm, Sweden: Samson & Wallin.

Sagan, C. (1977). *The dragons of Eden: Speculations on the evolution of human intelligence.* New York: Random House, Inc.

Santo Pietro, M.J., & Ostuni, E. (2003). *Successful communication with persons with Alzheimer's disease: An in-service manual.* St. Louis, MO: Mosby.

Schappert, S. (1992). *Office visits for otitis media: United States, 1975–90.* Compilation of Advance Data from Vital and Health Statistics: National Center for Health Statistics Series 16, No. 214, 1–18.

Schelp, A.O., Cola, P.C., Gatto, A.R., Goncalves da Silva, R., & de Carvalho, L.R. (2004). Incidence of oropharyngeal dysphagia associated with stroke in a regional hospital in Sao Paulo State-Brazil [article in Portuguese]. *Arquivos de Neuro-Psiquiatria, 62*, 503–506.

Schuknecht, H. (1974). *Pathology of the ear.* Cambridge, MA: Harvard University Press.

Seikel, A., King, D., & Drumright, D. (2005). *Anatomy and physiology for speech, language, and hearing* (3rd ed.). Clifton Park, NY: Thomson Delmar Learning.

Smith, K., & Kier, W. (1989). Trunks, tongues and tentacles: Moving with skeletons of muscle. *American Scientist, 77*, 28–35.

Smith, R., Green, G., & Van Camp, G. (1999). *Deafness and hereditary hearing loss.* Accessed July 1, 2009, from http://www.geneclinics.org/profiles/deafness-overview/details.html. Developed by the University of Washington, Seattle, WA.

Sohlberg, M.M., & Mateer, C.A. (1989). *Introduction to cognitive rehabilitation: Theory and practice.* New York: Guilford Press.

Sohlberg, M.M., & Mateer, C.A. (2001). *Cognitive rehabilitation: An integrative neuropsychological approach.* New York: Guilford Press.

Solomon, N., McCall, G., Trosset, M., & Gray, W. (1989). Laryngeal configuration and constriction during two types of whispering. *Journal of Speech and Hearing Research, 32*, 161–174.

Spoendlin, H. (1974). Neuroanatomy of the cochlea. In E. Zwicker & E. Terhardt (Eds.), *Facts and models in hearing.* New York: Springer.

Square-Storer, P.A., & Apeldoorn, S. (1991). An acoustic study of apraxia of speech in patients with different lesion loci. In C.A. Moore, K.M. Yorkston, & D.R. Beukelman (Eds.), *Dysarthria and apraxia of speech: Perspectives on management.* Baltimore, MD: Brookes Publishing.

Staecher, H., Praetorius, M., Kim, B., & Douglas, D.E. (2007). Vestibular hair cell regeneration and restoration of balance function induced by math 1 gene transfer. *Otology and Neurotology, 28*, 223–231.

Steel, K.P. (1983). The tectorial membrane of mammals. *Hearing Research, 9*, 327–359.

Stoel-Gammon, C. (1998). Phonological development in Down syndrome. *Mental Retardation and Developmental Disabilities Research Reviews, 3*, 300–306.

Stone, J., & Cotanche, D. (2007). Hair cell regeneration in the avian auditory epithelium. *International Journal of Developmental Biology, 51*, 633–647.

Strich, S.J. (1961). Shearing of nerve fibres as a cause of brain damage due to head injury. *Lancet, 2*, 443–448.

Tasaki, I., & Spiropoulos, C. (1959). Stria vascularis as source of endocochlear potential. *Journal of Neurophysiology, 22*, 149–155.

Taylor, W., Pearson, J., Mair, A., & Burns, W. (1965). Study of noise and hearing in jute weaving. *Journal of the Acoustical Society of America, 38*, 113–120.

Tilney, L., Tilney, M., & DeRosier, D. (1992). Actin filaments, stereocilia, and hair cells: How cells count and measure. *Annual Review of Cell Biology, 8*, 257–274.

Titze, I. (1994). *Principles of voice production.* Englewood Cliffs, NJ: Prentice-Hall, Inc.

Titze, I. (2006). *The myoelastic aerodynamic theory of phonation.* Iowa City, IA: National Center for Voice and Speech.

Troost, B.T., & Waller, M.A. (1998). Diagnostic principals in neuro-otology: The auditory system. In R.N. Rosenberg & D.E. Pleasure (Eds.), *Comprehensive neurology* (2nd ed., pp. 611–623). New York: Wiley & Sons, Inc.

Tucker, D.M., & Frederick, S.L. (1989). Emotion and brain lateralization. In H. Wagner & A. Manstead (Eds.), *Handbook of social psychophysiology* (pp. 27–70). New York: Wiley.

van den Berg, I. (1958). Myoelastic-aerodynamic theory of voice production. *Journal of Speech and Hearing Research, 1*, 227–244.

Wang, R., Earl, D., Ruder, R., & Graham, J. (2001). Syndromic ear anomalies and renal ultrasounds. *Pediatrics, 108*, 32.

Wertz, R.T., LaPointe, L.L., & Rosenbek, J.C. (1984). *Apraxia of speech in adults: The disorder and its management.* San Diego, CA: Singular Publishing.

Wever, E.G., & Lawrence, M. (1954). *Physiological acoustics.* Princeton, NJ: Princeton University Press.

Wilson, F.B. (1990). *Voice kit manual: A program of diagnosis and management for voice disorders.* Bellingham, WA: Voice Tapes, Inc.

Yorkston, K.M., Miller, R.M., & Strand, E.A. (1995). *Management of speech and swallowing in degenerative diseases.* Tucson, AZ: Communication Skill Builders.

Yorkston, K.M., Miller, R.M., & Strand, E.A. (2003). *Management of speech and swallowing in degenerative diseases* (2nd ed.). Austin, TX: Pro-Ed.

Yorkston, K.M., Spencer, K.A., & Duffy, J.R. (2003). Behavioral management of respiratory/phonatory dysfunction from dysarthria: A systematic review of the evidence. *Journal of Medical Speech-Language Pathology, 11*(2), xiii–xxxviii.

Yoshinaga-Itano, C., Sedey, A.L., Coulter, D.K., & Mehl, A.L. (1998). Language of early and later-identified children with hearing loss. *Pediatrics, 102,* 1161–1171.

Yost, W.A. (2000). *Fundamentals of hearing: An introduction* (4th ed.) San Diego, CA: Academic Press.

Young, W. (2003). *Acute spinal cord injury.* Retrieved February 28, 2008, from http://sci.rutgers.edu/index.php?page=viewarticle&afile=27_February_2003@AcuteSCI.htm.

Zemlin, W., Simmon, A., & Hammel, D. (1984). The frequency of occurrence of foramen thyroideum in the human larynx. *Folia Phoniatrica, 36,* 296–300.

Zeng, F.G., Oba, S., Garde, S., Sininger, Y., & Starr, A. (1999). Temporal and speech processing deficits in auditory neuropathy. *Neuroreport, 10,* 3429–3435.

Zwislocki, J.J. (1990). Active cochlear feedback: Required structure and response phase. In P. Dallos, C.D. Geisler, J.W. Matthews, M.A. Ruggero, & C.R. Steele (Eds.), *Mechanics and biophysics of hearing* (pp. 114–120). New York: Springer.

INDEX

Note: Page locators followed by f and t indicates figure and table respectively.